Lifestyle Medicine

Jeffrey I. Mechanick • Robert F. Kushner

Editors

Lifestyle Medicine

A Manual for Clinical Practice

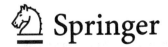

Editors
Jeffrey I. Mechanick
New York
USA

Robert F. Kushner
Chicago
USA

ISBN 978-3-319-79659-8
DOI 10.1007/978-3-319-24687-1

ISBN 978-3-319-24687-1 (eBook)

Springer Cham Heidelberg New York Dordrecht London

Printed on acid-free paper

Springer International Publishing AG Switzerland is part of Springer Science + Business Media (www.springer.com)

Foreword

Lifestyle: Back to the Future Medicine

Of all the haloed names tethered to the lore of medical practice—Maimonides, Osler, Harrison, Cushing—none looms so large as Hippocrates. We invoke his name when we first don the white coat and cross over into the rarefied privileges and responsibilities of patient care. Hippocrates' admonition on the topic of lifestyle is so often repeated as to be all but trite: "Let food be thy medicine, and medicine be thy food." We may perhaps presume that "food" was really a stand-in for lifestyle practices in general.

Lifestyle, then, was once salient to the practice of medicine. Here, on these carefully collated pages, we have the argument that it must be comparably so in the future.

The case is strong. A steady drumbeat of modern publications has attributed roughly 80% of all premature deaths and chronic diseases, in modern societies, to modifiable lifestyle practices. A reciprocal cadence of studies reveals the converse; when lifestyle practices are optimized, as much as 80% of chronic diseases and premature deaths indeed disappear. Perhaps even more compelling still, where salutary lifestyle practices prevail as the cultural norm, namely in the Blue Zones, there are, routinely, more years in life, more life in years, and a peaceful exit at the gentle close of such bounty.

That, then, is the luminous promise of lifestyle as medicine. But more than that it makes the case for the important contribution of these chapters, so, too, do the ominous projections of a doomed status quo. Should current epidemiologic trends persist, some 40% of Americans could be diabetic by mid-century, with related and even more dire projections elsewhere around the globe. Leaving aside the ghastly human cost of this, it is untenable on economic grounds alone. Lifestyle is the remedy.

This text willfully emphasizes lifestyle in clinical context, but views the relevant landscape through a suitably large window. Lifestyle is, implicitly if not explicitly, an aggregated set of choices; but the choices any of us makes are subordinate to the choices any of us has. The authors here recognize that, considering social and environmental determinants of, and influences on, the lifestyle practices that are, in turn, major determinants of health across the lifespan.

The content here is far ranging, as required to encompass the many ramifications of the topic. The particular emphasis on clinical practice invites the requisite attention to customary tools of that trade: biometrics, clinical evaluation tools, standardized measures, and risk analysis. An entire section of the book views the application of lifestyle medicine through the lens of disease specificity. Other chapters appropriately follow the implications of lifestyle medicine from clinic to community. Attention is given to cultural context, the built environment, policy and legislation, practice settings, and even the clearly important intangibles of this field, such as friendship and spirituality.

That the emphasis is on clinical practice is true to the declared mission, and thus only right. Readers are nonetheless well advised to consider that where lifestyle medicine is doing the most good for most members of a population, the delivery is far more a cultural than a clinical enterprise.

In the modern cultures shared by this book's authors, and presumably most readers, much of what accounts for them being "modern" conspires against health. Throughout most of human history, calories were relatively scarce and hard to come by, and physical activity was called survival and was unavoidable. We have devised new worlds where physical activity is scarce and hard to come by, and hyperpalatable calories, engineered to be irresistible, are unavoidable. Hectic schedules conspire against motion, propagate stress, and sabotage sleep. Social insularity, career-related itineracy, and the dissolution of the extended family erode the defense of social connections. Increasing preoccupation with glowing screens, perhaps at the expense of time-honored human connections as fundamental as eye contact, threatens our ambient empathy. The perils of toxic and addictive substances tempt as salves against the barrage of such assaults to which we are newly exposed and poorly adapted.

One would hope, then, that the needed transformation will begin in the clinics but not end there. The clinicians reading this book have the opportunity to ply the potent wares of lifestyle medicine more effectively on behalf of one patient at a time. That is progress. But in the aggregate, we clinicians have the potential to be the cutting edge of more expansive change at the level of culture. How much better, for instance, to counsel proficiently for good nutrition and daily activity, and send our patients out into an environment that facilitates these practices, rather than conspiring against them. This, too, is part of our mandate and implicit to the invitation of these pages.

This diversity of authorities looks at lifestyle medicine from both within and without. By so doing they offer the advantages of a sermon that is not of, by, and for the choir, but tailored to a large and comparably diverse congregation of clinicians. Lifestyle as medicine is not new, but many of the voices rallying to its support here are. The proposition is not new, but new data and new studies, populating these pages, validate its promise anew.

Lifestyle, once, figured among the salient imperatives of medical practice. It now figures again among the best, if not only, good options at the confluence of patient care, public health, human potential, environmental sustainability, and economic viability. Lifestyle is the best medicine we know for most of the people most of the time, and requires that we look ahead, and back, to the future. With expertise, authority, insight, and hybrid vigor, the authors here do just that and light the way forward.

-fin

President, American College of Lifestyle Medicine   David L. Katz
Drafted: July 14, 2015   MD, MPH, FACPM, FACP

Preface

Lifestyle—the manner in which people live—is fundamental to health, wellness, and prevention of disease. It follows that attention to lifestyle is critically important to effective and successful health care. But here is the challenge: Health-care professionals receive very little, if any, formal training about lifestyle counseling and, therefore, are ill equipped to incorporate lifestyle issues into clinical practice.

In response, "lifestyle medicine" is evolving as a means to fill this knowledge gap. Strictly speaking, lifestyle medicine approaches health and wellness by harnessing the power of lifestyle-related behaviors and influencing the environment we live in. In more colloquial terms, lifestyle medicine addresses how we should live in order to be healthy. This is more than a trite semantic, more than just conjoining two words *lifestyle* and *medicine* to create yet another discipline to learn in an already overburdened system of health care. Rather, it is a formal approach that promises to enhance and strengthen a reinvigorated health-care system that is still outpaced by the epidemic proportions and complexity of chronic disease: obesity, diabetes, depression, hypertension, and cancer, among others.

Lifestyle Medicine—A Manual for Clinical Practice presents this formal approach in a pragmatic context. This is a manual that provides clear and succinct text on nearly all aspects of lifestyle medicine. The approach is both explanatory and pragmatic, providing case studies and bulleted translation of academic information into clinical practice recommendations. There is an emphasis on scientific evidence wherever possible as well as expert opinion by those who practice lifestyle medicine. There is a "how to" rationality to the book, consistent with a premise that any and all health-care professionals should, and perhaps must, incorporate lifestyle medicine. We include a checklist at the end of the book that summarizes key points and provides a practical tool for routine patient encounters.

The book begins with a set of introductory chapters that detail the why's, what's, and wherefore's of lifestyle medicine in current clinical practice. Next, a portfolio of paradigms, tools, models, and programs that are critical to this formal approach are provided. These chapters begin with generalized discussions but then migrate into specific descriptions on healthy eating, physical activity, sleep hygiene, behavior, smoking cessation, managing substance abuse, and alcohol moderation. To complete these discussions, chapters are included on integrative medicine, transculturalization for adapting recommendations to different regions and ethnicities, and the need for community engagement. Finally, specific disease states are presented within a lifestyle medicine context to provide clear explanations and examples of how to implement lifestyle medicine, including cardiometabolic risk reduction (obesity, diabetes, hypertension, and dyslipidemia), cancer, depression, musculoskeletal disorders, neurodegenerative conditions, chronic kidney disease, liver disease, gastrointestinal disorders, chronic pulmonary disease, and AIDS. We suggest that the reader not only spend time on each chapter in succession but also prepare to refer to relevant chapters when needed for specific patient management issues.

Will this book enhance and improve your clinical practice? Yes, we believe it will, by better understanding key principles and implementing the proposed formal approach.

What can be expected as a result of this enriched clinical practice? With widespread implementation of lifestyle medicine, we anticipate better clinical outcomes in chronic disease processes, introduction and facilitation of lifestyle education and training, more lifestyle-centered research with practical metrics and findings, and an overall improvement in the epidemiology of chronic diseases across local, national, and perhaps even global scales. We hope you share our vision for the future of medicine and need to optimize health care by actualizing principles of lifestyle medicine, for your own personal benefit, for the benefit of your patients, and for the aggregate benefit of a society in need.

Jeffrey I. Mechanick, MD

Robert F. Kushner, MD

Contents

1   Why Lifestyle Medicine? 1
Jeffrey I. Mechanick and Robert F. Kushner

2   The Importance of Healthy Living and Defining Lifestyle Medicine 9
Robert F. Kushner and Jeffrey I. Mechanick

3   Communication and Behavioral Change Tools: A Primer for Lifestyle
Medicine Counseling 17
Robert F. Kushner and Jeffrey I. Mechanick

4   Paradigms of Lifestyle Medicine and Wellness 29
Robert Scales and Matthew P. Buman

5   Composite Risk Scores 41
Ruth E. Brown and Jennifer L. Kuk

6   Clinical Assessment of Lifestyle and Behavioral Factors During Weight
Loss Treatment 55
David B. Sarwer, Kelly C. Allison and Rebecca J. Dilks

7   Anthropometrics and Body Composition 65
Dympna Gallagher, Claire Alexander and Adam Paley

8   Physical Activity Measures 77
David R. Bassett and Kenneth M. Bielak

9   Metabolic Profiles—Based on the 2013 Prevention Guidelines 83
Neil J. Stone, John Wilkins and Sakina Kazmi

10 The Chronic Care Model and the Transformation of Primary Care 89
Thomas Bodenheimer and Rachel Willard-Grace

11 Guidelines for Healthy Eating 97
Linda Van Horn

12 A Review of Commercial and Proprietary Weight Loss Programs 105
Nasreen Alfaris, Alyssa Minnick, Patricia Hong and Thomas A. Wadden

13 Physical Activity Programs 121
Damon Swift, Neil M. Johannsen and Timothy Church

14 Behavior Modification and Cognitive Therapy 129
John P. Foreyt and Craig A. Johnston

15 Treating Tobacco Use in Clinical Practice 135
Allison J. Carroll, Anna K. Veluz-Wilkins and Brian Hitsman

16 Alcohol Use and Management 151
Evan Goulding

17 Sleep Management 161
Kelly Glazer Baron and Leland Bardsley

18 Integrative Medicine 171
Melinda Ring and Leslie Mendoza Temple

19 Transcultural Applications to Lifestyle Medicine 183
Osama Hamdy and Jeffrey I. Mechanick

**20 Community Engagement and Networks: Leveraging Partnerships
to Improve Lifestyle** 191
Juliette Cutts, Mary-Virginia Maxwell, Robert F. Kushner
and Jeffrey I. Mechanick

21 Lifestyle Therapy as Medicine for the Treatment of Obesity 199
Jamy D. Ard and Gary D. Miller

22 Lifestyle Therapy for Diabetes Mellitus 221
W. Timothy Garvey and Gillian Arathuzik

**23 Lifestyle Therapy in the Management of Cardiometabolic Risk:
Diabetes Prevention, Hypertension, and Dyslipidemia** 245
W. Timothy Garvey, Gillian Arathuzik, Gary D. Miller and Jamy Ard

24 Cancer 269
Elaine Trujillo, Barbara Dunn and Peter Greenwald

25 Lifestyle Medicine for the Prevention and Treatment of Depression 281
Jerome Sarris and Adrienne O'Neil

26 Promoting Healthy Lifestyle Behaviors in Patients with Persistent Pain 291
Patricia Robinson, David Bauman and Bridget Beachy

27 Forestalling Age-Related Brain Disorders 299
Mark P. Mattson

28 Chronic Kidney Disease 311
Girish N. Nadkarni and Joseph A. Vassalotti

29 Nonalcoholic Fatty Liver Disease and Steatohepatitis 321
Erin M. McCarthy and Mary E. Rinella

30 Gastroenterology Disease and Lifestyle Medicine 333
Gerald Friedman

31 Lifestyle Medicine and Chronic Pulmonary Disease 341
Glen B. Chun and Charles A. Powell

32 Lifestyle Medicine and HIV-Infected Patients 349
Vani Gandhi, Tiffany Jung and Jin S. Suh

Appendix: Lifestyle Medicine Checklist 357

Index 359

Contributors

Claire Alexander Department of Medicine and Institute of Human Nutrition, Columbia University, New York, NY, USA

Nasreen Alfaris Center for Weight and Eating Disorders, University of Pennsylvania Perelman School of Medicine, Philadelphia, PA, USA

Kelly C. Allison Center for Weight and Eating Disorders and Stunkard Weight Management Program, Perelman School of Medicine, University of Pennsylvania, Philadelphia, PA, USA

Gillian Arathuzik Lahey Outpatient Center, Danvers, MA, USA
Addison Gilbert Hospital, Gloucester, MA, USA

Jamy Ard Department of Epidemiology and Prevention, Wake Forest University, Winston-Salem, NC, USA
Weight Management Center, Winston-Salem, NC, USA

Leland Bardsley Illinois Institute of Technology, Chicago, IL, USA

Kelly Glazer Baron Department of Neurology, Feinberg School of Medicine, Northwestern University, Chicago, IL, USA

David R. Bassett Department of Kinesiology, Recreation, and Sport Sciences, University of Tennessee, Knoxville, TN, USA

David Bauman Central Washington Family Medicine Residency Program, Yakima, WA, USA

Bridget Beachy Central Washington Family Medicine Residency Program, Yakima, WA, USA

Kenneth M. Bielak Department of Family Medicine, University of Tennessee Medical Center, Knoxville, TN, USA

Thomas Bodenheimer Department of Family and Community Medicine, University of California, San Francisco, San Francisco, CA, USA

Ruth E. Brown School of Kinesiology and Health Science, York University, Toronto, Canada

Matthew P. Buman School of Nutrition and Health Promotion, Arizona State University, Phoenix, AZ, USA

Allison J. Carroll Department of Preventive Medicine, Northwestern University Feinberg School of Medicine, Chicago, IL, USA

Glen B. Chun Division of Pulmonary, Critical Care and Sleep Medicine, Icahn School of Medicine at Mount Sinai, New York, NY, USA

Timothy Church Preventive Medicine Laboratory, Pennington Biomedical Research Center, Baton Rouge, LA, USA

Juliette Cutts Yakima Valley Farm Workers Clinic, Salud Medical Center, Woodburn, OR, USA

Rebecca J. Dilks Center for Weight and Eating Disorders, Perelman School of Medicine, University of Pennsylvania, Philadelphia, PA, USA

Barbara K. Dunn NIH/National Cancer Institute/Division of Cancer Prevention/Chemopreventive Agent Development Research Group, NIH Clinical Center, Bethesda, MD , USA

John P. Foreyt Behavioral Medicine Research Center, Baylor College of Medicine, Houston, TX, USA

Gerald Friedman Division of Gastroenterology, Icahn School of Medicine at Mount Sinai, New York, NY, USA

Dympna Gallagher Department of Medicine and Institute of Human Nutrition, Columbia University, New York, NY, USA

Body Composition Unit, New York Obesity Research Center, Columbia University Medical Center, New York, NY, USA

Vani Gandhi Spencer Cox Center for Health, Institute for Advanced Medicine, Mount Sinai St. Luke's and Mount Sinai Roosevelt Hospitals, Icahn School of Medicine at Mount Sinai, New York, NY, USA

W. Timothy Garvey Department of Nutrition Sciences, University of Alabama at Birmingham, GRECC, Birmingham VA Medical Center, UAB Diabetes Research Center, Birmingham, AL, USA

Evan Goulding Department of Psychiatry and Behavioral Sciences, Feinberg School of Medicine, Northwestern University, Chicago, IL, USA

Peter Greenwald Division of Cancer Prevention at the National Cancer Institute (NCI), Bethesda, MD, USA

Osama Hamdy Joslin Diabetes Center, Harvard Medical School, Boston, MA, USA

Brian Hitsman Department of Preventive Medicine, Northwestern University Feinberg School of Medicine, Chicago, IL, USA

Patricia Hong Departments of Medicine and Psychiatry, University of Pennsylvania Perelman School of Medicine, Philadelphia, PA, USA

Linda Van Horn Department of Preventive Medicine, Northwestern University Feinberg School of Medicine, Chicago, IL, USA

Neil M. Johannsen School of Kinesiology, LSU College of Human Sciences and Education, Baton Rouge, LA, USA

Craig A. Johnston Department of Medicine, Department of Pediatrics-Nutrition, USDA/ARS Children's Nutrition Research Center, Baylor College of Medicine, Houston, TX, USA

Tiffany Jung Spencer Cox Center for Health, Institute for Advanced Medicine, Mount Sinai St. Luke's and Mount Sinai Roosevelt Hospitals, Icahn School of Medicine at Mount Sinai, New York, NY, USA

Sakina Kazmi Department of Cardiology, Feinberg School of Medicine, Northwestern University, Chicago, IL, USA

Jennifer L. Kuk School of Kinesiology and Health Science, York University, Toronto, 4700 Keele StreetON, Canada

Robert F. Kushner Northwestern Comprehensive Center on Obesity, Northwestern University Feinberg School of Medicine, Chicago, IL, USA

Mark P. Mattson Laboratory of Neurosciences, National Institute on Aging Intramural Research Program, Baltimore, MD, USA

Mary-Virginia Maxwell Catholic Family and Child Service, Yakima, WA, USA

Erin M. McCarthy Center for Lifestyle Medicine, Northwestern Medicine, Chicago, IL, USA

Jeffrey I. Mechanick Division of Endocrinology, Diabetes and Bone Disease, Icahn School of Medicine at Mount Sinai, New York, NY, USA

Gary D. Miller Department of Health and Exercise Science, Wake Forest University, Winston-Salem, NC, USA

Alyssa Minnick Departments of Medicine and Psychiatry, University of Pennsylvania Perelman School of Medicine, Philadelphia, PA, USA

Girish N. Nadkarni Division of Nephrology, Department of Medicine, Icahn School of Medicine at Mount Sinai, New York, NY, USA

Adrienne O'Neil IMPACT Strategic Research Centre, Deakin University, Geelong, VIC, Australia

Adam Paley Department of Medicine and Institute of Human Nutrition, Columbia University, New York, NY, USA

Charles A. Powell Division of Pulmonary, Critical Care and Sleep Medicine, Icahn School of Medicine at Mount Sinai, New York, NY, USA

Mary E. Rinella Department of Gastroenterology and Hepatology, Northwestern University Feinberg School of Medicine, Chicago, IL, USA

Melinda Ring Osher Center for Integrative Medicine at Northwestern University, Northwestern Feinberg School of Medicine, Chicago, IL, USA

Patricia Robinson Mountainview Consulting Group, Inc., Zillah, USA

Jerome Sarris Department of Psychiatry & The Melbourne Clinic, University of Melbourne, Parkville, VIC, Australia

Centre for Human Psychopharmacology, Swinburne University of Technology, Hawthorn, VIC, Australia

David B. Sarwer Center for Weight and Eating Disorders and Stunkard Weight Management Program, Perelman School of Medicine, University of Pennsylvania, Philadelphia, PA, USA

Robert Scales Division of Cardiovascular Diseases, Mayo Clinic-Arizona, Scottsdale, AZ, USA

Neil J. Stone Feinberg School of Medicine, Northwestern University, Chicago, IL, USA

Jin S. Suh Department of Medicine, Mount Sinai St. Luke's and Mount Sinai Roosevelt Hospitals, New York, NY, USA

Damon Swift Preventive Medicine Laboratory, Pennington Biomedical Research Center, Baton Rouge, LA, USA

Leslie Mendoza Temple NorthShore University HealthSystem Integrative Medicine Program, University of Chicago Pritzker School of Medicine, Glenview, IL, USA

Elaine Trujillo Bethesda, MD, USA

Joseph A. Vassalotti Division of Nephrology, Department of Medicine, Icahn School of Medicine at Mount Sinai, New York, NY, USA

National Kidney Foundation, Inc., New York, NY, USA

Anna K. Veluz-Wilkins Department of Preventive Medicine, Northwestern University Feinberg School of Medicine, Chicago, IL, USA

Thomas A. Wadden Departments of Medicine and Psychiatry, University of Pennsylvania Perelman School of Medicine, Philadelphia, PA, USA

John Wilkins Department of Preventive Medicine, Feinberg School of Medicine, Northwestern University, Chicago, IL, USA

Department of Cardiology, Feinberg School of Medicine, Northwestern University, Chicago, IL, USA

Rachel Willard-Grace Department of Family and Community Medicine, University of California, San Francisco, San Francisco CA, USA

Why Lifestyle Medicine?

1

Jeffrey I. Mechanick and Robert F. Kushner

Abbreviations

CDC	Centers for Disease Control and Prevention
CVD	Cardiovascular disease
DALY	Disability-adjusted life year
GBD	Global burden of disease
HBT	Health-based target
MMWR	Morbidity and Mortality Weekly Report
NCD	Noncommunicable diseases
QALY	Quality-adjusted life year

Introduction

Medicine has witnessed exponential growth and successes over a long history spanning millennia. Throughout this time, physicians and other health-care professionals have accepted a primarily reductionist philosophy. As more information has been discovered, learned, and then categorized, medical specialization became an expedient solution to the challenges of effective clinical practice, research, and education. Moreover, as pathophysiological states have been interpreted as complex, the emergent nature of disease management prompted newer humanistic patient care models. This evolution in medical care will be explored in the context of lifestyle.

The question "Why Lifestyle Medicine?" will be addressed by focusing on two key components: chronic disease and risk reduction. This chapter intends to provide not only sufficient rationale for the existence of lifestyle medicine but

J. I. Mechanick (✉)
Division of Endocrinology, Diabetes and Bone Disease,
Icahn School of Medicine at Mount Sinai, 1192 Park Avenue,
New York, NY 10128, USA
e-mail: jeffreymechanick@gmail.com

R. F. Kushner
Northwestern Comprehensive Center on Obesity,
Northwestern University Feinberg School of Medicine,
750 North Lake Shore Drive Rubloff 9-976, Chicago, IL 60611, USA
e-mail: rkushner@northwestern.edu

an imperative for the routine practice and teaching of lifestyle medicine throughout medical and allied health education.

The Problem: Chronic Disease

Lifestyle medicine can be broadly defined as the non-pharmacological and nonsurgical management of chronic disease. Chronic disease is a pathophysiological state lasting beyond an acute insult and initial physiological response, consisting of adaptive and maladaptive processes, and evolving toward a steady state, which may never be achieved. In general, chronic disease states are those lasting for more than 3 months (though this metric is not uniformly accepted; [12, 13]), often lasting a lifetime, and since they involve multiple interacting factors (hormones, neurons, organs, drugs, behaviors, psychosocial factors, etc.), they are often described as complex.

Historically, chronic disease was viewed as merely the prolongation of signs and symptoms related to an underlying, discrete disease process that oftentimes, but not exclusively, presents acutely. Thus, the management strategy, in this traditional framework, was to continue treatment directed to the dominant signs and symptoms, as well as the underlying known pathophysiological state. Over time, and concurrent with technological advances in pharmacotherapy (including molecular-targeted therapy) and device manufacturing (including surgery and other noninvasive interventions), the management of chronic disease became focused on interventions and complication management.

What changed? There are three principal drivers for a new chronic disease model:

- Awareness of epidemiological dimensions that expose flaws in our current biomedical paradigm
- Creation of global and domestic messaging and campaigns about the significance of chronic disease, in terms of mortality, morbidity, and economic cost

© Springer International Publishing Switzerland 2016
J. I. Mechanick, R. F. Kushner (eds.), *Lifestyle Medicine,* DOI 10.1007/978-3-319-24687-1_1

- Synthesis of a systems-based understanding of disease complexity and the need for new management strategies

Once this nature of chronic disease is reenvisioned, a call for action can be fashioned. This mandate may take the form of a modified medical model that clarifies the roles for lifestyle medicine while also recognizing shortcomings and directions for improvement.

Driver 1: Epidemiologic Dimensions

Chronic diseases afflict about half of all Americans (in 2012), account for 84% of health-care spending (in 2006), and in general can be prevented [14]. The Centers for Disease Control and Prevention (CDC) regularly updates and publishes epidemiological data and statistics for chronic diseases on their Healthy People 2020 website and in their Morbidity and Mortality Weekly Report (MMWR; [15]. Prevalence rates for selected chronic diseases among adults were extracted from these and other sources and are provided in Table 1.1. Pediatric prevalence rates are not depicted, but, particularly in the case of obesity, the prevalence rate of children with features of metabolic syndrome is alarming. However, early evidence demonstrating effectiveness of preventive programs among this population is encouraging [16, 17]. The increasing prevalence rates and socioeconomic impact of prediabetes are also concerning and bring into focus the role of prevention [18–21]. Due to multiple ill-defined factors, dynamic modeling of the US obesity epidemic indicates that prevalence rates are stabilizing, although confounded by racial disparities and still burdened by increased costs [22–24].

Cardiometabolic risk factors account for many of the high-prevalence-rate statistics in Table 1.1. Each of these chronic disease states poses great threats to individual and population-based health. These numbers likely underestimate the prevalence of total chronic disease since one specific disease may increase the risk for other chronic diseases. For instance, in a study by Tarleton et al. [25], adult cancer survivors in California from 2009 to 2010 had a greater chance of having obesity, or having a diagnosis of asthma or arthritis. Chronic disease prevalence rates have, for the most part, increased over time and have not been sufficiently impacted by the current high-technology and high-cost care models in the USA. There are several implications of this statement: (a) chronic disease prevalence rates may in fact be increasing due to unknown and/or changing drivers, (b) current intervention strategies are appropriate but inadequately implemented, and/or (c) simply put, current knowledge and conceptualization of chronic disease processes are critically incomplete and therefore, in theory, can never bend the curve. In order to better understand this problem to effectively synthesize an improved chronic disease care model, two metrics require discussion: the disability-adjusted life year (DALY) and the quality-adjusted life year (QALY).

The DALY unites mortality and morbidity into a representation of healthy life lost due to disability and/or premature death. Simply put, DALY can be described:

- As a measure of disease burden,
- In terms of years of healthy life lost, and
- As equal to "years of life lost" *plus* "years lived with disability" [26].

An example of DALY is the effect of diet and exercise on disease burden in overweight/obese patients.

This metric can be modified to improve performance. For instance, DALY computations include both disability and social weighting; details may be found in Devleesschauwer

Table 1.1 Summary of prevalence rates of selected chronic diseases in the USA

Chronic disease	Year(s)	Prevalence rate (%)	Comments	Ref.
Obesity/overweight	2010	68.2	Based on BMI ≥ 30 kg/m^2	[1]
≥ 1 of 3 heart disease risk factors	2007–2008	49.7	Uncontrolled BP, LDL-C, smoking	[2]
Hypertension	2007–2010	33.0	Higher in African-Americans	[1]
Arthritis	2010–2012	22.7	Doctor diagnosed	[3]
Hypercholesterolemia	2012	13.8	Total cholesterol ≥ 240 mg/dl	[1]
Kidney disease	1999–2004	13.1	Stages 1–4 only	[4]
Alzheimer's disease	2014	12.0	Estimates, age ≥ 65 years	[5]
Osteoporosis	2010	10.3	Adults ≥ 50 years old	[6]
Diabetes	2012	9.3	Increased from 8.3% in 2010	[7]
Depression	2006, 2008	9.1	4.1% major depression	[8]
Asthma	2012	8.9	Adults	[9]
COPD	2012	6.4	Adults	[9]
Cancer survivors	2012	4.4	13.7 million/312.8 million total US population	[10]
HIV	2011	0.37	CDC estimates, age ≥ 13 years	[11]

BMI body mass index, *BP* blood pressure, *CDC* Centers for Disease Control and Prevention, *COPD* chronic obstructive pulmonary disease, *LDL-C* low-density lipoprotein cholesterol

et al. [27] and Larson [28]. In addition, computation methodologies vary and are prone to error, especially with low-quality data, which is why more transparency is needed in DALY studies [29, 30]. The DALY metric is more appropriate than incidence rates or mortality figures since, in general, life expectancies are rising [31]. Based on the premise that each person is born with a certain number of life years spent in optimal health, one DALY would correspond to one lost year of healthy life. Moreover, the number of DALYs correlates with overall public health impact and has been a principal metric in global burden of disease (GBD) studies [27] and determination of health-based targets (HBTs; [32]). By extension, DALY and HBT can be used to prioritize disease severities, relativize positive and negative outcomes, and optimize public health interventions [28]. Collectively, the top chronic diseases in four GBD studies in 1990 [33], 2001 [34], 2004 [35], and 2010 [36] are lower respiratory infections, diarrheal diseases, ischemic heart disease, unipolar depression, and stroke [27]. In cancer patients from 184 countries in 12 world regions, the GBD correlates with degrees of human development and country resources [37].

The economic dimension of chronic disease management is important but somewhat elusive. On the one hand, nearly 80% of preventive options add to medical costs [38]. On the other hand, it is the downstream, anticipated cost savings, along with improved quality-of-life measures, longevity, and drug adherence, as well as reduced doctor visits and adverse events, which prompt this medical investment [39]. Cost-benefit analyses are useful in the assessment of chronic disease prevention, as exemplified by the positive effects of the Expanded Food and Nutrition Education Program on prevention of diet-related chronic disease [40]. The QALY metric unites quality and quantity of life into a representation of healthy life years gained or lost by a specific medical intervention in the context of cost for each life year. Simply put, QALY can be described:

- As a measure of disease burden,
- In terms of economic impact of a specific medical intervention on life years, and
- Where cost-utility analysis is based on the ratio of cost to QALY saved for an intervention [41].

An example of QALY is the monetary cost of lifestyle intervention and primary prevention in patients with prediabetes.

The QALY metric imparts relevance of an intervention in a setting of limited resources, and similar to DALY, incorporates a weighting calculus to optimize performance. Economic burden of chronic disease can also be reflected by measures of annual medical expenditures or annual productivity losses [42]. Regarding the former, Medicare payments for all chronic conditions in 2005 amounted to US$2.5 trillion with the following breakdown:

- Cardiovascular disease: US$442 billion in 2011,
- Diabetes: US$245 billion in 2012,
- Lung diseases: US$174 billion in 2010,
- Obesity: US$147 billion in 2008,
- Joint diseases: US$128 billion in 2003, and
- Alzheimer's disease: US$183 billion in 2011 [43].

This problem is further highlighted by Parekh et al. [44] who point out that more than one third of Americans have *multiple* chronic conditions, prompting a more aggressive stance and multi-platform approach by the US Department of Health and Human Services. In short, epidemiological data indicate that chronic diseases are becoming more prevalent and complex, exceeding our current workforce numbers, and resistant to our current care models; therefore, action is needed.

Driver 2: Campaigns and Messaging

The dimensions of any solution to chronic diseases need to be scalable. That is, the new medical model will need to grow and address chronic care problems across geographies, socioeconomic classes, ethnicities, and genetic makeups. For instance, social determinants of poor health outcomes (e.g., disparities in access to health care [45]) and cost barriers in low-income individuals [46] would need to enrich the current care model for better results at a population-based scale. Patient expectations for a new chronic disease model also contribute to the need for effective communication and messaging. Thus, a prerequisite to this approach is an effective social marketing messaging strategy or campaign that can disseminate valuable information and successfully motivate and inform patients, health professionals, and other stakeholders.

Campaigns on a global scale were boosted by "Disability-adjusted life years (DALYs) for 291 diseases and injuries in 21 regions, 1990–2010: a systematic analysis for the Global Burden of Disease Study 2010", which investigated DALYs for 291 diseases and injuries in 21 regions [36]. The key finding was that GBD was transitioning from communicable to noncommunicable diseases (NCDs; mental and behavioral disorders, musculoskeletal disorders, and diabetes) and from premature death to disability [36]. In 2012, 68% of deaths worldwide were due to NCDs (up from 60% in 2000; [47]). Thus, it is not surprising that the United Nations created the draft resolution "Political Declaration of the High-level Meeting of the General Assembly on the Prevention and Control of Non-communicable Diseases" (A/66/L.1; agenda item 117, 66th session, September 16, 2011) [48]. This was followed by the World Health Organization's "2008–2013 Action Plan for the Global Strategy for the Prevention and Control of Noncommunicable Diseases"; the four NCDs were cardiovascular, diabetes, cancer, and chronic respiratory [49].

At the domestic level in the USA, tobacco smoking, poor diet, physical inactivity, and alcohol use top the list of leading causes of preventable deaths [50]. A recent analysis of the problem of chronic disease in the USA, specifically addressing why obesity prevalence, related morbidity, and mortality rates are not responding as hoped to a wide range of interventions, identified health literacy, messaging, and ascribing "value" to a preventive care model as important focal points [51]. In other words, people are not placing sufficient value on receiving preventive medicine care, are therefore not asking for or purchasing insurance policies (or the medical care itself), and as a result, not receiving necessary lifestyle medicine services.

Driver 3: Synthesis That Addresses Chronic Disease Complexity

Process terms [52] often interfere with communication and comprehension, but here the concept of complexity and non-linear thinking requires some discussion. Chronic diseases are complex due to multimorbidities, interactions with the external environment, effects on health perceptions and behaviors, and changes induced by various interventions [53]. There is also a defined level of uncertainty implicit to all complex systems, and in the case of chronic disease, this applies to both the biomedical and social spaces [54]. Traditional therapeutic strategies involve one intervention, one target, and an evidence base to support the action. This type of linear approach works very well when there is a clear dominant driver for the pathology, typically found in acute illness. However, in chronic disease states, where there are multiple drivers, many of which are networked without a clear dominant node, nonlinear approaches involving multiple interventions concurrently or in a special sequence may be optimal [55].

If chronic diseases are to be addressed in a manner that is associated with better outcomes, and this is now deemed to require complex event processing strategies, then a new mind-set is required. This new approach should capture not only disease-oriented and technologically obtained data but as many parts as possible pertaining to a patient's life, their story, and their needs. It is this synthesis of the individual parts, recognition of the holistic partnerships among pathophysiology, behavior, and environment, and detection of relevant, emergent properties that now allow us to create a new chronic disease model to improve health care.

A key aspect of the emergent nature of chronic disease is the notion of residual risk. This is a quantification of the risk occurring after evidence-based interventions for specific risk-reduction indications [56]. In other words, even after taking into consideration all of the specific risk-reduction strategies (e.g., lipid lowering, blood pressure lowering, weight loss, et al.) for cardiovascular disease (CVD), there is still a residual risk for developing CVD due to unknown variables. The notion of residual risk stems primarily from the statin intervention studies in patients with cardiometabolic risk factors where secondary predictors and classifiers are discovered. Residual risk has also been described in a variety of cancer models where there is relapse after optimal primary therapies, arguing for genomic signatures to guide molecular-targeted therapies [57] or broader nutritional medicine approaches [58]. In depression, factors contributing to residual risk may be unhealthy eating patterns, other adverse lifestyle habits, and socioeconomics [59]. The concept of residual risk can be viewed as risk emanating from pathology that is still unrecognized (or under-recognized) relative to the known risks targeted by evidence-based guidelines and standards of care. (Of course, residual risk could also arise from flaws, shortcomings, and misinterpretations of evidence-based clinical practice guidelines or the risk engine employed.) Indeed, residual risk is a marker of complexity and incompleteness of medical knowledge and know-how; here, it is a hallmark of chronic disease and target for lifestyle medicine.

Call for Action: A Chronic Disease Care Model

The use of models to describe health-care activities is predicated on notions of "health," "disease," and their respective root causes. Chronic disease care models should be able to address the drivers and management goals of a chronic disease state in a safe, effective, and ethical manner within the societal constraints of cost factors, health-care policy, and a belief system of a target population. These models incorporate the aspects of clinical practice, research, and education. Moreover, recent advances in patient-centered care, behavioral medicine, and socioeconomics in health care have affirmed the biopsychosocial model.

From a systems standpoint, the biopsychosocial model is robust, especially with changing cultures, and can represent chronic disease more comprehensively in the context of multiple biological and environmental drivers with their complex interactions. In many cases, this type of chronic disease model can facilitate wellness visits and community engagement, promote interprofessional collaboration, include spirituality, and destigmatize illness [60–62].

Chronic disease management is distinctly challenging in the young and very elderly [63]. In Australia, an aging population, inadequate health-care workforce, and increased prevalence of chronic disease prompt collaborative chronic disease management, which has brought together the general practitioner and community pharmacist [64]. In Canada, efforts are under way to transition from embedded to dedicated chronic disease self-management programming [65]. Patient engagement and health coaching enhance knowledge, confidence, and concrete skills that are necessary in a comprehensive care model [66]. Other components of this model include genetic risk testing, medical specialties, nutritional counseling, physical activity, occupational and physiotherapy, behavioral therapy, and social support structures, including spirituality [67–70]. Prompt delivery, continuity of care, and easy access to health care are also necessary [71]. To facilitate these factors, traditional settings, such as the outpatient clinic, are supplemented by "telehealth" (the use of secure information and communication technologies), Accountable Care Organizations, and the Patient-Centered Medical Home [72].

From a research standpoint, high-quality prospective randomized controlled trials are necessary, though other methodologies remain valuable, such as surveillance studies to determine the social determinants for specific risk factors in specific populations [73]. These methodologies will need to be transparent about the details of the intervention. Clinical end points are another challenge in the chronic disease model, and future research designs will need to focus on clinically relevant, patient-oriented evidence that matters (symptom scores and quality-of-life measures) in addition to disease-oriented evidence (hard outcomes, biochemical, and other surrogate markers; [74, 75]). Additionally, the translation of the results into clinical practice will require standardization, diligent monitoring of performance, and agility to adapt to a variety of settings [75].

From an educational standpoint, chronic care models will need to be taught to health-care professionals, as well as patients (as part of a patient-centered approach) and other stakeholders in the social space. Teachers are not limited to physicians and should include all participants in the health professional team [76]. Programs are designed to be transfor-

mational and range from traditional professional school settings to continuing educational curriculum, and to workplace events. Programs contain baseline content, on-the-job training, and interactive follow-up, utilizing direct interpersonal contact, interprofessional team teaching and group learning, community projects, and web-based materials [77, 78]. Any potential progress with implementing a chronic disease care model will depend on effective education and expansion of a well-trained health-care workforce [79].

Each of these model components contends with challenges in prevention, diagnosis, and management. All in all, there are many shortcomings in the current approach to chronic care; therefore, a new approach is needed.

The Response: A Lifestyle Medicine Care Model

A lifestyle medicine care model finds its roots in the preventive medicine care model of the 1960s. The promotion of lifestyle change was among several initiatives in these early preventive care model versions, along with population screening, safety initiatives, and vaccinations [80]. However, despite the obvious virtues of these tactics, the existing health-care system was unable to effectively fund and implement them. Contemporary responses to this dilemma have concluded that a cultural change is needed in order to reboot these initiatives [80].

There is a conspicuous paucity of peer-reviewed publications on chronic disease and lifestyle in the medical literature, but a cursory analysis of PubMed citations provides some insight into recent trends (Table 1.2). More specifically, there are only 1% of intervention papers on lifestyle (denominator = "drugs" + "surgery" + "lifestyle" as keywords) and only 16% of articles on "disease" (as a keyword) also including "chronic disease" (as a keyword). However, the growth rate of lifestyle medicine publications (225% increase from 1999–2004 to 2009–2014) is greater than the growth rates for publications on drugs (134%) or surgery (152%). Of note,

Table 1.2 Emerging literature on "lifestyle medicine"[a]

Keyword	Citations				Growth (%)[b]
	1999–2004	2004–2009	2009–2014	Total	
Drug	624,461	783,070	838,969	4,467,766	134
% non-English				14	
Surgery	451,497	579,030	686,508	3,496,431	152
% non-English				22	
Disease	458,415	629,504	807,286	3,149,692	176
% non-English				16	
Chronic disease	72,362	103,403	130,618	504,240	181
% non-English				20	
Lifestyle	15,738	26,307	35,467	104,592	225
% non-English				11	

[a] PubMed computerized literature search was performed on July 13, 2014. The ratio of total "chronic disease" citations divided by total "disease" citations = 16%. The ratio of total "lifestyle" citations divided by total ("drug" + "surgery" + "lifestyle") management citations = 1%
[b] Growth (%) = ("2009–2014" citations divided by "1999–2004" citations) × 100

Fig. 1.1 Rationale for a lifestyle medicine model.Multiple drivers create a chronic pathophysiological state. The current biomedical model addresses single risk factors with single pharmaceutical or surgical interventions. The chronic disease model is created based on epidemiological data, messaging to patients and health-care professionals, and complexity. Residual risk is depicted by the *closed dots* with single interventional successes in risk reduction depicted by the two *open dots*. Lifestyle interventions target residual risk factors to create a healthy physiological state, promote wellness, and prevent disease progression or new disease

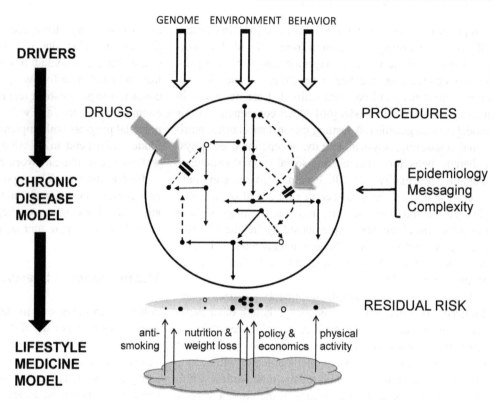

the percentage of non-English articles on lifestyle (11%) is relatively low compared with the other categories (14–20%), suggesting a lag in recognizing lifestyle medicine on a global scale. This is a simple bird's eye view of the problem and further analyses would need to address individual components (practice, research, education, public health, and economics), scope (organ systems, disease states, functional status, and ethnicities), and scales (local, regional, national, and global) to yield the necessary information to advance this new field. Thus, as a response to recognizing chronic disease models as a significant advance, lifestyle medicine, although nascent right now, is gaining popularity and poised for concrete, evidence-based imperatives for implementation.

The reasons to implement lifestyle medicine can be broken down into the following:

1. increased prevalence of chronic disease and synthesis of chronic disease models suitable for the current healthcare climate;
2. recognition of the importance of a preventive care paradigm to reverse trends and lower prevalence rates for chronic disease; this provides benefit in terms of quality of life, longevity, economics and productivity, and overall health of a society;
3. awareness of a specific role for wellness and health promotion within the preventive care paradigm; this investment of health-care dollars translates in the aforementioned benefits;
4. addressing residual risk factors in complex pathologies, such as cancer and metabolic syndrome, using tools not generally learned in traditional medical training; and
5. addressing specific risk management problems, such as tobacco cessation, weight management, healthy eating, physical activity, and glycemic control, using tools, metrics, and methods not traditionally taught (Fig. 1.1).

Conclusions

In this chapter, the mandate for lifestyle medicine finds its roots in the high prevalence rates of chronic disease and the vast adverse downstream effects on quality of life, longevity, and societal burdens. As greater knowledge accrues regarding the complexity of chronic disease and the roles for nonpharmacological and nonsurgical interventions, especially within a preventive care paradigm, implementation strategies need to be assembled into a coherent framework amenable to our current health-care landscape. The challenges are formidable. The solution resides in creating a suitable infrastructure and philosophy that merges traditional aspects of medicine with nuanced individualized care.

Conflict of Interest JM discloses that he has received honoraria from Abbott Nutrition International for lectures and program development; RK discloses that he has received honoraria from Novo Nordisk, Vivus, Takeda, Eisai, and Retrofit for participation on advisory board.

References

1. Go AS, Mozaffarian D, Roger VL, et al. Heart disease and stroke statistics—2014 update: a report from the American Heart Association. Circulation. 2014. doi:10.1161/01.cir.0000441139.02102.80. Accessed 22 June 2014.
2. CDC. Million hearts: strategies to reduce the prevalence of leading cardiovascular disease risk factors—United States, 2011. MMWR Morb Mortal Wkly Rep. 2011;60:1248–51.
3. Centers for Disease Control and Prevention. Prevalence of doctor-diagnosed arthritis and arthritis-attributable activity limitation—United States, 2010–2012. MMWR Morb Mortal Wkly Rep. 2013;62:869–92.
4. Coresh J, Selvin E, Stevens LA, et al. Prevalence of chronic kidney disease in the United States. JAMA. 2007;298:2038–47.
5. Alzheimer's Association. Alzheimer's facts and figures. 2015. http://www.alz.org/alzheimers_disease_facts_and_figures. asp#prevalence. Accessed 22 June 2014.
6. Wright NC, Looker AC, Saag KG, et al. The recent prevalence of osteoporosis and low bone mass in the United States based on bone mineral density at the femoral neck or lumbar spine. J Bone Mineral Res. 2014. doi:10.1002/jbmr.2269.
7. CDC. National Diabetes Statistics Report. 2014. http://www.cdc. gov/diabetes/pubs/statsreport14/national-diabetes-report-web.pdf. Accessed 22 June 2014.
8. CDC. Current depression among adults—United States, 2006 and 2008. MMWR Morb Mortal Wkly Rep. 2010;59:1229–35.
9. American Lung Association, Epidemiology and Statistics Unit. Estimated prevalence and incidence of lung disease. 2014. http://www.lung.org/finding-cures/our-research/trend-reports/estimated-prevalence.pdf. Accessed 22 June 2014.
10. De Moor JS, Mariotto AB, Parry C, et al. Cancer survivors in the United States: prevalence across the survivorship trajectory and implications for care. Canc Epidemiol Biomark Prev. 2013;22:561–70.
11. CDC. Diagnoses of HIV infection in the United States and Dependent Areas. 2011. http://www.cdc.gov/hiv/library/reports/surveillance/2011/surveillance_Report_vol_23.html#3. Accessed 22 June 2014.
12. Perrin EC, Newacheck P, Pless IB, et al. Issues involved in the definition and classification of chronic health conditions. Pediatrics. 1993;91:787–93.
13. O'Halloran J, Miller GC, Britt H. Defining chronic conditions for primary care with ICPC-2. Fam Pract. 2004;21:381–6.
14. CDC. Chronic disease and health promotion. 2015. http://cdc.gov/chronicdisease/overview/index.htm. Accessed 18 July 2014.
15. CDC. Healthy people 2020. 2011. http://www.cdc.gov/nchs/healthy_people/hp2020.htm. Accessed 22 June 2014.
16. CDC. CDC grand rounds: childhood obesity in the United States. MMWR Morb Mortal Wkly Rep. 2011;60:42–6.
17. Chung A, Backholer K, Wong E, et al. Trends in child and adolescent obesity prevalence according to socioeconomic position: protocol for a systematic review. Systematic Rev. 2014;3:52–6.
18. CDC. Awareness of prediabetes—United States, 2005–2010. MMWR. 2013;62:209–12.
19. Guariguata L, Whiting DR, Hambleton I, et al. Global estimates of diabetes prevalence for 2013 and projections for 2035. Diab Res Clin Pract. 2014;103:137–49.
20. Slack T, Myers CA, Martin CK, et al. The geographic concentration of US adult obesity prevalence and associated social, economic, and environmental factors. Obesity. 2014;22:868–74.
21. Eilerman PA, Herzog CM, Luce BK, et al. A comparison of obesity prevalence: military health system and United States populations, 2009–2012. Military Med. 2014;179:462–70.
22. Thomas DM, Weedermann M, Fuenmeler BF, et al. Dynamic model predicting overweight, obesity, and extreme obesity prevalence trends. Obesity. 2014;22:590–7.
23. CDC. Obesity—United States, 1999–2010. MMWR Surveill Summ. 2013;62:120–8.
24. Ostbye T, Stroo M, Eisenstein EL, et al. Is overweight and class I obesity associated with increased health claims costs? Obesity. 2014;22:1179–86.
25. Tarleton HP, Ryan-Ibarra S, Induni M. Chronic disease burden among cancer survivors in the California behavorial risk factor surveillance system, 2009–2010. J Cancer Surviv. 2014. doi:10.1007/s11764-014-0350-x.
26. Forster M, Veeman JL, Barendregt JJ, et al. Cost-effectiveness of diet and exercise interventions to reduce overweight and obesity. Int J Obes (Lond). 2011;35:1071–8.
27. Devleesschauwer B, Havelaar AH, Maertens de Noordhout C, et al. Calculating disability-adjusted life years to quantify burden of disease. Int J Public Health. 2014;59:565–9.
28. Larson BA. Calculating disability-adjusted-life-years lost (DALYs) in discrete time. Cost Eff Res Alloc. 2013;11:18–24.
29. Polinder S, Haagsma JA, Stein C, et al. Systematic review of general burden of disease using disability-adjusted life years. Popul Health Metr. 2012;10:21–36.
30. Schroeder SA. Incidence, prevalence, and hybrid approaches to calculating disability-adjusted life years. Popul Health Metr. 2012;10:19–26.
31. Struijk EA, May AM, Beulens JWJ, et al. Development of methodology for disability-adjusted life years (DALYs) calculation based on real-life data. PloS ONE. 2014;8:e74294. doi:10.1371/journal.pone.0074294.
32. Gibney K, Sinclair M, O'Toole J, et al. Using disability-adjusted life years to set health-based targets: a novel use of an established burden of disease metric. J Public Health Policy. 2013;34:439–46.
33. Murray CJ, Lopez AD. The global burden of disease: a comprehensive assessment of mortality and disability from diseases, injuries and risk factors in 1990 and protected to 2020. Cambridge: Harvard University Press; 1996.
34. Lopez AD, Mathers CD, Ezzati M, et al. Global burden of disease and risk factors. New York: Oxford University Press; 2006.
35. World Health Organization. The global burden of disease: 2004 update. 2015. http://www.who.int/healthinfo/global_burden_disease/2004_report_update/en/index.html. Accessed 12 July 2014.
36. Murray CJ, Vos T, Lozano R, et al. Disability-adjusted life years (DALYs) for 291 diseases and injuries in 21 regions, 1990–2010: a systematic analysis for the Global Burden of Disease Study 2010. Lancet. 2013;380:2197–223.
37. Soerjomataram I, Lortet-Tieulent J, Parkin DM, et al. Global burden of cancer in 2008: a systematic analysis of disability-adjusted life-years in 12 world regions. Lancet. 2012;380:1840–50.
38. Russell LB. Preventing chronic disease: an important investment, but don't count on cost savings. Health Aff. 2009;28:42–5.
39. Zhang NJ, Wan THT, Rossiter LF, et al. Evaluation of chronic disease management on outcomes and cost of care for Medicaid beneficiaries. Health Policy. 2008;86:345–54.
40. Rajgopal R, Cox RH, Lambur M, et al. Cost-benefit analysis indicates the positive economic benefits of the Expanded Food and Nutrition Education Program related to chronic disease prevention. J Nutr Educ Behav. 2002;34:26–37.
41. Irvine L, Barton GR, Gasper AV, et al. Cost-effectiveness of a lifestyle intervention in preventing type 2 diabetes. Int J Technol Assess Health Care. 2011;27:275–82.
42. Guy GP, Yabroff KR, Ekwueme DU, et al. Estimating the health and economic burden of cancer among those diagnosed as adolescents and young adults. Health Aff. 2014;33:1024–31.

43. Erdem E, Prada SI, Haffer SC. Medicare payments: how much do chronic conditions matter? Medicare Medicaid Res Rev. 2013;3:E1–15.

44. Parekh AK, Kronick R, Tavenner M. Optimizing health for persons with multiple chronic conditions. JAMA. 2014. doi:10.1001/jama.2014.10181.

45. Ryan JG. Race, risk, and behaviors: race and disproportionate burdens of chronic disease. Clin Therapeutics. 2014;36:464–8.

46. Campbell DJT, Ronksley PE, Manns BJ, et al. The association of income with health behavior change and disease monitoring among patients with chronic disease. PloS One. 2014;9:e94007. doi:10.1371/journal.pone.0094007.

47. World Health Organization. The top 10 causes of death. http://www.who.int/mediacentre/factsheets/fs310/en/index2.html. Accessed 18 July 2014.

48. President of the General Assembly, United Nations. Draft political declaration of the high-level meeting on the prevention and control of non-communicable diseases. http://www.un.org/en/ga/ncdmeeting2011/pdf/NCD_draft_political_declaration.pdf. Accessed 15 July 2014.

49. World Health Organization. Non-communicable diseases and mental health. http://www.who.int/nmh/publications/9789241597418 en/. Accessed 15 July 2014.

50. Mokdad AH, Marks JS, Stroup DF, et al. Actual causes of death in the United States, 2000. JAMA. 2004;29:1238–45.

51. American Association of Clinical Endocrinologists. 2014 AACE/ACE Consensus Conference of Obesity. http://mms.businesswire.com/media/20140325006164/en/408761/1/aace.pdf [see EC.5. in document]. Accessed 18 July 2014.

52. Harmon P. A glossary of commonly used business process terms. http://www.ispi.org/archives/Glossary/PHarmon.pdf. Accessed 7 Sept 2014.

53. Sturmberg JP. Multimorbidity and chronic disease: an emergent perspective. J Eval Clin Pract. 2014. doi:10.1111/jep.12126.

54. McGrath JW, Winchester MS, Kaawa-Mafigiri D, et al. Challenging the paradigm: anthropological perspectives on HIV as a chronic disease. Med Anthropol. 2014. doi:10.1080/01459740.2014.892483.

55. Higgins JP. Nonlinear systems in medicine. Yale J Biol Med. 2001;75:247–60.

56. Vanuzzo D. The epidemiological concept of residual risk. Intern Emerg Med. 2011;6(Suppl 1):S45–51.

57. Dieci MV, Arnedos M, Delaloge S, et al. Quantification of residual risk of relapse in breast cancer patients optimally treated. Breast. 2013;22:S92–5.

58. Bradbury KE, Appleby PN, Key TJ. Fruit, vegetable, and fiber intake in relation to cancer risk: findings from the European Prospective Investigation into Cancer and Nutrition (EPIC). Am J Clin Nutr. 2014;100(suppl 1):394S–8S.

59. Jacka FN, Cherbuin N, Anstey KJ, et al. Dietary patterns and depressive symptoms over time: examining the relationships with socioeconomic positions, health behaviours and cardiovascular risk. PloS One. 2014;9:e87657. doi:10.1371/journal.pone.0087657.

60. Riley TA, Janosky JE. Moving beyond the medical model to enhance primary care. Popul Health Manage. 2012;15:189–93.

61. Sadler LS, Newlin KH, Johnson-Spruill I, et al. Beyond the medical model: interdisciplinary programs of community-engaged health research. Clin Transl Sci. 2011;4:285–97.

62. Dyer AR. The need for a new "New Medical Model": a bio-psychosocial-spiritual model. South Med J. 2011;104:297–8.

63. Buja A, Damiani G, Gini R, et al. Systematic age-related differences in chronic disease management in a population-based cohort study: a new paradigm of primary care is required. PloS One. 2014;9:e91340. doi:10.1371/journal.pone.0091340.

64. Rieck AM. Exploring the nature of power distance on general practitioner and community pharmacist relations in a chronic disease management context. J Interprof Care. 2014. doi:10.3109/1356182 0.2014.906390.

65. Liddy C, Mill K. An environmental scan of policies in support of chronic disease self-management in Canada. Chr Dis Inj Can. 2014;34:55–63.

66. Simmons LA, Wolever RQ, Bechard EM, et al. Patient engagement as a risk factor in personalized health care: a systematic review of the literature on chronic disease. Genome Med. 2014;6:16–29.

67. Mackenzie L. Can chronic disease management plans including occupational therapy and physiotherapy services contribute to reducing falls risk in older people? Austr Fam Phys. 2014;43:211–5.

68. Brooks AT, Andrade RE, Middleton KR, et al. Social support: a key variable for health promotion and chronic disease management in Hispanic patients with rheumatic diseases. Clin Med Insights Arthr Musculoskel Dis. 2014;7:21–6.

69. Drutchas A, Anandarajah G. Spirituality and coping with chronic disease in pediatrics. Rhode Island Med J. 2014;97:26–30.

70. Vorderstrasse AA, Ginsberg GS, Kraus WE, et al. Health coaching and genomics—potential avenues to elicit behavior change in those at risk for chronic disease: protocol for personalized medicine effectiveness study in Air Force primary care. Global Adv Health Med. 2013;2:26–38.

71. Hussey PS, Schneider EC, Rudin RS, et al. Continuity and the costs of care for chronic disease. JAMA Intern Med. 2014;174:742–8.

72. Jones A, Hedges-Chou J, Bates J, et al. Home telehealth for chronic disease management: selected findings of a narrative synthesis. Telemed e-Health. 2014;20:346–80.

73. Owen N, Salmon J, Koohsari MJ, et al. Sedentary behavior and health: mapping environmental and social contexts to underpin chronic disease prevention. Br J Sports Med. 2014;48:174–7.

74. Shaughnessy AF. Focusing on patient-oriented evidence that matters in the care of patients with diabetes mellitus. Pharmacotherapy. 2004;24:295–7.

75. Wigg AJ, Chinnaratha MA, Wundke R, et al. A chronic disease management model for chronic liver failure. Hepatology. 2014. doi:10.1002/hep.27152.

76. Ritsema TS, Bingenheimer JB, Scholting P, et al. Differences in the delivery of health education to patients with chronic disease by provider type, 2005–2009. Prev Chronic Dis. 2014;11:130175. doi:10.5888/pcd11.130175.

77. Bloem BR, Munneke M. Revolutionising management of chronic disease: the ParkinsonNet approach. BMJ. 2014;348:g1838. doi:http://dx.doi.org/10.1136/bmj.g1838.

78. Bain L, Kennedy C, Archibald D, et al. A training program designed to improve interprofessional knowledge, skills and attitudes in chronic disease settings. J Interprof Care. 2014. doi:10.3109/13 561820.2014.898622.

79. Patel KK. Practical and policy implications of a changing health care workforce for chronic disease management. J Ambul Care Manage. 2013;36:302–4.

80. Clarke JL. Preventive medicine: a ready solution for a health care system in crisis. Popul Health Manage. 2010;10:S3–11.

The Importance of Healthy Living and Defining Lifestyle Medicine

Robert F. Kushner and Jeffrey I. Mechanick

Abbreviations

AHA	American Heart Association
ARIC	Atherosclerosis Risk in Communities Study
BMI	Body mass index
CVD	Cardiovascular diseases
DALY	Disability-adjusted life year
DASH	Dietary Approaches to Stop Hypertension
DSE	Diabetes support and education
EPIC	European Prospective Investigation into Cancer and Nutrition
ILI	Intensive lifestyle-based weight loss intervention
NCD	Noncommunicable diseases
NHANES	National Health and Nutrition Examination Survey
NIH	National Institutes of Health
OR	Odd ratios
PURE	Prospective Urban Rural Epidemiology
SCD	Sudden cardiac death
T2D	Type-2 diabetes
WOH	World Health Organization
YLDs	Years lived with disabilities
YLL	Years of life lost

R. F. Kushner (✉)
Northwestern Comprehensive Center on Obesity, Northwestern University Feinberg School of Medicine, 750 North Lake Shore Drive Rubloff 9-976, Chicago, IL 60611, USA
e-mail: rkushner@northwestern.edu

J. I. Mechanick
Division of Endocrinology, Diabetes and Bone Disease, Icahn School of Medicine at Mount Sinai, 1192 Park Avenue, New York, NY 10128, USA
e-mail: jeffreymechanick@gmail.com

Introduction

The background and rationale for development of lifestyle medicine as a new model of care was reviewed in Chap. 1. In this chapter, we revisit the burden of noncommunicable diseases (NCD) in greater detail, the associated risk factors and contributing influences that heighten risk, the rarity of good health, and the difference between lifestyle medicine and other closely aligned specialty areas.

Rationale for Development of a New Discipline

Lifestyle medicine is a nascent discipline that has recently emerged as a systematized approach for management of chronic disease. The individual elements and skillsets that define lifestyle medicine are determined, in large part, by the primary contributors to NCD. Unhealthy lifestyle behaviors are among the leading risk factors for increased disability-adjusted life years (DALYs) in the USA [1] and around the world [2]. DALYs have become an important metric to assess health outcome and are defined as the sum of years of life lost (YLLs) due to premature mortality and years lived with disabilities (YLDs). Globally, NCD account for about 63 % of all deaths. By 2030, it is estimated that NCD may account for 52 million deaths worldwide [3]. One of the primary aims of the 2011 United Nations High-Level Meeting of the General Assembly on Non-communicable Diseases was "reducing the level of exposure of individuals and populations to the common modifiable risk factors for NCD, namely, tobacco use, unhealthy diet, physical inactivity, and the harmful use of alcohol, and their determinants, while at the same time strengthening the capacity of individuals and populations to make healthier choices and follow lifestyle patterns that foster good health" [4]. More recently, the World Health Organization (WHO) published the *2008–2013 Action Plan for the Global Strategy for the Prevention and Control of Noncommunicable Diseases* to prevent and control four NCD—car-

J. I. Mechanick, R. F. Kushner (eds.), *Lifestyle Medicine*, DOI 10.1007/978-3-319-24687-1_2

Table 2.1 Individual risk factors contributing to the five leading causes of death in the USA, 2010. [6]

	Heart disease	Cancer	Lower respiratory disease	Stroke	Unintentional injuries
Tobacco	✓	✓	✓	✓	
Poor diet	✓	✓		✓	
Physical inactivity	✓	✓		✓	
Overweight	✓	✓		✓	
Alcohol		✓		✓	✓

Table 2.2 Common themes in current dietary and lifestyle recommendations

	USDA Dietary Guidelines (2010)	American Heart Association (AHA) (2006)	American Diabetes Association (2014)	American Cancer Society (2012)	AHA/ACC guideline on lifestyle management to reduce cardiovascular risk (2014)
Healthy body weight	✓	✓	✓	✓	✓
Engage in physical activity	✓	✓	✓	✓	✓
Increase fruits and vegetables	✓	✓	✓	✓	✓
Choose whole grains (high fiber foods)	✓	✓	✓	✓	✓
Limit salt	✓	✓	✓	✓	✓
Limit saturated fat, *trans* fat, and cholesterol	✓	✓	✓		✓
Limit consumption of alcoholic beverages	✓	✓	✓	✓	
Minimize intake of added sugars	✓	✓	✓		✓
Limit consumption of processed meat and meat products				✓	✓
Consume fish, especially oily fish		✓			
Limit consumption of refined grains	✓				

USDA US Department of Agriculture, *ACC* American College of Cardiology

diovascular diseases (CVD), diabetes, cancers, and chronic respiratory diseases and four shared risk factors—tobacco use, physical inactivity, unhealthy diets, and the harmful use of alcohol [5]. These diseases are preventable. It is estimated that up to 80 % of heart disease, stroke, and type-2 diabetes (T2D) and over a third of cancers could be prevented by eliminating these four shared risk factors. The four types of diseases and their risk factors are considered together in the WHO action plan in order to emphasize common causes and highlight potential synergies in prevention and control.

In the USA, the five leading causes of death in 2010 were diseases of the heart, cancer, chronic lower respiratory diseases, cerebrovascular disease (stroke), and unintentional injuries [6]. Among persons aged 80 years, these five diseases represented 66 % of all deaths. Selected modifiable lifestyle risk factors for these diseases are displayed in Table 2.1. Other modifiable risk factors associated with these diseases include hypertension, hypercholesterolemia, and T2D (heart diseases); sun exposure, ionizing radiation, and hormones (cancer); and air pollutants, occupational exposure, and allergens (lower respiratory disease).

The similarity of modifiable lifestyle risk factors for the five leading causes of death is striking. The strength of the evidence regarding the impact of daily habits on health outcomes is further supported by comparing the leading clinical guidelines on prevention and treatment of disease [7–11] (Table 2.2).

Individual lifestyle behaviors are among the five multiple determinants of health as defined by Healthy People 2020, the science-based, 10-year national objectives for improving the health of all Americans [12]. The other four determinants are environment, social, health care, and genetics and biology. In reality, the occurrence or reduction of individual risk factors are closely aligned with the other major determinants. For example, whether an individual consumes an unhealthy diet or is physically inactive will depend, in part, on social, demographic, environmental, economic, and geographical attributes of the neighborhood where the person lives and works [6].

Impact of a Healthy Lifestyle on Chronic Disease

There is a strong body of evidence that practicing healthy lifestyle behaviors reduces the risk of chronic disease. In 2009, the American College of Preventive Medicine published a comprehensive review of the scientific evidence for lifestyle medicine both for the prevention and treatment of chronic disease [13]. Twenty-four chronic diseases were reviewed in this publication, highlighting the impact of a healthy lifestyle on improving the root causes of disease.

Recently, multiple systematic reviews and meta-analyses have been published that demonstrate the beneficial impact of lifestyle interventions in reducing T2D incidence in patients with impaired glucose tolerance [14, 15], management of T2D [16, 17], hypercholesterolemia [18], CVD [11], and the metabolic syndrome [19, 20]. In the National Institutes of Health (NIH)-AARP Diet and Health Study population-based cohort study among 207,449 men and women, the 11-year risk for incident T2D for men and women whose diet score, physical activity, smoking status, and alcohol use were all in the low-risk group had odd ratios (OR) for T2D of 0.61 and 0.43, respectively, compared to the high-risk group [21]. T2D and obesity are among the two most significant NCDs that currently affect 366 and 500 million people worldwide, respectively [22, 23]. Often called "diabesity" because of their close association, one of the most effective targets for T2D treatment is management of excess body weight by diet and physical activity. The beneficial impact of weight loss on glycemic control and reduction of cardiovascular risk factors has been recently demonstrated in the Look AHEAD (Action for Health in Diabetes) trial. In this prospectively controlled, randomized study conducted at 16 US research centers, 5145 overweight adults aged 45–76 years with T2D were randomized to either an intensive lifestyle-based weight loss intervention (ILI) or a diabetes support and education (DSE) intervention [24]. Although 4-year results showed statistically significant improvements in fitness, glycemic control, and cardiovascular risk factors [25, 26], the trial was discontinued in September, 2012 after a median follow-up of 9.6 years on the basis of a futility analysis [27]. The probability of observing a significant positive result at the planned end of follow-up was estimated to be 1%. Proposed explanations for the lack of significant difference in rates of cardiovascular events between the ILI and DSE groups include a 2.5% difference in weight loss between groups at year 10, intensification of medical management of cardiovascular risk factors, and low event rate [28].

Over the past several years, there has been an increased interest in evaluating the benefit of adhering to "low-risk lifestyle" behaviors on the development of morbidity and mortality. Although the criteria for defining "low-risk lifestyle" factors vary, these studies have shown that adherence to a healthy lifestyle is associated with improved health outcomes. The following population studies are notable for their size and magnitude in demonstrating the potential impact of fostering lifestyle medicine as a new discipline.

In the European Prospective Investigation into Cancer and Nutrition (EPIC) study, 23,153 German participants aged 35–65 years were followed-up for a mean of 7.8 years. Adherence to four health behaviors (not smoking, exercising 3.5 h per week, eating a healthy diet (high intake of fruits, vegetables, and whole-grain bread and low meat consumption), and having a body mass index (BMI) of 30 kg/m^2) at baseline was associated with 78% lower risk of developing chronic disease (T2D 93%, myocardial infarction 81%, stroke 50%, and cancer 36%) than participants without the healthy factors [29].

In the Nurses' Health Study, a prospective cohort study of 81,722 US women from 1984 to 2010, a low-risk lifestyle was defined as not smoking, BMI of less than 25 kg/m^2, exercise duration of 30 min/day or longer, and top 40% of the alternate Mediterranean diet score, which emphasizes high intake of vegetables, fruits, nuts, legumes, whole grains, and fish and moderate intake of alcohol. Compared with women with no low-risk factors, the multivariate relative risk of sudden cardiac death (SCD) decreased progressively for women with 1, 2, 3, and 4 low-risk factors to 0.54, 0.41, 0.33, and 0.08, respectively. The proportion of SCD attributable to smoking, inactivity, overweight, and poor diet was 81% [30].

The Atherosclerosis Risk in Communities Study (ARIC), a prospective epidemiological study of 15,792 men and women aged 44–64 years at enrollment, demonstrated that adopting a healthy lifestyle after age 45 results in substantial benefits after only 4 years compared to people with less healthy lifestyles, reducing mortality and CVD risk by 40 and 35%, respectively [31].

To further explore the relationship between change in health behaviors, socioeconomic status, and mortality, Stringhini et al. [32] followed a cohort of 10,308 civil servants from baseline examination (1985–1988) to phase 7 (2002–2004) in the British Whitehall II study. After adjusting for sex and year of birth, those with the lowest socioeconomic position had 1.60 times higher risk of death from all causes than those with the highest socioeconomic position. However, this association was attenuated by 72% when four health behaviors (smoking, alcohol consumption, diet, and physical activity) were entered in the statistical model.

In a population-based, prospective cohort of 20,721 Swedish men aged 45–79 years without history of chronic disease followed for 11 years, five low-risk behaviors (a healthy diet, moderate alcohol consumption, no smoking, being physically active, and having a healthy waist circumference) were associated with 86% lower risk of myocardial infarction events compared with the high-risk group with no low-risk factors [33].

Table 2.3 Definitions of poor, intermediate, and ideal cardiovascular health for each American Heart Association (AHA) metric for adults 20 years of age

Goal/metric	Poor health	Intermediate health	Ideal health
Current smoking	Yes	Former ≤ 12 months	Never or quit > 12 months
Body mass index (kg/m^2)	≥ 30	25–29.9	< 25
Physical activity	None	1–149 min/week moderate intensity or 1–74 min/week vigorous intensity or 1–149 min/week moderate + vigorous	≥ 150 min/week moderate intensity or ≥ 75 min/week vigorous intensity or ≥ 150 min/week moderate + vigorous intensity
Healthy Diet Score[a]	0–1 components	2–3 components	4–5 components
Total cholesterol (mg/dl)	> 240	200–239, or treated to goal	< 200
Blood pressure (mm Hg)	SBP ≥ 140 or DBP ≥ 90	SBP 120–139 or DBP 80–89 or treated to goal	< 120/< 80
Fasting plasma glucose (mg/dl)	≥ 126	100–125 or treated to goal	< 100

SBP systolic blood pressure, *DBP* diastolic blood pressure

[a] Healthy Diet Score is based on an overall dietary pattern that is consistent with a Dietary Approaches to Stop Hypertension (DASH)-type eating plan. Individual components are: fruits and vegetables: ≥ 4.5 cups per day; fish: ≥ two 3.5-oz servings per week; fiber-rich whole grains: ≥ three 1-oz equivalent servings per day; sodium: < 1500 mg per day; sugar-sweetened beverages: ≤ 450 kcal (36 oz) per week; nuts, legumes, and seeds: ≥ four servings per week; processed meats: none or ≤ two servings per week; saturated fat: < 7 % of total energy intake. Adapted from reference [36].

Another approach used to assess the burden of disease is to combine lifestyle and physiological risk factors. This has been extensively applied to CVD. In the INTERHEART study, a case–control study of acute myocardial infarction across 52 countries, 15,152 cases and 14,820 controls were enrolled between 1999 and 2003 to assess the effect of risk factors on development of coronary disease [34]. The study showed that over 90 % of the proportion of risk for an initial myocardial infarction is collectively attributable to nine measured and potentially modifiable risk factors: cigarette smoking, raised ApoB/Apo A1 ratio, hypertension, abdominal obesity, psychosocial factors, daily consumption of fruits and vegetables, regular alcohol consumption, and regular physical activity.

The concept of "cardiovascular health metrics" has also emerged as a method to assess cardiovascular risk and coined as "Life's Simple 7" by the American Heart Association (AHA) in their 2020 Strategic Impact Goals to target a 20 % relative improvement in overall cardiovascular health in all Americans [35]. The AHA combines four health behaviors (smoking, diet, physical activity, and body weight) with three health factors (plasma glucose, cholesterol, and blood pressure) as their metrics and assesses adherence as poor, intermediate, or ideal by distinct definitions (Table 2.3) [36]. The AHA also recently published 11 comprehensive articles in a themed series entitled "Recent Advances in Preventive Cardiology and Lifestyle Medicine" that emphasize the multiple determinants of cardiovascular health [37]. Finally, Yang et al. [38] analyzed the associations between the number of ideal cardiovascular health metrics and mortality over a median follow-up of 14.5 years using data from the National Health and Nutrition Examination Survey (NHANES). Compared with individuals with 0 or 1 metric at ideal levels, those with six or more metrics at ideal levels had 51, 76, and 70 % lower adjusted hazards for all-cause, CVD, and ischemic heart disease mortality, respectively.

The Rarity of Good Health

Despite the importance of following a healthy life, multiple population studies have shown that only a minority of individuals adhere to healthy lifestyle behaviors. In a comparative analysis of middle-aged adults aged 40–74 years participating in the NHANES III 1988–1994 and 2001–2006 surveys, the proportion of adults who adhered to all five healthy habits (≥ 5 fruits and vegetables/day, regular exercise 12 times/month, maintaining a BMI between 18.5 and 29.9 kg/m^2, moderate alcohol consumption, and not smoking) decreased from 15 to 8 % [39]. Adherence to the ideal health metrics was also analyzed by Ford et al. [40] using data from NHANES 1999 to 2002. Overall, about 1.5 % of participants met none of the seven ideal cardiovascular health metrics, and 1.1 % of participants met all seven metrics; most adults met two, three, or four ideal health metrics. Based on an analysis of the NHANES data, Huffman et al. [41] projects that the AHA goal of reducing CVD by 20 % by 2020 will not be reached.

Poor health behaviors are not confined to the USA. Akesson et al. [33] (discussed above) identified five low-risk behaviors (a healthy diet, moderate alcohol consumption, no smoking, being physically active, and having a healthy waist circumference) that were associated with a 86 % lower risk of myocardial infarction events compared with the high-risk group with no low-risk factors. Despite the impact of healthy living, only 1 % of the population comprised the low-risk group and followed all five healthy lifestyle practices.

In the Prospective Urban Rural Epidemiology (PURE) study, 153,996 adults, aged 35–70 years, from 17 low-, middle-, and high-income countries of the world were surveyed for their health behaviors after a median of 5 years and 4 years after sustaining a coronary heart disease event or stroke, respectively [42]. Despite having known CVD, less

Table 2.4 Current definitions of lifestyle medicine

American College of Life-style Medicine 2011 [50]	Lifestyle medicine is the therapeutic use of evidence-based lifestyle interventions to treat and prevent lifestyle related diseases in a clinical setting. It empowers individuals with the knowledge and life skills to make effective behavior changes that address the underlying causes of disease
Egger et al. 2012 [51]	The application of environmental, behavioral, medical, and motivational principles to the management of lifestyle-related health problems (including self-care and self-management) in a clinical setting
Lianov and Johnson [52]	Evidence-based practice of assisting individuals and families to adopt and sustain behaviors that can improve health and quality of life
Rippe 1999, 2014 [53]	The integration of lifestyle practices into the modern practice of medicine both to lower the risk factors for chronic disease and/or, if disease already present, serve as an adjunct in its therapy. Lifestyle medicine brings together sound, scientific evidence in diverse health-related fields to assist the clinician in the process of not only treating disease, but also promoting good health

than 1 in 20 individuals adhered to the three healthy lifestyle behaviors of avoiding cigarette smoking, undertaking regular physical activity, and eating a healthy diet. The investigators also noted that, overall, individuals from upper-middle-income and low-income countries had a lower prevalence of three of the healthy lifestyle behaviors than those from high-income and lower-middle-income countries.

Defining Lifestyle Medicine

The literature reviewed in the chapter presents a strong argument for the benefits of healthy living and a need to increase the number of people engaging in those health behaviors. However, it is important to consider how a proposed new discipline of lifestyle medicine differs from other closely aligned fields in medicine, such as preventive medicine, individualized or personalized medicine, or integrative medicine. Certainly, there is overlap in the targets of intervention but there are also important differences in philosophy and scope of practice. *Preventive medicine* focuses on the health of individuals, communities, and defined populations. Its goal is to protect, promote, and maintain health and well-being and to prevent disease, disability, and death [43]. *Individualized or Personalized Medicine* tries to tailor medical interventions in terms of stratifying care by genetic characteristics [44]. A recently suggested definition was offered by Schleidgen et al. [45] as a discipline that "seeks to improve tailoring and timing of preventive and therapeutic measures by utilizing biological information and biomarkers on the level of molecular disease pathways, genetics, proteomics as well as metabolomics."

Integrative medicine is closely aligned with lifestyle medicine in its core tenets. It has multiple definitions that describe a specialty that incorporates both conventional and alternative therapies. Rakel [46] defines it as "healing-oriented medicine that takes account of the whole person (body, mind, and spirit), including all aspects of lifestyle. It emphasizes the therapeutic relationship and makes use of all appropriate therapies, both conventional and alternative." According to Rees and Weil [47], "integrated medicine selectively

incorporates elements of complementary and alternative medicine into comprehensive treatment plans alongside solidly orthodox methods of diagnosis and treatment. It focuses on health and healing rather than disease and treatment." The core competencies in integrated medicine for medical school curricula defines integrative medicine as "an approach to the practice of medicine that makes use of the best available evidence, taking into account the whole person (body, mind, and spirit), including all aspects of lifestyle" [48]. Finally, Snyderman and Weil [49] define integrative medicine as "preventive maintenance of health by paying attention to all relative components of lifestyle, including diet, exercise, and well-being."

Similar to integrative medicine, several definitions of *lifestyle medicine* have been proposed and are listed in Table 2.4 [50–53]. Common elements in all of these definitions are the application of evidence-based lifestyle interventions that promote self-management for promotion of well-being, prevention of illness, and management of chronic disease. To support this new initiative, the *American Journal of Lifestyle Medicine* was launched in 2007 along with creation of a new academic medical society (the American College of Lifestyle Medicine, http://lifestylemedicine.org/) and an educational track in lifestyle medicine at the American College of Preventive Medicine's annual meeting. Societies promoting lifestyle medicine have also been formed in Europe (ESLM, https://eu-lifestylemedicine.org/) and Australia (ALMA, http://lifestylemedicine.com.au/). For the purposes of this book, we define lifestyle medicine as "the nonpharmacological and nonsurgical prevention and/or management of chronic disease."

Conclusion

There is a significant body of literature that demonstrates that adoption of low-risk lifestyle behaviors and ideal cardiovascular health metrics are associated with reduced mortality. However, there is also considerable evidence that healthy lifestyle behaviors are incorporated by a minority of the population. Lifestyle medicine presents a new and challenging approach to address the prevention and treatment of NCD, the most important and prevalent causes for increased morbidity and mortality worldwide.

References

1. US Burden of Diseases Collaborators. The state of US health, 1990–2010. Burden of diseases, injuries, and risk factors. JAMA. 2013;310(6):591–608.

2. Lim SS, Vos T, Flaxman AD, et al. A comparative risk assessment of burden of disease and injury attributable to 67 risk factors and risk factor clusters in 21 regions, 1990–2010: a sysmematic analysis for the Global Burden of Disesae Study 2010. The Lancet. 2012;380:2224–2163.

3. Marrero SL, Bloom DE, Adashi EY. Noncommunicable diseases. A global health crisis in a new world order. JAMA. 2012;307:2037–8.

4. United Nations General Assembly. Political declaration of the high-level meeting of the General Assembly on the prevention and control of non-communicable diseases. 16 September, 2011. http://www.globalhealth.gov/global-health-topics/non-communicable-diseases/ncdmeeting2014.html. Accessed 6 Oct 2014.

5. World Health Organization. 2008–2013 action plan for the global strategy for the prevention and control of noncommunicable diseases: prevent and control cardiovascular diseases, cancers, chronic respiratory diseases and diabetes. Geneva: WHO Document Production Services; 2008.

6. Yoon PW, Bastian B, Anderson RN, et al. Potentially preventable deaths from the five leading causes of death—United States, 2008–2010. MMWR. 2014;63(17):369–74.

7. U.S. Department of Agriculture and U.S. Department of Health and Human Services. Dietary guidelines for Americans. 7th ed. Washington, DC: U.S. Government Printing Office; 2010. http://health.gov/dietaryguidelines/2010.asp. Accessed 6 Oct 2014.

8. Lichtenstein AH, Appel LJ, Brands M, et al. Diet and lifestyle recommendations revision 2006. A scientific statement from the American Heart Association Nutrition Committee. Circulation 2006;114:82–96.

9. Evert A, Boucher JL, Cypress M, American Diabetes Association, et al. Nutrition therapy recommendations for the management of adults with diabetes. Diab Care. 2014;37(Suppl 1):S120–43.

10. Kushi LH, Doyle C, McCullough M, et al. American Cancer Society Guidelines on nutrition and physical activity for cancer prevention. Reducing the risk of cancer with healthy food choices and physical activity. CA Cancer J Clin. 2012;62:30–67.

11. Eckel RH, Jakicic JM, Ard JD, et al. 2013 AHA/ACC Guideline on lifestyle management to reduce cardiovascular risk. J Am Coll Card 2014;63(25):2960–84.

12. Healthy People 2020. 2010. http://www.healthypeople.gov/. Accessed 6 Oct 2014.

13. American College of Preventive Medicine. *Lifestyle Medicine—Evidence Review*. 30 June 2009. http://c.ymcdn.com/sites/www.acpm.org/resource/resmgr/lmi-files/lifestylemedicine-literature.pdf. Accessed 24 Sept 2014

14. Yoon U, Kwok LL, Magkidis A. Efficacy of lifestyle interventions in reducing diabetes incidence in patients with impaired glucose tolerance: a systematic review of randomized controlled trials. Metab Clin Exp. 2013;62:303–14 (Review of trials demonstrated that lifestyle intervention can have a beneficial effect on the incidence of diabetes in patients with impaired glucose tolerance).

15. Ali M, Echouffo-Tcheugul JB, Williamson DF. How effective were lifestyle interventions in real-world settings that were modeled on the diabetes prevention program? Health Aff. 2012;31(1):67–75 (Review concludes that the costs associated with diabetes prevention can be lowered without sacrificing effectiveness).

16. Avery L, Flynn D, van Wersch A, et al. Changing physical activity behavior in type 2 diabetes. A systematic review and meta-analysis of behavioral interventions. Diab Care. 2012;35:2681–9 (Review concludes that behavioral interventions that increase physical activity produce clinically significant improvements in long-term glucose control).

17. Umpierre D, Ribeiro PAB, Kramer CK, et al. Physical activity advice only or structured exercise training and association with HbA1c levels in type 2 diabetes. A systemic review and meta-analysis. JAMA. 2011;305(17):1790–9.

18. Mannu GS, Zaman MJS, Gupta A, et al. Evidence of lifestyle modification in the management of hypercholesterolemia. Curr Cardiol Rev. 2013;9:2–14.

19. Yamaoka K, Tango T. Effects of lifestyle modification on metabolic syndrome: a systematic review and meta-analysis. BMC Med. 2012;10:138.

20. Pattyn N, Cornelissen VA, Toghi Eshghi SR, Vanhees L. The effect of exercise on the cardiovascular risk factors constituting the metabolic syndrome. Sports Med. 2013;43:121–33.

21. Reis J, Loria CM, Sorlie PD, et al. Lifestyle factors and risk for new-onset diabetes. A population-based cohort study. Ann Intern Med. 2011;155:292–9.

22. IDF Diabetes Atlas. 2014. http://www.idf.org/diabetesatlas/5e/the-global-burden. Accessed 6 Oct 2014.

23. World Health Organization. 2015. http://www.who.int/topics/obesity/en/. Accessed 6 Oct 2014.

24. Wing RR, Lang W, Wadden TA, et al. Benefits of modest weight loss in improving cardiovascular risk factors in overweight and obese individuals with type 2 diabetes. Diab Care. 2011;34:1481–6.

25. The Look AHEAD Research Group. Long-term effects of a lifestyle intervention on weight and cardiovascular risk factors in individuals with type 2 diabetes mellitus. Four-year results of the Look AHEAD Trial. Arch Intern Med. 2010;170(17):1566–75.

26. Gregg EW, Chen H, Wagenknecht LE, et al. Association of an intensive lifestyle intervention with remission of type 2 diabetes. JAMA. 2012;308(23):2489–96.

27. Weight loss does not lower heart disease risk from type 2 diabetes. NIH News. 2012. http://www.nih.gov/news/health/oct2012/niddk-19.htm. Accessed 6 Oct 2014.

28. The Look AHEAD Research Group. Cardiovascular effect of intensive lifestyle intervention in type 2 diabetes. N Engl J Med 2013;369(2):145–54.

29. Ford ES, Bergmann MM, Kroger J, et al. Healthy living is the best revenge. Findings from the European prospective investigation into cancer and nutrition-Potsdam study. Arch Intern Med. 2009;169(15):1355–62.

30. Chiuve SE, Fung TT, Rexrode KM, et al. Adherence to a low-risk, healthy lifestyle and risk of sudden cardiac death among women. JAMA. 2011;306(1):62–9.

31. King DE, Mainous AG, Geesey ME. Turning back the clock: adopting a healthy lifestyle in middle age. Am J Med. 2007;120:598–603.

32. Stringhini S, Sabia S, Shipley M, et al. Association of socioeconomic position with health behaviors and mortality. JAMA. 2010;303(12):1159–66.

33. Akesson A, Larsson SC, Discacciati A, Wolk A. Low-risk diet and lifestyle habits in the primary prevention of myocardial infarction in men. A population-based prospective cohort study. J Am Coll Card. 2014;64(13):1299–1306.

34. Yusuf S, Hawkins S, Oumpuu S, et al. Effect of potentially modifiable risk factors associated with myocardial infarction in 52 countries (the INTERHEART study): case-control study. The Lancet. 2004;364:937–52.

35. American Heart Association. My life check. Live better with life's simple 7. 2015. http://mylifecheck.heart.org/Default.aspx?NavID=1&CultureCode=en-us. Accessed 1 May 2013.

36. Lloyd-Jones DM, Hong Y, Labarthe D, et al. Defining and setting national goals for cardiovascular health promotion and disease prevention: the American Heart Association's strategic impact goal through 2020 and beyond. Circulation. 2010;121:586–613.

37. Franklin BA, Cushman M. Recent advances in preventive cardiology and lifestyle medicine. A themed series. Circulation. 2011;123:2274–83.

38. Yang Q, Cogswell ME, Flanders WD, et al. Trends in cardiovascular health metrics and associations with all-cause and CVD mortality among US adults. JAMA. 2012;307(12):1273–83.

39. King DE, Mainous AG, Carnemolla M, Everett CJ. Adherence to healthy lifestyle habits in US adults, 1988–2006. Am J Med. 2009;122:528–34.

40. Ford ES, Greenlund KJ, Hong Y. Ideal cardiovascular health and mortality from all causes and diseases of the circulatory system among adults in the United States. Circulation. 2012;125:987–95.

41. Huffman MD, Capewell S, Ning H, et al. Cardiovascular health behavior and health factor changes (1988–2008) and projections to 2020. Results from the National Health and Nutrition Examination Surveys. Circulation. 2012;125:2595–602.

42. Teo K, Lear S, Islam S, et al. Prevalence of a healthy lifestyle among individuals with cardiovascular disease in high-, middle- and low-income countries. The Prospective Urban Rural Epidemiology (PURE) study. JAMA. 2013;309(15):1613–21.

43. American College of Preventive Medicine. http://www.acpm.org/. Accessed 9 Oct 2014.

44. Hatz MHM, Schremser K, Rogowski WH. Is individualized medicine more cost-effective? A systematic review. Pharmacoeconomics. 2014;32:443–55.

45. Schleidgen S, Klingler C, Bertram T, Rogowski WH, Marckmann G. What is personalized medicine: sharpening a vague term based on a systematic literature review. BMC Med Ethics. 2013;14:55.

46. Rakel D, Weil A. Philosophy of integrative medicine. In: Rakel D, editor. Integrative medicine. 3rd ed. Philadelphia: Elsevier; 2012. pp. 2–11.

47. Rees L, Weil A. Integrated medicine. Imbues orthodox medicine with the values of complementary medicine. BMJ. 2001;322:119–20.

48. Kligler B, Maizes V, Schachter S, Park CM, Gaudet T, Benn R, Lee R, Remen RN. Core competencies in integrated medicine for medical school curricula: a proposal. Acad Med. 2004;79:521–31.

49. Snyderman R, Weil AT. Integrative medicine: bringing medicine back to its roots. Arch Intern Med. 2002;162:395–7.

50. American College of Lifestyle Medicine Standards. 2015. http://www.lifestylemedicine.org/standards. Accessed 10 Oct 2014.

51. Egger GJ, Binns AF, Rossner SR. The emergence of "lifestyle medicine" as a structured approach for management of chronic disease. Med J Aust. 2009;190(3):143–5.

52. Lianov L, Johnson M. Physician competencies for prescribing lifestyle medicine. JAMA. 2010;304(2):202–3.

53. In: Rippe JM, editor. Lifestyle medicine. 2nd ed. New York, CRC Press; 2013. pp. xix–xxii.

Communication and Behavioral Change Tools: A Primer for Lifestyle Medicine Counseling

Robert F. Kushner and Jeffrey I. Mechanick

Abbreviations

CBT   Cognitive behavioral therapy
IOM   Institute of Medicine
MI   Motivational interviewing
SCT   Social cognitive theory
SDM   shared decision-making
SOC   Stages of change
TPB   Theory of planned behavior

Introduction

The practice of lifestyle medicine is dependent upon the provider's ability to implement behavior change in his/her patients regardless of the target behavior, for example, smoking cessation, reduction in alcohol use, increasing consumption of fruits and vegetables, engagement in physical activity, or reducing body weight. Although personal responsibility is important, there are multiple reasons why patients may have difficulty adhering to medical recommendations. In the preceding chapter, the five determinants of health are reviewed, which are defined by Healthy People 2020 [1] as influencing health outcomes: individual behavior, environment, social, health care, and genetics and biology. The term "behavioral" refers to the underlying processes, such as cognition, emotion, temperament, personality, and motivation. The term "social" encompasses sociocultural, socioeconomic, and sociodemographic status [2]. Attention to these and other contextualizing factors is important to further understand the barriers that patients face when implementing lifestyle changes. How we help patients change behavior represents a set of cognitive tools that are grounded in behavioral science. This chapter provides a primer on the importance of communication as well as the most commonly used theories and approaches for behavior change. Examples of dialogues between the clinician and patient are included throughout the chapter to illustrate how the principles and theories of behavior change are applied in clinical practice.

Contextualization of Care

Contextualization of care refers to those elements of a patient's environment or behavior that are relevant to their care, including their economic situation, access to care, social support, and skills and abilities [3]. Recently, the Institute of Medicine (IOM) [4] published their recommendation for a candidate list of 17 domains that represent the social and behavioral determinants of health data that are best suited to capture in the electronic health record (Table 3.1). These factors are intended to offer useful information to health-care providers for the provision of more targeted patient care.

The social determinants of health, that is, the economic and social conditions that influence the health of people and communities, are particularly important in the practice of lifestyle medicine and present several considerations that must be incorporated when providing effective counseling. The first is health disparities, which encompass an appreciation of the racial, ethnic, and cultural factors that impact treatment decision-making. Cultural competence refers to having the capacity to function effectively as a health-care provider within the context of the cultural beliefs, practices, and needs presented by patients and their communities [5]. In contrast, cultural humility implies having an attitude that acknowledges that a patient's culture can only be appreciated by learning from the patient. The second consideration is health literacy, which is often defined as a set of skills that

R. F. Kushner (✉)
Northwestern Comprehensive Center on Obesity, Northwestern University Feinberg School of Medicine, 750 North Lake Shore Drive, Rubloff 9-976, Chicago, IL 60611, USA
e-mail: rkushner@northwestern.edu

J. I. Mechanick
Division of Endocrinology, Diabetes and Bone Disease, Icahn School of Medicine at Mount Sinai, 1192 Park Avenue, New York, NY 10128, USA
e-mail: jeffreymechanick@gmail.com

© Springer International Publishing Switzerland 2016
J. I. Mechanick, R. F. Kushner (eds.), *Lifestyle Medicine*, DOI 10.1007/978-3-319-24687-1_3

Table 3.1 Institute of Medicine candidate domains for inclusion in the electronic health record [4]

Individual factors		
Sociodemographic	*Psychological*	*Behavioral*
Sexual orientation	Health literacy	Dietary patterns
Race/ethnicity	Stress	Physical activity
Country of origin/US born or non-US born	Negative mood and affect: depression and anxiety	Nicotine use and exposure
Education	Psychological assets: conscientiousness, patient engagement/activation, optimism, and self-efficacy	Alcohol use
Financial resources strain: food or housing insecurity		
Individual-level social relationships and living conditions	*Neighborhoods/communities*	
	Geocodable domains: socioeconomic and race/ethnic characteristics	
Social connections and social isolation		
Exposure to violence		

people need in order to function effectively in the health-care environment [6]. It represents the capacity of individuals to obtain, communicate, process, and understand health information and services in order to make appropriate decisions [7]. The skills include the ability to read and understand text, interpret information, and speak and listen effectively. These skills are particularly important when we ask patients to track their diet, read food labels, incorporate behavioral advice, or take prescribed medication. Low health literacy is associated with poorer health outcomes and poorer use of health-care services [6].

The Patient–Physician Encounter

The cornerstone of effective treatment for lifestyle behavior change is grounded in skillful and empathetic provider–patient communication. This vital interaction is affirmed by Balint's assertion [8] that "the most frequently used drug in medical practice is the doctor himself." From the patient's perspective, a caring provider is compassionate, supportive, trustworthy, open-minded, and nonjudgmental. He or she takes into account the patient's needs, values, beliefs, goals, personality traits, and fears [8]. In a review of the literature, Stewart [9] found that the quality of communication between the physician and patient directly influenced patient health outcomes. Since the primary aim of lifestyle counseling is to influence what the patient does *outside* the office, the time spent *in* the office needs to be structured and effective.

Effective counseling begins with establishing rapport and soliciting the patient's agenda. Attentively listening to the patient to understand his or her goals and expectations is the first essential step. Asking the patient, "How do you hope that I can help you?" is an information-gathering, open-ended question that directly addresses his or her concerns. Among 28 identified elements of care that were inquired about with patients before the office visit, Kravitz [10] found that "discussion of own ideas about how to manage condi-

tion" was ranked as the highest pre-visit physician expectation. This is not always done in the primary care office. In a survey of 264 patient–physician interviews, patients completed their statement of concern only 28% of the time, being interrupted by the physician after an average duration of 23 s [11]. Physicians were found to redirect the patient and focus the clinical interviews before giving patients the opportunity to complete their statement of concern. Lifestyle interviewing and counseling should be patient centered, allowing the patient to be an active participant in setting the agenda and having his or her concerns heard. This requires skillful management by the provider to structure the interview within the time allocated.

Communication

The style of communication used by the provider refers to the approach taken when interacting with and counseling patients. Emanuel and Emanuel [12] describe four models of the physician–patient relationship: *paternalistic*—the physician acts as the patient's guardian, articulating and implementing what is best for the patient; *informative*—the physician is a purveyor of technical expertise, providing the patient with the means to exercise control; *interpretive*—the physician is a counselor, supplying relevant information and engaging the patient in a joint process of understanding; and *deliberative*—the physician acts as a teacher or friend, engaging the patient in a dialogue on what course of action would be best. In practice, the style of communication may change from patient to patient and depend upon the provider's personality.

Roter et al. [13] define four similar prototypes of doctor–patient relationships using a "power" balance sheet. In this model, power relates to who sets the agenda, whether the patient's values are expressed and considered, and what role the physician assumes. As illustrated in Table 3.2, high provider and high patient power (A) depicts a relationship of mutuality, balance, and shared decision-making (SDM).

Table 3.2 Provider–physician communication relationships [4]

PHYSICIAN POWER

		HIGH	LOW
PATIENT POWER	HIGH	Mutuality (A)	Consumerism (C)
	LOW	Paternalism (B)	Dysfunctional (D)

High provider and low patient power (B) is consistent with Emanuel's paternalistic model where the provider sets the agenda and prescribes the treatment. In the low provider and high patient power relationship (C), the patient sets the agenda and takes sole responsibility for decision-making; Roter et al. [13] term relationship C as "consumerism." Lastly, in a low provider and low patient power relationship (D), the role of the provider and patient is unclear and undefined. This is a dysfunctional relationship. According to Roter et al. [13], the optimal relationship is that of mutuality (relationship A) or what they call "relationship-centered medicine" or "patient centeredness." In the course of providing lifestyle medical care, it is likely that more than one of these relationships is used among patients. Another important communication style that is related to patient satisfaction is caring. Verbal displays of caring include expressing empathy, statements of reassurance and support, positive reinforcement, and courtesy [14].

Depending on the patient's course of treatment and response, various strategies and techniques are used during the visit. The interaction is directed toward keeping the patient motivated and providing a sense of control. This interaction boosts patient empowerment, which is often defined as a process by which people gain mastery over their lives [15]. A fundamental objective in lifestyle medicine is for patients to take increased responsibility for and a more active role in decision-making regarding their own health. According to Spreitzer [16], four key components of patient empowerment are: (a) meaningfulness (or relevance)—the change is worth investing energy in; (b) self-efficacy—the belief in one's capabilities to achieve a desired result by one's actions; (c) impact—the accomplishment of a task is perceived to make a difference in the scheme of things; and (d) self-determination (or choice)—a decision that is characterized by self-initiation.

Regardless of whether an appropriate therapeutic and supportive relationship is established, many patients will not achieve their behavioral goals. In this case, it is extremely important not to label these patients as noncompliant. The word "compliance" suggests that a submissive patient should obey the authoritative providers' instructions. "Noncompliance" denotes failure or refusal to cooperate. This description is consistent with the paternalistic provider–patient relationship model discussed above. Some authors have suggested that the word "adherence" is a better alternative to compliance, emphasizing the patient's role as an active decision-maker [17, 18]. Still others have abandoned both terms because they exaggerate the importance of the clinician and do not aid in helping the patient overcome behavioral obstacles [19]. Simply asking the patient what is hard about a particular behavioral change is more productive in problem-solving than giving them purposeless labels.

Structuring the Encounter: Using the Five As

The five As is an organizational construct for clinical counseling that has been used for smoking cessation [20], alcohol dependence [21], and weight management [22], among other lifestyle behaviors. It provides a structured framework for the clinician when engaging a patient in behavior change. The five As are *Ask, Advise, Assess, Assist*, and *Arrange*. An example of how to apply the five As for weight management is shown in Table 3.3. An abbreviated version of the five As *(Ask, Advise, and Refer)* [23] can be utilized for the busy clinician who does not have the time or resources to implement lifestyle medicine in the office. An example would be to *ask* about the importance and impact of stress in the patient's life, *advise* the patient that stress reduction would help improve the patient's health, and *refer* the patient to a meditation program in the community.

Shared Decision-Making

The concept of SDM is stipulated in the Affordable Care Act to ensure that medical care better aligns with patients' preferences and values [24]. SDM describes a collaboration process between patients and their clinicians to reach agreement about a health decision that may involve multiple treatment options and targets or therapy [25, 26]. Clinicians and patients work together to clarify the patients' values and concerns, select a preference-sensitive decision, and agree on a follow-up plan. This process is consistent with the "agree" and "arrange" components of the five As model described above. Intrinsic to SDM is the use of patient decision aids, which are written materials, videos, or interactive electronic presentations designed to inform patients about care options [24]. An example of SDM using a patient decision aid is smoking cessation counseling. The pros and cons of gradual reduction in the number of cigarettes smoked versus abrupt

Table 3.3 Application of the five A's to weight management

Five As	Purpose	Example dialogue
Ask	Ask permission to discuss weight; take a weight, history, and assess impact on health	"Can we talk about your weight?" "What approaches have you used in the past to control your weight?"
Advise	Provide feedback and information about impact of excess weight and benefits of weight reduction	"The excess weight around your belly is very likely making your GERD symptoms worse." "As little as a 5–10% weight loss will improve your diabetes"
Assess	Measure body mass index and waist circumference and assess obesity-related comorbidities; assess readiness for weight reduction	"How confident are you that you can tackle your weight at this time?" "Can you see yourself getting at least 30 min of brisk walking on most days of the week?"
Assist	Decide with patient where to begin making changes and which behaviors to focus on	"Tracking your diet using an electronic program will allow you to monitor your diet and caloric intake"
Arrange	Arrange for a follow-up appointment; make referrals to other resources	"I would like to schedule an appointment for you to see our dietitian." "A good option for you is to sign up for the Weight Watchers class at your worksite"

GERD gastroesophageal reflux disease

cessation can be discussed along with the options of which (if any) of the multiple pharmacotherapy treatments to choose.

Motivational Interviewing

How do clinicians assess motivation and facilitate lifestyle behavior change? Simply asking patients, "Are you motivated to make a change?" is likely to yield mixed results ranging from "yes, no, or maybe," which is difficult to interpret. Motivational interviewing (MI) is a client-centered, directive method for enhancing intrinsic motivation to change by exploring and resolving ambivalence [27]. It focuses on what the patient wants and how the patient thinks and feels. According to MI, motivation to change is viewed as something that is evoked in the patient rather than imposed. It is the patient's task (not the clinician's) to articulate and resolve his or her own ambivalence [28]. Readiness is viewed

as the balance of two opposing forces: [1] motivation, or the patient's desire to change and [2] resistance, or the patient's resistance to change [29]. Readiness for change is seen as the extent to which the patient has contemplated the need for change, having considered the pros and cons of change.

Intrinsic to this model is the concept that most patients are ambivalent about changing long-standing lifestyle behaviors, fearing that change will be difficult, uncomfortable, or depriving. The result of initiating a change plan when the patient is not ready often leads to frustration and disappointment. Patients frequently misattribute their lack of success to a failure of effort (low willpower). Patients who are ready and have thought about the benefits and difficulties of changing a behavior are more likely to succeed. One helpful, simple, and rapid method to begin a readiness assessment is to "anchor" the patient's interest and confidence to change on a numerical scale. Figure 3.1 displays an example of this technique for a patient with diabetes using a 10-point Lik-

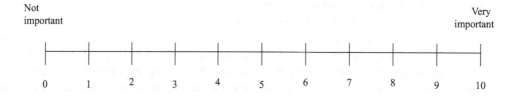

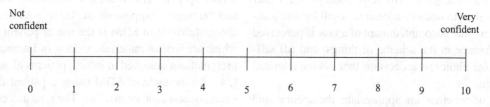

Fig. 3.1 Using motivational interviewing (MI) to assess level of importance and confidence to change behavior

ert scale. To assess readiness, simply ask the patient, "On a scale from 0 to 10, with 0 being not important and 10 being very important, how *important* is it for you get your diabetes under control at this time?" and "Also on a scale from 0 to 10, with 0 being not confident and 10 being very confident, how *confident* are you that you get your diabetes under control at this time?" [30]. This is a very useful method to initiate further discussion.

The following dialogue about weight management further demonstrates the use of this technique:

> Clinician: "G, you've told me M has been encouraging you to lose weight. On a scale from 0 to 10 with 0 being not important and 10 being very important, how interested are you in losing weight?"
>
> G: "I'm about an 8."
>
> Clinician: "Ok, now I'd like to know how confident you are, again on a scale from 0 to 10 with 0 being not confident and 10 being very confident, that you can make the changes necessary to lose weight."
>
> G: "I'm about a 3."
>
> Clinician: "That's interesting. You rate the importance pretty high, at an 8, but your confidence is much lower, at a 3. What would need to happen to raise your confidence score to a 5 or 6?"
>
> G: "Boy, I can think of a few things. First, M needs to get off my back. She constantly reminds me of what I should and should not be eating. That just makes me eat more. Second, Sundays are always difficult. We have the entire family over after church for a huge lunch. I can't seem to control myself. Maybe if I had some ideas on how to control myself I wouldn't feel so bad about dieting."
>
> Clinician: "Those are two very important concerns and seem like a good place to start. Have you talked to M about her comments and how they make you feel?"
>
> G: "Not really. I guess I just get so mad I shut her out."
>
> Clinician: "What can you say that would be helpful?"
>
> G: "I guess I could ask her not to comment on my eating and that I am trying to make better choices...."

In this example, the clinician was able to quickly identify two targets of opportunity to deal with behavior change.

MI uses four general principles to explore and resolve ambivalence [27]:

- Express empathy. Empathy refers to understanding the patient's feelings and perspectives without judging, criticizing, or blaming.
- Develop discrepancy. The second principle is to create and amplify the discrepancy between present behavior

and the patient's broader goals and values. Discrepancy has to do with the importance of change and the distance that the patient's behavior would need to travel in order to reach the desired level. This is called the "behavioral gap". The general approach is one that results in the patient reflecting on the actions and reasons for change. The dialogue below illustrates this principle.

> Clinician: "F, we've discussed how important it is for you to reduce your fat intake. We've also discussed strategies and options you can use at dinner, the most difficult time for you. However, it still sounds like your fat intake is too high, you're adding butter to your dinner rolls and you're using fatty salad dressing. I know you want to bring your cholesterol down. Help me understand what is making it difficult for you to choose a healthier dinner?"
>
> F: "I know I need to get my dinner under better control. If I did better planning before dinner, like avoiding the dinner rolls completely and ordering balsamic vinaigrette, I would do a better job."
>
> Clinician: "That sounds right on target. I'd like you to focus on those strategies this week."

In this example, the clinician laid out the behavioral discrepancy for the patient in clear terms. The patient was able to articulate the problem and a solution. In this case, dinner rolls were a trigger to use butter.

- Support self-efficacy. Self-efficacy refers to a person's belief in his or her ability to carry out and succeed with a specific task. Other common terms are hope and faith. A general goal of MI is to enhance the patient's confidence in her capacity to cope with obstacles and to succeed in change. The confidence scale used above quickly assesses the patient's level of confidence for a particular behavioral change.
- Roll with resistance. Although reluctance to change is to be expected in lifestyle behaviors, resistance (denial, arguing, putting up objections, and/or yes-but statements) arises from the interpersonal interaction between the clinician and patient. In this case, the therapeutic relationship is endangered and the counseling process becomes dysfunctional. It is a signal that the patient–clinician rapport is damaged. If this occurs, the clinician's task is to double back, understand the reason for resistance behavior, and redirect counseling. Rolling with resistance means not to confront the patient but allow them to express themselves. Using a reflective response serves to acknowledge the person's feelings or perceptions. The following dialogue illustrates this technique:

D: "I'm trying as hard as I can but I'm not losing weight!"

Clinician: "It's frustrating to work hard and not see the results you expect."

D: "That is so true. It's hard to imagine how I can work any harder. I lost 40 pounds the last time I went on a diet and I can't seem to lose a pound now. What's the use?"

Clinician: "I can see how you are discouraged and even a bit confused about what is going on. Let's take a closer look at your food logs and see if we can find some answers."

Self-Determination

One of the most frustrating and distressing situations in clinical care is when a patient seems to lack motivation for change. Even after the clinician has addressed all of the benefits and obstacles to change and has laid out specific strategies to take action, the patient appears to be having an inability or unwillingness to move or act, or in other words, is in a state of inertia. It is therefore not surprising that one of the most frequently asked questions by clinicians is, "How do I motivate my patient?" The theory of self-determination and the counseling process of MI (discussed above) are particularly useful for these patients who seem to lack motivation for change.

According to the theory of self-determination, people are motivated to act by very different types of factors, either because they value a particular activity (internal motivation) or because there is strong external coercion (external motivation) [31]. People will be internally motivated only when a change holds personal interest for them, that is, enjoyment, satisfaction, and intrinsic reward.

Although powerful in its own right, intrinsic motivation requires supportive conditions (e.g., people and an environment that are positive influences on behavior change as intrinsic motivation can be readily disrupted by various less supportive conditions). For example, let us look at a patient who wants to reduce the size of his dinner meal but whose wife serves family style (all food is presented in large serving dishes on the table), uses large plates, and encourages him to finish the food so there are no leftovers. In this case, the non-supportive condition (the way dinner meals are served) will trump intrinsic motivation. Therefore, patients must not only be ready, willing, and able to make change, there must also be a supportive condition. At the other end of the spectrum are non-motivated patients who do not see any value in changing, do not feel competent to change, or are not expecting the change to yield a desired outcome. The basic skill of the clinician is to identify whether patients' motivation is internal or external and to help patients find supportive conditions for health behavior change.

In between these two extremes is a continuum of externally motivated patients who are prompted to change by their significant others or their need to feel a connectedness with or valued by others. The more one is externally motivated, the less he or she shows interest, value, and movement toward the achievement of change, and then as a result, the more he or she tends to blame others for a negative outcome. One end of this continuum is the patient who presents himself for changing a particular behavior, for example, cigarette smoking, solely based on the prompting of his physician or wife. He will likely just "go through the motions" to satisfy these external demands. The other end of the continuum is an externally motivated patient who makes changes to avoid guilt or anxiety or to achieve pride in oneself. An example would be a binge eater who feels bad about herself whenever she binges alone. Although an externally motivated patient can make positive behavior changes, the ultimate goal is to help patients become self-determined, that is, to internalize and assimilate the changes to the self so that they experience greater autonomy in their action.

According to Watson and Tharp [32], all behaviors pass through the following sequence—control by others, control by self, and automatization. When the patient achieves internal motivation, changes become more automatic and patients are authentic to their own goals. For example, a patient gains the assertiveness to say "no" to many of the peripheral demands asked of her and learns to prioritize her time to exercise on a regular schedule. This new acquired sense of autonomy and control reinforces her internal motivation to carve out precious time for herself.

Stages of Change (SOC)

When counseling patients, it is also important to assess whether the patient is ready to make changes in their behavior. One model, the transtheoretical or stages of change model clarifies this process. It proposes that at any specific time, patients change problem behaviors by moving through a series of stages representing several levels of readiness to change. There are five discrete stages of change: precontemplation, contemplation, preparation, action, and maintenance [33, 34]. Patients move from one stage to the next in the process of change and it is likely that they may repeat stages several times before lasting change occurs. Within the SOC model, the clinician's tasks include both assessing the patient's stage of change and using behavioral counseling strategies to help advance the patient from one stage to the next. Table 3.4 shows samples of how to assess stages of change for a patient with obesity, describes the characteristics of each, identifies appropriate cognitive and behavioral coun-

Table 3.4 Stages of change (SOC) model using diabetes as an example

Stage	Characteristics	Patient verbal cues	Appropriate intervention	Sample of dialogue
Precontemplation	Unaware of problem, no interest in change	"I'm not really concerned about my diabetes. I feel fine. It's not a problem"	Provide information about health risks and benefits of controlling elevated blood pressure	"Would you like to read some information about the problems associated with diabetes?"
Contemplation	Aware of problem, beginning to think of changing	"I need to get my diabetes under better control but with all that's going on in my life right now, I'm not sure I can"	Help resolve ambivalence; discuss barriers	"Let's look at the benefits of improved diabetes control, as well as what you may need to change"
Preparation	Realizes benefits of making changes and thinking about how to change	"I have to get my diabetes under better control, and I'm planning to do that"	Teach behavior modification; provide education	"Let's take a closer look at how you can reduce some of the simple carbohydrates in your diet and how to increase your activity during the day"
Action	Actively taking steps toward achieving the behavioral goal, but only for a brief period (less than 6 months)	"I'm doing my best. This is harder than I thought"	Provide support and guidance with a focus on the long term (relapse control)	"It's terrific that you're working so hard. What problems have you had so far? How have you solved them?"
Maintenance	Initial treatment and behavioral goals reached and sustained for a longer period of time (e.g., more than 6 months)	"I've learned a lot through this process"	Relapse control	"What situations continue to tempt you to over consume sweets? What can be helpful for the next time you face such a situation?

seling strategies, and provides helpful dialogues for each stage.

It is important to remember that stages of change often reflect discrete behaviors. For instance, a patient may be in the preparation stage for making changes to her diet, for example, adding more fruits and vegetables to each meal, but remains in the precontemplation stage for engaging in more physical activity. In this case, you would praise the patient and provide specific advice about adding more fruits and vegetables while encouraging the patient to think about how to add small bouts of physical activity in the course of the day.

The SOC model incorporates ten specific processes of change, which are activities and experiences that individuals engage in when they attempt to modify problem behaviors. Successful changers employ different processes at each particular stage of change. The basic skill of the clinician is to listen for these experiential verbal statements to determine where a patient is in the six stages of change. Four of the most useful processes of change with examples specific to lifestyle medicine are as follows [35]:

Example: In her counseling session, S explains that she has talked to people who have been successful in reducing their stress level and that this has made her a bit more hopeful that she can reduce her stress level too. The clinician determines that S is moving from precontemplation to contemplation.

Example: J remarks that he almost always grabs some candy every time he passes his secretary's desk—and he is not even hungry! The clinician determines that J is moving from contemplation to preparation.

Example: K explains that talking to a friend, someone she can count on, has been very important when she feels depressed—the time when she often turns to food for comfort. K explains that her friend has helped her to control her emotional urges for eating for the past 4 months. The clinician determines that K has moved from preparation to action.

- Consciousness raising: patients actively seek new information and gain understanding and feedback about behavior change.
  - Example: In her counseling session, S explains that she has talked to people who have been successful in reducing their stress level and that this has made her a bit more hopeful that she can reduce her stress level too. The clinician determines that S is moving from precontemplation to contemplation.
- Environmental reevaluation: patients consider and assess how diet, physical activity, and coping are affected by their physical and social environments.
  - Example: J remarks that he almost always grabs some candy every time he passes his secretary's desk—and he is not even hungry! The clinician determines that J is moving from contemplation to preparation.
- Helping relationships: patients trust, accept, and utilize the support of others in their attempts to change behavior.
  - Example: K explains that talking to a friend, someone she can count on, has been very important when she

feels depressed—the time when she often turns to food for comfort. K explains that her friend has helped her to control her emotional urges for eating for the past 4 months. The clinician determines that K has moved from preparation to action.

- Self-reevaluation: patients conduct emotional and cognitive reappraisal of individual values with respect to their behavior change goals.
  - Example: P explains that despite losing and keeping off 10 % of her body weight, she still struggles with her body shape. She has learned to replace negative self-talk with more positive statements, for example, "I am 16 pounds lighter now and have a new wardrobe that looks pretty darn good. Even though I still want to take off another 15 pounds, I'm going to celebrate my success along the way. I'm going to continue the healthy eating and physical activity plan I have been on for the past 8 months." The clinician determines that P is moving from action to maintenance.

Many of these processes are embedded in other behavior change models. The role of the clinician is to guide the patient through these behavioral or thought processes, depending on their particular stage of change for a specific behavior.

Part of the decision for individuals to move from one stage to the next is based on the relative weight given to the *pros* and *cons* of changing behavior. The pros represent positive aspects of changing behavior, while the cons represent negative aspects of changing behavior, which may be thought of as barriers to change [36]. The following clinician–patient dialogue illustrates weighing of the pros and cons of beginning an exercise routine:

Clinician: "B, do you think you can exercise at least two times this week?"
B: "I'd like to, but time has always been a major issue."
Clinician: "Ok, I know that you want to exercise since we have talked about this before. And I know that you have a treadmill in the basement. What are the factors that make it hard for you to get started?"
B: "It's really all about time. Knowing myself, I would need to exercise in the morning. That means getting up a half hour earlier."
Clinician: "Is that doable?"
B: "Yes, it is. If I took my workout clothes out the night before and laid them on the chair, it would be even easier. I guess I could also make a point of going to sleep on time the night before."
Clinician: "Well the benefits are pretty clear—feel better during the day, get off to a good start, and burn more calories. Is there any downside to the plan?"
B: "The only downside is losing a half hour of sleep twice a week, and making sure I get my workout clothes ready the night before. I can do this."

In this example, B moved from the preparation stage to the action stage with the help of the clinician.

Health Belief Model

What about the patient who does not seem to understand the need to change a health behavior? This is another situation that can arise when counseling patients. The model that describes this, the health belief model, holds the principle that health behavior change is a function of the individual's perceptions regarding his or her vulnerability to illness and perceived effectiveness of treatment [37, 38]. Behavior change is determined by individuals who:

- Perceive themselves to be susceptible to a particular health problem,
- See the problem as serious,
- Are convinced that treatment/prevention is effective and not overly costly in regard to money, effort, or pain,
- Are exposed to a cue to take health action, and
- Have confidence that they can perform a specific behavior (self-efficacy).

The basic skill of the clinician is to help patients understand these behavioral change factors. This model is particularly useful when a patient is perceived to be in the precontemplation stage of change making behavioral changes. The following dialogue illustrates use of the health belief model:

Clinician: "J, what do you know about the health risks of having an elevated blood sugar?"
J: "Everybody is telling me that I should be concerned about my blood sugar, but I feel alright as I am. My dad's sugar was high and he lived to be 85 years old!"
Clinician: "I see. While it is true that everyone may be different, your blood sugar does concern me. You do meet the criteria for diabetes and your elevated sugar puts you at higher risk for developing blindness, kidney failure, and heart disease. This is a serious problem."
J: "I didn't know that. But I think having a high blood sugar just runs in my family."
Clinician: "J, you've never tried bring your blood sugar down. I think you can make a difference by modifying your eating and physical activity levels. We know that making small changes can make a big difference in your health problems and will likely lower your risk for heart disease. What do you think about our developing a plan for you together?"
J: "If it's that serious and you can help me, I'll give it a try."

When using the health belief model for behavior change, it is important to give feedback to the patient and continuously link the patient's behavior changes to positive internal cues of health by pointing out that the changes the patient is making are directly leading to improved physical or mental well-being. In a weight loss or management setting, examples of improved physical or mental well-being include lower blood pressure or cholesterol levels, climbing a flight of stairs with less breathlessness, or improved mood. These positive attributions are intended to strengthen the "cause and effect" relationship between behavior and health and reinforce motivation.

Social Cognitive Theory (SCT)/Ecological Models

It is important to know the supportive resources and barriers patients have to changing their behaviors. Social cognitive theory emphasizes the interactions between the person and his or her environment. Behavior, therefore, is a function of aspects of both the environment and the person, all of which are in constant reciprocal interaction [39]. The behavioral choices we make regarding what we eat or what we do are determined, in part, by accessibility, affordability, and available resources. Ecological models expand our definition of environmental influences to include interpersonal relationships, family, community, and city. The "built environment," meaning the environment that humans built, is an important concept in viewing behavior [40]. For example, our patients may be more likely (or less likely) to take a walk depending on neighborhood safety, lighting, sidewalks, traffic, and if there is an enjoyable route. Diet may be determined, in part, by whether the patient has access to neighborhood grocery stores versus large supermarkets, fast-food chains versus sit-down restaurants, fresh versus processed foods, and the price of food. These are essential questions to ask the patient prior to establishing behavior-change goals.

Two central concepts of social learning theory are self-efficacy and outcome expectations:

- Self-efficacy or confidence, previously mentioned under the health belief model and MI, refers to a patient's belief in his or her ability to change or maintain a specific behavior under a variety of circumstances. It is not a general belief about oneself, but a specific belief that is tied to a particular task [32]. Higher levels of self-efficacy are predictive of improved treatment outcomes [41]. Low self-efficacy may be due to either perceived or actual deficits in personal knowledge, skills, resources, or environmental supports [42].
- Outcome expectancies are the degree to which a patient believes that a given course of action will lead to a particular outcome. This is also a central feature of the health belief model. Outcome expectations must be favorable for behavior change to occur. Expectations are typically described as an individual's anticipation of the effects of future experiences. The following dialogue illustrates the assessment of self-efficacy and outcome expectation:

> Clinician: "K, you need to reduce your salt intake to less than 2300 mg daily. Based on what I have learned about your diet so far, there are many changes you can make to affect this reduction. Do you have any thoughts on what you can do?"
>
> K: "Well, although restaurant eating is probably my biggest problem, that's going to be tough. It's really hard for me to cut back when I'm entertaining all the time."
>
> Clinician: "Ok, where do you think you can make a change?"
>
> K: "Starting at home would be better. I can count on my wife to help me. I can ask her to use less salt in cooking, put the salt shaker away, and don't buy salty snacks."
>
> Clinician: "Sounds like a plan."
>
> K: "So if I consistently reduce my salt intake to less than 2300 mg daily, how much lower will my blood pressure be?"
>
> Clinician: "It's hard to predict exactly, but I would expect it to drop about 5 points or so. We'll see what it is when I see you back in a month."

Theory of Planned Behavior (TPB)

The patient's perceived control over behavioral change is also considered important; this is where the theory of planned behavior (TPB) comes in. According to the TPB, the intention to act is guided by three belief considerations—behavioral beliefs, normative beliefs, and control beliefs [43]. Behavioral beliefs refer to the patient's perceived outcomes (benefits and rewards) and attitudes toward engaging in the behavior. Normative beliefs refer to the subjective norms or pressure of others in the family or community regarding the behavioral change. Control beliefs refer to the presence of factors that may facilitate or impede performance of the behavior and the perceived power of these factors. In combination, these three beliefs lead to the formation of a behavioral *intention* to take action, similar to the support provided by a three-legged stool. A key principle of the TPB is that behavioral change (an observed action) is immediately preceded by intention. Applying this model, the more favorable the attitude and subjective norm, and the greater the perceived control, the stronger should be the patient's intention to change behavior. This concept is illustrated in Fig. 3.2.

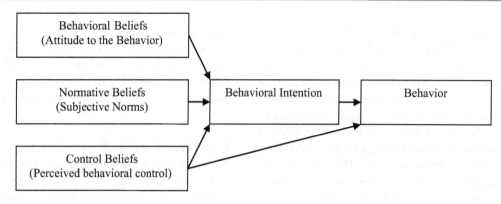

Fig. 3.2 Theory of planned behavior (TPB) [43]

But intention may not be enough. Behavioral change will only occur if the patient has a sufficient degree of perceived *and* actual control over the behavior. This is illustrated by an additional direct arrow between perceived behavioral control and behavior. Multiple studies have identified the importance of the TPB in explaining intended behavior change [44–47]. The following dialogue illustrates the importance of identifying normative beliefs and perceived and actual behavioral control:

> Clinician: "We've talked about how the food around the office and on everyone's desk is problematic for you. By keeping food diaries over the past 2 weeks, we've identified that you are consuming simple sugars in candy and other munch food every day. What's the likelihood that you can change the office environment?"
>
> P: "That's going to be problem. First of all, my coworkers like having food around. None of them seem to care about simple sugars. My boss is the one who fills up the candy dish every Monday morning. I've already talked to the coworkers immediately around me and they said they would try to be more conscious about the treats. I'm thinking about this all day long. I can't tell people what they can or cannot do."
>
> Clinician: "Here's an idea. Perhaps you can help change what people bring into the office. Instead of a candy dish, what about a fruit bowl? You can make it a community effort where everyone who wants to contribute can. At least there would be an alternative to the candy and nuts. Who knows, maybe it will catch on."
>
> P: "That's really a good idea. I'm going to try it."

Cognitive Behavioral Therapy (CBT)

When it comes to helping patients take action, CBT is a most common behavioral therapy employed. It incorporates various strategies intended to help change and reinforce new dietary and physical activity behaviors as well as thoughts and attitudes [48, 49]. Rather than exploring the psychological underpinning for behavior that may be rooted in childhood (the past), CBT focuses on short-term, problem-oriented treatments that address the present and future. The primary aim of CBT is to produce cognitive change, that is, attention to inner thoughts, attitudes, and emotions as well as to the events that both trigger and result from our actions [50].

Behavior is a function of the person in interaction with the environment; this is in contrast to "willpower," which implies that some entity, inner strength, or psychological make-up is all that is needed to change a behavior. CBT is based on the need to cultivate skills that are developed through knowledge and practice versus just needing good intentions to succeed. Patients may present for treatment interested in cutting down on their alcohol intake (contemplation stage of change) but need to consciously apply learned techniques and strategies in order to succeed. The key traditional CBT techniques are self-monitoring, stimulus control, problem-solving, stress management, social support, and cognitive restructuring. CBT is explained in detail in Chap. 14.

Conclusions

Good communication between the provider and patient is paramount in eliciting behavior change. Rather than simply educating and instructing patients on what to do, behavior change counseling should be a guiding and collaborative process. Behavior change theories are intended to explain the biological, cognitive, behavioral, psychological, environmental, and motivational determinants of human behavior. They also provide interventions to produce changes in knowledge, attitudes, motivation, self-confidence, skills, and social support required for behavior change and maintenance [51]. A skilled clinician mixes and matches all of these behavior change principles, strategies, and techniques during counseling. Often, several methods are used with the same patient depending on the targeted behavior and course of treatment.

References

1. Healthy People 2020. 2014. http://www.healthypeople.gov/. Accessed 25 Dec 2014.
2. The Office of Behavioral and Social Sciences Research (OBSSR). 2014. http://obssr.od.nih.gov/about_obssr/BSSR_CC/BSSR_definition/definition.aspx. Accessed 25 Dec 2014.
3. Weiner SJ, Schwartz A, Weaver F, et al. Contextual errors and failures in individualizing patient care. A multicenter study. Ann Intern Med. 2010;153:69–75.
4. Institute of Medicine. Capturing social and behavioral domains and measures in electronic health records: phase 2. 2014. http://www.nap.edu/catalog/18951/capturing-social-and-behavioral-domains-and-measures-in-electronic-health-records. Accessed 25 Dec 2014.
5. Association of American Medical Colleges. Cultural competence education. Cultural competence for medical students. 2014. https://www.aamc.org/download/54338/data/. Accessed 25 Dec 2014.
6. Berkman ND, Sheridan SL, Donahue KE, et al. Low health literacy and health outcomes: an updated systematic review. Ann Intern Med. 2011;159:97–107.
7. Coleman CA, Hudson S, Maine L. Health literacy practices and educational competencies for health professionals: a consensus study. J Health Commun. 2013;18:82–102.
8. Balint M. The doctor, his patient and the illness. New York: International University Press; 1972.
9. Stewart MA. Effective physician-patient communication and health outcomes: a review. Can Med Assoc J. 1995;152:1423–33.
10. Kravitz RL. Measuring patients' expectations and requests. Ann Intern Med. 2001;134:881–8.
11. Marvel MK, Epstein RM, Flowers K, Beckman HB. Soliciting the patient's agenda. Have we improved? JAMA. 1999;281:283–7.
12. Emanuel EJ, Emanuel LL. Four models of the physician-patient relationship. JAMA. 1992; 267:2221–2226.
13. Roter D. The enduring and evolving nature of the patient-physician relationship. Patient Educ Couns. 2000;39:5–15.
14. Cousin G, Schmid Mast M, Roter DL, Hall JA. Concordance between physician communication style and patient attitudes predicts patient satisfaction. Patient Educ Couns. 2012;87:193–7.
15. Schulz PJ, Nakamoto K. Health literacy and patient empowerment in health communication: the importance of separating conjoined twins. Patient Educ Couns. 2013;90:4–11.
16. Spreitzer CM. Psychological empowerment in the workplace: dimensions, measurement, and validation. Acad Manage J. 1995;18:1442–65.
17. Luftey KE, Wishner WJ. Beyond "compliance" is "adherence." Improving the prospect of diabetes care. Diabetes Care. 1999;22:635–9.
18. Jaret P. 10 ways to improve patient compliance. Hippocrates. 2001; Feb/Mar: 22–28.
19. Steiner JF, Earnest MA. The language of medication-taking. Ann Intern Med. 2000;132:926–30.
20. The Tobacco Use and Dependence Clinical Practice Guideline Panel. A clinical practice guideline for treating tobacco use and dependence. JAMA. 2000;283:3244–54.
21. Fleming M, Manwell LB. Brief intervention in primary care settings. A primary treatment method for at-risk, problem, and dependent drinkers. Alcohol Res Health. 1999;23:128–37.
22. Vallis M, Piccinini-Vallis H, Sharma AM, et al. Modified 5 As. Minimal intervention for obesity counseling in primary care. Can Fam Physician. 2013;59:27–31.
23. Fiore MC, Balley WC, Cohen SJ, et al. Treating tobacco use and dependence: clinical practice guideline. Rockville: US Dept of Health and Human Services (USDHHS), Public Health Service (PHS); 2000. Report 1-58763-007-9.
24. Oshima Lee E, Emanuel EJ. Shared decision making to improve care and reduce costs. N Engl J Med. 2013;368:6–8.
25. Politi MC, Wolin KY, Legarie F. Implementing clinical practice guidelines about health promotion and disease prevention through shared decision making. J Gen Intern Med. 2013;28:838–44.
26. Sonntag U, Wiesner J, Fahrenkrog S, et al. Motivational interviewing and shared decision making in primary care. Patient Educ Couns. 2012;87:62–6.
27. Miller WR, Rollnick S. Motivational interviewing.In: Preparing people for change. 2nd ed. New York: Guilford; 2002. p. 25. (3rd ed).
28. Britt E, Hudson SM, Blampied NM. Motivational interviewing in health settings: a review. Patient Educ Couns. 2004;53:147–55.
29. Katz DL. Behavior modification in primary care: the pressure system model. Prev Med. 2001;32:66–72.
30. Rollnick S, Mason P, Butler C. Health behavior change: a guide for practitioners. London: Churchill Livingstone; 1999.
31. Ryan RM, Deci EL. Self-determination theory and the facilitation of intrinsic motivation, social development, and well-being. Am Psych. 2000;55(1):68–78.
32. Watson DL, Tharp RG. Self-directed behavior. In: Watson DL, Tharp RG, editors. Self-modification for personal adjustment. 8th ed. Belmont: Wadsworth Group; 2002.
33. Prochaska J, DiClemente C. Stages and processes of self-change of smoking. Toward an integrative model of change. J Consult Clin Psych. 1983;51:390–5.
34. Prochaska JO, DiClimente CC. Toward a comprehensive model of change. In: Miller WR, editor. Treating addictive behaviors. New York: Plenum; 1986. pp. 3–27.
35. Prochaska JO, Velicer WF. The transtheoretical model of health behavior change. Am J Health Promot. 1997;12(1):38–48.
36. Levenson W, Cohen MS, Brandy D, Duffy ED. To change or not to change: "Sounds like you have a dilemma". Ann Intern Med. 2001;135(5):386–90.
37. Becker MH. The health belief model and sick-role behavior. Health Ed Monogr. 1974;2:409–19.
38. Janz NK, Champion VL, Strecher VJ. The health belief model. In: Glanz K, Rimer BK, Lewis FM, editors. Health behavior and health education: theory, research, and practice. 3rd ed. San Francisco: Jossey-Bass; 2002. pp. 45–66.
39. Barnanowski T, Cullen KW, Nicklas T, et al. Are current health behavioral change models helpful in guiding prevention of weight gain efforts? Obes Res 2003;11(Suppl):23–43.
40. Booth KM, Pinkston MM, Poston WSC. Obesity and the built environment. JADA. 2005;105:S110–S7.
41. Witkiewitz K, Marlatt GA. Relapse prevention for alcohol and drug problems. That was zen, this is tao. Am Psych. 2004;59(4):224–35.
42. Rosal MC, Ebbeling CB, Lofgren I, et al. Facilitating dietary change: the patient-centered counseling model. JADA. 2001;101:332–338,341.
43. Aizen I Theory of planned behavior. 2015. http://people.umass.edu/aizen/. Accessed 25 Dec 2015.

44. Brickell TA, Chatzisarantis NL, Pretty GM. Autonomy and control: augmenting the validity of the theory of planned behaviour in predicting exercise. J Health Psychol. 2006;11:51–63.

45. Rhodes RE, Bianchard CM, Matheson DH. A multicomponent model of the theory of planned behaviour. Br J Health Psychol. 2006;11(pt 1):119–37.

46. Brug J, De Vet E, de Nooijer J, Verplanken B. Predicting fruit consumption; cognitions, intention, and habits. J Nutr Educ Behav. 2006;38:73–81.

47. Armitage CJ, Conner M. Efficacy of the theory of planned behaviour: a meta-analytic review. Br J Soc Psychol. 2001;40:471–99.

48. Foreyt JP, Poston WSC. What is the role of cognitive-behavior therapy in patient management? Obesity Res. 1998;6(Suppl 1):18–22.

49. Wadden TA, Foster GD. Behavioral treatment of obesity. Med Clin North Am. 2000;84:441–61.

50. Williamson DA, Perrin LA. Behavioral therapy for obesity. Endocrinol Metab Clin. 1996;25(4):943–54.

51. Whitlock EP, Orleans CT, Pender N, Allan J. Evaluating primary care behavioral counseling interventions. An evidence-based approach. Am J Prev Med. 2002;22(4):267–84.

Paradigms of Lifestyle Medicine and Wellness

Robert Scales and Matthew P. Buman

Abbreviations

ACSM	American College of Sports Medicine
AHRQ	Agency for Healthcare Research and Quality
AMA	American Medical Association
BHC	Behavioral health consultant
CAD	Coronary artery disease
CMA	Canadian Medical Association
DALYs	Disability-adjusted life years
EIM	Exercise is medicine
FCTC	Framework Convention on Tobacco Control
GBDS	Global Burden of Disease Study
HAPO	Hyperglycemia and Adverse Pregnancy Outcome
PCBH	Primary Care Behavioral Health
PCMH	Patient-Centered Medical Home
PCPCC	Patient-Centered Primary Care Collaborative
PPACA	Patient Protection and Affordable Care Act
QOL	Quality of life
T2D	Type-2 diabetes
US	United States
USPSTF	US Preventive Services Task Force
WHO	World Health Organization
YLD	Years lived with a disability
YLL	Years of life lost

A Physician's Description of the Dilemma of the Modern Practice of Medicine

"There I am standing by the shore of a swiftly flowing river and I hear a cry of a drowning man. So I jump into the river, put my arms around him, pull him to shore and apply ar-

tificial respiration. Just when he begins to breathe, there is another cry for help. So I jump into the river, reach him, pull him to shore, apply artificial respiration, and then just as he begins to breathe, another cry for help. So back in the river again, reaching, pulling, applying, breathing and then another yell. Again and again, without end, goes the sequence. You know, I am so busy jumping in, pulling them to shore, applying artificial respiration, that I have no time to see who the hell is upstream pushing them in" [1].

Preventive Medicine

This story was told by a physician to describe a dilemma that exists within the modern practice of medicine. The current practice has been built on a fee-for-service model of treating disease rather than disease prevention and health promotion [1]. The US health-care system is inundated with people coming to the clinic or emergency department with some type of acute or worsening chronic medical condition. Health-care professionals work together to stabilize the patient, diagnose the cause, and then prescribe appropriate treatment. However, there are limitations in a health-care system that predominantly relies on reactive "downstream" endeavors with a focus on illness or injury [1]. Health-care spending within the US remains higher than any other nation, but health-care outcomes continue to rank lower than any of the other developed countries [2]. A health-care system that includes preventive medicine offers a proactive "upstream" solution to prevent illness and promote wellness through services of health promotion.

Affordable Healthcare Act

The Patient Protection and Affordable Care Act (PPACA) requires Medicare and commercial health plans to pay for preventive services that are graded highest by the US Preventive Services Task Force (USPSTF), with no expense to patients [3–5]. The USPSTF consists of an independent panel of non-

R. Scales (✉)
Division of Cardiovascular Diseases, Mayo Clinic-Arizona, 13400 East Shea Boulevard, Scottsdale, AZ 85259, USA
e-mail: Scales.Robert@mayo.edu

M. P. Buman
School of Nutrition and Health Promotion, Arizona State University, Phoenix, AZ, USA

© Springer International Publishing Switzerland 2016
J. I. Mechanick, R. F. Kushner (eds.), *Lifestyle Medicine,* DOI 10.1007/978-3-319-24687-1_4

federal experts in prevention and primary care who ranked 64 clinical preventive services based on a rigorous review of the scientific literature. A range of specific services (e.g., immunization vaccines, screenings, behavioral counseling and education, pharmacotherapy) were selected with the capacity to prevent or reduce cardiovascular disease, cancer, infectious disease, and other conditions that impact the health of children, adolescents, adults, and pregnant women. This evidenced-based grading system provides a guideline for physicians as they consider the best options for integrating preventive services into their practice. The USPSTF recognizes that clinical decisions by a physician are individualized to the patient. However, the guide may help physicians prioritize the various preventive services. In this new model of health-care delivery, financial incentives will be available to health-care professionals who embrace disease prevention and health promotion. Updated recommendations of the USPSTF guide are available along with the supporting scientific evidence at www.USPreventiveServicesTaskForce. org. Recommendations for specific age groups and clinical characteristics can be accessed by smart phone or on the web at www.epss.ahrq.gov.

Chapter Purpose Statement

This chapter defines a paradigm for preventive medicine and offers a framework for physicians and allied health-care professionals to apply lifestyle medicine and wellness in the clinic. Strategies are identified to improve the physician's ability to provide effective lifestyle medicine within a busy clinical practice. This includes education in preventive medicine and ongoing support for the physician that begins in medical school and prepares them to deliver team-based models of wellness.

Natural History of Disease

Chronic disease, which may last years or decades, has a natural life history [6]. Exposure to factors favoring the development of disease occurs in early life and extends over time. This may include factors associated with the environment, occupation, and the society in which we live. Other factors include our personal physiological and genetic profile and the lifestyle we adopt [7]. Consequently, disease may exist within a progressive sequence of stages prior to a clinical diagnosis. Prevention simply means inhibiting the development of a disease before it occurs. However, the term has been expanded to include measures that interrupt or slow down the progression of disease. Therefore, there are different levels of disease prevention that can be applied throughout the natural life history of disease development.

Levels of Disease Prevention

Figure 4.1 describes a contemporary paradigm for disease prevention and has been adapted from work by the National Public Health Partnership [8].

In *primary prevention*, proactive interventions focus on altering a person's susceptibility to disease or reducing exposure to the factors that cause disease in susceptible individuals. Here, no disease is present. A prenatal and postnatal educational intervention that promotes and supports breast-feeding in new mothers is an example of primary prevention. Breastfeeding decreases the likelihood of breast and ovarian cancer in the mother; it reduces ear, lower respiratory tract, and gastrointestinal infections in infants, and it lowers the risk of asthma, type-2 diabetes (T2D) and obesity in younger children [4].

Secondary prevention is the early detection and treatment of early-stage disease and related risk factors. Here, disease may be present without symptoms. A blood test to screen for T2D is an example of an appropriate secondary prevention measure in asymptomatic adults with a sustained blood pressure >135/80 mmHg [4]. The early identification of at-risk individuals (fasting plasma glucose ≥100 mg/dl) may prompt additional health promotion strategies, including lifestyle education and counseling [9, 10].

Tertiary prevention is the alleviation of disability and illness that can be the consequence of a diagnosed disease. Here, rehabilitative efforts may focus on restoring effective functioning. For some, there may be symptoms associated with the disease, but this is not always the case. At this level of prevention, interventions also aim to slow down, stabilize, or reverse the disease process before it becomes more serious and disabling. There is typically more evidence of chronic disease in aging adults. This is a scenario familiar to physicians as they provide care for these patients. Therefore, tertiary level prevention is appropriate in this patient population. Using diagnosed heart disease as an example, the survivor of a myocardial infarction is still susceptible to a second attack, and someone living with heart failure remains vulnerable to ongoing medical complications and hospital readmission. Surgical intervention and optimal medical management will be crucial to patient care. However, a physician referral to a medically directed, supervised cardiac rehabilitation program is an example of a tertiary preventive service that compliments standard care and enhances clinical outcomes. Mortality rates for patients with coronary artery disease (CAD) are up to 34% lower in those who participate in outpatient cardiac rehabilitation compared with nonparticipants [11]. Hospitalizations for a recurrent cardiac event are also decreased [12, 13]. Clearly, there is a rationale to

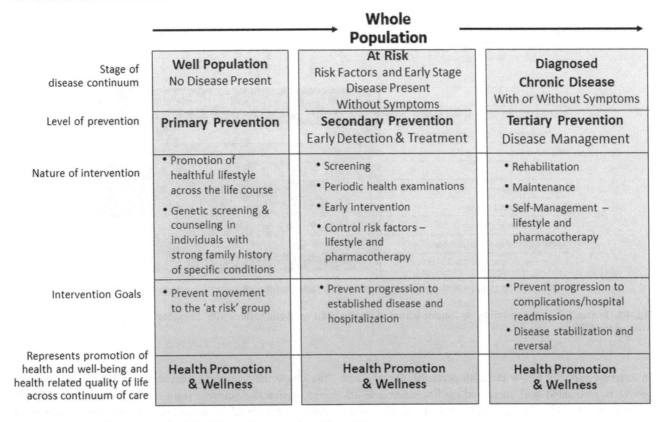

	Well Population No Disease Present	**At Risk** Risk Factors and Early Stage Disease Present Without Symptoms	**Diagnosed Chronic Disease** With or Without Symptoms
Stage of disease continuum			
Level of prevention	**Primary Prevention**	**Secondary Prevention** Early Detection & Treatment	**Tertiary Prevention** Disease Management
Nature of intervention	• Promotion of healthful lifestyle across the life course • Genetic screening & counseling in individuals with strong family history of specific conditions	• Screening • Periodic health examinations • Early intervention • Control risk factors – lifestyle and pharmacotherapy	• Rehabilitation • Maintenance • Self-Management – lifestyle and pharmacotherapy
Intervention Goals	• Prevent movement to the 'at risk' group	• Prevent progression to established disease and hospitalization	• Prevent progression to complications/hospital readmission • Disease stabilization and reversal
Represents promotion of health and well-being and health related quality of life across continuum of care	**Health Promotion & Wellness**	**Health Promotion & Wellness**	**Health Promotion & Wellness**

Fig. 4.1 Levels of disease prevention in healthcare. (Source: Adapted from [8])

support preventive measures prior to the diagnosis of disease. However, this example shows there is a place for all the levels of disease prevention within the paradigm of lifestyle medicine and wellness. A nationwide directory of cardiac and pulmonary rehabilitation programs is available at www.aacvpr.org as a resource for physicians as they consider the best interest of the patient.

Where Does Lifestyle Medicine Fit Within this Paradigm?

The Global Burden of Disease Study (GBDS) 2010 is the largest and most current population-based analysis of the influence of risk factors on the burden of disease and injury in 187 countries and 21 regions of the world. The burden of disease was quantified by the estimated sum of years of life lost (YLL) and the years lived with a disability (YLD), otherwise known as the deaths and disability-adjusted life years (DALYs). Lifestyle factors ranked high among 67 identified risk factors that were considered attributable to the burden of disease and injury in all parts of the world [7]. High blood pressure, tobacco use including secondhand smoke, household air pollution, a diet low in fruits, and alcohol use were ranked as the leading risk factors globally for men and women combined. These were considered the main causes of

chronic disease, especially cardiovascular disease and cancers. Other lifestyle factors that were ranked in the top 20 included physical inactivity (10th), diet high in sodium (11th), diet low in nuts and seeds (12th), suboptimal breast feeding (14th), diet low in whole grains (16th), diet low in vegetables (17th), diet low in seafood omega-3 fatty acids (18th), and drug use (19th) (Fig. 4.2). Dietary risk factors and physical inactivity collectively accounted for 10% of global DALYs in 2010. These findings underline the importance of integrating a lifestyle medicine approach within a wellness model of health-care delivery. The burden attributed to each risk factor varies across regions and subpopulations. The contribution of any given risk factor may also change across the lifespan. For example, the Australian Longitudinal Study on Women's Health used the same methodology adopted in the GBDS to identify that among women >30 years of age, the population risk of heart disease attributed to physical inactivity outweighed all other risk factors, including high blood pressure, smoking, or body mass index [14]. In women ≤30 years of age, the highest population risk was attributed to smoking. Contextualized information such as this is critical to the tailored design and implementation of lifestyle medicine and health promotion initiatives within a region or country.

The importance of a physically active lifestyle is underlined by evidence from the Aerobics Center Longitudinal Study and subsequent research, which have identified that

Risk factor	Global	High-income Asia Pacific	Western Europe	Australasia	High-income North America	Central Europe	Southern Latin America	Eastern Europe	East Asia	Tropical Latin America	Central Latin America
High blood pressure	1	1	2	3	3	1	2	2	1	1	4
Tobacco smoking, including second-hand smoke	2	2	1	2	1	2	3	3	2	4	5
Household air pollution from solid fuels	3	42	–	–	–	14	23	20	5	18	11
Diet low in fruits	4	4	7	6	6	5	6	5	3	6	7
Alcohol use	5	5	6	9	7	4	4	1	8	2	2
High body-mass index	6	8	3	1	2	3	1	4	9	3	1
High fasting plasma glucose	7	7	5	5	4	7	5	10	7	5	3
Childhood underweight	8	39	38	37	39	38	38	38	38	32	23
Ambient particulate matter pollution	9	9	11	26	14	12	24	14	4	27	19
Physical inactivity and low physical activity	10	3	4	4	5	6	7	7	10	8	6

Ranking legend

■ 1–5　■ 6–10　□ 11–15　□ 16–20　□ 21–25　□ 26–30　□ 31–35　■ 36–40　■ > 40

Regions are ordered by mean life expectancy. No data = attributable disability-adjusted life-years were not quantified.

Fig. 4.2 Top ten risk factors ranked by attributable burden of disease in the ten world regions with the highest life expectancy, 2010. (Source: Adapted from [7])

an exercise capacity below the 20th percentile for age and gender is associated with increased cardiac death and all-cause mortality [15–17]. In a meta-analysis of 33 studies involving 103,000 participants who were followed for an extended period, age-adjusted mortality rates were lowest among the most cardiovascular fit individuals and highest among the least fit [17]. In a 6.2-year follow-up of 6213 US veteran men, maximal graded exercise testing classified into five categorical cardiovascular fitness gradients identified that the least fit had > 4 times the risk of all-cause mortality compared with those with the highest cardiovascular fitness level in both apparently healthy individuals and those with cardiovascular disease. Cardiovascular fitness level was also a stronger predictor of mortality than the more traditional risk factors, which included smoking, hypertension, high cholesterol, and T2D [18]

In randomized controlled studies of individuals already diagnosed with CAD, those who adhered to a lifestyle involving multiple healthful behaviors (i.e., low-fat diet, structured exercise, stress management, and tobacco avoidance) more readily controlled symptoms, stabilized or reversed the atherosclerosis based on angiographic evaluations, and reduced the chance of recurrent cardiac events compared with a control group over a 4–6-year period [13, 19–22].

The 4-year follow-up results of the Diabetes Prevention Program demonstrated that compared with medications and a control group, lifestyle intervention was more effective in preventing the new onset of diabetes in a population with early signs of risk [9]. In the Nurses Health Study, a prospective observational study of 84,941 apparently healthy female nurses followed over a 16-year period, there were 3300 (26%) new cases of T2D. Overweight or obesity was

the single most important predictor of T2D. Lack of exercise, a poor diet, current smoking, and abstinence from alcohol use were all associated with a significantly increased risk of T2D, even after adjusting for the body mass index. Those with limited alcohol consumption were classified as lower risk. It was concluded that more than 90% of T2D cases could have been prevented with the adoption of a more healthful lifestyle [9, 23]. In summary, physicians who promote the medicinal qualities of a healthful lifestyle will not only prevent premature death (i.e., increase lifespan) but they will also alleviate prolonged periods of illness (i.e., increase healthspan) in the individuals they serve.

The Influence of Lifestyle on Gene Expression and Primordial Prevention

Lifestyle behaviors can also modify gene expression [24–27]. For example, in a study of 126 men and women with CAD or ≥ 2 cardiac risk factors, peripheral blood profiles showed changes in the expression of 143 genes in a group electing to adopt a rigorous heart healthful lifestyle (i.e., low-fat diet, structured exercise, stress management, tobacco avoidance) for a 1-year period. Controls showed little change in gene expression. Lifestyle modification effectively reduced expression of proinflammatory genes associated with neurophil activation and molecular pathways important to vascular function, including cytokine production, carbohydrate metabolism, and steroid hormones [28]. Encouraging findings such as this have resulted in the evolution of individualized medicine, where it may be feasible to identify and prevent disease from occurring in individuals with a strong family history of a specific medical condition. This concept has been termed primordial prevention, and it adds a new dimension to prevention at the primary level. For example, genetic screening and counseling has been recommended as a high priority preventive service for adult women with a family history of breast, ovarian, tubal, or peritoneal cancer [5]. The Hyperglycemia and Adverse Pregnancy Outcome (HAPO) Study underlined the importance of glucose metabolism biomarkers during pregnancy as a predictor of fetal health [29]. Consequently, the USPSTF now recommend screening for gestational diabetes mellitus in asymptomatic pregnant women after 24 weeks of gestation [5]. This is an example of a primordial prevention strategy that focuses on the health of a prospective mother and her unborn child. Additional examples of primordial prevention strategies that are beyond the scope of this chapter include the use of the epigenome and genetic imprinting to prevent the development of disease risk factors [30, 31].

How Much Time Do Physicians Spend on Prevention and Lifestyle Counseling?

An analysis of a large dataset of primary care visits using the National Ambulatory Medical Care Survey, identified physicians incorporate priority USPSTF preventive services within their practice. However, the study investigators concluded, that generally an inadequate amount of time was devoted to prevention, including lifestyle counseling [32]. This was consistent with an earlier evaluation that calculated > 50 % of the visit time focused on the medical history and only 20 % on health education. Almost no time was spent on nutrition (3 %), exercise (2 %), and smoking cessation (1 %) [33]. Direct observation of a community family practice setting with audiotaping of physician–patient interactions identified that exercise counseling was provided in 22 % of visits with an average time allocation of 49 s [34]. In a larger study of 10,000 patients, 34 % were counseled about exercise during their previous physician visit [35]. However, in a survey of primary care physicians, 87 % reported that they frequently advised patients to be physically active [36].

In a survey of patients that were overweight or affected by obesity, 30 and 42 %, respectively, reported that they were advised by their physician to lose weight within the past year [37]. In a more recent study, 40 primary care physicians were audiotaped during 461 consultations with a similar patient population. In this study, all physicians discussed weight loss with at least some of their patients for an average of 3.3 min [38]. However, in those that received this discussion, there was no additional weight loss compared with those that did not. Further analysis of the audiotaped sessions revealed that patients lost weight at 3 months if the physician used a collaborative method of communication that respected the

patient's freedom of choice regarding behavior change. Consequently, it appears that physicians cannot always rely on advice giving and persuasive tactics to effectively promote lifestyle medicine.

Clearly, it is not a simple task to provide optimal disease prevention to every patient in the clinical setting. There may be numerous factors to explain a less than ideal delivery of services. It has been documented that this may include factors associated with the health-care system (e.g., time-pressured appointments and reimbursement), the patient (e.g., personal motivation, health literacy, and complex comorbidities), and the physician (e.g., knowledge of guidelines, limited training and confidence in preventive medicine and health communication, low patient expectations, and poor physician self-care) [38–42]. The remainder of this chapter will focus on the identification of supportive solutions for the physician and potential models that can be used to deliver wellness in the clinic.

How Much Behavior Change Counseling Is Taught in Medical School?

Effective physician communication increases the likelihood of patients adhering to treatment recommendations and the adoption of healthful behaviors [43, 44]. However, many physicians in clinical practice have received little to no formal training in behavior change counseling. In the study of physician communication to promote weight loss, only 38 % of physicians reported prior training in health communication [38]. Traditionally, formal training in physician–patient communication has not been a major component of the medical school curriculum [45]. However, an increasing number of new medical school graduates are now entering the profession with at least some rudimentary skills in health communication [46].

In a recent 10-year follow-up cross-sectional survey of all existing medical schools ($N=2090$) in 171 countries (32 % response rate), it was identified that 27 % of schools taught a specific module on tobacco control compared with 11 % reported a decade earlier [47]. Seventy-seven percent integrated tobacco education teaching into other areas of the curriculum compared with 40 % in the original survey. A lecture format was the most popular teaching method (78 %), while others used patient-centered approaches such as role-playing (31 %). This report showed an encouraging trend towards tobacco education in medical schools worldwide, and it concluded that ongoing efforts were required for this to be a routine component of the curriculum.

The World Health Organization (WHO) Framework Convention on Tobacco Control (FCTC) is an international treaty that was adopted in 2003, with the aim to reduce the health consequences of tobacco use by promoting the initiation of evidence-based tobacco control interventions worldwide

[48]. In a web-based cross-sectional survey completed by a stratified convenient sample of key informants in 69 countries (70% response rate), it was identified that there were 61 current tobacco treatment training programs available in 37 of the 48 countries that responded [49]. Three quarters of them began in 2000 or later, and 40% began after 2003 when the FCTC was adopted. Programs estimated training approximately 14,000 health-care professionals in clinical practice, mostly physicians and nurses. Most programs used evidence-based guidelines and reported adherence to core tobacco treatment competencies. The median training duration was 16 h, but this varied widely, most notably in low-income countries. At least in the example of tobacco control, there appears to be a trend towards more education and/or training in medical school and clinical practice. The opportunity to learn about behavior change counseling in medical school and the provision of ongoing in-service education will help better prepare physicians for preventive medicine.

What Is the Wellness of Physicians?

Medical school and residency training are formative periods in a physician's professional and personal development. Physicians are encouraged to assume work habits that are in the best interest of the patient, which may supersede self-interest [50]. Consequently, the demands of balancing work and personal life starts early in a physician's career and appears to remain a hazard of the profession [51, 52]. In a survey to determine the personal and clinical exercise-related attitudes and behaviors of 1906 freshmen US medical students (mean age=24 years) at 17 medical schools, students reported exercising a median of 45 min/day. Nearly all students (98%) engaged in some moderate or vigorous exercise in a typical week, with 64% meeting national physical activity recommendations. In addition, 79% of respondents believed it would be highly relevant to their future practice to counsel patients about exercise [51].

In a survey to evaluate levels of burnout, depression, stress, mental quality of life (QOL), physical QOL, and fatigue in 2246 medical students in the midst of studying at seven US medical schools, 82% had at least one form of distress, and 58% had ≥3 of these characteristics [53]. In another study, the Empathy, Spirituality, and Wellness in Medicine Survey was used to compare the self-care behaviors of 963 medical students, residents, and attending physicians and identified that residents scored the lowest for adequate hours of sleep, exercise, and seatbelt use. Residents used tobacco and alcohol less than medical students, but they reported higher depression and anxiety with less time spent in social activities outside of their profession [54]. It is a sad irony that prospective physicians start out with healthful self-care practices and intentions to promote preventive medicine, but

this appears to become eroded shortly after entering a professional life in medicine. Studies show physicians continue to practice poor self-care throughout their career. Long work hours, job-related stress, and a reluctance to seek help from others often results in burnout [41, 52, 55].

Why Is Physician's Wellness Important?

The Women Physician's Health Study evaluated a large representative sample of US female physicians ($N = 4501$) by questionnaire to identify self-reported determinants of physician prevention-related counseling and screening practice. Physicians reported that they tended to preach what they practiced in their personal life. Those that adopted preventive health behaviors, or were at least trying to improve their self-care habits, reported that they were more likely to practice preventive services: lifestyle assessment, education and counseling, administration of flu vaccinations, screening for breast and skin cancer or abnormal cholesterol, and promoting hormone replacement therapy [56].

A review of the literature on physician wellness showed that when physicians are unwell, the performance of health-care can be suboptimum [41]. Physician responses to patient concerns are more abrupt and less compassionate, medical errors become more frequent, patient satisfaction declines, and malpractice suits increase [57–59]. Consequently, physician wellness might not only benefit the physician personally, it could also be vital to the delivery of high-quality health-care.

A culture change is needed within the medical profession to support physician wellness. The Canadian Medical Association (CMA) has taken a step in this direction by developing a national strategic plan to improve the mental health of physicians, residents, and medical students [60]. The plan involves recommendations to promote physician wellness on multiple levels, which includes targeting individuals, structures and systems. The CMA challenges the medical schools and residency programs to create a culture change within their environment that strives to shape the attitudes of students towards self-care and wellness. In this process, students are encouraged to recognize the early warning signs of distress and know how to seek help. This concept also extends to practicing physicians with a particular emphasis on individuals that have already experienced emotional distress or burnout. The CMA plan includes a campaign to support wellness within the health-care systems and organizations where the physicians practice. This includes the provision of resources and the elimination of punitive and discriminatory responses that can be associated with physician mental health and treatment. Efforts to support physician wellness within the US can learn from the Canadian experience.

Models of Wellness

Team-Based Medicine

A primary care physician is expected to manage approximately 2300 patients with an average visit time of 15 min. It has been estimated that it would take the physician 7.4 h in a workday to provide all of the services recommended by preventive services guidelines and even more time to adequately manage chronic conditions [61, 62]. Therefore, it is imperative that there is an effective organizational structure to reduce the physician's burden of responsibility while maintaining high-quality care. To meet this challenge, the majority of physician practices now rely on a team-based approach to patient care that utilizes nonphysician team members to provide clinical tasks, patient education, and monitoring under the guidance of the physician. There will be an increased reliance on teams that can function at a high level with an anticipated increase in patient volume with the introduction of the Affordable Healthcare Act. Team-based primary care will also be important as insurance carriers offer financial incentives based on patient outcomes with a goal of improving the quality of patient care. The California Healthcare Foundation have identified key elements of cohesive team building based on lessons learned from a study of high-functioning teams in the primary care setting [42, 63]. The practices studied encompassed the spectrum of primary care, from a one-physician private office to large integrated multispecialty groups with numerous health-care professionals, including primary care clinicians, nurses, medical assistants, health educators, social workers, community health workers, pharmacists, practice managers, and clerical assistants. A common theme was the expansion of the traditional 15-min visit to involve other team members to provide direct patient care, which included pre-visit and post-visit consultations, between-visit contacts, and community care away from the clinical site [42]. The health coach is a title that is more readily being used in primary care to describe a team member that assists the physician by providing these types of duties, which may include planning for behavior change [64, 65]. Another option for the physician is to provide additional patient support with a referral to specialty services such as behavioral health, nutrition counseling physical therapy, cardiac rehabilitation, individualized medicine, integrative medicine, or complementary and alternative medicine.

Primary Care Behavioral Health

The primary care physician routinely encounters a broad range of mental health issues in the clinic, including depression, anxiety, suicidal tendencies, substance abuse, and psychiatric disorders [66, 67]. Time-pressured consultations, complex medical histories, a reluctance or failure by both the physician and patient to recognize a psychosocial issue exists, and limited resources or training in mental health have resulted in less than optimal behavioral health services in the primary care clinic [68]. It is perhaps no surprise that for those who receive treatment, psychotropic medications are more readily prescribed than specialty behavioral health services [69]. As a result, new models of health-care delivery have emerged to bring mental health services into the clinic and help reduce the burden of responsibility on the physician [67, 70].

Primary Care Behavioral Health is one model of care that has been proposed to meet this challenge by positioning a mental health specialist within the primary care clinic to work as a behavioral health consultant (BHC) in collaboration with the physician and other members of the health-care team. In this model, the BHC is available to address not only the mental health needs of the patient but also provides a specialized service that promotes preventive strategies such as smoking cessation, weight control, and stress management education in an effort to manage chronic disease (e.g., chronic pain, headaches, hypertension, T2D, and obesity). A guide is available to describe how this integrated model of care is being utilized in clinics within the US Air Force and Army, the Veterans Administration, and private health-care institutions such as Kaiser Permanente [68]. The Agency for Healthcare Research and Quality (AHRQ) conducted a comprehensive review of the evidence associated with practice models that integrated behavioral health into primary care and concluded that, at least in the case of psychiatric problems, integrated care generally improved clinical outcomes [71].

Patient-Centered Medical Home

With a new model of health-care delivery that requires more coordination, preventive services, and patient self-management, a less fragmented and collaborative model of care is needed [3, 72]. The Patient-Centered Medical Home (PCMH) model of care "facilitates partnerships between patients, their families, and the health-care team to take into account patient preferences and needs that promote better coordination and delivery of care" [73]. The PCMH is being adopted by a number of physician organizations and focuses on enhancing the patient experience by integrating improvements that are both "high-tech" (e.g., electronic medical records, registries to promote population-based disease management, and connected health interventions) and "high-touch" (e.g., cultivating the physician–patient relationship). Here, there is an emphasis on interventions that keep the patient well between visits and reduce the need to come into the clinic. The promotion of lifestyle medicine and wellness is integral to the success of the PCMH.

Currently, there are more than 90 commercial health plans, 42 states and 3 federal initiatives testing the PCMH model. The Patient-Centered Primary Care Collaborative (PCPCC) is one group that has reviewed 46 medical home initiatives across the US and identified preliminary evidence that the PCMH model improves the quality of care and population health and reduces health-care costs [74]. While these findings are encouraging, the Commonwealth Fund's Patient-Centered Medical Home Evaluator's Collaborative recognizes there is an urgent need for high-quality evaluations that measure the impact of the PCMH and improve its implementation. The collaborative consists of more than 75 researchers, divided into 5 workgroups, with a focus on the key dimensions of PCMH evaluation: cost/utilization, clinical quality, patient experience, clinician/staff experience, and process/implementation. The collaborative anticipates that a consensus on optimal standardized measures to evaluate cost, utilization, and quality outcomes will help strengthen medical home research and help influence primary care policy [75].

Connected Health

Connected Health is a model of health-care delivery supported by electronic processes and communication in order to deliver health services remotely. Connected Health applications use various technology platforms such as the Internet (e.g., eHealth), telephone and interactive voice response systems (e.g., telehealth), mobile and smartphone-based applications (e.g., mHealth), and computer-tailored print [76]. Connected Health applications to lifestyle medicine have the potential to enhance clinical care and the self-management of healthful behaviors between clinical encounters.

The growth of Connected Health interventions has mirrored the ubiquitous and global growth of personal technology. Internet use in the USA has grown from 14% in 1995 to 87% in 2014. Ninety percent of adults own a cell phone and 58% own a smartphone [77]. African-Americans and Hispanics have the highest rates of smartphone adoption (64 and 60%, respectively), and individuals with a low household income (US$ 30,000/year) and education (high school completion) are adopting smartphones at rates faster than any other population subgroup. It is estimated that 72% of Internet users and 31% of cell phone owners have accessed health information using these technologies.

Considerable evidence suggests that Internet and telemanagement interventions are efficacious at delivering a host of lifestyle interventions, including cancer prevention and control [78], the management of gastrointestinal disease [79], diabetes [80], and heart failure [81]. Compared with usual care, enrollment in a heart failure telemanagement service more effectively prevented hospital readmission and

reduced related costs in this patient population [81, 82]. A reduction in early hospital readmission has been identified by the US government as a national priority in an effort to improve the quality of care and minimize unnecessary health-care expense [83].

Recent attention has shifted to developing smartphone-based health interventions given the ubiquity of this technology and the potential for widespread dissemination through existing channels such as the Apple and Google app stores [84]. However, most developers to date have not used evidence-based strategies [85]; efficacy has been modest [86, 87], and a recent comprehensive review indicated few interventions have been empirically evaluated [88]. A great amount of research is currently underway in this area.

A promising area of growth in Connected Health is the advent of wearable and portable medical technology. Wearable sensors can monitor various health parameters (e.g., physical activity, sleep, heart rate, blood pressure, and glucose level), improve symptom management, and enhance communication between the patient and physician. There are limited examples of these technologies being integrated into clinical practice. One recent example was the implementation of a digital health-feedback system in patients with hypertension [89]. Patients were given a wearable sensor and poppy-sized ingestible sensors, which collectively monitored activities of daily living, physical activity, and compliance and timing of antihypertensive treatment. Data was automatically transmitted to a provider. The system provided support for clinical decisions and management by helping to discriminate between inadequate medication utilization, pharmacologic unresponsiveness, and the need for patient counseling. While the opportunities for wearable and portable technologies are exciting, challenges remain, including sensor validation, the protection of patient privacy, and the successful integration into existing clinical practice settings.

Lifestyle Medicine in Practice

Some national associations for health professionals have begun to recognize the important role of lifestyle medicine in clinical practice. For example, Exercise is Medicine™ (EIM) is a recent initiative that is being promoted by the American College of Sports Medicine (ACSM) and the American Medical Association (AMA) to address the low-level physical activity counseling that exists in a clinical setting. The vision for this initiative calls on all primary care physicians to promote physical activity and exercise to every patient at every outpatient visit [90]. Recognizing the time constraints of patient consultations, these national associations recommend that physicians consider a menu of four options in the promotion of EIM.

- Option 1 consists of asking the patient about their current level of physical activity with two short closed-ended questions and assigning a numerical score similar to the other recognized vital signs [91, 92].
- Option 2 includes the provision of an optimistic recommendation to exercise. This could happen during the same consultation as option 1 or be revisited at a future appointment.
- Option 3 invites the physician to budget more time to counseling and prescribing the specifics of an exercise plan.
- Option 4 consists of referring the patient to an exercise professional and/or program such as cardiac rehabilitation or physical therapy for more specialized guidance.

The physician is not obligated to change their practice in anyway. However, it is anticipated that giving the physician practical suggestions such as these will make the task of promoting EIM less daunting during time-pressured consultations. This example shows how a physician can be strategic in the application of lifestyle medicine in the clinic and elect the best option that suits any given situation.

Kaiser Permanente Southern California is one organization that has taken steps to apply this wellness model within their practice by incorporating questions about exercise within the routine measurement of traditional vital signs. Over a 1.5-year period from when this quality improvement process was implemented, it was observed that 86% of all eligible patients ($N=1,537,798$) had the exercise vital sign in the electronic medical record [92]. The ACSM has developed online resources to assist the physician in the promotion of EIM, including a list of certified exercise professionals that can provide patients further guidance with physical activity out in the community [90]. A review of the physical activity counseling literature in primary care has identified that a physician partnership with an allied professional results in better long-term patient adherence to physical activity [93].

Behavior Change Counseling and Motivational Interviewing

Behavior change counseling in the medical setting has progressed from simple advice giving to structured brief interventions, [94] to strategic patient-centered methods of communication, such as motivational interviewing [95, 96]. This latter approach has gained substantial empirical support as an effective option for physicians to counsel patients that are ambivalent or not ready to change behavior [97, 98]. It has been described as a teachable, collaborative, goal-oriented style of communication for eliciting and strengthening a person's own motivation to change [95, 96]. The distinct style, skills, and strategies that characterize the approach differ

from traditional persuasive methods by enabling patients to discover their own intrinsic motivation for change, which is supported with strategic empathic listening. Patients are given the opportunity to partner with their health-care professional to interpret personalized health information and identify solutions rather than being told what they must do. In the negotiation of a treatment plan, the health-care professional acknowledges the patient's freedom to decide what, if anything, they will change when they leave the clinic. In a systematic review and meta-analysis of 72 randomized controlled trials, motivational interviewing outperformed traditional advice giving in approximately 80% of the studies [97].

Motivational interviewing first demonstrated its efficacy in the treatment of substance abuse and addictions [99], but the evidence-base has continued to grow with successful applications to variety of clinical populations in health-care settings [97, 100]. Although grounded in psychology, the approach is not exclusive to counselors or psychologists. When effectively delivered, patients are more receptive to treatment recommendations, which makes consultations less frustrating for the physician. Improved behavioral and clinical outcomes have even been observed in brief consultations. Therefore, it lends itself well to the primary care setting, where time is often a limiting factor [97, 101]. The USPSTF has recommended the systematic use of motivational interviewing or brief interventions that include its key components in primary care practice [102, 103].

An investigation of motivational interviewing training methods identified significant short-term gains in competency with participation in an interactive workshop. Longer-term improvements in proficiency were observed with ongoing feedback and supervision [104, 105]. Experienced trainers are available in the US and other regions of the world to provide this type of professional training to clinicians [106]. In addition, there are now several medical schools that have included motivational interviewing training in their academic program [107].

Conclusion

Niccolo Machiavelli, the sixteenth-century philosopher stated that "at the beginning a disease is easy to cure but difficult to diagnose; but as time passes, not having been recognized or treated at the outset, it becomes easy to diagnose but difficult to cure" [101]. This reminds us that preventive medicine is not a new concept. Historically, preventive services have not been at the forefront of mainstream health care in the US. However, the health-care system is on the cusp of a paradigm shift towards disease prevention and health promotion with the introduction of the Affordable Healthcare Act. Preventive medicine will be part of the solution as physicians consider the best options to lower the burden of chronic disease at a time when patient volumes will reach a record high. There is compelling evidence to support the inclusion of lifestyle medicine and wellness within clinical practice. When delivered effectively, physicians will not only add years to a patient's life, but more importantly life to those years.

References

1. McKinley JB. A case for refocusing upstream: the political economy of illness. In: Conrad P, editor. The sociology of health and illness: critical perspectives. 8th ed. New York: Worth Publishers; 2010. p. 578–91.
2. Muennig PA, Glied SA. What changes in survival rates tell us about US health care. Health Aff (Millwood). 2010;29(11):2105–13.
3. Koh HK, Sebelius KG. Promoting prevention through the affordable care act. N Engl J Med. 2010;363(14):1296–9.
4. Agency for Healthcare Research and Quality. The guide to clinical preventive services 2012: recommendations of the U. S. Preventive Services Task Force. 2012. http://www.ahrq.gov/professionals/clinicians-providers/guidelines-recommendations/guide/guide-clinical-preventive-services.pdf. Accessed 6 May 2014.
5. Agency for Healtcare Research and Quality. U. S. Preventive Services Task Force A and B recommendations: U. S. Preventive Task Force. 2014. http://www.uspreventiveservicestaskforce.org/uspstf/uspsabrecs.htm. Accessed 6 May 2014.
6. Mausner JS, Mausner KS, Epidemiology B. Epidemiology: an introductory text. Philadelphia: WB Saunders Co; 1985.
7. Lim SS, Vos T, Flaxman AD, Danaei G, Shibuya K, Adair-Rohani H, et al. A comparative risk assessment of burden of disease and injury attributable to 67 risk factors and risk factor clusters in 21 regions, 1990–2010: a systematic analysis for the Global Burden of Disease Study 2010. Lancet. 2013;380(9859):2224–60.
8. National Public Health Partnership. The language of prevention. Melbourne: NPHP; 2006.
9. Knowler WC, Barrett-Connor E, Fowler SE, Hamman RF, Lachin JM, Walker EA, et al. Reduction in the incidence of type 2 diabetes with lifestyle intervention or metformin. N Engl J Med. 2002;346(6):393–403.
10. Grundy SM, Cleeman JI, Daniels SR, Donato KA, Eckel RH, Franklin BA, et al. Diagnosis and management of the metabolic syndrome: an American Heart Association/National Heart, Lung, and Blood Institute scientific statement. Circulation. 2005;112(17):2735–52.
11. Suaya JA, Stason WB, Ades PA, Normand S-LT, Shepard DS. Cardiac rehabilitation and survival in older coronary patients. J Am Coll Cardiol. 2009;54(1):25–33.
12. Witt BJ, Jacobsen SJ, Weston SA, Killian JM, Meverden RA, Allison TG, et al. Cardiac rehabilitation after myocardial infarction in the community. J Am Coll Cardiol. 2004;44(5):988–96.
13. Haskell WL, Alderman EL, Fair JM, Maron DJ, Mackey SF, Superko HR, et al. Effects of intensive multiple risk factor reduction on coronary atherosclerosis and clinical cardiac events in men and women with coronary artery disease. The Stanford Coronary Risk Intervention Project (SCRIP). Circulation. 1994;89(3):975–90.
14. Brown WJ, Pavey T, Bauman AE. Comparing population attributable risks for heart disease across the adult lifespan in women. Br J Sports Med. 2014;49:1069–76. doi:0.1136/bjsports-2013-093090.
15. Blair SN, Kohl HW, Barlow CE, Paffenbarger RS, Gibbons LW, Macera CA. Changes in physical fitness and all-cause mortality: a prospective study of healthy and unhealthy men. JAMA. 1995;273(14):1093–8.
16. Blair SN, Kampert JB, Kohl HW, Barlow CE, Macera CA, Paffenbarger RS, et al. Influences of cardiorespiratory fitness and other precursors on cardiovascular disease and all-cause mortality in men and women. JAMA. 1996;276(3):205–10.
17. Kodama S, Saito K, Tanaka S, Maki M, Yachi Y, Asumi M, et al. Cardiorespiratory fitness as a quantitative predictor of all-cause mortality and cardiovascular events in healthy men and women: a meta-analysis. JAMA. 2009;301(19):2024–35.
18. Myers J, Prakash M, Froelicher V, Do D, Partington S, Atwood JE. Exercise capacity and mortality among men referred for exercise testing. N Engl J Med. 2002;346(11):793–801.
19. Ornish D, Brown SE, Billings J, Scherwitz L, Armstrong W, Ports T, et al. Can lifestyle changes reverse coronary heart disease?: the Lifestyle Heart Trial. Lancet. 1990;336(8708):129–33.
20. Ornish D, Scherwitz LW, Billings JH, Gould KL, Merritt TA, Sparler S, et al. Intensive lifestyle changes for reversal of coronary heart disease. JAMA. 1998;280(23):2001–7.
21. Hambrecht R, Niebauer J, Marburger C, Grunze M, Kälberer B, Hauer K, et al. Various intensities of leisure time physical activity in patients with coronary artery disease: effects on cardiorespiratory fitness and progression of coronary atherosclerotic lesions. J Am Coll Cardiol. 1993;22(2):468–77.
22. Niebauer J, Hambrecht R, Velich T, Hauer K, Marburger C, Kälberer B, et al. Attenuated progression of coronary artery disease after 6 years of multifactorial risk intervention role of physical exercise. Circulation. 1997;96(8):2534–41.
23. Hu FB, Manson JE, Stampfer MJ, Colditz G, Liu S, Solomon CG, et al. Diet, lifestyle, and the risk of type 2 diabetes mellitus in women. N Engl J Med. 2001;345(11):790–7.
24. Hietaniemi M, Jokela M, Rantala M, Ukkola O, Vuoristo JT, Ilves M, et al. The effect of a short-term hypocaloric diet on liver gene expression and metabolic risk factors in obese women. Nutr Metab Cardiovasc Dis. 2009;19(3):177–83.
25. Lin DW, Neuhouser ML, Schenk JM, Coleman IM, Hawley S, Gifford D, et al. Low-fat, low-glycemic load diet and gene expression in human prostate epithelium: a feasibility study of using cDNA microarrays to assess the response to dietary intervention in target tissues. Cancer Epidemiol Biomarkers Prev. 2007;16(10):2150–4.
26. Ornish D, Magbanua MJM, Weidner G, Weinberg V, Kemp C, Green C, et al. Changes in prostrate gene expression in men undergoing an intensive nutrition and lifestyle intervention. Proc Natl Acad Sci U S A. 2008;105(24):8369–74.
27. Hagberg JM, Rankinen T, Loos R, Perusse L, Roth SM, Wolfarth B, et al. Advances in exercise, fitness, and performance genomics in 2010. Med Sci Sports Exerc. 2011;43(5):743–52.
28. Ellsworth DL, Croft DT, Weyandt J, Sturtz LA, Blackburn HL, Burke A, et al. Intensive cardiovascular risk reduction induces sustainable changes in expression of genes and pathways important to vascular function. Circulation: Cardiovascular Genetics. 2014: CIRCGENETICS. 113.000121.
29. Coustan DR, Lowe LP, Metzger BE, Dyer AR. The Hyperglycemia and Adverse Pregnancy Outcome (HAPO) study: paving the way for new diagnostic criteria for gestational diabetes mellitus. Am J Obstet Gynecol. 2010;202(6):654, e1–e6.
30. Feil R, Fraga MF. Epigenetics and the environment: emerging patterns and implications. Nat Rev Genet. 2012;13(2):97–109.
31. Foraker RE, Olivo-Marston SE, Allen NB. Lifestyle and primordial prevention of cardiovascular disease: challenges and opportunities. Curr Cardiovasc Risk Rep. 2012;6(6):520–7.
32. Pollak KI, Krause KM, Yarnall KS, Gradison M, Michener JL, Østbye T. Estimated time spent on preventive services by primary care physicians. BMC Health Serv Res. 2008;8(1):245.
33. Yawn B, Goodwin MA, Zyzanski SJ, Stange KC. Time use during acute and chronic illness visits to a family physician. Fam Pract. 2003;20(4):474–7.

34. Podl TR, Goodwin MA, Kikano GE, Stange KC. Direct observation of exercise counseling in community family practice. Am J Prev Med. 1999;17(3):207–10.

35. Wee CC, McCarthy EP, Davis RB, Phillips RS. Physician counseling about exercise. JAMA. 1999;282(16):1583–8.

36. College of Family Physicians of Canada. Physical activity report: results from the 2001 National Family Physician Workforce Survey. 2001. http://www.cfpc.ca/research/janus/janushome.asp. Accessed 21 April 2014.

37. Sciamanna CN, Tate DF, Lang W, Wing RR. Who reports receiving advice to lose weight?: results from a multistate survey. Arch Intern Med. 2000;160(15):2334–9.

38. Pollak KI, Alexander SC, Coffman CJ, Tulsky JA, Lyna P, Dolor RJ, et al. Physician communication techniques and weight loss in adults: project CHAT. Am J Prev Med. 2010;39(4):321–8.

39. Cabana MD, Rand CS, Powe NR, Wu AW, Wilson MH, Abboud P-AC, et al. Why don't physicians follow clinical practice guidelines? A framework for improvement. JAMA. 1999;282(15):1458–65.

40. Walsh JM, McPhee SJ. A systems model of clinical preventive care: an analysis of factors influencing patient and physician. Health Educ Behav. 1992;19(2):157–75.

41. Wallace JE, Lemaire JB, Ghali WA. Physician wellness: a missing quality indicator. Lancet. 2009;374(9702):1714–21.

42. Bodenheimer T. Building teams in primary care: lessons learned. Oakland: California HealthCare Foundation; 2007.

43. Emmons KM, Rollnick S. Motivational interviewing in health care settings: opportunities and limitations. Am J Prev Med. 2001;20(1):68–74.

44. Maguire P, Pitceathly C. Key communication skills and how to acquire them. Br Med J. 2002;325(7366):697.

45. Anderson M, Cohen J, Hallock J, Kassebaum D, Turnbull J, Whitcomb M. Learning objectives for medical student education-Guidelines for medical schools: report I of the Medical School Objectives Project. Acad Med. 1999;74(1):13–8.

46. Association of American Medical Colleges. Medical School Graduation Questionnaire. 2013. All Schools Summary Report 2013.

47. Richmond R, Zwar N, Taylor R, Hunnisett J, Hyslop F. Teaching about tobacco in medical schools: a worldwide study. Drug Alcohol Rev. 2009;28(5):484–97.

48. Yach D. WHO framework convention on tobacco control. Lancet. 2003;361(9357):611.

49. Rigotti NA, Bitton A, Richards AE, Reyen M, Wassum K, Raw M. An international survey of training programs for treating tobacco dependence. Addiction. 2009;104(2):288–96.

50. Accreditation Council for Graduate Medical Education. Common program requirements. 2013. http://www.acgme.org/acgmeweb/Portals/0/PFAssets/ProgramRequirements/CPRs2013.pdf. Accessed 10 July 2014.

51. Frank E, Galuska DA, Elon LK, Wright EH. Personal and clinical exercise-related attitudes and behaviors of freshmen US medical students. Res Q Exerc Sport. 2004;75(2):112–21.

52. Dyrbye LN, Varkey P, Boone SL, Satele DV, Sloan JA, Shanafelt TD. Physician satisfaction and burnout at different career stages. Mayo Clin Proc. 2013;88:1358–67.

53. Dyrbye LN, Harper W, Durning SJ, Moutier C, Thomas MR, Massie FS Jr, et al. Patterns of distress in US medical students. Med Teach. 2011;33(10):834–9.

54. Hull SK, DiLalla LF, Dorsey JK. Prevalence of health-related behaviors among physicians and medical trainees. Acad Psychiatry. 2008;32(1):31–8.

55. Sotile WM, Sotile MO. The resilient physician: effective emotional management for doctors & their medical organizations. Chicago: American Medical Association Press; 2002.

56. Frank E, Rothenberg R, Lewis C, Belodoff BF. Correlates of physicians' prevention-related practices: findings from the Women Physicians' Health Study. Arch Fam Med. 2000;9(4):359.

57. Stewart MA. Effective physician-patient communication and health outcomes: a review. Can Med Assoc J. 1995;152(9):1423.

58. Shanafelt TD, Bradley KA, Wipf JE, Back AL. Burnout and self-reported patient care in an internal medicine residency program. Ann Intern Med. 2002;136(5):358–67.

59. Haas JS, Cook EF, Puopolo AL, Burstin HR, Cleary PD, Brennan TA. Is the professional satisfaction of general internists associated with patient satisfaction? J Gen Intern Med. 2000;15(2):122–8.

60. Jones JW, Barge BN, Steffy BD, Fay LM, Kunz LK, Wuebker LJ. Stress and medical malpractice: organizational risk assessment and intervention. J Appl Psychol. 1988;73(4):727.

61. Yarnall KS, Pollak KI, Østbye T, Krause KM, Michener JL. Primary care: is there enough time for prevention? Am J Public Health. 2003;93(4):635–41.

62. Østbye T, Yarnall KS, Krause KM, Pollak KI, Gradison M, Michener JL. Is there time for management of patients with chronic diseases in primary care? Ann Fam Med. 2005;3(3):209–14.

63. Bodenheimer T. Building teams in primary care: 15 case studies. Oakland: California HealthCare Foundation; 2007.

64. Handley M, MacGregor K, Schillinger D, Sharifi C, Wong S, Bodenheimer T. Using action plans to help primary care patients adopt healthy behaviors: a descriptive study. J Am Board Fam Med. 2006;19(3):224–31.

65. Ammentorp J, Uhrenfeldt L, Angel F, Ehrensvärd M, Carlsen EB, Kofoed P-E. Can life coaching improve health outcomes? A systematic review of intervention studies. BMC Health Serv Res. 2013;13(1):428.

66. Regier DA, Narrow WE, Rae DS, Manderscheid RW, Locke BZ, Goodwin FK. The de facto US mental and addictive disorders service system: epidemiologic catchment Area prospective 1-year prevalence rates of disorders and services. Arch Gen Psychiatry. 1993;50(2):85–94.

67. Gatchel RJ, Oordt MS, Association AP. Clinical health psychology and primary care: practical advice and clinical guidance for successful collaboration. Washington, DC: American Psychological Association; 2003.

68. Gray GV, Brody DS, Johnson D. The evolution of behavioral primary care. Prof Psychol Res Pract. 2005;36(2):123.

69. Robinson P, Reiter J. Behavioral consultation and primary care: a guide to integrating services. New York: Springer; 2007.

70. Stosahl K. Integrating behavioral health and primary care services: the primary mental health model. In: Blount A, editor. Integrated primary care: the future of medical and mental health collaboration. New York, NY: W. W. Norton; 1998. p. 139–66.

71. Butler M, Kane RL, McAlpine D, Kathol RG, Fu SS, Hagedorn H, et al. Integration of mental health/substance abuse and primary care. Rockville: Agency for Healthcare Research and Quality; 2008.

72. Culliton BJ. Extracting knowledge from science: a conversation with Elias Zerhouni. Health Aff (Millwood). 2006;25(3):w94–103.

73. Hesse BW, Nilsen WJ, M Hunter C. News from NIH: the patient-centered medical home. Transl Behav Med. 2012;2:1–2.

74. Nielsen M, Langner B, Zema C, Hacker T, Grundy P. Benefits of implementing the Primary Care Medical Home: a review of cost & quality results. Washington, DC: Patient-Centered Primary Care Collaborative; 2012.

75. Rosenthal MB, Abrams AK. Measuring the success of medical homes: recommendations from the PCMH Evaluators' collaborative. 2012. http://www.commonwealthfund.org/publications/blog/2012/may/measuring-the-success-of-medical-homes-blog. Accessed 22 Aug 2014.

76. Rabin B, Glasgow R. Dissemination of interactive health communication programs. In: Routledge, editor. Interactive health com-

munication technologies: promising strategies for health behavior change. 1st ed. New York: Routledge; 2012.

77. Pew Internet Research. Pew internet: mobile. 2014. http://www.pewinternet.org/fact-sheets/mobile-technology-fact-sheet/. Accessed 23 May 2014.

78. Sanchez MA, Rabin BA, Gaglio B, Henton M, Elzarrad MK, Purcell P, et al. A systematic review of eHealth cancer prevention and control interventions: new technology, same methods and designs? Transl Behav Med. 2013;3(4):392–401.

79. Knowles SR, Mikocka-Walus A. Utilization and efficacy of internet-based eHealth technology in gastroenterology: a systematic review. Scand J Gastroenterol. 2014;49(4):387–408.

80. Glasgow RE, Strycker LA, King DK, Toobert DJ. Understanding who benefits at each step in an Internet-Based Diabetes Self-Management Program: application of a Recursive Partitioning Approach. Med Decis Mak. 2014;34(2):180–91.

81. Giordano A, Scalvini S, Zanelli E, Corrà U, GL L, Ricci V, et al. Multicenter randomised trial on home-based telemanagement to prevent hospital readmission of patients with chronic heart failure. Int J Cardiol. 2009;131(2):192–9.

82. Leppin AL, Gionfriddo MR, Kessler M, Brito JP, Mair FS, Gallacher K, et al. Preventing 30-day hospital readmissions: a systematic review and meta-analysis of randomized trials. JAMA Intern Med. 2014;174:1095–107.

83. Joynt KE, Jha AK. A path forward on Medicare readmissions. N Engl J Med. 2013;368(13):1175–7.

84. Bennett GG, Glasgow RE. The delivery of public health interventions via the Internet: actualizing their potential. Annu Rev Public Health. 2009;30:273–92.

85. Pagoto S, Schneider K, Jojic M, DeBiasse M, Mann D. Evidence-based strategies in weight-loss mobile apps. Am J Prev Med. 2013;45(5):576–82.

86. Fanning J, Mullen SP, McAuley E. Increasing physical activity with mobile devices: a meta-analysis. J Med Internet Res. 2012;14(6):e161.

87. Hekler EB, Klasnja P, Froehlich JE, Buman MP, editors. Mind the theoretical gap: interpreting, using, and developing behavioral theory in HCI research. Proceedings of the SIGCHI Conference on Human Factors in Computing Systems; ACM; 2013.

88. Bender JL, Yue RYK, To MJ, Deacken L, Jadad AR. A lot of action, but not in the right direction: systematic review and content analysis of smartphone applications for the prevention, detection, and management of cancer. J Med Int Res. 2013;15(12):e287.

89. Godbehere P, Wareing P. Hypertension assessment and management: role for digital medicine. J Clin Hypertens. 2014;16(3):235.

90. American College of Sports Medicine. Exercise is medicine. 2013. http://www.exerciseismedicine.org. Accessed 6 May 2014.

91. Greenwood JL, Joy EA, Stanford JB. The physical activity vital sign: a primary care tool to guide counseling for obesity. J Phys Act Health. 2010;7(5):571–6.

92. Sallis RE. Exercise is medicine and physicians need to prescribe it! Br J Sports Med. 2009;43(1):3–4.

93. Tulloch H, Fortier M, Hogg W. Physical activity counseling in primary care: who has and who should be counseling? Patient Educ Couns. 2006;64(1):6–20.

94. Goldstein MG, DePue J, Kazura A, Niaura R. Models for provider–patient interaction: applications to health behavior change. In: Shumaker S, Schron E, Ockene J, McBee W, editors. The handbook of health behavior change. 2nd ed. New York: Springer; 1998. p. 85–113.

95. Rollnick S, Miller WR, Butler C. Motivational interviewing in health care: helping patients change behavior. New York: Guilford; 2008.

96. Miller WR, Rollnick S. Motivational interviewing: helping people change. New York: Guilford; 2013.

97. Rubak S, Sandbæk A, Lauritzen T, Christensen B. Motivational interviewing: a systematic review and meta-analysis. Br J Gen Pract. 2005;55(513):305–12.

98. Söderlund LL, Madson MB, Rubak S, Nilsen P. A systematic review of motivational interviewing training for general health care practitioners. Patient Educ Couns. 2011;84(1):16–26.

99. Lundahl B, Burke BL. The effectiveness and applicability of motivational interviewing: a practice-friendly review of four meta-analyses. J Clin Psychol. 2009;65(11):1232–45.

100. Lundahl B, Moleni T, Burke BL, Butters R, Tollefson D, Butler C, et al. Motivational interviewing in medical care settings: a systematic review and meta-analysis of randomized controlled trials. Patient Educ Couns. 2013;93(2):157–68.

101. Scales R, Miller JH. Motivational techniques for improving compliance with an exercise program: skills for primary care clinicians. Curr Sports Med Rep. 2003;2(3):166–72.

102. McTigue KM, Harris R, Hemphill B, Lux L, Sutton S, Bunton AJ, et al. Screening and interventions for obesity in adults: summary of the evidence for the US Preventive Services Task Force. Ann Intern Med. 2003;139(11):933–49.

103. Whitlock EP, Polen MR, Green CA, Orleans T, Klein J. Behavioral counseling interventions in primary care to reduce risky/harmful alcohol use by adults: a summary of the evidence for the US Preventive Services Task Force. Ann Intern Med. 2004;140(7):557–68.

104. Madson MB, Loignon AC, Lane C. Training in motivational interviewing: a systematic review. J Subst Abuse Treat. 2009;36(1):101–9.

105. Miller WR, Yahne CE, Moyers TB, Martinez J, Pirritano M. A randomized trial of methods to help clinicians learn motivational interviewing. J Consult Clin Psychol. 2004;72(6):1050.

106. Motivational Interviewing Network of Trainers. 2013. http://www.motivationalinterviewing.org. Accessed 23 May 2014.

107. Daeppen J-B, Fortini C, Bertholet N, Bonvin R, Berney A, Michaud P-A, et al. Training medical students to conduct motivational interviewing: a randomized controlled trial. Patient Educ Couns. 2012;87(3):313–8.

Composite Risk Scores

5

Ruth E. Brown and Jennifer L. Kuk

Abbreviations

ACC	American College of Cardiology
AHA	American Heart Association
ARIC	Atherosclerosis risk in communities
AS	Atherosclerotic
BMI	Body mass index
CARDIA	Cardiovascular Health Study, Coronary Artery Risk Development in Young Adults
CHD	Coronary heart disease
CMDS	Cardiometabolic disease staging system
CVD	Cardiovascular disease
DASH	Dietary approaches to stop hypertension
EGIR	European Group for the Study of Insulin Resistance
EOSS	Edmonton obesity staging system
GLP-1	Glucagon-peptide 1
HDL-C	High-density lipoprotein cholesterol
HIV	Human immunodeficiency virus
hs-CRP	High-sensitivity C-reactive protein
IDF	International Diabetes Federation
IGT	Imaired glucose tolerance
LDL-C	Low-density lipoprotein cholesterol
MetS	Metabolic syndrome
MI	Myocardial infarction
NCEP ATP III	National Cholesterol Education Program Adult Treatment Program III
SBP	Systolic blood pressure
T2D	Type-2 diabetes
TC	Total cholesterol
WC	Waist circumference
WHO	World Health Organization

J. L. Kuk (✉)
School of Kinesiology and Health Science, York University, 4700 Keele Street, Toronto, ON M3J 1P3, Canada
e-mail: jennkuk@yorku.ca

R. E. Brown
School of Kinesiology and Health Science, York University, Toronto Canada

Introduction

Cardiovascular disease (CVD) remains the leading cause of death worldwide [1]. The most prominent risk factors for CVD include age, gender, obesity, smoking, diabetes, hypertension, and dyslipidemia [2]. During the past several decades, there have been major advances in treating CVD and its associated risk factors; it is now internationally accepted that the initiation and intensity of pharmacological therapy for CVD prevention should be based on a patient's baseline absolute CVD risk [3]. Absolute CVD risk can be determined through composite risk scores, which assess multiple risk factors simultaneously to predict disease onset or outcomes and to help guide treatment. In order to be clinically useful, it is important to first understand the origin of the risk score in terms of the population and outcome that it was developed for and second that the risk model is updated when new evidence arises. Within the past several decades, there have been numerous updates to older risk scores as well as the development of new risk scores that assess several chronic conditions. Thus, choosing the most appropriate risk assessment model for patients can be difficult. Furthermore, no single risk algorithm can account for all relevant risk factors for CVD, and therefore patients may still exhibit residual cardiovascular risk, which is the risk of experiencing a cardiovascular event even when patients achieve target levels of metabolic risk factors [4]. Conversely, they may not experience CVD even though their predicted risk level is high. Lifestyle management, including diet, physical activity, smoking cessation, and weight management, remains the cornerstone of both CVD prevention and residual cardiovascular risk reduction [3, 4]. Further, several pharmacological agents have been identified that may help alleviate the burden of absolute and residual cardiovascular risk [5]. Importantly, risk assessment is only useful if a patient understands what their risk means and what they need to do to improve their risk. Therefore, optimal risk communication between health professional and patient is necessary for optimal patient care.

© Springer International Publishing Switzerland 2016
J. I. Mechanick, R. F. Kushner (eds.), *Lifestyle Medicine,* DOI 10.1007/978-3-319-24687-1_5

This review will describe the development and clinical utility of the Framingham Risk Score, the Reynolds Risk Score, the Pooled Cohort Equations, lifetime risk scores, the metabolic syndrome (MetS), the Edmonton Obesity Staging System, and the Cardiometabolic Disease Staging System. Residual cardiovascular risk and patient communication will also be discussed.

Framingham Risk Score

Some of our greatest understanding of the underlying causes of CVD derives from the Framingham Heart Study. The Framingham Heart Study was developed in Framingham, MA, in 1948, and the original cohort included 5209 adults, ages 30–62 years, who initially did not have CVD. This cohort has been followed since 1948 and has provided rich epidemiological data on the development of CVD [6]. From these data, the Framingham Risk Score was developed to estimate absolute CVD risk and is the oldest and most widely used and studied CVD risk score available [7]. To date, multiple risk scores for coronary heart disease (CHD) and CVD have been developed and modified over time using data from the Framingham original cohort as well as the offspring cohort.

Due to the ongoing nature of the Framingham Heart Study, the algorithm has been revised over time to reflect the latest evidence (Table 5.1). The very first risk equation for CHD from the Framingham Heart Study was developed in 1967; [8] however, this equation was not validated and for the most part was not used clinically [9]. Subsequently, an 8-year risk of general CVD and specific subtypes of CVD was developed in 1976 [10]. This demonstrated that CVD is actually a heterogeneous condition, wherein some CVD risk factors are more relevant for certain subcomponents of CVD. For example, systolic blood pressure (SBP) is particularly important for stroke risk, whereas smoking and glucose intolerance may be more important for risk of intermittent claudication. This study also highlighted that certain risk factors have a risk continuum that should not be simply dichotomized into high and low. For example, CVD risk is proportional to the level of SBP and cholesterol, and there is no threshold for where risk begins to increase. Finally, this study demonstrated that an individual with a clustering of multiple subclinical risk factors might be more at risk than an individual with a single high-risk factor. In 1991, a new algorithm for 10-year risk of CHD was developed, and it was the first time that a points system was developed in order for clinicians to do a simple assessment of absolute CHD risk [11]. In 1998, a simplified sex-specific 10-year CHD prediction model that included age, diabetes status, smoking status, blood pressure, total cholesterol (TC), and high-density lipoprotein cholesterol (HDL-C) was developed (Table 5.1) [12]. This Framingham CHD risk score was adapted and incorporated into the National Cholesterol Edu-

cation Program Expert Panel on Detection, Evaluation, and Treatment of High Blood Cholesterol in Adults (NCEP ATP III) as part of their updated recommendations for screening and treatment of dyslipidemia in 2001 [13]. According to the ATP III, the intensity of risk reduction therapy should be adjusted to reflect an individual's level of absolute risk. One of the changes in this version of the Framingham CHD risk score by the ATP III was that it did not include diabetes but considered the presence of diabetes as the equivalent of having CHD.

The most recent adaptation of the Framingham Risk Score is a general cardiovascular risk profile that predicts risk of developing general CVD and the individual CVD components (CHD, stroke, peripheral artery disease, and heart failure; comparable to disease-specific algorithms) for use in primary care (Table 5.1) [2]. The risk factors included in the algorithm are age, TC, HDL-C, SBP, blood pressure treatment, smoking status, and diabetes status. Importantly, for the first time, a simple CVD risk score was developed for when blood measures are not available, allowing the physician to immediately assess the 10-year CVD risk of the patient by using age, body mass index (BMI), SBP, antihypertensive medication use, current smoking, and diabetes status.

A limitation to the Framingham Risk Score was that it was derived from a single community in the USA that was predominantly middle-aged and white. Others have also criticized the Framingham Risk Score because the Framingham population tended to be "high risk" to begin with, having high levels of hypercholesterolemia, dietary intake of saturated fat, smoking, and other CVD risk factors [9]. A systematic review of studies that compared predicted Framingham 10-year CHD or CVD risk scores with observed risk reported that the accuracy of the risk score varied widely between populations and that the more high-risk the population, the greater the degree of underestimation [14]. Furthermore, a recent review observed that the majority of cross-sectional and cohort studies that have used the Framingham Risk Score applied it to populations (e.g., human immunodeficiency virus (HIV) or rheumatoid arthritis) and outcomes (non-CHD events) for which the scores were not originally developed [15]. Others have reported that the Framingham Risk Score overestimate CHD risk in populations from the UK, Belfast, and France [16] as well as in African Caribbean adults [17], while underestimating risk in white European and South Asian women [17]. There is also evidence that the Framingham Risk Score may grossly underestimate CVD mortality rate in low socioeconomic populations [18]. Among different ethnic cohorts in the USA, the Framingham Risk Score performed reasonably well in black and white men and women but overestimated risk in Japanese American and Hispanic men and Native American women. However, recalibrating the scores to take into consideration the prevalence of risk factors and underlying rates of developing CHD within different populations improves the predictive

Table 5.1 Comparisons among the Framingham Risk Score for coronary heart disease (CHD) and cardiovascular disease (CVD), the Reynolds Risk Score for CVD, and the Pooled Cohort Equations

	Framingham 12-year CHD risk score (1967) [8]	Framingham 8-year CVD risk score (1976) [10]	Framingham 10-year CVD risk score (1991) [11]	Framingham 10-year CHD risk score (1998) [12]	Framingham ATP-III CHD risk score (2001) [13]	Framingham 10-year general CVD risk score (2008) [2]	Reynolds Risk Score for CVD (2007, 2008) [28, 29]	Pooled Cohort Equations 10-year atherosclerotic CVD risk score [3]
Variables	Age	Age	Age	Age	Age	Age	Age	Age
	TC	TC	TC	TC	TC	TC	TC	TC
	SBP	SBP	SBP	SBP	SBP	SBP	SBP	SBP
	Smoking	Smoking	Smoking	Smoking	Smoking	Smoking	Smoking	Smoking
	ECG-LVH	ECG-LVH	ECG-LVH					
			HDL-C	HDL-C	HDL-C	HDL-C	HDL-C	HDL-C
	Relative weight				HBP medication	HBP medication		HBP medication
						Diabetes		Diabetes
	A1C	Glucose intolerance	Diabetes	Diabetes				
							hs-CRP	
							Family history of premature MI	
							A1C (women with T2D only)	
End-point	MI, coronary insufficiency, angina pectoris, death from CHD	CHD, congestive heart failure, cerebrovascular disease, intermittent claudication	MI, CHD, death from CHD, stroke, CVD, death from CVD	Angina pectoris, MI, coronary insufficiency, CHD death	MI, CHD death	CHD, cerebrovascular events, peripheral artery disease, heart failure	MI, ischemic stroke, coronary revascularization, cardiovascular death	CHD death, nonfatal MI, fatal stroke, non-fatal stroke
Population derived	Framingham original cohort	Framingham original cohort	Framingham original and offspring cohorts	Framingham original and offspring cohorts	Modified Framingham CHD risk score	Framingham original and offspring cohorts	Women's health study and physician's health study II	ARIC study, Cardiovascular Health Study, CARDIA study Framingham original and offspring cohorts
	N=2187	N=5209	N=5573	N=5345		N=8491	N=24 558 women Age: 45+ year	N=24,626
	Age: 30–62 years	Age: 35–64 years	Age: 30–74 years	Age: 30–74 years		Age: 30–74 years	N=10 724 men Age: 50–80 years	Age: 40–79 years

ATP III Adult Treatment Program III, *TC* cardiovascular disease, *SBP* systolic blood pressure, *ECG-LVH* electrocardiogram left ventricular hypertrophy, *MI* myocardial infarction, *HDL-C* high-density lipoprotein cholesterol, *HBP* high blood pressure, *hs-CRP* high-sensitivity C-reactive protein, *A1C* hemoglobin A1c, *ARIC* Atherosclerosis risk in communities study, *CARDIA* coronary artery risk in young adults study

accuracy [19]. Therefore, when utilizing the Framingham Risk Score in populations that are not similar to the Framingham cohort, recalibration should be considered.

Despite the demonstrated ability of Framingham to predict CVD risk, some individuals who have low CVD risk will still experience a cardiac event, just as some persons with high risk will never develop CVD. This is termed residual risk and is the individual risk that is not accounted for by the risk algorithms. Residual risk exists for all algorithms and may be due to factors that are associated with CVD, but not included in the models, or they result from suboptimal assessment of predictive factors. Accordingly, some investigators have attempted to determine if the clinical utility and residual risk of the Framingham Risk Score could be improved by adding additional variables to the model. Wang et al. (2006) reported that the addition of nontraditional biomarkers, such as high-sensitivity C-reactive protein (hs-CRP), to conventional risk factors in the Framingham CHD risk scores had only small improvements for classifying risk [20]. However, another study reports that less than 50% of patients who presented with myocardial infarction (MI) would be classified as high risk and be considered for intensive lipid-lowering therapy using common CVD risk scores (Framingham, Reynolds, PROCAM, ASSIGN, QRISK, and SCORE). However, within these algorithms, Framingham tended to classify patients as higher risk than the other algorithms. The study suggests that additional measures, such as high coronary artery calcium score or carotid artery plaques, may improve discrimination and that adding these risk factors to current algorithms may improve the classification of CVD risk [21]. Others have suggested that adding carotid intima thickness, ankle brachial index, or hs-CRP to the Framingham models could potentially improve classifying CVD risk in individuals [22–24]. However, the cost-effectiveness or clinical feasibility of testing these biomarkers in practice is not known.

Another commonly cited CVD risk factor that is not currently used in the Framingham Risk Score is history of premature parental CVD, even though this variable was reported to be an independent predictor of future CVD in the Framingham Offspring Cohort [25]. Accordingly, the Update of the Canadian Cardiovascular Society for the Diagnosis and Treatment of Dyslipidemia proposed that the Framingham CVD risk score be doubled when an individual has a family history of premature CVD [26]. However, Stern et al. [27] stated that clinicians should not use this modified score as there is no hard evidence to justify including family history in the algorithm, and besides, Framingham researchers reported that inclusion of parental data in the model increases predictive accuracy only to a small extent.

Finally, lifestyle modification behaviors, particularly diet and physical activity, are also associated with CVD risk and play a large role in CVD prevention [3]. However, none of the Framingham models, or any other CVD risk equation, include diet or physical activity in their risk algorithms. This may be because information for diet and physical activity is assessed using many different methods and is often considered unreliable as it is assessed using self-reported data. Nonetheless, information about a patient's current diet and physical activity should be obtained during initial risk assessment and may be particularly important for estimating residual CVD risk.

In summary, the Framingham Heart Study has provided a wealth of knowledge about the major risk factors for CVD. Although some have challenged the clinical utility of the Framingham Risk Score in certain populations, these scores have been used in many different countries and populations to assess CVD risk and help guide treatment. Whether or not additional variables beyond the traditional risk factors could be used to better discriminate individuals at high risk of CVD is currently not known and requires further investigation.

Reynolds Risk Score

Like the Framingham Risk Score, the Reynolds Risk Score is an algorithm that predicts 10-year risk of CVD but includes hs-CRP and family history of MI in its algorithm. Dr. Paul Ridker and colleagues developed and validated the model for women in 2007 [28] and for men in 2008 [29]. Prediction algorithms were derived using data from 24,558 female health professionals in the Women's Health Study aged 45 years and older and 10,724 men from the Physicians Health Study II aged 50–80 years old. The variables used in the Reynolds Risk Score are hs-CRP, parental history of premature MI, SBP, TC, HDL-C, current smoker, and hemoglobin A1c (HbA1C; for females with diabetes only; Table 5.1).

The Reynolds Risk Score was derived using data from predominantly white adults from a high socioeconomic background. Therefore, as with the Framingham Risk Score, extrapolation to more ethnically and socioeconomically diverse populations, populations under 45 years for women, and under 50 years for men should be interpreted with caution. Another limitation is that the algorithm is based on self-report data for blood pressure in females and self-report BMI in males. Both the Framingham ATP-III CHD risk score and the Reynolds Risk Score are recommended for use by the American College of Cardiology (ACC) and the American Heart Association (AHA) and are also used as part of the national guidelines for CVD prevention in Canada. However, the few studies that have compared the Framingham and Reynolds scores often show that predicted CVD risk varies widely between the models. For example, the Reynolds Risk Score reclassified a number of adults into more appropriate risk categories and was reported to be a better predictor of CHD compared to the Framingham ATP-III model [28, 29]. However, this analysis may have been biased as it used the same population that was used to originally develop the Reynolds Risk Score. Another study reported that among a large multiethnic cohort of women, the ATP-III and Framingham CVD score overestimated risk for CHD and CVD, while the Reynolds Risk Score was better at classifying risk in black and white women [30]. Furthermore, another US study suggests that 4.7% of US women would require more intense lipid management if the Reynolds Risk Score was used instead of the Framingham Risk Score. Conversely, 10.5% of US men would require less intense lipid management if the Reynolds Risk Score was used in place of the Framingham Risk Score [31]. Thus, the relative clinical utility of Reynolds versus Framingham is unclear.

In summary, the best approach for CVD evaluation and prevention is to routinely test the patient for CVD risk factors and to use a risk score assessment. Although neither the Framingham Risk Score nor the Reynolds Risk Score are without limitation, assessing CVD risk is important to optimize preventive treatments and to guide therapy. Clearly, more research is needed to compare the clinical utility between the two risk scores.

ACC/AHA Guidelines for Assessing Cardiovascular Risk (Pooled Cohort Equations)

In 2013, the ACC and AHA provided updated guidelines for the assessment of CVD risk [3]. These guidelines include new Pooled Cohort Equations that predict 10-year atherosclerotic CVD risk in non-Hispanic black and white adults age 40–79 years with no clinical signs or symptoms of atherosclerotic CVD (Table 5.1). The new Pooled Cohort Equations were derived using cohort data from Atherosclerosis Risk in Communities (ARIC), Cardiovascular Health Study, Coronary Artery Risk Development in Young Adults (CARDIA), and Framingham original and offspring study cohorts. The sex- and race-specific risk algorithms predict 10-year risk of initial hard atherosclerotic CVD events, including nonfatal MI or CHD death and fatal and nonfatal stroke [3]. The variables used in the algorithm are the same as those used in the Framingham CVD risk models and include age, TC, HDL-C, SBP, blood pressure treatment status, diabetes, and current smoking status. The guidelines recommend initiation of statin treatment in patients with high 10-year atherosclerotic (AS) CVD risk (≥7.5%) and consideration of statin treatment in patients with intermediate risk (5–7.5%). This translates into about one in three American adults being considered for statin therapy based on these guidelines [3]. These thresholds are considerably lower than the 20% high-risk and 10–20% intermediate-risk thresholds suggested in the ATP-III guidelines [13], and thus, more adults would be considered for statin therapy if these guidelines are implemented in clinical practice.

The guidelines also assessed the clinical utility of including novel risk factors for atherosclerotic CVD risk prediction, including family history of premature CVD, hs-CRP, coronary artery calcium, ankle-brachial index, coronary intima media thickness, apolipoprotein B, albuminuria, glomerular filtration rate, and cardiorespiratory fitness. It was recommended that if a risk-based treatment decision is still uncertain after initial risk assessment, a family history of premature CVD or measurement of hs-CRP, coronary artery calcium, or ankle-brachial index may be considered and that coronary artery calcium is likely the most clinically useful novel risk factor in adults with intermediate atherosclerotic CVD risk. However, the guidelines advise against measuring coronary intima media thickness in routine clinical practice due to concerns about measurement quality. Furthermore, there was insufficient evidence to recommend for or against measuring apolipoprotein B, albuminuria, glomerular filtration rate, or cardiorespiratory fitness for atherosclerotic CVD risk assessment [3].

The Pooled Cohort Equations have a demonstrated ability to estimate risk for both fatal and nonfatal MI and stroke and the ability to provide specific risk estimates for non-Hispanic blacks. Although not yet validated, the guidelines suggest that the equation for non-Hispanic whites may be used in other ethnic groups until ethnic-specific algorithms are developed. However, the Pooled Cohort Equations may overestimate atherosclerotic CVD risk in East Asian Americans and may underestimate risk in First Nation Americans and South Asian Americans [3]. Others have also criticized the new guidelines for excluding family history of premature CVD in the models, as well as including stroke as an endpoint, because it renders the algorithms much more sensitive to age and, additionally, because only ~40% of strokes are the result of large-vessel atherosclerotic CVD [32].

Attempts to examine the validity of the Pooled Cohort Equations in other cohorts have resulted in mixed findings. One study reported that the Pooled Cohort Equations accurately predicted 5-year incident atherosclerotic CVD in non-Hispanic white and black adults from the REGARDS study [33]. Conversely, the Pooled Cohort Equations overestimated 10-year CVD risk in non-Hispanic white and black adults from the MESA study, the REGARDS study, newer follow-up data from ARIC, and the Framingham study [34]. The Pooled Cohort risk equations were also found to overestimate 10-year atherosclerotic CVD risk by 75–150% in three large-scale US cohorts that were predominately made up of low-risk white individuals [34]. Moreover, among healthy European adults in the Rotterdam Study, the Pooled Cohort Equations greatly overestimated atherosclerotic CVD risk, and substantially more men and women would have been eligible for statin initiation based on these guidelines compared to the ATP-III guidelines or the European Society of Cardiology guidelines [35]. These results question the validity of the new Pooled Cohort risk equations, particularly in populations other than non-Hispanic white and black US adults. Clearly, more studies are needed to investigate if these risk equations are valid among individuals from other ethnic groups and countries and if they truly do provide better risk discrimination compared to more established CVD risk algorithms.

Lifetime Cardiovascular Risk

Lifetime cardiovascular risk is defined as the cumulative risk of developing CVD throughout the remainder of a person's life [36]. Recently, there has been much discussion on the clinical utility of assessing lifetime CVD risk. Some argue that because short-term risk equations are strongly age-dependent, many younger individuals with adverse risk profiles who have a high long-term risk are often "overlooked" when it comes to risk discussion and therapy initiation because their short-term risk is low [37]. As well, it has been reported that only assessing risk over 5–10 years restricts our appreciation of the true importance of the modifiable factors that cause CVD and, further, that lowering cholesterol has greater benefit if done earlier in life than later [38]. Indeed, life-time risk may be a clinically useful measure in those with low short-term but high long-term risk [39].

Several studies have attempted to assess the lifetime risk of CVD. In 2006, the first lifetime risk estimates for developing CVD at age 50 were estimated using Framingham data, and it was shown that lifetime risk is highly dependent on the number of elevated risk factors [40]. For example, men and women with an optimal risk factor profile at age 50 (only 3.2 % of men and 4.5 % of women) had a relatively low lifetime CVD risk, whereas those with at least two major risk factors had lifetime risks that exceeded 50 % [40]. Similar findings were confirmed in another study that also showed that the effect of risk factor burden on lifetime CVD risk was similar in black and white adults and across different birth cohorts [41]. In 2009, a 30-year model for risk of developing hard CVD was developed using Framingham data. This analysis demonstrated that 10-year CVD risk was very low for adults in their 20s and 30s, regardless of risk factors but that those with multiple elevated risk factors had 30-year risk profiles that were up to ten times higher [42]. Finally, Wilkins et al. (2012) reported that although middle-aged adults with an optimal risk factor profile have a lower absolute risk than middle-aged adults with one elevated risk factor, they still have a high absolute lifetime CVD risk of 30–40 % [43]. This reiterates the importance of maintaining a healthy lifestyle throughout life for CVD prevention.

Thus, although there is not yet a general consensus that lifetime CVD risk should be used in clinical practice, there is evidence that many adults have a high lifetime risk of CVD, particularly young adults with adverse risk factors, males, nonwhite adults, and those with a family history of premature CVD [37]. Assessing lifetime CVD risk may be beneficial in these populations as this could initiate discussion about lifestyle modification or consideration of early pharmacologic intervention that may not be apparent if using only short-term algorithms. However, a validated method of measuring lifetime risk that is applicable for different populations has yet to be established.

Residual Cardiovascular Risk

An important yet often under acknowledged concept to consider when assessing risk for any patient is that of residual risk. Residual risk is any difference in predicted risk that is not accounted for by the risk algorithm, which is why some individuals still experience a cardiac event even if metabolic targets are met or why some individuals will not have cardiac events even though their predicted risk is high [44]. All risk algorithms have an error component as no algorithm has

a perfect model fit. For most CVD risk algorithms, the c-statistic (measure of discrimination) is usually between 0.70 and 0.80, which means that the probability that the predicted absolute risk is higher in individuals who develop CVD versus those who do not is 70–80 %, meaning that there could be inaccurate risk ranking in up to a third of individuals. This error could be related to inappropriate cutoffs used for risk factors in the algorithm, error in assessment of the risk factors, or not including all relevant risk factors in the model for that individual. For example, factors such as diet and physical activity are associated with CVD and can modify the effects of other CVD risk factors, yet these variables are not included in CVD risk algorithms. Further, there is a host of measures for glucose control and metabolism or inflammation that could be included in algorithms, but due to cost and ease of assessment as opposed to biological relevance, the simpler measures are most often included.

Another possible reason for residual risk is that not all relevant risk factors may be targeted with statin therapy that specifically lowers LDL-C. Thus, atherogenic dyslipidemia, which is an imbalance of high triglycerides and low HDL-C, would not be improved by statin therapy and has been identified as a likely contributor to lipid-related residual cardiovascular risk even when LDL levels are normal [4]. Some clinical trials have shown that combining a statin with a fibrate, niacin, omega-3 fatty acid, or ezetimibe to lower triglyceride levels and increase HDL-C may better help to alleviate the burden of atherogenic dyslipidemia. However, there is little evidence for the effects of these agents on cardiovascular outcomes, and therefore large cardiovascular outcome trials are needed [5]. On the other hand, lifestyle modifications, including body weight reduction, healthy diet, and increased physical activity, are all associated with decreased triglycerides and increased HDL-C, and are important factors for decreasing residual cardiovascular risk [45]. However, results from the Look AHEAD trial recently showed that intensive lifestyle modification was not enough to decrease cardiovascular deaths or events in adults with T2D compared to a control group despite significant improvements in metabolic risk factors [46]. Therefore, lifestyle modification is important for improving the metabolic profiles of individuals at risk for CVD, but pharmacotherapy will likely also be necessary for preventing CVD deaths and events. Large cardiovascular outcome trials with novel lipid therapies for reducing atherogenic dyslipidemia and improving residual cardiovascular risk are eagerly awaited.

Metabolic Syndrome

MetS, sometimes referred to as syndrome X, insulin resistance syndrome, cardiometabolic syndrome, or dysmetabolic syndrome, is generally defined as a clustering of cardiometabolic factors [47]. This term first appeared in PubMed in 1952, with only sporadic reports until the Banting Lecture in 1988 when Dr. Gerald Reaven described "Syndrome X" [48]. In 2001, the National Cholesterol Education Program introduced the first diagnostic criteria for MetS, and research on this topic increased exponentially with now over 31,000 publications.

Despite the general consensus that MetS is a clustering of elevated fasting blood glucose and cardiovascular risk factors, there is debate as to which risk factors should be included in the diagnostic criteria, the thresholds for each criterion, and whether or not certain factors are central to the underlying pathology. Most commonly, increased waist circumference (WC), insulin resistance, dyslipidemia, and hypertension are included in the diagnostic criteria, with factors such as inflammation, kidney dysfunction [49], liver dysfunction, and ectopic fat deposition being suggested less frequently as features [50]. For example, both the World Health Organization (WHO) and the European Group for the Study of Insulin Resistance requires the presence of insulin resistance, but not necessarily obesity, to have the diagnosis of MetS [51, 52], while the International Diabetes Federation (IDF) requires the presence of abdominal obesity but not necessarily insulin resistance (Table 5.2) [53]. Of note, most

definitions include WC as a component of the syndrome, but not BMI, due to excess abdominal fat being more highly associated with other components of MetS and its greater importance in the etiology of the syndrome [54]. The numerous differing diagnostic criteria that include different factors and use various thresholds created confusion in the clinical community as to what MetS is and made research using the different criteria more difficult to compare. Differences in the factors and the thresholds used can alter the prevalence of MetS to range from 19 to 39 % [55] and how strongly it is associated with morbidity and mortality [56, 57]. Thus, in 2009, there was a new harmonized diagnostic criteria that was jointly published by the International Diabetes Federation Task Force on Epidemiology and Prevention; National Heart, Lung, and Blood Institute; American Heart Association; World Heart Federation; International Atherosclerosis Society; and International Association for the Study of Obesity. This criteria does not require the presence of any one component but, similar to past criteria, requires three of five of the factors for the diagnosis of MetS [47] (Table 5.2).

In youth and adolescents, the optimal diagnostic criteria for MetS are even less clear. Over the course of pubertal development, there are fluctuations in the metabolic profile that are not well understood. Clear thresholds for delineating

Table 5.2 Criteria for the metabolic syndrome according to the International Diabetes Federation (IDF), World Health Organization (WHO), European Group for the Study of Insulin Resistance (EGIR), National Cholesterol Education Program (NCEP), and the harmonized models

	IDF [53]	WHO [49]	EGIR [52]	NCEP [54]	Harmonized [47]
Required criteria	Central obesity or BMI >30 kg/m^2	IFG, IGT, or T2D/insulin resistance	Insulin resistance	None	None
Number of additional criteria	Any two of the following:	Two or more of the following:	Two or more of the following:	At least three of the following:	At least three of the following:
Central obesity	Ethnicity-specific	WHR >0.90 (males), WHR >0.85 (females), and/or BMI >30 kg/m^2	WC ≥ 94 cm (males) and WC ≥ 80 cm (females)	WC ≥ 102 cm (males) and WC ≥ 88 cm (females)	High WC (population- and country-specific)
Triglycerides	≥ 1.7 mM or drug treatment	>1.7 mM	>2.0 mM or drug treatment	≥ 1.7 mM or drug treatment	≥ 1.7 mM or drug treatment
HDL-C	Males <1.03 mM, females <1.29 mM, or drug treatment	<0.9 mM (males) and <1.0 mM (females)	<1.0 mM or drug treatment	<1.03 mM (males), <1.3 mM (females), or drug treatment	<1.0 mM (males), <1.3 mM (females), or drug treatment
Blood pressure	SBP ≥ 130 mm Hg or DBP ≥ 85 mm Hg or drug treatment	$\geq 140/90$ mm Hg	$\geq 140/90$ mm Hg or drug treatment	SBP ≥ 130 mm Hg or DBP ≥ 85 mmHg or drug treatment	SBP ≥ 130 mm Hg or DBP ≥ 85 mm Hg or drug treatment
Fasting plasma glucose	5.6 mM or T2D	IFG, IGT, or T2D: FGlu >6.1 mM or OGTT ≥ 7.8 mM	≥ 6.1 mM (but nondiabetic)	≥ 6.1 mM or drug treatment	≥ 6.1 mM or drug treatment
Insulin resistance	–	As measured by hyperinsulinemic euglycemic clamp	Top 25 % of the fasting insulin values among nondiabetic individuals	–	–
Microalbuminuria	–	Excretion rate ≥ 20 μg/min or albumin:creatinine ratio ≥ 30 mg/g	–	–	–

HDL-C high-density lipoprotein cholesterol, *SBP* systolic blood pressure, *DBP* diastolic blood pressure, *IGT* impaired glucose tolerance, *IFG* impaired fasting glucose, *WHR* waist to hip ratio, *OGTT* oral glucose tolerance test, *T2D* type-2 diabetes, *WC* waist circumference, *BMI* body mass index

healthy versus not healthy are not widely accepted. Consequently, it is not surprising that there are a variety of MetS criteria that have been developed using a mix of mainly age and sex percentiles or adult thresholds. These variations have resulted in a MetS prevalence that ranges between 6 and 39% [58]. Thus, as with adults, this has led some to question the clinical usefulness of MetS [59].

In addition to the problematic diagnosis of MetS, there is also a debate as to the central importance of insulin sensitivity versus obesity as reflected by the disparate diagnostic criteria by WHO and IDF that require the presence of one versus the other. In order for MetS to be a "syndrome," there must be an underlying pathology or cause [60]. In his Banting Lecture in 1988 [48], Reaven proposed that insulin resistance was central to the development of these cardiometabolic factors but did not include obesity as one of the factors in the syndrome. Interestingly, he did suggest that treatment for MetS should be weight maintenance (or weight loss) and physical activity [48]. To date, there have been several examinations into the relative importance of insulin resistance and obesity with varying conclusions. To date, research has demonstrated that most, but not all, individuals diagnosed with ATP III [61] or IDF [62] are insulin resistant. Similarly, most, but not all, individuals with MetS are obese [63, 64]. This may be due to suboptimal diagnostic criteria for MetS, suboptimal assessment of insulin resistance or obesity, or may reflect that MetS is not truly a syndrome but more simply an array of risk factors or conditions without clear relationships.

In addition, several investigations on the association between MetS and mortality risk place doubt on whether MetS is in fact a "syndrome" with a singular pathology and question whether MetS can uniquely identify risk beyond its individual factors [65]. MetS by most criteria is the compilation of 16 different metabolic factor combinations [63]. These combinations differ in their prevalence by age and sex and also in how they relate with mortality risk [63, 66]. Furthermore, some reports suggest that WC alone may be a better indicator of insulin resistance in young black South African women than ATP III MetS criteria [67]. Additionally, several reports indicate that MetS is much more strongly related to T2D risk than to CVD [68], largely owing to three of five factors (glucose, obesity, and triglycerides) being more predictive of T2D risk [69]. In fact, some studies demonstrate that certain MetS criteria are not predictive of all-cause or CVD morality risk [70]. Moreover, some studies indicate that MetS does not perform as well as traditionally used CVD risk algorithms, such as Framingham [71, 72]. This difference can be attributed to several mathematical as well as biological factors. Mathematically, the reduction of the five MetS criteria to a dichotomy reduces the information available and can only be used to provide relative risk estimates, as opposed to the Framingham algorithm that provides an absolute risk for CVD. From a biological standpoint, MetS does not consider clearly established non-metabolic CVD risk factors, such as age and smoking status, explaining why the relative risk estimates are inferior to Framingham. For these reasons, the clinical utility of MetS has been questioned [65] and may be why MetS is rarely diagnosed by clinicians [73].

Dysmetabolic syndrome is officially recognized as a medical diagnosis and is coded as ICD-9-CM 277.7. This code was replaced with ICD-10-CM E88.81 (metabolic syndrome) in October 2015. This is a billable medical code that can be used to specify a diagnosis on a reimbursement claim, formalizing the clinical diagnosis of this syndrome. However, Ford (2005) reported that 2 years after the release of the ICD-9-CM 277.7 code, very few patients had MetS listed as a diagnosis on medical records, suggesting that MetS is significantly underdiagnosed in patients [73]. The reasons for this are uncertain but may be related to the lack of pharmacological agents specifically for MetS.

Currently, the main lifestyle treatment goal of weight management and increasing physical activity for MetS has not changed from Dr. Reaven's Banting Lecture in 1988 [54]. Dietary approaches are also suggested for many MetS factors. However, the factors differ in the types of therapeutic dietary approaches used, though sharing some similar approaches. For example, the Dietary Approaches to Stop Hypertension (DASH) recommends restricting sodium intake as an important dietary intervention for hypertension [74], but less important for weight, glucose, or lipid management. Dietary management for T2D also has recommendations for sodium intake but will focus more on caloric reduction and glycemic index [75]. Similarly, pharmacological interventions are generally not tailored directly for MetS due to the heterogeneous presentation of risk factors. Thus, pharmacological interventions are generally targeted for each specific risk factor as opposed to "metabolic syndrome" as a whole. However, in understanding how MetS factors are interrelated in the same metabolic pathways, Ye et al. [76] have been able to design a unique pharmacotherapy that is able to simultaneously improve hypertension, hyperglycemia, obesity, and dyslipidemia in mice. Briefly, the antihypertensive alpha-2 adrenergic receptor agonist guanabenz activates a synthetic signal cascade that influences secretion of glucagon-peptide 1 (GLP-1) and leptin; these coordinated events attenuate blood pressure, blood glucose, blood lipids as well as reduced appetite and body weight [76].

Despite the limitations in comprehensively assessing, diagnosing, and treating MetS, the research on MetS has highlighted how T2D and CVD risk factors tend to cluster together, prompting assessment of other cardiometabolic risk factors when one is detected [77]. Nevertheless, although MetS is frequently the topic of research investigations, there is still debate on whether MetS can truly be called a "syndrome." In conjunction with the rare clinical diagnosis and the lack of pharmacological options, the clinical relevance of MetS has yet to be established.

Edmonton Obesity Staging System

The Edmonton Obesity Staging System (EOSS) is a model developed by Dr. Arya Sharma and Dr. Robert Kushner in 2009 that evaluates obesity-related health risk and recommends treatment according to the severity of risk [78]. The stages range from 0 to 4, indicating no obesity-related risk factors to severe end-stage disease. Unlike many of the other composite score models, EOSS considers not only metabolic risk factors (e.g., blood pressure) but also physical symptoms (e.g., aches and pains), psychopathology (e.g., depression), and functional ability and well-being in order to assess the overall health of the individual (Table 5.3).

The main reason why EOSS was developed was to individualize assessments since two people with similar levels of body fatness can have vastly different states of health. It was also proposed that a staging system would allow for the prioritization of treatment to patients who would most benefit from aggressive and resource-intensive weight management treatment. According to the current guidelines for weight management, all patients with obesity, regardless of their health risk profile, should be counseled to lose weight [79]. However, there exists a subgroup of obese individuals, commonly referred to as the "metabolically healthy obese," who are free from metabolic complications and may represent 6–32% of the obese population [80, 81]. There is also evidence that weight loss in the metabolically healthy obese may not improve cardiometabolic risk factors [82] and may even be detrimental to insulin sensitivity [83]. Therefore, a model such as the EOSS would allow proper counseling to

Table 5.3 Comparisons between the Cardiometabolic Disease Staging System and the Edmonton Obesity Staging System

	CDMS [88]	EOSS [78]	
	Description/criteria	Description/criteria	Management
Stage 0	Metabolically healthy: no risk factors	No apparent obesity-related risk factors, including physical symptoms, psychopathology, functional limitations, or impairments in well-being	Identification of factors contributing to increased body weight. Provide counseling to prevent further weight gain through lifestyle measures, such as healthy diet and physical activity
Stage 1	One or two of the following: WC $\geq$ 112 cm (males) or $\geq$ 88 cm (females) SBP $\geq$ 130 mm Hg or DBP $\geq$ 85 mm Hg or on antihypertensive medication HDL-C < 1.0 mM (males) or < 1.3 mM (females) or on lipid medication TG $\geq$ 1.7 mM or on lipid medication	Presence of obesity-related subclinical risk factors, mild physical symptoms, psychopathology, functional limitations, and/or impairment of well-being	Investigation for non-weight-related contributors to risk factors. Provide counseling for more intense lifestyle interventions, including diet and exercise to prevent further weight gain. Continuously monitor risk factors and health status
Stage 2	Metabolic syndrome or prediabetes: Only one of the following: Metabolic syndrome (>3): high WC high blood pressure low HDL-C high triglycerides IFG (fasting glucose $\geq$ 5.6 mM) IGT (2-h glucose $\geq$ 7.8 mM)	Presence of established obesity-related chronic disease and moderate limitations in activities of daily living and/or well-being	Initiation of obesity treatments including considerations of all behavioral, pharmacological, and surgical treatment options. Close monitoring and management of comorbidities as indicated
Stage 3	Metabolic syndrome + prediabetes: Any two of the following: Metabolic syndrome IFG IGT	Established end-organ damage such as myocardial infarction, heart failure, diabetic complications, incapacitating osteoarthritis, significant psychopathology, significant functional limitations, and/or impairment of well-being	More intensive obesity treatment including consideration of all behavioral, pharmacological, and surgical treatment options. Aggressive management of comorbidities as indicated
Stage 4	Presence of T2D and/or CVD: T2D: Glucose $\geq$ 7.0 mM or OGTT $\geq$ 11.0 mM or medication active CVD (angina pectoris, or status post a CVD event such as acute coronary artery syndrome, stent replacement, coronary artery bypass, thrombotic stroke, nontraumatic amputation due to peripheral vascular disease)	Severe (potentially end-stage) disabilities from obesity-related chronic diseases, including severe disabling psychopathology, functional limitations, and/or impairment of well-being	Aggressive obesity management as deemed feasible. Palliative measures including pain management, occupational therapy and psychosocial support

CDMS Cardiometabolic Disease Staging System, *CVD* cardiovascular disease, *DBP* diastolic blood pressure, *EOSS* Edmonton Obesity Staging System, *HDL-C* high-density lipoprotein cholesterol, *IFG* impaired fasting glucose, *IGT* impaired glucose tolerance, *OGTT* oral glucose tolerance test, *T2D* type-2 diabetes, *TG* triglyceride, *WC* waist circumference

these patients and more resource-intensive treatment to those who would benefit most from weight loss.

As EOSS is a relatively new model, few studies have investigated its clinical utility. The predictive ability of EOSS for mortality risk was investigated using data from the Aerobics Center Longitudinal Study. Compared to normal-weight adults, obese individuals in EOSS stage 0/1 had a similar all-cause mortality risk and a lower CVD and CHD mortality risk, whereas individuals in stage 2 or 3 had higher all-cause, CVD, and CHD mortality risks [84]. Similarly, using data from the National Health and Nutrition Examination Survey, adults in EOSS stage 2 or 3 were at higher mortality risk than EOSS stage 0 or 1, independent of BMI, presence of MetS, hypertriglyceridemia, and WC [85]. These results provide further support that the EOSS may be a more relevant measure of assessing obesity-related health risk, compared to traditional anthropometric measures alone, and may be more useful in determining a proper prognosis and guiding treatment [85].

An advantage of using EOSS to guide weight management is that it takes into consideration multiple aspects of health and not just body weight. A limitation to using EOSS is that not all of the risk factors may be directly caused by obesity (e.g., depression), which may make it difficult to determine which stage a patient should be in. As well, some of the risk factors may be subjective and diagnosis may differ depending on the clinician (e.g., physical functioning) or patient demographic (e.g., age, sex, or ethnicity). Furthermore, this staging system has yet to be validated in clinical practice or be investigated in the context of specificity, sensitivity, and reliability [78]. However, given that the widely used BMI tends to be a poor indicator of health status at the individual level, and that not all obese people present with comorbidities, the use of EOSS may prove to be a valuable clinical tool for the obese population.

Cardiometabolic Disease Staging System

Cardiometabolic risk is a ubiquitous term generally used to describe T2D and CVD risk factors. The term "cardiometabolic risk" was first used as a keyword in a single publication in PubMed in 1999 [86] and did not appear again until 2005. Since then, the use of the term "cardiometabolic risk" has increased exponentially and is now a keyword for over 1800 publications. In many of these publications, cardiometabolic risk is defined using MetS diagnostic criteria. However, unlike MetS, which is a dichotomous outcome, cardiometabolic risk is a spectrum of states that span from optimal health to prediabetes to MetS to overt T2D and CVD. The Cardiometabolic Disease Staging System (CMDS) was published by Dr. Timothy Garvey and colleagues in 2014 and is the first defined cardiometabolic risk algorithm [87]. CMDS grades risk on a scale from 0 to 4 (Table 5.3), ranging from metabolically healthy to T2D and/or CVD. As with EOSS,

CMDS is meant to help physicians objectively and systematically evaluate the severity of risk and balance the benefits versus the risks in deciding treatment interventions.

CMDS has been shown to predict incident 10-year T2D risk using data from CARDIA and CVD and all-cause mortality risk using data from NHANES III [88]. Further, they demonstrate that CMDS is able to predict risk independent of BMI. However, this is the only report to date using this algorithm, and it is unclear how this staging system performs in relationship to other algorithms.

CMDS is similar to EOSS [78] in its aim in developing a systematic treatment algorithm for many of the same chronic conditions but can be applied in all populations as opposed to only overweight and obese. Because the treatment therapy for many of the chronic conditions listed under CMDS and EOSS are the same, the patient will still likely receive a similar message in terms of increasing physical activity, improving dietary practices, and receiving consideration for pharmacological intervention. However, the stage at which intervention occurs, and whether or not weight loss is prescribed, may differ between the two models.

As with the various MetS criteria, there are differences in the centrality of the role of obesity versus insulin resistance in the etiology of cardiometabolic risk. The CMDS places insulin resistance at the center of the etiology of risk and places a secondary emphasis on obesity, whereas EOSS places obesity more centrally in the etiology of cardiometabolic, psychological, and physical impairments. These differences in the etiology can translate into differences in the suggested treatment decision-making strategy and specifically whether or not weight loss would be prescribed. Interestingly, CMDS stages 1, 2, and 3 would all fall under EOSS stage 1. Under EOSS stage 1, the physician is prompted to investigate other non-weight-related factors contributing to the patient's subclinically elevated risk profile, including the prescription of more intense lifestyle interventions to prevent further weight gain. What is currently unclear is whether the same individual under CMDS stage 1, 2, or 3 would be suggested to lose weight as opposed to prevent further weight gain and at what stage that distinction would occur, if at all.

Both EOSS and the CMDS are relatively new models that have yet to be validated. However, given the ever-increasing prevalence of obesity and cardiometabolic disease, the clinical utility of using either of these staging systems to assess and guide treatment seems promising and offers a more comprehensive treatment guide than body weight alone.

Patient Communication

Risk communication is defined as an open two-way exchange of information and opinion about risk, which leads to better understanding and decisions about clinical management [89]. Despite guidelines advocating absolute CVD risk assessment, some have expressed concerns that it is an unfamiliar concept to most people, that the equations are abstract constructs derived from mathematical equations, and that informing someone of their absolute risk is not very useful unless they are informed of how their risk would change if they improved their risk factors [90]. Evidence suggests that presenting risk in multiple ways is beneficial for patient understanding. Thus, presenting natural frequencies instead of relative risks [91] and using visual aids, such as graphs and pictures, may help to improve patient cognition of risk [92]. Recently, the "Your Heart Forecast" was developed as a way to convey to a patient through a series of graphs their 5-year CVD risk based on Framingham models, their 5-year CVD risk relative to a person of the same age with an optimal risk factor profile, their "cardiovascular age," their short-term risk over time, predicted age of drug initiation, and what their risk would be if they improved on their current risk factors [90]. A method such as this has the potential to convey meaningful information to a patient that would likely be more useful than simply informing them of their absolute short-term risk [93].

It is also important to acknowledge that terms that are often associated with risk discussions, such as" low-risk,", "high-risk," "likely," or "rare," are very subjective and can be interpreted in different ways depending on the patients' knowledge and past experiences [94]. Furthermore, there is evidence that both physicians and patients may struggle with interpreting statistical information, which, when poorly presented, can lead to inaccurate communication of risks [95]. Therefore, simplifying statistical information may also be helpful. For example, telling a patient that they have a 10% risk of developing CVD within the next 10 years may be less intuitive than telling them that if there were 100 patients just like them, 10 would develop CVD over the next 10 years. Furthermore, changing the population that they are being compared to will also influence their relative risk score. So, the same individual with a 10% 10-year risk may have a three-fold higher risk compared to an individual with an optimal risk factor profile. Thus, the reference population and the messaging used can have a large impact on patient understanding and interpretation of risk.

There is also evidence that general practitioners tailor the approach of risk communication depending on their perception of patient risk, motivation, and anxiety. For example, positive strategies that focus on achievable changes have been used when patients are at low risk and motivated to change lifestyle habits, whereas scare tactics have been used for high-risk patients or those who are dismissive about their health or unwilling to change their lifestyle habits [96]. As well, some practitioners may choose to mention CVD risk but not make it the main focus of a patient visit, particularly when patients are very resistant to discuss their CVD risk or when they have more important acute health issues to discuss [96].

With respect to obesity, it is important to acknowledge that body weight is a sensitive topic for most patients, with any insinuations of weight bias or weight stigma often affecting attempts at weight loss. Simply telling a patient to "eat less and move more" is far too simplistic of an approach and can lead to feelings of frustration for the patient. If the patient has obesity-related morbidities, the patient's readiness to change should be assessed and any barriers to weight loss should be addressed. The patient should be made aware of the increased risk of disease associated with obesity, such as CVD, T2D, and certain cancers, and the potential health benefits of losing 5–10% of body weight.

Thus, risk communication is not a simple "one size fits all" approach. A patient's risk should be presented in multiple ways that are simple and easy to understand. Health professionals may consider tailoring their risk communication approach based on the patient's attitudes towards their current health and motivations about changing lifestyle factors or beginning pharmacotherapy. It is important to consider that risk scores were designed for populations, not individuals, and therefore when considering a person's absolute risk, physician's discretion is critically needed [34]. Further, although risk estimates are intended to guide treatment, no risk score is perfect, and the patient should be informed of the residual cardiovascular risk that may persist even if metabolic goals are met and also that lifestyle modification is crucial for reducing residual risk and preventing CVD.

Conclusion

In conclusion, composite risk models advocate assessing health risk in order to prevent disease and to guide treatment. When selecting a composite risk model, it is important to be aware of the characteristics of the population and the specific outcomes the model was developed for, and to potentially recalibrate the model to improve applicability. Some models, such as the Framingham Risk Score and MetS, are continuously revised over time to reflect current evidence of relevant risk factors. Conversely, because many of the currently available risk scores are relatively new, there has been a paucity of research that has directly compared similar risk models or validated them in different populations, making the clinical utility of such models often difficult to determine. Although health agencies recommend that the intensity of treatment be based on initial risk assessment, more research that evaluates how risk assessment actually affects primary prevention or health outcomes is needed. Finally, risk assessment is only valuable if the patient understands their risk and what they need to do to improve their health. Patients should be made aware of the residual CVD risk that may persist even if they achieve treatment targets. More patient education on the benefits of lifestyle modification for reducing this risk is also needed. Thus, optimal risk communication between health care professionals and patients is vital for improving patient care.

References

1. Blaum CS, Xue QL, Michelon E, Semba RD, Fried LP. The association between obesity and the frailty syndrome in older women: the Women's Health and Aging Studies. J Am Geriatr Soc. 2005;53(6):927–34.
2. D'Agostino RB, Vasan RS, Pencina MJ, et al. General cardiovascular risk profile for use in primary care: the Framingham Heart Study. Circulation. 2008;117(6):743–53.
3. Goff DC, Lloyd-Jones DM, Bennett G, et al. 2013 ACC/AHA guideline on the assessment of cardiovascular risk: a Report of the American College of Cardiology/American Heart Association Task Force on Practice Guidelines. J Am Coll Cardiol. 2014;63(25 Pt B):2935–59.
4. Fruchart J-C, Sacks FM, Hermans MP, et al. The residual risk reduction initiative: a call to action to reduce residual vascular risk in dyslipidaemic patient. Diab Vasc Dis Res. 2008;5(4):319–35.
5. Fruchart J-C, Davignon J, Hermans MP, et al. Residual macrovascular risk in 2013: what have we learned? Cardiovasc Diabetol. 2014;13:26.
6. Dawber TR, Meadors GF, Moore FE. Epidemiological approaches to heart disease: the Framingham Heart Study. Am J Public Health Nations Health. 1951;41:279–86.
7. Bitton A, Gaziano T. The Framingham Heart Study's impact on global risk assessment. Prog Cardiovasc Dis. 2010;53(1):68–78.
8. Truett J, Cornfield J, Kannel W. A multivariate analysis of the risk of coronary heart disease in Framingham. J Chron Dis. 1967;20:511–24.
9. Bitton A, Gaziano T. The Framingham Heart Study's impact on global risk assessment. Prog Cardiovasc Dis. 2010;53(1):68–78.
10. Kannel B, McGee D, Gordon T. A general cardiovascular risk profile: the Framingham Study. Am J Cardiol. 1976;38:46–51.
11. Anderson KM, Wilson PW, Odell PM, Kannel WB. An updated coronary risk profile. A statement for health professionals. Circulation. 1991;83:356–62.
12. Wilson PWF, D'Agostino RB, Levy D, Belanger AM, Silbershatz H, Kannel WB. Prediction of coronary heart disease using risk factor categories. Circulation. 1998;97:1837–47.
13. Expert Panel on Detection, Evaluation and T of HBC in A. Executive summary of the third report of the National Cholesterol Education Program (NCEP) expert panel on detection, evaluation, and treatment of high blood cholesterol in adults (Adult Treatment Panel III). JAMA. 2001;285(19):2486–97.
14. Brindle P, Beswick A, Fahey T, Ebrahim S. Accuracy and impact of risk assessment in the primary prevention of cardiovascular disease: a systematic review. Heart. 2006;92(12):1752–9.
15. Tzoulaki I, Seretis A, Ntzani EE, Ioannidis JPA. Mapping the expanded often inappropriate use of the Framingham Risk Score in the medical literature. J Clin Epidemiol. 2014;67:571–7.
16. Empana J. Are the Framingham and PROCAM coronary heart disease risk functions applicable to different European populations? The PRIME Study. Eur Hear J. 2003;24:1903–11.
17. Tillin T, Hughes AD, Whincup P, et al. Ethnicity and prediction of cardiovascular disease: performance of QRISK2 and Framingham scores in a U.K. tri-ethnic prospective cohort study (SABRE–Southall And Brent REvisited). Heart. 2014;100:60–7.
18. Brindle PM, McConnachie A, Upton MN, Hart CL, Davey Smith G, Watt GCM. The accuracy of the Framingham risk-score in different socioeconomic groups: a prospective study. Br J Gen Pract. 2005;55:838–45.
19. D'Agostino RB, Grundy SM, Sullivan LM, Wilson P. Validation of the Framingham coronary heart disease prediction scores. JAMA. 2001;286(2):180–7.
20. Wang TJ, Gona P, Larson MG, et al. Multiple biomarkers for the prediction of first major cardiovascular events and death. N Engl J Med. 2006;355:2631–9.
21. Sposito AC, Alvarenga BF, Alexandre AS, et al. Most of the patients presenting myocardial infarction would not be eligible for intensive lipid-lowering based on clinical algorithms or plasma C-reactive protein. Atherosclerosis. 2011;214(1):148–50.
22. Pen A, Yam Y, Chen L, Dennie C, McPherson R, Chow BJW. Discordance between Framingham Risk Score and atherosclerotic plaque burden. Eur Heart J. 2013;34:1075–82.
23. Ferket BS, van Kempen BJH, Hunink MGM, et al. Predictive value of updating Framingham risk scores with novel risk markers in the U.S. general population. PLoS ONE. 2014;9(2):e88312.
24. Ridker PM, Cook N. Clinical usefulness of very high and very low levels of C-reactive protein across the full range of Framingham Risk Scores. Circulation. 2004;109(16):1955–9.
25. Lloyd-Jones D, Nam B-J, D'Agostino R, et al. Parental cardiovascular disease as a risk factor for cardiovascular disease in middle-aged adults: a prospective study of parents and offspring. JAMA. 2004;291(18):2204–11.
26. Anderson TJ, Grégoire J, Hegele R, et al. 2012 update of the Canadian Cardiovascular Society guidelines for the diagnosis and treatment of dyslipidemia for the prevention of cardiovascular disease in the adult. Can J Cardiol. 2013;29:151–67.
27. Stern RH. Problems with modified Framingham Risk Score. Can J Cardiol. 2014;30:248.e3.
28. Ridker P, Buring JE, Rifai N, Cook NR. Development and validation of improved algorithms for the assessment of global cardiovascular risk in women: the Reynolds risk score. JAMA. 2007;297(6):611–20.
29. Ridker PM, Paynter NP, Rifai N, Gaziano JM, Cook NR. C-reactive protein and parental history improve global cardiovascular risk prediction: the Reynolds Risk Score for men. Circulation. 2008;118:2243–51.
30. Cook NR, Paynter NP, Eaton CB, et al. Comparison of the Framingham and Reynolds risk scores for global cardiovascular risk prediction in the Multiethnic Women's Health Initiative. Circulation. 2012;125(14):1748–56.
31. Tattersall MC, Gangnon RE, Karmali KN, Keevil JG. Women up, men down: the clinical impact of replacing the Framingham Risk Score with the Reynolds Risk Score in the United States population. PLoS ONE. 2012;7(9):e44347.
32. Amin NP, Martin SS, Blaha MJ, Nasir K, Blumenthal RS, Michos ED. Headed in the right direction but at risk for miscalculation: a critical appraisal of the 2013 ACC/AHA risk assessment guidelines. J Am Coll Cardiol. 2014;63(25 Pt A):2789–94.
33. Muntner P, Colantonio LD, Cushman M, et al. Validation of the atherosclerotic cardiovascular disease Pooled Cohort risk equations. JAMA. 2014;311(14):1406–15.
34. Ridker PM, Cook NR. Statins: new American guidelines for prevention of cardiovascular disease. The Lancet. 2013;382(9907):1762–5.
35. Kavousi M, Leening MJG, Nanchen D, et al. Comparison of application of the ACC/AHA guidelines, Adult Treatment Panel III guidelines, and European Society of Cardiology guidelines for cardiovascular disease prevention in a European cohort. JAMA. 2014;311(14):1416–23.
36. Lloyd-Jones D, Larson M, Beiser A, Levy D. Lifetime risk of developing coronary heart disease. The Lancet. 1999;353:89–92.
37. Hippisley-cox J, Coupland C, Robson J, Brindle P. Derivation, validation, and evaluation of a new QRISK model to estimate lifetime risk of cardiovascular disease: cohort study using QResearch database. BMJ. 2010;341:c6624.

38. Sniderman AD, Furberg CD. Age as a modifiable risk factor for cardiovascular disease. The Lancet. 2008;371:1547–9.
39. Berry JD, Liu K, Folsom AR, et al. Prevalence and progression of subclinical atherosclerosis in younger adults with low short-term but high lifetime estimated risk for cardiovascular disease: the CARDIA and MESA studies. Circulation. 2009;119(3):382–9.
40. Lloyd-Jones DM, Leip EP, Larson MG, et al. Prediction of lifetime risk for cardiovascular disease by risk factor burden at 50 years of age. Circulation. 2006;113(6):791–8.
41. Berry J, Dyer A, Cai X, et al. Lifetime risks of cardiovascular disease. N Engl J Med. 2012;366(4):321–9.
42. Pencina MJ, D'Agostino RB, Larson MG, Massaro JM, Vasan RS. Predicting the 30-year risk of cardiovascular disease: the framingham heart study. Circulation. 2009;119:3078–84.
43. Wilkins JT, Ning H, Berry J, Zhao L, Dyer AR, Lloyd-jones DM. Lifetime risk and years lived free of total cardiovascular disease. JAMA. 2014;308(17):1795–801.
44. Libby P. The forgotten majority: unfinished business in cardiovascular risk reduction. J Am Coll Cardiol. 2005;46(7):1225–8.
45. Sampson U, Fazio S, Linton M. Residual cardiovascular risk despite optimal LDL cholesterol reduction with statins: the evidence, etiology, and therapeutic challenges. Curr Atheroscler Rep. 2012;14(1):1–10.
46. Wing RR, Bolin P, Brancati FL, et al. Cardiovascular effects of intensive lifestyle intervention in type 2 diabetes. N Engl J Med. 2013;369(2):145–54.
47. Alberti KGMM, Eckel RH, Grundy SM, et al. Harmonizing the metabolic syndrome: a joint interim statement of the International Diabetes Federation Task Force on Epidemiology and Prevention; National Heart, Lung, and Blood Institute; American Heart Association; World Heart Federation; International. Circulation. 2009;120(16):1640–5.
48. Reaven G. Banting lecture 1988. Role of insulin resistance in human disease. Diabetes. 1988;37:1595–607.
49. Alberti KG, Zimmet PZ. Definition, diagnosis and classification of diabetes mellitus and its complications. Part 1: diagnosis and classification of diabetes mellitus provisional report of a WHO consultation. Diabet Med. 1998;15:5395–53.
50. Després J-P. Is visceral obesity the cause of the metabolic syndrome? Ann Med. 2006;38(1):52–63.
51. Organization WH. Definition, diagnosis, and classification of diabetes mellitus and its complications: report of a WHO consultation. Part 1: diagnosis and classification of diabetes mellitus. 1999.
52. Balkau B, Charles M. Comment on the provisional report from the WHO. Diabet Med. 1999;16:442–3.
53. Zimmet P, Alberti G, Shaw J. A new IDF worldwide definition of the metabolic syndrome: the rationale and the results. Diabetes Voice. 2005;50(3):31–3.
54. Grundy SM, Cleeman JI, Daniels SR, et al. Diagnosis and management of the metabolic syndrome: an American Heart Association/National Heart, Lung, and Blood Institute Scientific Statement. Circulation. 2005;112(17):2735–52.
55. Cheung BMY, Ong KL, Man YB, Wong LYF, Lau C-P, Lam KSL. Prevalence of the metabolic syndrome in the United States National Health and Nutrition Examination Survey 1999–2002 according to different defining criteria. J Clin Hypertens. 2006;8:562–70.
56. Lakka H-M, Laaksonen DE, Lakka T, et al. The metabolic syndrome and total and cardiovascular disease mortality in middle-aged men. JAMA. 2002;288(21):2709–16.
57. McNeill AM, Rosamond WD, Girman CJ, et al. The metabolic syndrome and 11-year risk of incident cardiovascular disease in the atherosclerosis risk in communities study. Diabetes Care. 2005;28(2):385–90.
58. Marcovecchio ML, Chiarelli F. Metabolic syndrome in youth: chimera or useful concept? Curr Diab Rep. 2013;13:56–62.
59. Sabin M, Magnussen CG, Juonala M, Cowley M, Shield JPH. The role of pharmacotherapy in the prevention and treatment of paedi-
atric metabolic syndrome–Implications for long-term health: part of a series on Pediatric Pharmacology, guest edited by Gianvincenzo Zuccotti, Emilio Clementi, and Massimo Molteni. Pharm Res. 2012;65:397–401.
60. Shahar E. Metabolic syndrome? A critical look from the viewpoints of causal diagrams and statistics. J Cardiovasc Med. 2010;11(10):772–9.
61. Carr DB, Utzschneider KM, Hull RL, et al. Intra-abdominal fat is a major determinant of the National Cholesterol Education Program Adult Treatment Panel III criteria for the metabolic syndrome. Diabetes. 2004;53:2087–94.
62. Jennings CL, Lambert EV, Collins M, Levitt NS, Goedecke JH. The atypical presentation of the metabolic syndrome components in black African women: the relationship with insulin resistance and the influence of regional adipose tissue distribution. Metabolism. 2009;58:149–57.
63. Kuk J, Ardern C. Age and sex differences in the clustering association with mortality risk. Diabetes Care. 2010;33(11):2457–61.
64. Wildman RP, Muntner P, Reynolds K, Mcginn AP. The obese without cardiometabolic risk factor clustering and the normal weight with cardiometabolic risk factor clustering. Arch Intern Med. 2008;168(15):1617–24.
65. Kahn R, Buse J, Ferrannini E, Stern M. The metabolic syndrome: time for a critical appraisal. Joint statement from the American Diabetes Association and the European Association for the study of diabetes. Diabetes Care. 2005;28:2289–304.
66. Guize L, Thomas F, Pannier B, Bean K, Jego B, Benetos A. All-cause mortality associated with specific combinations of the metabolic syndrome according to recent definitions. Diabetes Care. 2007;30:2381–7.
67. Liao Y, Kwon S, Shaughnessy S, et al. Critical evaluation of adult treatment panel III criteria in identifying insulin resistance with dyslipidemia. Diabetes Care. 2004;27:978–83.
68. Ford E. Risks for all-cause mortality, cardiovascular disease, and diabetes associated with the metabolic syndrome. Diabetes Care. 2005;28(7):1769–78.
69. Sattar N. Why metabolic syndrome criteria have not made prime time: a view from the clinic. Int J Obes. 2008;32:S30–S4.
70. Benetos A, Thomas F, Pannier B, Bean K, Jégo B, Guize L. All-cause and cardiovascular mortality using the different definitions of metabolic syndrome. Am J Cardiol. 2008;102:188–91.
71. Wannamethee SG, Shaper a G, Lennon L, Morris RW. Metabolic syndrome vs Framingham Risk Score for prediction of coronary heart disease, stroke, and type 2 diabetes mellitus. Arch Intern Med. 2005;165:2644–50.
72. Stern M, Williams K, Gonzalez-Villalpando C, Hunt K, Haffner S. Does the metabolic syndrome improve identification of individuals at risk of type 2 diabetes and/or cardiovascular disease? Diabetes Care. 2004;27(11):2676–81.
73. Ford ES. Rarer than a blue moon: the use of a diagnostic code for the metabolic syndrome in the U.S. Diabetes Care. 2005;28(7):1808–9.
74. Zemel M. Dietary pattern and hypertension: the DASH study. Nutr Rev. 1997;55(8):303–5.
75. Bhattacharyya OK, Estey E, Cheng AYY. Update on the Canadian Diabetes Association 2008 clinical practice guidelines. Can Fam Physician. 2009;55:39–43.
76. Ye H, Charpin-El Hamri G, Zwicky K, Christen M, Folcher M, Fussenegger M. Pharmaceutically controlled designer circuit for the treatment of the metabolic syndrome. Proc Natl Acad Sci U S A. 2013;110(1):141–6.
77. Simmons RK, Alberti KGMM, Gale E a M, et al. The metabolic syndrome: useful concept or clinical tool? Report of a WHO Expert Consultation. Diabetologia. 2010;53(4):600–5.
78. Sharma a M, Kushner RF. A proposed clinical staging system for obesity. Int J Obes (Lond). 2009;33(3):289–95.

79. National Heart, Lung, and Blood Institute Obesity Education Initiative Expert Panel on the Identification, Evaluation and T of O and O in A. Clinical guidelines on the identification, evaluation, and treatment of overweight and obesity in adults. 1998.

80. Kuk J, Ardern C. Are metabolically normal but obese individuals at lower risk for all-cause mortality? Diabetes Care. 2009;32(12):2297–9.

81. Wildman RP, Muntner P, Reynolds K, et al. The obese without cardiometabolic risk factor clustering and the normal weight with cardiometabolic risk factor clustering. Arch Intern Med. 2008;168(15):1617–24.

82. Kantartzis K, Machann J, Schick F, et al. Effects of a lifestyle intervention in metabolically benign and malign obesity. Diabetologia. 2011;54(4):864–8.

83. Karelis a D, Messier V, Brochu M, Rabasa-Lhoret R. Metabolically healthy but obese women: effect of an energy-restricted diet. Diabetologia. 2008;51(9):1752–4.

84. Kuk J, Ardern C, Church T, et al. Edmonton Obesity Staging System: association with weight history and mortality risk. Appl Physiol Nutr Metab. 2011;36:570–6.

85. Padwal R, Pajewski N, Allison D, Sharma A. Using the Edmonton obesity staging system to predict mortality in a population-representative cohort of people with overweight and obesity. CMAJ. 2011;183(14):1059–66.

86. O'Connor KG, Harman SM, Stevens TE, et al. Interrelationships of spontaneous growth hormone axis activity, body fat, and serum lipids in healthy elderly women and men. Metabolism. 1999;48(11):1424–31.

87. Guo F, Moellering DR, Garvey WT. The progression of cardiometabolic disease: validation of a new cardiometabolic disease staging system applicable to obesity. Obesity (Silver Spring). 2014;22:110–8.

88. Guo F, Moellering DR, Garvey WT. The progression of cardiometabolic disease: validation of a new cardiometabolic disease staging system applicable to obesity. Obesity. 2014;22:110–8.

89. Edwards A, Elwyn G, Mulley A. Explaining risks: turning numerical data into meaningful pictures. BMJ. 2002;324:827–30.

90. Wells S, Kerr A, Eadie S, Wiltshire C, Jackson R. "Your Heart Forecast": a new approach for describing and communicating cardiovascular risk? Heart. 2010;96(9):708–13.

91. Gigerenzer G, Edwards A. Simple tools for understanding risks: from innumeracy to insight. BMJ. 2003;327:741–4.

92. Goodyear-Smith F, Arrol B, Chan L, Jackson R, Wells S, Kenealy T. Patients prefer pictures to numbers to express cardiovascular benefit. Ann Fam Med. 2008;6:213–7.

93. Jackson R. Lifetime risk: does it help to decide who gets statins and when? Curr Opin Lipidol. 2014;25(4):247–53.

94. Edwards A, Elwyn G, Mulley A. Explaining risks: turning numerical data into meaningful pictures. BMJ. 2002;324:827–30.

95. Gigerenzer G, Edwards A. Simple tools for understanding risks: from innumeracy to insight. BMJ. 2003;327:741–4.

96. Bonner C, Jansen J, McKinn S, et al. Communicating cardiovascular disease risk: an interview study of General Practitioners' use of absolute risk within tailored communication strategies. BMC Fam Pract. 2014;15:106.

Clinical Assessment of Lifestyle and Behavioral Factors During Weight Loss Treatment

David B. Sarwer, Kelly C. Allison and Rebecca J. Dilks

Abbreviations

BAI	Beck Anxiety Index
BED	Binge eating disorder
BDI-II	Beck Depression Inventory-II
BN	Bulimia nervosa
DSM-5	Diagnostic and Statistical Manual of Mental Disorders, Fifth Edition
EDE	Eating disorder examination
EMR	Electronic medical record
HAMD	Hamilton Depression Rating Scale
HRQOL	Health-related quality of life
IWQOL	Impact of weight on quality of life
NES	Night eating syndrome
PCOS	Polycystic ovary syndrome
QEWP-R	Questionnaire on Eating and Weight Patterns-Revised
SSBs	Sugar sweetened beverages
STAI	State-Trait Anxiety Index
WALI	Weight and Lifestyle Inventory

Introduction

The clinical assessment of lifestyle and behavioral factors that contribute to obesity can be performed by a number of health-care professionals and by a number of methods. Some physicians offering weight management treatment may wish to evaluate these factors personally. Other physicians, particularly those working in a multidisciplinary team, may have physician extenders—nurse practitioners, nurses, dietitians,

or behaviorists—evaluate patients' lifestyles. Many of those extenders may eventually serve as the primary treatment coordinators. Thus, asking patients about these issues provides an opportunity to begin to develop rapport and a strong clinical relationship. Much of the assessment involves direct questioning of the patients' history and current behavioral factors that have contributed to the development of excess weight. Specific domains, such as eating behavior, physical activity, and psychosocial status, can also be assessed by patient-reported outcome measures. Many of these are psychometrically validated tools that have been published in the academic literature and can be scored and evaluated against population norms; others may be "home-grown" measures that provide relevant clinical information to the practitioner but do not have psychometric support.

An "Obesity-Focused" History

A logical first step in initiating obesity care is to take a comprehensive history that addresses the lifestyle and behavioral issues specific to weight loss [1–3]. In our program, we routinely use the Weight and Lifestyle Inventory (WALI) with new patients [4]. (Table 6.1 provides a description of all of the psychosocial and behavioral measures discussed in the chapter, including information on where to obtain the measures.) Patients are asked to complete the questionnaire prior to the appointment. The WALI takes approximately 60–90 min to complete, and the responses are then reviewed in detail during the clinical assessment. The inventory provides a wide breadth of information that would likely take several hours to complete through direct questioning. By reviewing selected elements with patients in person, more in-depth discussions of particularly salient issues can take place. Many weight management programs or individual providers have created similar assessment tools that meet their individual needs.

Whether or not an inventory like the WALI is used, patients should be asked to describe their chronological history of weight gain. Patients should be prompted to identify

D. B. Sarwer (✉) · K. C. Allison
Center for Weight and Eating Disorders and Stunkard Weight Management Program, Perelman School of Medicine, University of Pennsylvania, Philadelphia, PA, USA
e-mail: dsarwer@mail.med.upenn.edu

R. J. Dilks
Center for Weight and Eating Disorders, Perelman School of Medicine, University of Pennsylvania, Philadelphia, PA, USA

© Springer International Publishing Switzerland 2016
J. I. Mechanick, R. F. Kushner (eds.), *Lifestyle Medicine,* DOI 10.1007/978-3-319-24687-1_6

Table 6.1 Commonly used measures of psychosocial functioning and eating behavior

Title	Description	Location
Weight and Lifestyle Inventory (WALI)	Provides a comprehensive assessment of psychosocial and behavioral factors which contribute to the development of obesity	Available from authors
Questionnaire on Eating and Weight Patterns-Revised (QWEP-R)	Allows for the assessment of symptoms of binge eating disorder and bulimia nervosa; based on DSM-5 diagnostic criteria	See reference [26]
Eating Disorder Examination (EDE) interview and questionnaire	Assesses eating disorder symptomatology attitudes, and behaviors	See references [27] and [28]
Night Eating Questionnaire (NEQ)	Brief measures designed to assess symptoms of the night eating syndrome	See reference [29]
Night Eating Symptom History and Inventory	A more comprehensive measure of the clinical features of the night eating syndrome than provided by the NEQ	See reference [30]
College Alumnus Survey/Paffenbarger Survey	A comprehensive self-report measure of a full range of physical activities	See reference [31–32]
Modifiable Physical Activity Questionnaire	Assesses physical activity during occupational and leisure time as well as inactivity secondary to disability	See references [33–34]
Beck Depression Inventory -II (BDI-II)	Gold standard measure of depressive symptoms; widely used in obesity literature	See reference [40]
Hamilton Depression Rating Scale (HAM-D)	Alternative measure of depressive symptoms	See reference [41]
Patient Health Questionnaire -9 (PHQ-9)	Brief (nine-item) measure of depressive symptoms which align with diagnostic criteria of major depression	See reference [42]
Center for Epidemiological Studies-Depression (CES-D)	Measure of depressive symptoms widely used in large epidemiological studies	See reference [43]
Beck Anxiety Inventory (BAI)	Widely used measure of anxiety symptoms	See reference [45]
State-Trait Anxiety Inventory (STAI)	Measure of anxiety symptoms which allows evaluation of state (temporary) versus trait (characterological) symptoms of anxiety	See reference [46]
Medical Outcomes Short Form Survey (SF-36)	Gold standard measure of health-related quality of life; widely used in obesity literature	See references [49–50]
Impact of Weight on Quality of Life-Lite (IWQOL-Lite)	Measure of weight-related quality of life; often used in conjunction with SF-36	See reference [51]

DSM-5 Diagnostic and Statistical Manual of Mental Disorders, Fifth Edition

the age when they first realized they were overweight. Next, they should be asked to describe the subsequent trajectory of their weight to the current point, with specific focus on major life events that contributed to significant weight gains as well as major weight loss efforts. Some of this information potentially can be confirmed in the electronic medical record (EMR). Similarly, the patient can be asked to reflect on their weight graph that is captured in the EMR.

Common patterns of the history of weight gain include progressive weight gain, weight cycling or "yo-yo" dieting, and periods of weight stability (or loss) followed by weight gain. Rapid cycling of weight may reflect mood instability that may hint at the need for further assessment of mood, as detailed below. For many patients, the initial weight gain, or subsequent gains, may be precipitated by change in major life events, such as changes in employment, marital status, or illness. For others, the start of (a) new medication(s) or smoking cessation may lead to weight gain. For women, onset of adolescence, pregnancy, and menopause may correspond to a significant weight gain.

Discussion of patterns of weight gain will naturally lead to a discussion of weight loss efforts. This information also is collected in the WALI. Patients should be asked about their experience with self-directed diets, commercial weight loss programs, dietary counseling, portion-controlled or meal replacement programs, as well as over-the-counter and prescription weight loss medications. Some patients also choose complementary and alternative medicine approaches to weight loss, even in the absence of empirical support for these approaches.

Many patients who present for weight loss treatment are "dieting veterans" who have tried numerous weight loss programs sometimes for years prior to their current visit. Some of these approaches may have been appropriate and successful for a period of time, others may have been less appropriate and potentially unsafe or unhealthy. Patients should be asked why they felt specific programs were (or were not) successful, what elements of the programs were most useful or not helpful, and what led to eventual recidivism of behaviors and weight regain. This information may be particularly useful in tailoring the current treatment approach to patients' behavioral strengths and preferences.

This review of the patient's history may reveal several less common secondary causes that may warrant further medical evaluation and that could be missed in a more routine history and physical examination. While patients presenting for weight loss treatment often report having a "slow metabolism" or "endocrine problem," endocrine disorders contributing to obesity are rare. The exception is polycystic ovary syndrome (PCOS) [5]. PCOS is a common endocrine disorder that affects a substantial minority of women, perhaps as many 20 % [6]. PCOS is typically characterized by androgen excess or hyperandrogenism (with clinical features of acne, hirsutism, and/or male pattern balding, as well as elevated serum androgen concentrations), menstrual irregularities, and chronic anovulation. Currently, there are initiatives to subtype PCOS into primary ovarian morphology, hyperandrogenic, and insulin-resistant pathological forms, but diagnostic strategies continue to require consensus statements in lieu of definitive metrics and biochemical/molecular tests [7]. It is therefore important to recognize that at least 50 % of women with PCOS are obese, and insulin resistance (as a prediabetes condition) is common. Other endocrine problems associated with obesity include hypothyroidism, Cushing's syndrome, and hypothalamic tumors or compromise as a consequence of irradiation, infection, or trauma [8]. Hypothyroidism is more common in older women, and measurement of TSH is in this population a valuable diagnostic tool [9]. However, current guidelines do not recommend screening for hypothyroidism for all patients who present with obesity. Review of patients' medication history also may reveal drug-induced weight gain or the use of medications that interfere with weight loss [10–13]. When possible, patients should be switched to an alternative medication that is weight neutral.

Assessment of Environmental Factors and Eating Habits

As behaviorists who work in the area of obesity and eating disorders, we believe that environmental factors play a central role in the modern world's current obesity epidemic. Thus, environmental factors need to be considered and evaluated for the individual patient as well. Through direct questioning or use of a self-report questionnaire, patients should be asked about their eating habits—when and where they eat, who shops and cooks in the home, etc. Portion sizes, snacking, as well as beverage intake should be assessed. This information provides a sense of overall nutritional knowledge and also can be used to target specific problematic behaviors to be focused on during treatment.

A dietary history can be obtained either by having patients fill out a short questionnaire while in the waiting room or assessed as part of the clinical interview. A useful and convenient technique is to ask patients to describe a typical day of eating and drinking, what is also referred to as a 24-h dietary recall. As weekday dietary patterns are often different from weekend patterns, a brief dietary recall of both is recommended. Dietary behaviors, such as where food is eaten, what triggers eating, and whether the patient engages in binge eating, are also important information. For some pa-

tients, their habitual diet may be well managed but episodically uncontrolled due to stress or mood. More detailed information can be obtained by asking patients to keep a food and activity diary for several days to a week. The diary often provides more information as eating and physical activity habits that vary on different days of the week. The diary can be more accurate as patients can have difficulty recalling and including all foods consumed in a 24-h period. Keeping a food and activity diary can be easily accomplished with the use of one of the multiple electronic tracking programs that are available on the Internet. The use of electronic tracking programs can provide details about the diet by calculating certain nutritional values such as total intake of macronutrients, fiber, fluid, and sugar. Hand-written diaries are also helpful if patients are not able to use Internet-based tracking programs. The exercise of logging food and beverage intake also serves to increase the awareness of dietary habits and forms the basis for targeted changes. It also may provide clues about patients' ability and willingness to follow behavioral recommendations to be used during treatment.

The eating behavior and dietary intake of patients often range greatly. Many patients are likely consuming more than the 2000 kcal/day recommended by the US Department of Agriculture and other government agencies [14]. Some may report eating 3000–4000 kcal/day with many meals consisting of calorically dense foods from fast-food or take-out restaurants and including sugar sweetened beverages (SSBs). In contrast, some patients, often those working diligently to control their type-2 diabetes, will report quite healthy eating habits. Nevertheless, most, if not all, patients who present for weight loss report difficulties controlling their eating behavior over extended periods of time. When considered against the backdrop of our current food environment, where the presence of food is nearly ubiquitous, this is not surprising. Simply put, in the current food environment it is incredibly hard to "swim against the stream" and chronically practice restraint to maintain a healthy body weight over the course of a lifetime. At the same time, other individuals will report specific problems in controlling their food intake in response to emotional or social cues. Almost all cultures have customs related to eating as part of holidays, celebrations, and even death. Thus, the pairing of eating to social cues is taught early and often to most individuals. However, for some, these pairings can be symptomatic of more formal eating disorders.

Assessment of Disordered Eating

While obesity has never been recognized as an eating disorder, since its origins vary widely from person to person, the presence of disordered eating behavior should be assessed. (We use the term "disordered eating" here as an umbrella term that captures both symptoms of formal eating disorders as well as more disorganized eating patterns and habits that have likely contributed to the development and maintenance of obesity.) The disorder that warrants particular attention is binge eating disorder (BED), which is characterized by the consumption of an objectively large amount of food in a brief period of time (<2 h) with the patient's report of subjective loss of control during the overeating episode [15–17]. These episodes occur, on average, at least once per week over the previous 3 months to meet criteria for BED. Patients do not engage in a compensatory behavior, such as vomiting, laxative abuse, or excessive exercise, which distinguishes BED from bulimia nervosa (BN). BED is now fully recognized as a psychiatric disorder in the Diagnostic and Statistical Manual of Mental Disorders, Fifth Edition (DSM-5) [17]. Binge eating occurs in only about 2% of the general population but is found in approximately 15–20% of people with obesity treated in specialty clinics [18]. Binge eaters with obesity may require psychotherapeutic treatment or psychotropic medication either before or in addition to weight reduction. BN may also be present in people with obesity, as the compensatory behaviors do not typically correct perfectly for the energy consumed during binge episodes. BN also warrants mental health treatment independent of weight loss treatment.

Another condition to be assessed is night eating. Night eating syndrome (NES) is currently included under otherwise specified feeding and eating disorders in the DSM-5. NES is defined as a circadian delay in the pattern of eating, characterized by evening hyperphagia (i.e., the consumption of 25% or greater of total daily caloric intake after the evening meal) and/or two or more nocturnal ingestions per week (i.e., waking during the sleep period to eat) [19–21]. Other symptoms include lack of appetite for breakfast, initial or sleep maintenance insomnia, a strong urge to eat in the evening or upon awakening, the presence of the belief that one needs to eat to fall asleep, and depressed or worsening mood as the day progresses. Patients have awareness of their nocturnal ingestions, which differentiates NES from sleep-related eating disorder, where patients are sleepwalking and eating. The presence of night eating may also contribute to the development and maintenance of obesity as eating during this time may be adding additional daily calories, and the body may be processing this energy in a less efficient way during the night [22]. Persons with night eating may also benefit from psychotherapy or psychotropic medication to help reduce this behavior, either alone or in conjunction with weight loss treatment [23–25].

Assessment of BED, BN, and NES may include a structured interview or a validated screening questionnaire. The Questionnaire on Eating and Weight Patterns—Revised (QEWP-R) [26] assesses BED and BN based on DSM-5 criteria. Confirmation through interview is recommended to confirm that binge episodes are objectively large and that loss of control over the eating episodes is present. The frequency and intention of compensatory behaviors should also be checked through interviews. Another well-validated tool is the Eating Disorder Examination [27], which can be administered by interviews or questionnaires [28]. The Eating Disorder Examination (EDE) can be used to diagnose all of the eating disorders and assesses a fuller range of eating disordered attitudes and behaviors than the QEWP. It also takes longer to administer. The Night Eating Questionnaire [29] is a brief questionnaire that assesses night eating symptoms. The Night Eating Symptom History and Inventory [30] is a structured interview in which the NEQ is embedded; the instrument may be used to confirm the presence of NES based on the 2010 proposed diagnostic criteria [29, 31]. All of these measures have been primarily used in the context of clinical research studies. However, they may be useful for practitioners with specific interests or concerns in these areas.

Assessment of Physical Activity

Patients presenting for weight loss treatment also should be asked about their current level of physical activity. Participation in scheduled forms of exercise, such as jogging, biking/spinning, or exercise classes, as well as daily lifestyle activity, such as stair use and daily walking, should be assessed. Many individuals with obesity are quite sedentary, frequently due to the physical discomfort associated with activity. An informative open-ended question to begin the discussion around the issue of physical activity is, "What is the most physically active thing you do over the course of a week?" In today's society, walking to or from the car, train, or bus often represents the extent of daily physical activity for many individuals.

This discussion of physical activity can be augmented by the use of one of several questionnaires designed to assess physical activity. The College Alumnus Survey (commonly known as the Paffenbarger Survey) [32] is used to calculate self-reported leisure time physical activity kilocaloric expenditure per week. This survey has excellent reliability and validity, including predictive validity for cardiovascular disease outcomes, and compares favorably to a 7-day recall [32]. In addition, the survey allows patients to record modes of activity not well measured by the current generation of commercially available activity monitors or accelerometers (including strength training and swimming). While typically used in research settings, the measure can provide clinicians and patients with information on the entire range of physical activities that could be increased to promote additional activity. The Modifiable Physical Activity Questionnaire (MAQ) [33] assesses current (past year and past week) physical activity during occupational and leisure time as well as extreme levels of inactivity due to disability [34]. The MAQ was designed for easy modification of activities to maximize its use in a variety of populations [35].

Assessment of Psychiatric Status and History

The treating physician and/or physician extender who will be providing lifestyle modification treatment also should assess psychological, behavioral, and social factors that may have contributed to the development or maintenance of obesity and, as a result, may impact a weight loss effort. This includes an assessment of patients' psychiatric status and history, as should be done routinely during a history and physical examination. Particular attention should be paid to the presence of mood and anxiety disorders, which are the most common disorders in the general population and also occur in higher rates with more severe forms of obesity. Persons with an active substance abuse disorder and those with an active psychosis are inappropriate for weight loss treatment.

Mood Disorders

People with obesity are at higher risk for current and lifetime depression than people without obesity. For example, people with extreme obesity are almost five times more likely to have experienced an episode of major depression in the past year as compared to average weight individuals [36]. The prevalence of depression among adults over age 50 and with obesity is 14%, compared with 7.5% among healthy weight adults of the same age group [37]. Men with Class III obesity are 38% more likely to experience current depression and 40% more likely to have a lifetime history of depression than healthy-weight men. Women with Class III obesity are 31% more likely to experience current depression and 53% more likely to have a lifetime history of depression [38]. Further, women with obesity are more likely to experience a major depressive episode in the past year as compared with average weight women [39]. The relationship between obesity and depression appears to be stronger for women than men, perhaps because of our society's emphasis on female physical appearance. Across gender, the reasons for the link between depression and increasing weight are not fully understood but could include the experience of weight-related prejudice and discrimination, the presence of physical pain, or other impairments in quality of life.

The directionality of the relationship between obesity and depression is unclear. For many people with obesity, increased symptoms of depression may be a result, rather than a cause, of their obesity. The physical discomfort and challenges of being obese, as well as the associated health problems, may have a quite understandable impact on mood. Even as experts attempt to educate the public on the multifactorial nature of obesity, many individuals see obesity as a result of depression, an inability to control one's impulses, or even a moral failing. Unfortunately, some physicians and other medical professionals who work with people with obesity also hold these beliefs, which likely compromises their ability to establish strong rapport and effectively deliver treatment.

For all of these reasons, mood symptoms should be assessed. Attention should be paid to patients' appearance, speech, thought, mood, and appropriateness of affect in describing themselves and in responding to questions. If depression is suspected, patients should be asked about the frequency of crying or irritability. Patients who endorse the neurovegetative symptoms of depression—trouble sleeping, difficulty concentrating, or significant change in appetite or weight—should be referred for treatment for depression before the onset of a weight loss program. There are several brief depression screeners that may be used in practice. The Beck Depression Inventory-II (BDI-II) [40] is a 21-item survey and is the most widely used measure of depressive symptomatology. It is often used in the context of research studies. As several of the symptoms assessed by the BDI-II, such as disruption in sleep and physical discomfort, could be attributed to obesity as well as depression, the measure may yield some "false positives" for depression among persons with obesity. The Hamilton Depression Rating Scale (HAM-D) [41] is a multiple-item questionnaire used to provide an indication of depression and as a guide to evaluate improvements in symptoms. The Patient Health Questionnaire (PHQ-9) [42] is a nine-item depression scale based on the nine diagnostic criteria for major depressive disorder. Finally, the Center for Epidemiologic Studies of Depression Scale (CES-D) [43] is a 20-item, well-validated screening measure for depressed mood that is widely used. Both the PHQ-9 and CES-D have grown in popularity within the obesity-treating community and can be used for both research and clinical purposes.

Anxiety

Patients interested in weight loss treatment also may report issues with anxiety. The most common anxiety disorder is social anxiety disorder, which is found in less than 5% of the general population. However, it is a common condition in people with obesity and extreme obesity in particular [44]. In a society that puts such a premium on physical appearance and thinness, it is not surprising that a significant minority of those with extreme obesity report increased anxiety in social situations. In addition, intuitive thought and clinical experience suggests that uncontrolled anxiety may negatively impact the ability to adhere to weight loss programs and behavioral requirements. Thus, anxiety should be monitored closely. The Beck Anxiety Index (BAI) [45] or the State-Trait Anxiety Index (STAI) [46] can be used to assess anxiety symptoms. While both measures primarily have been used for research purposes, they can provide a clinician with valuable information about symptoms of anxiety. However, it should be noted that there is no evidence suggesting that the diagnosis of an anxiety disorder contraindicates weight loss treatment.

Substance Abuse

A minority of patients who present for weight loss will report a history of substance abuse. Approximately 5–10% of patients will have a history of illicit drug use or alcoholism [44]. Active use or abuse of illegal drugs or alcohol is widely considered a contraindication to weight loss treatment. Consumption of large amounts of alcohol, even in the absence of a formal diagnosis of alcohol abuse or dependence, is likely to have a negative impact on weight loss with any weight loss program.

Ongoing Mental Health Treatment

A sizable minority of patients who present for weight loss treatment will likely be engaged in some form of mental health treatment. The most common form of treatment is the use of antidepressants or antianxiety medications, typically prescribed by the patient's primary care physician. For many patients, these medications are appropriately controlling their symptoms. For patients whose symptoms do not appear to be well controlled, optimization of mental health status—either through the adjustment of the dosages of the psychiatric medications or with a referral to psychotherapy—is recommended prior to the onset of weight loss treatment.

Assessment of General Psychosocial Functioning

Prior to weight loss treatment, providers should assess other, more general, areas of psychosocial functioning. These areas include motivations and expectations for treatment, self-esteem, quality of life, body image, romantic and sexual relationships, and timing for weight loss treatment.

Motivations and Expectations

Improvements in overall health and longevity are likely the primary motivation for weight loss, given the comorbid medical problems associated with obesity in most patients. Without question, concerns about body image and physical appearance also motivate the pursuit of weight loss and may be the area of psychosocial functioning that patients "value" the most following weight loss. It is important that patients are "internally" motivated for weight loss—that they are seeking weight loss for improvements in their health and well-being. Patients who are "externally" motivated, interested in weight loss for some secondary gain, such as saving a troubled marriage, may struggle to adhere with treatment over time.

Individuals who present for all forms of weight loss treatment—from lifestyle modification to bariatric surgery—often have unrealistic expectations regarding the amount of weight they will lose. Individuals enrolled in lifestyle modification programs have been shown to have "goal" weight losses of 33% of their initial body weight, comparable to the weight losses seen with bariatric surgery [47]. While these unrealistic expectations were once thought to put individuals at risk for weight regain, it appears that they may be unrelated to the weight losses actually achieved. Nevertheless, individuals interested in weight loss are encouraged to set a modest, initial goal of losing approximately 5% of their body weight. As recently reviewed, losses of this magnitude are considered clinically significant as they are commonly associated with improvements in weight-related comorbidities [48].

Self-Esteem

For some individuals, the degree of obesity can dramatically impact their self-esteem, such that it is difficult for them to recognize and appreciate their other talents and abilities because of their struggles with their weight. For others, obesity has relatively little impact. These individuals may be quite comfortable with their work and home life, but their weight has been the one area where they have not been successful. Obesity may be more likely to impact the self-esteem of women, likely given our society's overemphasis on thinness as a criterion for physical beauty.

Quality of Life

Obesity also negatively impacts health-related quality of life (HRQOL). Numerous studies have shown a relationship between excess body weight and decreases in quality of life. Individuals often report significant difficulties with physical functioning (walking, climbing stairs) and often difficulties with occupational functioning. These impairments likely motivate many individuals to seek weight loss treatment.

HRQOL is most commonly assessed by the Medical Outcomes Study Short Form (SF-36). It is a self-report measure that assesses eight separate domains of HRQOL including physical functioning, role functioning related to physical and emotional problems, social functioning, pain, general mental health, vitality, and perception of general health. Higher scores on each scale indicate more positive HRQOL [49]. Not surprisingly, the most substantial reductions in HRQOL in persons with obesity are typically seen within the physical functioning domains of SF-36 [50]. While the SF-36 is the "gold standard" measure of HRQOL, other measures for assessing additional aspects of quality of life include the Impact of Weight on Quality of Life (IWQOL) and the shorter version, the IWQOL-Lite. These have been developed to examine the specific influence of weight on quality of life [51]. The IWQOL-Lite version contains 31 items and, in addition to a total score, provides subscores in physical functioning, self-esteem, sexual life, public distress, and work. A number of studies have identified a strong relationship between degree of obesity and impairments in HRQOL; more recent research has incorporated quality-of-life measures specifically tailored to assess the impact of excess body weight on quality of life [50]. The clinical utility of these measures is less clear.

Body Image Dissatisfaction

Individuals presenting for weight reduction may have expectations about the impact of weight loss on other areas of their lives. Many people hope that weight loss will improve not only their health but also their physical appearance and body image. Body image is an important aspect of quality of life for many individuals. Body image dissatisfaction is as common in people who are overweight or obese [52]. However, it is the *degree* of dissatisfaction that is directly related to excess weight, although people can report dissatisfaction concerning their entire bodies or just with specific features. Body image dissatisfaction is believed to have motivated many appearance-enhancing behaviors, including participation in physical activity, fashion purchases, and cosmetic surgery [53]. It also is believed to play an influential role in the decision to seek weight loss, even in the presence of other health problems.

People who are overweight or obese report greater body image dissatisfaction than average weight individuals [52]. Those who lose weight, whether by behavioral modification, weight loss medications, or surgery, report improvements in their body image. However, large weight losses may result in the development of loose and/or sagging skin of the abdomen, thighs, legs, and arms that may lead to body image dissatisfaction. This may lead some patients to present to a plastic surgeon for body contouring surgery.

Interpersonal and Romantic Relationships

Other individuals may have expectations about the impact of weight loss on their interpersonal relationships. Many people may intuitively think that as they lose weight, and feel better about themselves, their social and/or romantic relationships will improve. This does occur for many individuals. However, for some, the experience of a major weight loss becomes an unsettling experience. Some individuals may experience unwanted attention related to their weight loss and physical appearance that may make them uncomfortable. Others may be upset or angry that people who treated them as if they were "invisible" before now are friendly and sociable. Patients are encouraged to consider these issues prior to starting a weight loss effort and often may want to discuss them in visits with the health-care professional. In these cases, a referral to psychotherapy is often appropriate.

These challenges may be particularly salient for those individuals with a history of sexual abuse. There appears to be a modest association between sexual abuse and obesity [54]. Studies have suggested that between 16 and 32% of bariatric surgery candidates reported a history of sexual abuse, which appears to be higher than that seen in the general population [55, 56]. Interestingly, several studies have suggested that a history of previous sexual abuse is unrelated to weight loss following bariatric surgery. Nevertheless, patients with a history of sexual abuse often struggle with a range of psychological issues, including body image and sexual and romantic relationship issues, following bariatric surgery. While it may be impossible to predict which patients will struggle with these issues, the preoperative psychological evaluation presents an opportunity to discuss these issues with patients and inform them that they may experience some psychological distress related to this during the postoperative period.

Patients seeking bariatric surgery (regardless of sexual abuse history) often present with the expectation that weight loss will improve their sexual functioning and romantic relationships. Others fear that the weight loss may destabilize these relationships. In general, the few studies of this issue suggest that romantic relationship quality improves following bariatric surgery. The impact, however, seems to be a function of the quality of the existing relationship. That is, stable, functional relationships may improve, while unstable, dysfunctional relationships appear to be at risk of deteriorating.

Patients should consider the potential impact of their weight loss on their marital and sexual relationships. Body weight can play a complex role in some relationships. Some partners may feel threatened or jealous witnessing a partner's weight loss. Some patients may be uncomfortable with additional romantic or sexual attention, particularly those with a history of sexual abuse. In these cases, a spouse may engage in behaviors, such as bringing high-calorie foods into the home repeatedly, that may sabotage the weight loss efforts of the other partner. Couples are encouraged to discuss these issues prior to the onset of a weight loss effort. Clinicians who identify discord between partners on these issues can recommend couples counseling as a strategy to help the couple understand these patterns of behavior and develop strategies to work together on weight control efforts.

One important aspect of quality of life often overlooked among persons with obesity is sexual functioning. The relationship between obesity and sexual functioning is complex and requires an understanding of the relationship between obesity and reproductive hormones (male hypogonadism), the impact of weight-related comorbidities (type-2 diabetes and hypertension), and the psychosocial factors that may lead to impairments in sexual functioning [50]. For example, sex drive, or libido, may be decreased with the increased medical burden and self-consciousness about one's appearance. Additionally, the physical exertion required to engage in sexual activity may become difficult. These factors alone, or in combination with obesity, lead to impairments in sexual functioning [50].

Little is known about the effects of surgically induced weight loss on sexual functioning. People with extreme obesity report greater impairments in sexual quality of life than those with lesser amounts of obesity [57]. Given our society's emphasis on thinness as a sign of physical beauty and sexuality, it is not surprising that women with obesity are often stigmatized as potential sexual partners. Obesity-related metabolic abnormalities, and the medications often used to treat them, are also associated with problems in sexual functioning. Intuitive thought suggests that the physical and psychological benefits associated with bariatric surgery will lead to improvements in sexual functioning; however, these issues have been the object of little study to date [58] but with some evidence suggesting that the massive weight loss seen with surgery is associated with significant improvements in sexual function.

Timing Factors

Another important part of the assessment is the timing of the weight loss effort. Ideally, patients are motivated to engage in weight loss at a time that is relatively free of major life stressors. Thus, the presence of these stressors, such as changes in employment, living situation, and health of close relatives, should be assessed by the clinician. It is probably easiest to do this by direct questioning; interest in these areas also may promote the development of rapport with the patient. Increased stress is associated with attrition from weight reduction treatment [59]. Thus, the patient should be relatively free of stressors for the months of treatment. Weight maintenance rather than weight loss should be encouraged during periods of high stress. An understanding of patient's motivation and stress level will help both the patient and practitioner determine the patient's readiness to change maladaptive behaviors.

Conclusion

The clinical assessment of behavioral and lifestyle variables is a central element of the delivery of effective weight management interventions. A comprehensive assessment requires the clinician to proceed well beyond the basic elements of a history and physical examination. The health-care professional must inquire about a wide range of behaviors and interpersonal variables that have contributed to weight gain and that may interfere with the ability to successfully engage in weight management treatment. Much of this can be done in the context of a clinical interview. However, given the emotionally sensitive nature of body weight and eating behavior, the questioning must be done in a sensitive, empathetic, and non-pejorative manner that allows for the development of rapport between patient and provider. Psychometrically validated measures also can be used to provide additional information that can be used to guide treatment. Thorough assessment and attention to these behavioral and lifestyle variables is critical to the successful delivery of the entire spectrum of weight loss interventions.

Conflicts of Interest Dr. Sarwer reports that he has consulting relationships with the following companies: BARONova, EnteroMedics, Ethicon, Kythera, and Neothetics. These relationships have had no influence on the contents of this chapter. Dr. Allison and Ms. Dilks report no potential conflicts of interest.

References

1. Sarwer DB, Allison KC, Berkowitz RI. Obesity: assessment and treatment. In: Hass LI, editor. Handbook of primary care psychology. New York: Oxford University Press; 2004. pp. 435–53.
2. Kushner RF, Sarwer DB. Medical and behavioral evaluation of patients with obesity. Psychiatr Clin North Am. 2011;34(4):797–812.
3. Wadden TA, Sarwer DB. Behavioral assessment of candidates for bariatric surgery: a patient-oriented approach. Surg Obes Relat Dis. 2006;2(2):171.
4. Wadden TA, Foster GD. Weight and lifestyle inventory (WALI). Surg Obes Relat Dis. 2006;2(2):180–99.
5. Linné Y. Effects of obesity on women's reproduction and complications during pregnancy. Obes Rev. 2004;5(3):137–43. (Review).
6. Sarwer DB, Allison KC, Gibbons LM, Markowitz JT, Nelson DB. Pregnancy and obesity: a review and agenda for future research. J Womens Health (Larchmt). 2006;15(6):720–33. (Review).
7. Setji TL, Brown AJ. Polycystic ovary syndrome: update on diagnosis and treatment. Am J Med. 2014;127(10):912–9.
8. Gambineri A, Vicennati V, Pagotto U, Pasquali R. Obesity and the polycystic syndrome. Int J Obesity 2002;26:883–96.
9. Garber JR1, Cobin RH, Gharib H, Hennessey JV, Klein I, Mechanick JI, et al. Clinical practice guidelines for hypothyroidism in adults: cosponsored by the American Association of Clinical Endocrinologists and the American Thyroid Association. Endocr Pract. 2012;18(6):988–1028.

10. Aronne LJ, editor. A practical guide to drug-induced weight gain. Minneapolis: McGraw-Hill; 2002. pp. 77–91.
11. Zimmermann, Kraus T, Himmerich H, et al. Epidemiology, implications and mechanisms underlying drug-induced weight gain in psychiatric patients. J Psychiatr Res. 2003;37:193–220.
12. American Diabetes Association, American Psychiatric Association, American Association of Clinical Endocrinologists, and North American Association for the Study of Obesity. Consensus development conference on antipsychotic drugs and obesity and diabetes. Obes Res. 2004;12:362–8.
13. Fontaine KR, Heo M, Harrigan EP et al. Estimating the consequences of anti-psychotic induced weight gain on health mortality rate. Psychiatry Res. 2001;101:277–88.
14. Wright JD, Wang CY. Trends in intake of energy and macronutrients in adults from 1999–2000 through 2007–2008: NCHS Data Brief. 2010;(49).
15. American Psychiatric Association. Diagnostic and statistical manual of mental disorders. 4th edn, text revision. Washington, DC: American Psychiatric Association; 2000.
16. Spitzer RL, Devlin MJ, Walsh BT et al. Binge eating disorder: a multisite field trial of the diagnostic criteria. Int J Eat Disord 1993;11:191–204.
17. American Psychiatric Association. Diagnostic and statistical manual of mental disorders. 5th edn. Washington, DC: APA; 2013.
18. Allison KC, Stunkard AJ. Obesity and eating disorders. Psychiatr Clin North Am. 2005;28:55–67.
19. Allison KC, Lundgren JD, O'Reardon, et al. Proposed diagnostic criteria for night eating syndrome. Int J Eat Disord 2010;43:241–7.
20. Allison KC, Stunkard AJ, Their SL. Overcoming night eating syndrome. Oakland: New Harbinger; 2004.
21. Allison KC, Lundgren JD, O'Reardon JP, Geliebter A, Gluck ME, Vinai P, et al. Proposed diagnostic criteria for night eating syndrome. Int J Eat Disord. 2010;43(3):241–7.
22. Gluck ME, Venti CA, Salbe AD, Krakoff J. Nighttime eating: commonly observed and related to weight gain in an inpatient food intake study. Am J Clin Nutr 2008;88:900–5.
23. Allison KC, Lundgren JD, Moore RH, O'Reardon JP, Stunkard AJ. Cognitive behavior therapy for night eating syndrome: a pilot study. Am J Psychother. 2010;64:91–106.
24. O'Reardon JP, Allison KC, Martino NS, Lundgren JD, Heo M, Stunkard AJ. A randomized placebo-controlled trial of sertraline in the treatment of the night eating syndrome. Am J Psychiatry 2006; 163(5):893–8. (Wander Wal review').
25. Vander Wal JS. Night eating syndrome: a critical review of the literature. Clin Psychol Rev 2012;32:49–59.
26. Spitzer RL, Yanovski S, Marcus MD. The questionnaire on eating and weight patterns-revised (QEWP-R). New York: New York State Psychiatric Institute.
27. Fairburn CG, Cooper Z, O'Connor ME. The eating disorder examination. 16th Edn. In: Fairburn CG, editor. Cognitive behavior therapy and eating disorders. New York: Guilford; 2008. pp. 265–308.
28. Fairburn CG, Beglin SJ. Assessment of eating disorders: interview or self-report questionnaire. Int J Eat Disord. 1994;16:363–70.
29. Allison KC, Lundgren JD, O'Reardon JP, Martino NS, Sarwer DB, Wadden TA, et al. The night eating questionnaire (NEQ): predictive properties of a measure of severity of the night eating syndrome. Eat Behav 2008;9(1):62–72.
30. Lundgren JD, Allison KC, Vinai P, Gluck ME. Assessment instruments for night eating syndrome. In: Lundgren JD, Allison KC, Stunkard AJ, editors. Night eating syndrome: research, assessment, and treatment. New York: Guilford; 2012. pp. 197–217.
31. Allison KC, Lundgren JD, O'Reardon JP, Geliebter A, Gluck ME, Vinai P et al. Proposed diagnostic criteria for night eating syndrome. Int J Eat Disord 2010;43:241–7.
32. Paffenbarger RS, Wing AL, Hyde RT. Physical activity as an index of heart attack risk in college alumni. Am J Epidemiol 1978;108:161–75.
33. Kriska, AM, Knowler, WC, LaPorte RE et al. Development of questionnaire to examine relationship of physical activity and diabetes in Pima Indians. Diabetes Care 1990;13:401–11.
34. Vuillemin A, Oppert JM, Guillemin F, Essermeant L, Fontvieille AM, Galan P, et al. Self-administered questionnaire compared with interview to assess past-year physical activity. Med Sci Sports Exerc. 2000;32(6):1119–24.
35. Kriska AM. Modifiable activity questionnaire. Med Sci Sports Exerc.1997;29(6 Suppl):S73–8.
36. Onyike CU, Crum RM, Lee HB, Lyketsos CG, Eaton WW. Is obesity associated with major depression? Results from the third national health and nutrition examination survey. Am J Epidemiol. 2003;158(12):1139–47.
37. Roberts RE, Kaplan GA, Shema SJ, Strawbridge WJ. Are the obese at greater risk for depression? Am J Epidemiol. 2000;152(2):163–70.
38. Zhao G, Ford ES, Dhingra S, Li C, Strine TW, Mokdad AH. Depression and anxiety among US adults: associations with body mass index. Int J Obes (Lond). 2009;33(2):257–66.
39. Carpenter KM, Hasin DS, Allison DB, Faith MS. Relationships between obesity and DSM-IV major depressive disorder, suicide ideation, and suicide attempts: results from a general population study. Am J Public Health. 2000;90(2):251–7.
40. Beck AT, Steer RA. BDI beck depression inventory manual. San Antonio: Harcourt Brace & Company; 1993.
41. Hedlund JL, Viewig BW. The Hamilton rating scale for depression: a comprehensive review. J Oper Psychiatry. 1979;10:149–65.
42. Kroenke K, Spitzer RL, Williams JBW. The PHQ-9—validity of a brief depression severity measure. J Gen Intern Med. 2001;16:606–13.
43. Radloff LS. The CES-D scale: a self report depression scale for research in the general population. Appl Psychol Meas. 1977;1:385–401.
44. Mitchell JE, Selzer F, Kalarchian MA, Devlin MJ, Strain GW, Elder KA, et al. Psychopathology before surgery in the longitudinal assessment of bariatric surgery-3 (LABS-3) psychosocial study. Surg Obes Relat Dis. 2012;8(5):533–41.
45. Beck AT, Epstein N, Brown G, Steer RA. An inventory for measuring clinical anxiety: psychometric properties. J Consult Clin Psychol 1988;56:893–7.
46. Spielberger CD, Sydeman, SJ. State-trait anxiety inventory and state-trait anger expression inventory. In: Maruish M.E., editor. The use of psychological testing for treatment planning and outcome assessment. Hillsdale: Lawrence Erlbaum Associates; 1994. pp. 292–321.
47. Foster GD, Wadden TA, Swain RM, Stunkard AJ, Platte P, Vogt RA. The Eating Inventory in obese women: clinical correlates and relationship to weight loss. Int J Obes Relat Metab Disord. 1998;22(8):778–85.
48. Jensen MD, Ryan DH, Apovian CM, Ard JD, Comuzzie AG, Donato KA, et al. 2013 AHA/ACC/TOS guideline for the management of overweight and obesity in adults: a report of the American college of cardiology/American heart association task force on practice guidelines and the obesity society. J Am Coll Cardiol. 2014;63(25 Pt B):2985–3023.
49. Ware JE Jr, Sherbourne CD. The MOS 36-item short-form health survey (SF-36). I. Conceptual framework and item selection. Med Care. 1992;30(6):473–83.
50. Sarwer DB, Lavery M, Spitzer JC. A review of the relationships between extreme obesity, quality of life, and sexual function. Obes Surg. 2012;22(4):668–76.

51. Kolotkin RL, Crosby RD, Kosloski KD, Williams GR. Development of a brief measure to assess quality of life in obesity. Obes Res. 2001;9(2):102–11.

52. Sarwer DB, Dilks RJ, Spitzer JC. Weight loss and changes in body image. In: Cash TF, Smolak L, editors. Body image: a handbook of science, practice, and prevention. 2nd Edn. New York: Guilford; 2011, 369–77.

53. Sarwer DB, Magee L, Clark V. Physical appearance and cosmetic medical treatments: physiological and socio-cultural influences. J Cosmet Dermatol. 2003;2(1):29–39.

54. Gustafson TB, Sarwer DB. Childhood sexual abuse and obesity. Obes Rev. 2004;5(3):129–35.

55. Grilo CM, Masheb RM, Brody M, Toth C, Burke-Martindale CH, Rothschild BS. Childhood maltreatment in extremely obese male and female bariatric surgery candidates. Obes Res. 2005;13(1):123–30.

56. Gustafson TB, Gibbons LM, Sarwer DB, Crerand CE, Fabricatore AN, Wadden TA, et al. History of sexual abuse among bariatric surgery candidates. Surg Obes Relat Dis. 2006;2(3):369–74. (discussion 375–6).

57. Sarwer DB, Spitzer JC, Wadden TA, Rosen RC, Mitchell JE, Lancaster K, et al. Sexual functioning and sex hormones in persons with extreme obesity and seeking surgical and nonsurgical weight loss. Surg Obes Relat Dis. 2013;9(6):997–1007.

58. Sarwer DB, Spitzer JC, Wadden TA, Mitchell JE, Lancaster K, Courcoulas A, et al. Changes in sexual functioning and sex hormone levels in women following bariatric surgery. JAMA Surg. 2014;149(1):26–33.

59. Enzi G. Socioeconomic consequences of obesity: the effect of obesity on the individual Pharmacoeconomics.1994;5(Suppl 1):54–7.

Anthropometrics and Body Composition

7

Dympna Gallagher, Claire Alexander and Adam Paley

Abbreviations

AA	African-American
ASM	Appendicular skeletal muscle
BD	Body density
BH	Body height
BIA	Bioimpedance analysis
BMI	Body mass index
BW	Body weight
C	Caucasian
CAG	Corrected arm girth
CCG	Corrected calf girth
CT	Computed tomography
CTG	Corrected thigh girth
CVD	Cardiovascular disease
DXA	Dual-energy X-ray absorptiometry
EA	European-American
HA	Hispanic-American
IMAT	Intermuscular adipose tissue
MRI	Magnetic resonance imaging
NIH	National Institutes of Health
R	Resistance
S	Stature
SM	Skeletal muscle
TBBM	Total body bone mineral
TBW	Total body water
VAT	Visceral adipose tissue
WHR	Waist–hip ratio
WHO	World Health Organization

This work was supported by Grants RO1-DK72507, UO1-DK094463, and P30-DK26687 from the National Institutes of Health.

D. Gallagher (✉)
Department of Medicine and Institute of Human Nutrition, Columbia University, New York, NY, USA

Body Composition Unit, New York Obesity Research Center, Columbia University Medical Center, 21 Audubon Ave, New York, NY 10032, USA
e-mail: dg108@cumc.columbia.edu

C. Alexander
Department of Psychology, Gettysburg College, 300 North Washington St., Gettysburg, PA, 17325

A. Paley
James Clack School of Engineering, University of Maryland, 1131 Glenn Martin Hall University of Maryland, College Park, MD, 20742

Introduction

Understanding how lifestyle interventions, commonly used in the treatment of chronic diseases, influence body composition is important for understanding the effects (beneficial or negative) of such interventions. For example, the treatment of type-2 diabetes (T2D), metabolic syndrome, coronary heart disease, hypertension, obesity, osteoporosis, or some forms of cancer by nutritional, physical activity, or medication interventions may impact the loss or gain of body tissues. Under some circumstances, it can be clinically important and meaningful to quantify the specific changes as a means of monitoring the effects of the intervention.

There is no one body composition measurement method that provides information on all body tissues. Body composition measurement methods vary in complexity, cost and precision, and range from simple field-based methods (e.g., anthropometry, bioimpedance analysis [BIA]) to more technically challenging laboratory-based methods (e.g., dual-energy X-ray absorptiometry (DXA), air plethysmography, and magnetic resonance imaging (MRI)). Table 7.1 lists some of the available methods of measuring body composition.

Body Composition Methods

Anthropometry The assessment of body composition in an individual can occur at a simple level where anthropometric measures, such as weight, height, waist, and hip circumference as well as skinfold thickness are obtained. For routine

© Springer International Publishing Switzerland 2016
J. I. Mechanick, R. F. Kushner (eds.), *Lifestyle Medicine*, DOI 10.1007/978-3-319-24687-1_7

Table 7.1 Available measurement methods of body composition

Method /main result(s)	Advantages	Disadvantages	Prediction equation
Anthropometry/ Body weight, height, skinfolds, body circumferences, and dimensions	Inexpensive, simple to acquire, safe, and can be used in settings that range from the research laboratories to field	The need for trained observers, relatively high between-measurement technical error for some measurements, mechanical limitations of some instruments for the very obese, "errors" in some geometric prediction models assuming stable between-subject anatomic proportions, and population and population specificity of component prediction formulas	*Predicting skeletal muscle mass* [12]: Skeletal Muscle (kg) = BH (cm) X (0.00744 x CAG2+0.00088 x CTG2+9.9941 x CCG2) + 2.4 x sex − 0.048 x age + race+7.8 CAG = corrected arm girth; CTG = corrected thigh girth; CCG = corrected calf girth; Sex: 0 for female; 1 for male; Race: 0= white/Hispanic, 1.1 for African-American, −0.2 for Asian Skeletal Muscle (kg) = 0.244 x BW + 7.80 x BH + 6.6 x Sex −0.098 x age + race − 3.3 Sex =0 for female and 1 for male, race =−1.2 for Asian, 1.4 for African-American, and 0 for white and Hispanic

Study	Age (yr)	Gender	Race	Equation
Peterson et al. [36]	Adult	Males	Not specified	$\%BF = 20.94878 + (\text{age} \times 0.1166) - (\text{Ht} \times 0.11666) + (\text{sum of 4 skinfolds} \times 0.42696) - ((\text{sum of 4 skinfolds})^{2 \times} 0.00159)$ Sum of triceps + subscapular + suprailiac upmidthigh
	Adult	Females		$\%BF = 22.18945 + (\text{age} \times 0.06368) + (\text{BMI} \times 0.60404) - (\text{Ht} \times 0.14520) + (\text{sum of 4 skinfolds} \times 0.30919) - ((\text{sum of 4 skinfolds})^2 \times 0.00099562)$ Sum of triceps subscapular + suprailiac + midthigh
Durnin and Wormersley [9]	17–72	Males $n=209$	Not specified	$BD = 1.1765 - 0.0744(\log_{10}X)$ X(mm)=Σ4 skinfolds (triceps, biceps, subscapular, iliac crest)
	16–68	Females $n=272$		$BD = 1.1567 - 0.0717(\log_{10}X)$ X(mm)=Σ4 skinfolds (triceps, biceps, subscapular, iliac crest)
Forsyth and Sinning [37]	19–22	Males $n=50$	Not specified	$BD = 1.10647 - 0.00162(X_1) - 0.00144(X_2) - 0.00077(X_3) + 0.00071(X_4)$ X_1 = subscapular skinfold (mm) X_2 = abdominal skinfold (mm) X_3 = triceps skinfold (mm) X_4 = mid-axilla skinfold (mm)

Table 7.1 (continued)

Method /main result(s)	Advantages	Disadvantages	Prediction equation		Sample	Age	Equation
			Jackson et al. [38]	Not specified	Females $n=249$	18–55	$BD = 1.24374 - 0.03162(\log_{10} \times x_1) - 0.00066 (X_4)$ $BD = 1.24389 - 0.04057(\log_{10} \times x_2) - 0.00016 (X_3)$ $X_1 = \Sigma4$ skinfolds (triceps, abdominal, front thigh, iliac crest in mm) $X_2 = \Sigma3$ skinfolds (triceps, front thigh, iliac crest in mm) $X_3 =$ age (yrs) $X_4 =$ gluteal circumference (cm)
			Katch and McArdle [39]	Caucasian	Males $n=53$	19.3 ± 1.5	$BD = 1.09665 - 0.00103(X_1) - 0.00056(X_2) - 0.00054(X_3)$ $X_1 =$ triceps skinfold (mm) $X_2 =$ subscapular skinfold (mm) $X_3 =$ abdominal skinfold (mm)
					Females $n=69$	20.3 ± 1.8	$BD = 1.09246 - 0.00049(X_1) - 0.00075(X_2) - 0.00710(X_3) - 0.00121(X_4)$ $X_1 =$ subscapular skinfold (mm) $X_2 =$ iliac crest skinfold (mm) $X_3 =$ biepicondylarhumerus breadth (cm) $X_4 =$ thigh girth (cm)
			Wilmore and Behnke [40]	Not specified	Males $n=133$	22.04 ± 3.10	$BD = 1.08543 - 0.000886(X_1) - 0.00040(X_2)$ $X_1 =$ abdominal skinfold (mm) $X_2 =$ front thigh skinfold (mm)
					Females $n=128$	21.41 ± 3.76	$BD = 1.06234 - 0.00068(X_1) - 0.00039(X_2) - 0.00025(X_3)$ $X_1 =$ subscapular skinfold (mm) $X_2 =$ triceps skinfold (mm) $X_3 =$ front thigh skinfold (mm)

Selected single-frequency BIA equations for predicting fat-free mass

Method /main result(s)	Advantages	Disadvantages	Prediction equation		Sample	Age	Equation
Bioelectrical impedance analysis/resistance, stature	Inexpensive portable simple, safe, quick	All variables should be considered: hydration status, consumption of food or beverages, ambient air and skin temperatures, recent physical activity and bladder activity	Baumgartner et al. [41]	White /USA	35M 63F	65–94	$0.28(S^2/R)+0.27(W)+4.5(S)+0.31(\text{Thigh C}) - 1.732$
			Deurenberg et al. [42]	Unknown / Netherland	661	16–83	$0.34(S^2/R) - 0.127(\text{Age}) + 0.273(W)+4.56(\text{Sex})+15.34(S)-12.44$
			Segal et al. [43]	Unknown /USA	1069M	17–59	$0013(S^2) - 0.044(R)+0.305(W) - 0.168(\text{Age})+22.668$
			Segal et al. [44]	Unknown /USA	498F	17–62	$0.0011(S^2) - 0.021(R)+0.232(W) - 0.068(\text{Age})+14.595$

Table 7.1 (continued)

Method /main result(s)	Advantages	Disadvantages	Prediction equation			

Two and three-compartment body composition models for measuring percentage fat (%Fat)

Method /main result(s)	Advantages	Disadvantages	Model	Equations for %Fat	Population	Reference
Air displacement plethysmography/ total body volume	Relatively high accuracy fast	Many individuals with BMI 60 kg/m² will not fit within the instrument	2C	$100 \times (4.95/D_b - 4.50)$	General population	Siri [45]
			2C	$100 \times (4.570/D_b - 4.142)$	Lean and obese	Brozek et al. [46]
			2C	$100 \times (4.374/D_b - 3.928)$	African-American males	Schutte et al. [47]
			2C	$100 \times (4.83/D_b - 4.37)$	African-American females	Ortiz et al. [48]

D_b= Weight/total body volume, body density (in kg/L)

Four-compartment body composition models for measuring percentage fat (%Fat)

Method /main result(s)	Advantages	Disadvantages	Model	Equations for %Fat	Reference
DXA/total body bone mineral (TBBM)	Easy to use, low X-ray radiation exposure, accurate for limb lean and fat	Bias: body size, sex, fatness. Many individuals with BMI 40 kg/m² will not fit within the field-of-view for soft tissue. Expensive equipment and specialized cannot be used in pregnant women	3C	$100 \times [6.386/D_b - 3.961 \times \text{TBBM} - 6.090]$	Lohman [49]
			4C	$100 \times [2.747/D_b - 0.714 \times (\text{TBW/W}) + 1.129 \times \text{TBBM/W}) - 2.037]$	Selinger [50]
			4C	$100 \times [2.748/D_b - 0.6744 \times (\text{TBW/W}) + 1.4746 \times (\text{TBBM/W}) - 2.051]$	Heymsfield et al. [51]
			4C	$100 \times [2.513/D_b - 0.739 \times (\text{TBW/W}) + 0.947 \times (\text{TBBM/W}) - 1.790]$	Withers et al. [52]

D_b= Weight/total body volume, body density (in kg/L)
TBW, total body water (in kg)
W, body weight (in kg)
TBBM, total body bone mineral (osseous + nonosseous; in kg)

Regression equations to predict total visceral adipose tissue (VAT) volume from VAT area imaged at L4-L5 and at 6 cm above
$L4\text{-}L5\ (L4\text{-}L5 + 6)$ [53]

Method /main result(s)	Advantages	Disadvantages	Variables in model	R^2
MRI	High accuracy and reproducibility for whole body and regional adipose tissue and skeletal muscle	Many individuals with BMI 40 kg/m² will not fit within the field-of-view for soft tissue. Expensive instrument access and the need for trained image analysis technicians may limit routine imaging method use to specialized research studies and centers	L4-L5*	0.8269
			L4-L5* + sex* + race*	0.8678
			L4-L5* + sex* + race* + age group†	0.8674
			L4-L5* + sex* + race* + BMI*	0.8777
			L4-L5* + sex* + race* + waist*	0.8843
			L4-L5* + sex* + race* + age group* + BMI† + waist* + (race x L4-L5)* + (sex x L4-L5)*	0.8983
			(L4-L5+6)*	0.9737
			(L4-L5+6)* + sex* + race*	0.9741
			(L4-L5+6) *+ sex* + race* + age group*	0.9745
			(L4-L5+6)* + sex* + race* + age group* + BMI*	0.9750
			(L4-L5+6)* + sex* + race* + age group* + BMI* + waist*	0.9756
			(L4-L5+6)* + sex* + race† + age group* + BMI† + waist* + (race x 6 cm)* + (sex x 6 cm)*	0.9766

R^2, percentage of variance explained by the regression variables
*Term is significant in the model
†Term is not significant in the model.

BH body height, *BW* body weight, *BMI* body mass index, *R* resistance, *S* stature, *W* body weight, *DXA* dual-energy X-ray absorptiometry, *MRI* magnetic resonance imaging, *TBBM* total body bone mineral

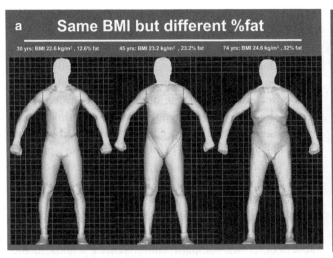

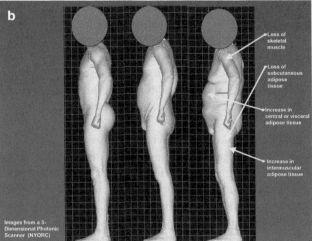

Fig. 7.1 **a** and **b** Three-dimensional whole-body scans of three males with similar height, weight, and BMI (23–24 kg/m^2), but differing in age (25, 45, and 78 years) and percentage body fat (12 %, 23 %, and 32 %). **a** Despite BMI being similar, the corresponding percent body fat is significantly different across the three individuals. **b** The difference in body morphology between the three males indicates differences in adipose tissue distribution and skeletal muscle distribution, neither of which can be detected from visual inspection of body shape. With advancing age, there are increases in central adiposity and in intermuscular adipose tissue with corresponding losses in subcutaneous adipose tissue and skeletal muscle mass.

clinical use, anthropometric measurements have been preferred due to the ease of measurement and low cost. Waist circumference and the waist–hip ratio (WHR) measurements are commonly used surrogates of fat distribution, especially in epidemiology studies. Waist circumference is highly correlated with visceral fat and is included as a clinical risk factor in the definition of the metabolic syndrome [1]. Specifically, waist circumferences greater than 102 cm (40 in.) in men and 88 cm (35 in.) in women are suggestive of elevated risk. Lower circumference measurements have been suggested for Asian (As) populations, for example 85 cm and 75 cm for Chinese men and women, respectively [2].

Body Mass Index The National Institutes of Health (NIH) and the World Health Organization (WHO) [3, 4] adopt similar body weight (BW; adjusted for height) guidelines for overweight and obesity. The body mass index (BMI=weight kg/height m^2) continues to be the most commonly used index of weight status, where normal weight is a BMI 18.5–25.9 kg/m^2; overweight is a BMI 25.0–29.9 kg/m^2; and obese is a BMI > 30.0 kg/m^2 although the true ranges may differ across ethnic groups. Despite BMI not being a direct measure of body composition, it is commonly considered as an index of fatness due to the high correlation between BMI and percent body fat in children [5] and adults [6]. The prediction of percent body fat in African-American (AA), As, and Caucasian (C) adults was found to vary with age (higher in older persons), sex (higher in males), and race (higher in As compared to AA and C). The following Eq. [7] is proposed to estimate the percent body fat:

$$\textit{Percent Body Fat} = 76.0 - 1097.8 \times (1/\text{BMI})$$
$$-20.6 \times \text{SEX} + 0.053 \times \text{Age} + 95.0 \times \text{Asian}$$
$$\times (1/\text{BMI}) - 0.044 \times \text{Asian} \times \text{Age} + 154$$
$$\times \text{SEX} \times (1/\text{BMI}) + 0.034 \times \text{SEX} \times \text{Age},$$

where multiple R=0.90; SEE =4.31 %; sex =0 for female and 1 for male; race =1 for As, 2 for other races.

In an analysis including Hispanic-American (HA) adults, no differences in the prediction of percent fat from BMI were observed between HA, European-American (EA), and AA men. In women, differences in percent body fat predicted by BMI were observed between HA and EA ($P < 0.002$) and AA and HA ($P=0.020$), but not between AA and EA ($P=0.490$). At BMIs < 30 kg/m^2, HA tended to have more body fat than EA and AA, and at BMIs > 35 kg/m^2, EA tended to have more body fat than the other groups [8].

Figure 7.1a, b shows the three-dimensional whole-body scans of three males with similar height, weight, and BMI (23–24 kg/m^2), but differing in age (25, 45, and 78 years) and percentage body fat (12, 23, and 32 %). Despite BMI being similar, the corresponding percent body fat is significantly different across the three individuals. The latter serves to demonstrate that BMI is a poor indicator of percentage body fat.

Prediction of Percent Fat and/or Fat-Free Mass (FFM) Skinfold thickness, which estimates the thickness of the subcutaneous fat layer, is highly correlated with percent body fat. Since the subcutaneous fat layer varies in thickness throughout the body, a combination of site measures is recommended reflecting upper and lower body distribution. Predictive percent body fat equations based on skinfold measures are age, sex, and ethnicity specific in adults. Examples of predictive equations in adults include Durnin and Womersley [9], Jackson et al. [10], and Davidson et al. [11].

Prediction of Skeletal Muscle Mass Arm, thigh, and calf muscle areas can be estimated based on skinfold thickness and limb circumference measures [12]. In one study, a skinfold-circumference model was found to have a higher accuracy than a BW and height model in predicting total body skeletal muscle in healthy adult populations [12]. The following two equations are proposed to estimate skeletal muscle (with whole-body MRI as the reference method), and these models were developed and cross-validated in nonobese adults (BMI < 30 kg/m^2).

Model 1

$$SM = Ht \times \left(\begin{array}{l} 0.00744 \text{ x } CAG^2 + 0.00088 \\ \times CTG^2 + 0.00441 \times CCG^2 \end{array} \right)$$
$$+ 2.4 \times sex - 0.048 \times age + race + 7.8$$

$R^2 = 0.91$; $P: < 0.0001$; SEE $= 2.2$ kg; sex $= 0$ for female and 1 for male; race $= -2.0$ for As, 1.1 for AA, and 0 for C and Hispanic. Ht is height in meters; CAG = skinfold corrected upper arm girth; CTG = skinfold corrected thigh girth; CCG = skinfold corrected calf girth); all girths in cm.

Model 2

$$SM = Ht \times \left(\begin{array}{l} 0.00744 \text{ x } CAG^2 + 0.00088 \\ \times CTG^2 + 0.00441 \times CCG^2 \end{array} \right)$$
$$+ 2.4 \times sex - 0.048 \times age + race + 7.8$$

$R^2 = 0.86$, $P: < 0.0001$, and SEE $= 2.8$ kg; sex $= 0$ for female and 1 for male, race $= -1.2$ for As, 1.4 for AA, and 0 for C and Hispanic; BW is the body weight in kilograms, and Ht is the height in meters.

Additional anthropometric equations were recently developed [13] that report sufficient accuracy for the prediction of skeletal muscle (SM) mass in groups and for research and survey purposes, but not for use in individuals or for clinical purposes. The variables identified for men were BW, waist, hip, and age, and for women were BW, hip, age, and height.

Bioimpedance Analysis (BIA) BIA is a simple, low-expense, noninvasive body composition measurement method. It is based on the electrical conductive properties

of the human body [14]. Measures of bioelectrical conductivity ar proportional to total body water (TBW) and the body's components with high water concentrations such as fat-free and SM mass. BIA assumes that the body consists of two compartments, fat and FFM (BW = Fat + FFM). It is best known as a technique for the measurement of percent body fat. Compared to multi-compartment body composition models, a two-compartment model approach (BIA and anthropometry being two examples) produces greater errors when estimating percent body fat in children and adults. A recent study [15] reported on a new eight-electrode, segmental multifrequency BIA device developed to estimate body composition in healthy and euvolemic adults. The results reported validity and precision comparable to other two-compartment reference methods, including air displacement plethysmography, deuterium dilution, and DXA.

It is reported that there is a strong correlation between BIA resistance and skeletal muscle measurements in the arms and legs. Janssen et al. [16] reported that MRI-measured SM mass is strongly correlated to the BIA resistance index (Ht^2/R), and the following SM prediction equation was developed from a multiethnic group (C, Hispanic, and AA) of females ($n = 158$) and males ($n = 230$).

$$SM \text{ mass (kg)} = [(Ht^2 / R \times 0.401) + (sex \times 3.825) + (age \times -0.071)] + 5.102$$

Ht is height in centimeters; R is BIA resistance in ohms; sex $= 0$ for female and 1 for male; age in years. $R^2 = 0.86$; SEE $= 2.7$ kg (9 %). The advantages of BIA include its portability, ease of use, relatively low initial cost and cost per use, minimal subject participation requirement, and its safety, thus making it attractive for large-scale studies or use in the office. Depending upon the device used, measurements are commonly obtained by tetrapolar or bipedal placement of electrodes while the subject lies supine or remains standing. Measurements are obtained in seconds. The accuracy of body fat measures is considered to be within 3.5–5.0 % [14] when conditions such as ambient temperature, participant hydration status, position of participant, correct electrode placement, use of appropriate equations, and eating and drinking that can affect TBW are regulated. Thus, subjects are typically asked to refrain from exercise and be well hydrated on the day of measurement. The aforementioned conditions represent the standard measurement conditions recommended for all BIA systems. BIA is not ideal for circumstances where typical hydration of lean mass may not be as assumed, such as during growth, pregnancy and lactation, weight loss, marked obesity, or certain disease states, for example, congestive heart failure, peripheral edema or ascites; it is also not recommended for participants with a pacemaker. Standard measurement conditions should follow the instrument-specific manufacturer guidelines.

Dual-Energy X-ray Absorptiometry (DXA) DXA provides an important means of quantifying total body and regional fat mass, SM mass, and bone mineral mass and density. Using specific anatomic landmarks, the trunk, legs, and arms are identified. The fat-free soft tissue (i.e., nonfat and non-bone mineral mass) of the extremities is largely ($\sim 76\%$) skeletal muscle and is considered appendicular skeletal muscle (ASM) mass. DXA- and MRI-measured lower limb SM mass have been shown to be highly correlated ($r = 0.94$, $P < 0.001$) in adults [17], and high correlations have been found between DXA-measured ASM and MRI-derived total body SM mass in adults ($r = 0.98$) [18].

Baumgartner et al. [19] were the first to develop an anthropometric equation for predicting ASM mass in elderly Hispanic and non-Hispanic white men and women. Sarcopenia was defined as an ASM (kg)/height^2 (m^2) less than two standard deviations below the mean of the young reference group. In the elderly men, the mean ASM/height^2 was approximately 87% of the young group. The corresponding value in women was approximately 80%. Obese and sarcopenic persons are reported as having worse outcomes including higher levels of metabolic disorders and poorer physical function than those who are nonobese and sarcopenic [20, 21]. These individuals demonstrate a relative increase in fat mass and a reduction in lean mass. How best to define sarcopenia and sarcopenic obesity continues to be debated [22]. The definitions for sarcopenia based on muscle mass alone and elevated fatness for obesity have produced conflicting results with regards to the relationship between "sarcopenic obesity" and impaired physical function [23]. What is clear is that the combination of low-muscle mass and weakness are contributors to disability in older ages.

Air Displacement Plethysmography Air displacement plethysmography uses air displacement to measure body volume from which an estimate of FFM and fat can be derived using a two-compartment model [24]. A commercially available system, the BOD POD (Life Measurement Instruments Inc., Concord, CA), can be used in persons weighing between 35 and 200 kg. To measure body volume accurately, it is necessary to account for the effects of air trapped in clothing, hair, and lungs. The measured body volume is corrected for these effects. The advantages of air plethysmography are its quickness and relative ease for the subject. The disadvantages of air plethysmography are the cost of the equipment and the need for technically trained staff. In addition, the breathing maneuver required for the purpose of predicting lung volume may be difficult for some: Claustrophobic persons may be unable to tolerate the small chamber dimensions; size limitations exclude individuals from the BOD POD who are > 200 or < 35 kg.

Magnetic Resonance Imaging (MRI) Whole-body MRI is increasingly being used as a reference method for evaluating and monitoring changes over time in whole-body and regional-body composition. Due to the expense associated with this technique, it does not present as a practical measurement method for use in clinical screening. However, it needs to be acknowledged that human in vivo measurements of SM mass, total adipose tissue mass and its distribution, and masses of several organs is possible. Subjects are placed on the scanner platform (1.5 or 3.0 T) with their arms extended above their heads. The protocol involves the acquisition of approximately 40 axial images, 10 mm thickness, and at 40 mm intervals across the whole body, with an acquisition time of 20 min [25]. Image analysis software is used to analyze images. This protocol allows for the quantification of adipose tissue distribution, specifically total-body visceral, subcutaneous, and intermuscular adipose tissue (IMAT) depots in children and adults. The limitations of MRI include the high costs for scan acquisition and processing of data, inability of large subjects to fit within the field-of-view, and problems scanning claustrophobic persons.

Visceral Adipose Tissue (VAT) Excess abdominal or VAT is recognized as an important risk factor in the development of coronary heart disease and T2D. The most accurate measurement of VAT requires MRI, which is impractical in a clinical setting. Figure 7.2a shows the three-dimensional reconstruction images of VAT in two females with similar weight, height, and BMI, but differing in age (25 and 78 years). VAT mass is four times greater in the older woman (Fig. 7.3).

Female A 25 years, weight 54.0 kg, height 1.6 m, BMI 21 kg/m^2, total adipose tissue 14.0 kg, subcutaneous adipose tissue 13.0 kg, VAT 0.5 kg, IMAT 0.6 kg, and skeletal muscle 20.0 kg.

Female B 78 years, weight 54.0 kg, height 1.6 m, BMI 21.4 kg/m^2, total adipose tissue 20.0 kg, subcutaneous adipose tissue 15.3 kg, VAT 2.1 kg, IMAT 2.6 kg, and skeletal muscle 15.0 kg.

Before Bariatric Surgery 66 years, weight 135.4 kg, height 1.8 m, BMI 43 kg/m^2, total adipose tissue 62.6 kg, subcutaneous adipose tissue 47.0 kg, VAT 11.1 kg, IMAT 4.6 kg, and skeletal muscle 33.4 kg.

Following Bariatric Surgery
At 12 months: 67 years, weight 93.4 kg, height 1.8 m, BMI 29.6 kg/m^2, total adipose tissue 33.3 kg, subcutaneous adipose tissue 26.7 kg, VAT 3.7 kg, IMAT 3.0 kg, and skeletal muscle 25.9 kg.

At 24 months: 68 years, weight 98.5 kg, height 1.8 m, BMI 31.6 kg/m^2, total adipose tissue 39.7 kg, subcutaneous adipose tissue 29.3 kg, VAT 6.5 kg, IMAT 3.9 kg, and skeletal muscle 23.3 kg.

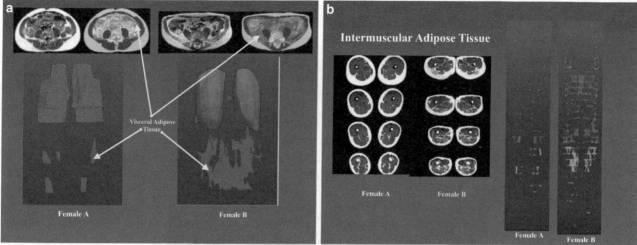

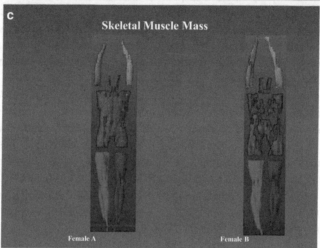

Fig. 7.2 **a** Three-dimensional reconstruction images of visceral adipose tissue (VAT) in two females with similar weight, height, and BMI, but differing in age (25 and 78 years). Total VAT mass is four times greater in the older woman. The upper panels show a single cross-sectional slice in grey scale *(left)* acquired at approximately the lumbar vertebrae L4–L5, with analyzed slice using colors *(right)* to identify VAT *(purple)*, skeletal muscle *(red)*, organs and intestines *(yellow)*, and subcutaneous adipose tissue *(green)*. The lower panel shows the quantity of VAT at its location in relation to the lungs *(orange)*. *Yellow arrows* point to the VAT. **b** Cross-sectional grey scale images of midthigh *(left)* and the three-dimensional reconstruction images of intermuscular adipose tissue (IMAT) across the body in the same two females with similar weight, height, and BMI but differing in age (25 and 78 years). IMAT mass is four times greater in the older woman. **c** Three-dimensional reconstruction images of whole-body SM mass in the same two females with similar weight, height, and BMI but differing in age (25 and 78 years). SM mass was 25 % lower in the older woman

At approximately 60 months: 70 years, weight 103.0 kg, height 1.8 m, BMI 32.3 kg/m², total adipose tissue 48.6 kg, subcutaneous adipose tissue 35.8 kg, VAT 8.1 kg, IMAT 4.8 kg, and skeletal muscle 24.1 kg.

Waist circumference and the WHR are commonly used to predict visceral fat accumulation in epidemiological studies and the office setting. Several investigators have argued that simple waist circumference is a better index of variation in VAT than WHR. Abdominal fat estimated by DXA does not differentiate between the intra-abdominal and subcutaneous abdominal depots. DXA has some advantages over MRI as a means of estimating fat distribution, including relative ease of access to systems, simplicity of measurements, and relatively low cost.

Intermuscular Adipose Tissue The adipose tissue located between muscle bundles and visible by MRI is referred to here as IMAT. Previous reports [26] suggest that adipose tissue located below the muscle fascia is significantly negatively correlated with insulin sensitivity, whereas subcutaneous adipose tissue (SAT) located above the muscle fascia is not correlated with insulin sensitivity. In elderly, greater IMAT (as suggested by lower skeletal muscle attenuation by computed tomography (CT) is associated with lower specific force production [27]. The most accurate measurement of IMAT requires imaging techniques, which are impractical in a clinical setting. Currently, there is no surrogate measure of IMAT. Figure 7.2b shows cross-sectional grey scale images of midthigh (left) and the three-dimensional reconstruction

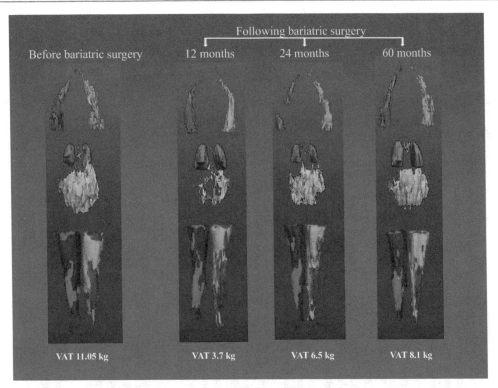

Fig. 7.3 Three-dimensional reconstructed images of visceral adipose tissue (VAT) in one male before having bariatric surgery, and following surgery, at 12 months, 24 months, and at approximately 60 months. Shown are the amounts of VAT at each time point

images of IMAT across the body in two females with similar weight, height, and BMI but differing in age (25 and 78 years). IMAT mass is four times greater in the older woman.

Skeletal Muscle Mass During the adult life span, BW generally increases slowly and progressively until about the seventh decade, and thereafter, declines in old age. An increased incidence of physical disabilities and comorbidities are likely linked to aging associated body composition changes that includes but not limited to losses in muscle mass, force, and strength. Skeletal muscle mass (SM) represents ~40% of the BW in young adults. With increasing age, SM mass decreases to ~30% of the young values at elderly ages. SM mass is one of the more difficult components to quantify. Common measurement methods include anthropometry, DXA-derived ASM, and MRI. Figure 7.2c shows the three-dimensional reconstruction images of whole-body SM mass in two females with similar weight, height, and BMI but differing in age (25 and 78 years). SM mass was 25% lower in the older woman.

Clinical Implications

The measurement of body composition in patient care is useful to predict clinical outcomes and to guide and determine response to therapeutic interventions. Practical examples including those listed in Table 7.2 are: sarcopenia with implications for frailty and immobility; sarcopenic obesity with

implications for metabolic risk; cachexia related to wasting diseases; excess adiposity with implications for cardiovascular morbidity; increased visceral adiposity (independent of total adiposity) that plays a pathophysiological role in many chronic diseases; lipodystrophy reflecting fat accumulation in one or more locations (e.g., abdomen, dorsocervical spine, breasts) or fat loss on the face, buttocks, and extremities (e.g., secondary to antiretroviral therapy) that is strongly associated with insulin resistance, diabetes, and dyslipidemia.

Conclusion

The measurement of body composition in the truest sense allows for the estimation of body tissues, organs, and their distributions in living persons without inflicting harm. It is important to recognize that there is no single measurement method in existence that is error free. Furthermore, bias can be introduced if a measurement method makes assumptions related to body composition proportions and characteristics that are inaccurate across different populations.

Some methodological concerns include the following: hydration of fat-free body mass changes with age and differs across ethnic groups [28]; the density of fat-free body mass changes with age and differs between men and women [29]; total body potassium decreases with age [28] and fatness [30] and differs between blacks and whites [31]; the mass of skeletal muscle differs across race group [32]; and VAT differs across sex [33] and race [34, 35] groups, inde-

Table 7.2 Clinical correlates of body composition components

Clinical condition	Population	Finding(s)	Reference
Normal glucose tolerant Prediabetes Diabetes	Ages 45–80 years, Caucasian females and males	Abdominal SAT is more strongly associated with cardiovascular risk factors (triglycerides and HDL-cholesterol) in women. Visceral adipose tissue (VAT) is more strongly associated with CV risk factors (total cholesterol and triglycerides) in men	Scheuer et al. [54]
Pediatric hematopoietic stem cell transplantation survivors	Survivors (aged 12–25 years); median 9.7 (4.3–19.3) years after transplantation compared to age-, race-, and sex-matched healthy controls	Increased marrow adipose tissue, abnormal bone microarchitecture, higher VAT, higher muscle fat infiltration	Mostoufi-Moab et al. [55]
Acromegaly before and after pituitary surgery	Untreated acromegaly patients (n = 23) before and 2 years following surgery	VAT and SAT mass were lower than predicted in active acromegaly and increased after surgery in males and females (concomitant with lowering of GH, IGF-1 and insulin resistance). IMAT was higher in active acromegaly and decreased in women after surgery. Intrahepatic lipid increased with no change in intramyocellular lipid after surgery. Skeletal muscle mass decreased in men	Reyes-Vidal et al. [56]
Adipose tissue depots by gender and metabolic health	Review	Gluteal-femoral adipose tissues of women may provide a safe lipid reservoir for excess energy or they may directly regulate systemic metabolism via release of metabolic products or adipokines	Karastergiou et al. [57]
HIV-related lipodystrophy and increased cardiovascular disease (CVD) risk	586 HIV-infected individuals and 280 controls	Great VAT in HIV-infected individuals and CVD risk is higher in HIV-infected compared to controls at every level of VAT. Peripheral lipoatrophy (as measured by leg SAT) associated with increased CVD risk in HIV-infected patients even after controlling for VAT	Lake et al. [58]
Aging related sarcopenia (loss of muscle mass and decline in muscle strength, strongly associated with physical disability, poor quality of life and frailty)	Review	Sarcopenia with obesity is associated with higher levels of metabolic disorders and an increased risk of mortality than obesity or sarcopenia alone	Wannamethee and Atkins [21]
Asian Indians have lower BMI and higher central adiposity with higher prevalence of type-2 diabetes than the general US population	Asian Indians (40–84 years) living in India and 757 Asian Indians (40–84 years) living in the USA	Age-adjusted diabetes prevalence was higher in India (38 %) than in the USA (24 %). Age-adjusted prediabetes prevalence was lower in India (24 %) than in the USA (33 %). Asian Indians in India had lower BMI and waist circumference measurements than those living in the USA; they still had a higher prevalence of type-2 diabetes even at normal levels of BMI and in both sexes	Gujral et al. [59]
Malnutrition and different types of cachexia: recognizing when to nutritionally intervene	Review	There is a need for a widely accepted definition of cachexia, validated to predict successful and meaningful outcomes, which can be used to identify patients most likely to benefit from early intervention	Baldwin [60]

CVD cardiovascular disease, *VAT* visceral adipose tissue

pendent of total adiposity. These between-group differences influence the absolute accuracy of methods for estimating fatness or FFM involving the two-compartment model approach. The clinical significance of the body compartment to be measured should first be determined before a measurement method is selected since the more advanced techniques are less accessible and more costly.

References

1. Grundy SM, Brewer HB Jr, Cleeman JI, Smith SC Jr, Lenfant C; American Heart Association; National Heart, Lung, and Blood Institute. Definition of metabolic syndrome: report of the National Heart, Lung, and Blood Institute/American Heart Association conference on scientific issues related to definition. Circulation. 2004;109(3):433–8. (Review. PubMed PMID:14744958).

2. Zeng Q, He Y, Dong S, Zhao X, Chen Z, Song Z, Chang G, Yang F, Wang Y. Optimal cut-off values of BMI, waist circumference and waist:height ratio for defining obesity in Chinese adults. Br J Nutr. 2014;112(10):1735–44. doi:10.1017/S0007114514002657. (Epub 2014 Oct 10. PubMed PMID: 25300318).

3. World Health Organization (editor). Obesity: preventing and managing the global epidemic. Report of a WHO consultation on obesity. Geneva, June 3–5, 1997. Geneva: WHO; 1998.

4. US Department of Health and Human Services (editor). Clinical guidelines on the identification, evaluation, and treatment of overweight and obesity in adults: the evidence report. Washington, DC: US DHHS; 1998. pp. 98–4083.

5. Mei Z, Grummer-Strawn LM, Pietrobelli A, Goulding A, Goran MI, Dietz WH. Validity of body mass index compared with other body-composition screening indexes for the assessment of body fatness in children and adolescents. Am J Clin Nutr. 2002;75(6):978–85.

6. Gallagher D, Visser M, Sepulveda D, Pierson RN, Harris T, Heymsfield SB. How useful is body mass index for comparison of body fatness across age, sex, and ethnic groups? Am J Epidemiol. 1996;143(3):228–39.

7. Gallagher D, Heymsfield SB, Heo M, Jebb SA, Murgatroyd PR, Sakamoto Y. Healthy percentage body fat ranges: an approach for developing guidelines based on body mass index. Am J Clin Nutr. 2000;72(3):694–701.

8. Fernández JR, Heo M, Heymsfield SB, Pierson RN Jr, Pi-Sunyer FX, Wang ZM, Wang J, Hayes M, Allison DB, Gallagher D. Is percentage body fat differentially related to body mass index in Hispanic Americans, African Americans, and European Americans? Am J Clin Nutr. 2003;77(1):71–5. (PubMed PMID: 12499325).

9. Durnin JV, Womersley J. Body fat assessed from total body density and its estimation from skinfold thickness: measurements on 481 men and women aged from 16 to 72 years. Br J Nutr. 1974;32:77–97.

10. Jackson AS, Ellis KJ, McFarlin BK, Sailors MH, Bray MS. Cross-validation of generalised body composition equations with diverse young men and women: the Training Intervention and Genetics of Exercise Response (TIGER) Study. Br J Nutr. 2009;101(6):871–8. (PubMed: 18702849).

11. Davidson LE, Wang J, Thornton JC, Kaleem Z, Silva-Palacios F, Pierson RN, Heymsfield SB, Gallagher D. Predicting fat percent by skinfolds in racial groups: Durnin and Womersley revisited. Med Sci Sports Exerc. 2011;43(3):542–9. doi:10.1249/MSS.0b013e3181ef3f07. (PubMed PMID: 20689462; PMCID: PMC3308342).

12. Lee RC, Wang Z, Heo M, Ross R, Janssen I, Heymsfield SB. Total-body skeletal muscle mass: development and cross-validation of anthropometric prediction models. Am J Clin Nutr. 2000;72(3):796–803. (Erratum in: Am J Clin Nutr 2001 May;73(5):995. PubMed PMID: 10966902).

13. Al-Gindan YY, Hankey C, Govan L, Gallagher D, Heymsfield SB, Lean ME. Derivation and validation of simple equations to predict total muscle mass from simple anthropometric and demographic data. Am J Clin Nutr. 2014;100(4):1041–51. doi:10.3945/ajcn.113.070466. (Epub 2014 Aug 13. PubMed PMID: 25240071).

14. Baumgartner RN. Electrical impedance and total body electrical conductivity. In: Roche AF, Heymsfield SB, Lohman TG, editors. Human body composition. Champaign: Human Kinetics; 1996. pp. 79–102.

15. Bosy-Westphal A, Schautz B, Later W, Kehayias JJ, Gallagher D, Müller MJ. What makes a BIA equation unique? Validity of eight-electrode multifrequency BIA to estimate body composition in a healthy adult population. Eur J Clin Nutr. 2013;67(Suppl 1):S14–21. doi:10.1038/ejcn.2012.160. (PubMed PMID: 23299866).

16. Janssen I, Heymsfield SB, Baumgartner RN, Ross R. Estimation of skeletal muscle mass by bioelectrical impedance analysis. J Appl Physiol. 1985, 2000;89(2):465–71. (PubMed PMID: 10926627).

17. Shih R, Wang Z, Heo M, Wang W, Heymsfield SB. Lower limb skeletal muscle mass: development of dual-energy X-ray absorptiometry prediction model. J Appl Physiol. 2000;89(4):1380–6.

18. Kim J, Wang Z, Heymsfield SB, Baumgartner RN, Gallagher D. Total-body muscle mass: estimation by new dual-energy X-ray absorptimetry method. Am J Clin Nutr. 2002;76(2):378–83.

19. Baumgartner RN, Koehler KM, Gallagher D, Romero L, Heymsfield SB, Ross RR, Garry PJ, Lindeman RD. Epidemiology of sarcopenia among the elderly in New Mexico. Am J Epidemiol. 1998;147(8):755–63. (Erratum in: Am J Epidemiol 1999 Jun 15;149(12):1161. PubMed PMID: 9554417).

20. Atkins JL, Whincup PH, Morris RW, Lennon LT, Papacosta O, Wannamethee SG. Sarcopenic obesity and risk of cardiovascular disease and mortality: a population-based cohort study of older men. J Am Geriatr Soc. 2014;62(2):253–60. doi:10.1111/jgs.12652. (Epub 2014 Jan 15. PubMed PMID: 24428349; PubMed Central PMCID: PMC4234002).

21. Wannamethee SG, Atkins JL. Muscle loss and obesity: the health implications of sarcopenia and sarcopenic obesity. Proc Nutr Soc. 2015;27:1–8. ((Epub ahead of print) PubMed PMID: 25913270).

22. Studenski SA, Peters KW, Alley DE, Cawthon PM, McLean RR, Harris TB, Ferrucci L, Guralnik JM, Fragala MS, Kenny AM, Kiel DP, Kritchevsky SB, Shardell MD, Dam TT, Vassileva MT. The FNIH sarcopenia project: rationale, study description, conference recommendations, and final estimates. J Gerontol A Biol Sci Med Sci. 2014;69(5):547–58. doi:10.1093/gerona/glu010. (PubMed PMID: 24737557; PMCID: PMC3991146).

23. Dam TT, Peters KW, Fragala M, Cawthon PM, Harris TB, McLean R, Shardell M, Alley DE, Kenny A, Ferrucci L, Guralnik J, Kiel DP, Kritchevsky S, Vassileva MT, Studenski S. An evidence-based comparison of operational criteria for the presence of sarcopenia. J Gerontol A Biol Sci Med Sci. 2014;69(5):584–90. doi:10.1093/gerona/glu013. (PubMed PMID: 24737561; PMCID: PMC3991139).

24. Dempster P, Aitkens S. A new air displacement method for the determination of human body composition. Med Sci Sports Exerc. 1995;27:1692–7.

25. Gallagher D, Kovera AJ, Clay-Williams G, Agin D, Leone P, Albu J, Matthews DE, Heymsfield SB. Weight loss in postmenopausal obesity: no adverse alterations in body composition and protein metabolism. Am J Physiol Endocrinol Metab. 2000;279(1):E124–31. (PubMed PMID: 10893331).

26. Goodpaster BH, Thaete FL, Simoneau JA, Kelley DE. Subcutaneous abdominal fat and thigh muscle composition predict insulin sensitivity independently of visceral fat. Diabetes. 1997;46(10):1579–85. (PubMed PMID: 9313753).

27. Goodpaster BH, Carlson CL, Visser M, Kelley DE, Scherzinger A, Harris TB, Stamm E, Newman AB. Attenuation of skeletal muscle and strength in the elderly: the Health ABC Study. J Appl Physiol. 1985, 2001;90(6):2157–65. (PubMed PMID: 11356778).

28. Mazariegos M, Wang ZM, Gallagher D, Baumgartner RN, Allison DB, Wang J, Pierson RN Jr, Heymsfield SB. Differences between young and old females in the five levels of body composition and their relevance to the two-compartment chemical model. J Gerontol 1994;49(5):M201–8.

29. Heymsfield SB, Wang Z, Baumgartner RN, Dilmanian FA, Ma R, Yasumura S. Body composition and aging: a study by in vivo neutron activation analysis. J Nutr. 1993;123(2 Suppl):432–7.

30. Pierson RN Jr, Lin DH, Phillips RA. Total-body potassium in health: effects of age, sex, height, and fat. Am J Physiol. 1974;226(1):206–12.

31. Cohn SH, Abesamis C, Zanzi I, Aloia JF, Yasumura S, Ellis KJ. Body elemental composition: comparison between black and white adults. Am J Physiol. 1977;232(4):E419–22.

32. Gallagher D, Visser M, De Meersman RE, Sepulveda D, Baumgartner RN, Pierson RN, et al. Appendicular skeletal muscle mass: effects of age, gender, and ethnicity. J Appl Physiol. 1997;83(1):229–39.

33. Shen W, Punyanitya M, Silva AM, Chen J, Gallagher D, Sardinha LB, Allison DB, Heymsfield SB. Sexual dimorphism of adipose tissue distribution across the lifespan: a cross-sectional whole-body magnetic resonance imaging study. Nutr Metab (Lond). 2009;6:17. doi:10.1186/1743-7075-6-17. (PMID: 19371437; PMCID: PMC2678136).

34. Gallagher D, Kuznia P, Heshka S, Albu J, Heymsfield SB, Goodpaster B, Visser M, Harris TB. Adipose tissue in muscle: a novel depot similar in size to visceral adipose tissue. Am J Clin Nutr. 2005;81(4):903–10. (PubMed PMID: 15817870; PubMed Central PMCID: PMC1482784).

35. Gallagher D, Kelley DE, Yim JE, Spence N, Albu J, Boxt L, Pi-Sunyer FX, Heshka S; MRI Ancillary Study Group of the Look AHEAD Research Group. Adipose tissue distribution is different in type 2 diabetes. Am J Clin Nutr. 2009;89(3):807–14. doi:10.3945/ajcn.2008.26955. (Epub 2009 Jan 21. PubMed PMID: 19158213; PubMed Central PMCID: PMC2714397).

36. Peterson MJ, Czerwinski SA, Siervogel RM. Development and validation of skinfold-thickness prediction equations with a 4-compartment model. Am J Clin Nutr. 2003;77(5):1186–91. (PubMed PMID: 12716670).

37. Forsyth HL, Sinning WE. The anthropometric estimation of body density and lean body weight of male athletes. Med Sci Sports. 1973;5(3):174–80. (PubMed PMID: 4747639).

38. Jackson AS, Pollock ML, Ward A. Generalized equations for predicting body density of women. Med Sci Sports Exerc. 1980;12:175–82.

39. Katch FI, McArdle WD. Prediction of body density from simple anthropometric measurements in college-age men and women. Hum Biol. 1973;45(3):445–55. (PubMed PMID: 4750412).

40. Wilmore JH, Behnke AR. An anthropometric estimation of body density and lean body weight in young men. J Appl Physiol. 1969;27(1):25–31. (PubMed PMID: 5786965).

41. Baumgartner RN, Heymsfield SB, Lichtman S, Wang J, Pierson RN Jr. Body composition in elderly people: effect of criterion estimates on predictive equations. Am J Clin Nutr. 1991;53(6):1345–53. (PubMed PMID: 2035461).

42. Deurenberg P, van der Kooy K, Leenen R, Weststrate JA, Seidell JC. Sex and age specific prediction formulas for estimating body composition from bioelectrical impedance: a cross-validation study. Int J Obes. 1991;15(1):17–25. (PubMed PMID: 2010255).

43. Segal KR, Gutin B, Presta E, Wang J, Van Itallie TB. Estimation of human body composition by electrical impedance methods: a comparative study. J Appl Physiol. 1985;58(5):1565–71. (PubMed PMID: 3997721).

44. Segal KR, Van Loan M, Fitzgerald PI, Hodgdon JA, Van Itallie TB. Lean body mass estimation by bioelectrical impedance analysis: a four-site cross-validation study. Am J Clin Nutr. 1988;47(1):7–14. (PubMed PMID: 3337041).

45. Siri WE. The gross composition of the body. Adv Biol. Med Phys. 1956;4:239–80. (PubMed PMID: 13354513).

46. Brozek J, Grande F, Anderson JT, Keys A. Densitometric analysis of body composition: revision of some quantitative assumptions. Ann NY Acad Sci. 1963;110:113–40.

47. Schutte JE, Townsend EJ, Hugg J, Shoup RF, Malina RM, Blomqvist CG. Density of lean body mass is greater in blacks than in whites. J Appl Physiol Respir Environ Exerc Physiol. 1984;56(6):1647–9. (PubMed PMID: 6735823).

48. Ortiz O, Russell M, Daley TL, Baumgartner RN, Waki M, Lichtman S, et al. Differences in skeletal muscle and bone mineral mass between black and white females and their relevance to estimates of body composition. Am J Clin Nutr. 1992;55(1):8–13.

49. Lohman TG. Human body composition. Champaign: Human Kinetics; 1996.

50. Selinger A. The body as a three component system. PhD thesis. Urbana: University of Illinois; 1977.

51. Heymsfield SB, Lichtman S, Baumgartner RN, Wang J, Kamen Y, Aliprantis A, Pierson RN Jr. Body composition of humans: comparison of two improved four-compartment models that differ in expense, technical complexity, and radiation exposure. Am J Clin Nutr. 1990;52(1):52–8. (PubMed PMID: 2360552).

52. Withers RT, Smith DA, Chatterton BE, Schultz CG, Gaffney RD. A comparison of four methods of estimating the body composition of male endurance athletes. Eur J Clin Nutr. 1992;46(11):773–84. (PubMed PMID: 1425531).

53. Demerath EW, Sun SS, Rogers N, Lee M, Reed D, Choh AC, Couch W, Czerwinski SA, Chumlea WC, Siervogel RM, Towne B. Anatomical patterning of visceral adipose tissue: race, sex, and age variation. Obesity (Silver Spring). 2007;15(12):2984–93. doi:10.1038/oby.2007.356. (PubMed PMID: 18198307; PubMed Central PMCID: PMC2883307).

54. Scheuer SH, Færch K, Philipsen A, Jørgensen ME, Johansen NB, Carstensen B, Witte DR, Andersen I, Lauritzen T, Andersen GS. Abdominal fat distribution and cardiovascular risk in men and women with different levels of glucose tolerance. J Clin Endocrinol Metab. 2015;100(9):3340–7 (JC20144479). ((Epub ahead of print) PubMed PMID: 26120787).

55. Mostoufi-Moab S, Magland J, Isaacoff EJ, Sun W, Rajapakse CS, Zemel B, Wehrli F, Shekdar K, Baker J, Long J, Leonard MB. Adverse fat depots and marrow adiposity are associated with skeletal deficits and insulin resistance in long-term survivors of pediatric hematopoietic stem cell transplantation. J Bone Miner Res. 2015. doi:10.1002/jbmr.2512. ((Epub ahead of print) PubMed PMID: 25801428).

56. Reyes-Vidal CM, Mojahed H, Shen W, Jin Z, Arias-Mendoza F, Fernandez JC, Gallagher D, Bruce JN, Post KD, Freda PU. Adipose tissue redistribution and ectopic lipid deposition in active acromegaly and effects of surgical treatment. J Clin Endocrinol Metab. 2015;100(8):2946–55 (jc20151917). ((Epub ahead of print) PubMed PMID: 26037515).

57. Karastergiou K, Smith SR, Greenberg AS, Fried SK, Sex differences in human adipose tissues—the biology of pear shape. Biol Sex Differ. 2012;3(1):13. doi:10.1186/2042-6410-3-13. (PubMed PMID: 22651247; PMCID: PMC3411490).

58. Lake JE, Wohl D, Scherzer R, Grunfeld C, Tien PC, Sidney S, Currier JS. Regional fat deposition and cardiovascular risk in HIV infection: the FRAM study. AIDS Care. 2011;23(8):929–38. doi:10.1080/09540121.2010.543885. (Epub 2011 Jun 24. PubMed PMID: 21767228; PubMed Central PMCID: PMC3249238).

59. Gujral UP, Narayan KM, Pradeepa RG, Deepa M, Ali MK, Anjana RM, Kandula NR, Mohan V, Kanaya AM. Comparing type 2 diabetes, prediabetes and their associated risk factors in Asian Indians in India and in the US: the CARRS and MASALA studies. Diabetes Care. 2015;38(7):1312–8. doi:10.2337/dc15-0032. (Epub 2015 Apr 15. PubMed PMID: 25877810; PubMed Central PMCID: PMC4477335).

60. Baldwin C. The effectiveness of nutritional interventions in malnutrition and cachexia. Proc Nutr Soc. 2015;19:1–8. ((Epub ahead of print) PubMed PMID: 26087760).

Physical Activity Measures

David R. Bassett and Kenneth M. Bielak

Abbreviations

ACT	Activity Counseling Trial
ACSM	American College of Sports Medicine
CDC	Centers for Disease Control and Prevention
DHHS	Department of Health and Human Services
EVS	Exercise vital sign
HCPs	Health-care professionals
NIH	National Institutes of Health
PACE	Physician-based Assessment and Counseling for Exercise
PAEE	Physical activity energy expenditure
PAR-Q	Physical Activity Readiness Questionnaire
TDEE	Total daily energy expenditure
USPSTF	US Preventative Services Task Force

Introduction

Physical inactivity is a major public health problem in the USA and other countries [1, 2]. In 2008, less than half of Americans obtained the recommended levels of physical activity [3, 4]. Regular physical activity is associated with decreased all-cause mortality, as well as decreased risks of developing obesity, diabetes, heart disease, stroke, dementia, and other chronic diseases [5]. Both epidemiological studies and randomized clinical trials point to the health benefits of acquiring rather modest volumes of moderate-intensity physical activity.

The 2008 Physical Activity Guidelines by the US Department of Health and Human Services (DHHS) recommended that all US adults should perform at least 150 min/week of moderate activity, 75 min of vigorous activity, or a combination of both [6]. In addition, the guidelines recommended that adults engage in 8–10 exercises that strengthen the major muscle groups, on 2 days/week. For US youth (ages 6–19 years), the guidelines recommended 60 min/day of aerobic activity to include muscle-strengthening and bone-building activities [6].

Physical Activity Counseling in Primary Care

Physicians and other health-care professionals (HCPs) can encourage their patients to become more physically active. In 2012, 84 % of Americans visited a physician, with most of them having 1–3 health-care visits [7]. Therefore, physician-administered advice to engage in physical activity could have a broad population reach that would benefit the public health. However, only a small percentage of patients report that their primary care doctor counseled them on exercise [8].

The notion that physicians and other HCPs should counsel their patients to exercise has been around for a long time. In 1992, the Centers for Disease Control and Prevention (CDC) established a collaborative agreement with San Diego State University to develop a Physician-based Assessment and Counseling for Exercise (PACE) program. This was found to be feasible in clinical practice [9] and tested for efficacy in a 6-week intervention [10]. Twenty-seven physicians were randomly assigned to an intervention or control group. The intervention group delivered 3–5 min of counseling to their patients; 2 weeks later, a health educator followed up with a phone call. The effects of the program on physical activity were mixed; the intervention group reported greater increases in leisure-time walking than the control group, but not total walking.

In the late 1990s, the Activity Counseling Trial (ACT) was funded by the National Institutes of Health (NIH) to test the effectiveness of patient education and counseling in the primary care setting [11]. ACT was a 2-month randomized

D. R. Bassett (✉)
Department of Kinesiology, Recreation, and Sport Sciences, University of Tennessee, 1914 Andy Holt Ave., Knoxville, TN 37996, USA
e-mail: dbassett@utk.edu

K. M. Bielak
Department of Family Medicine, University of Tennessee Medical Center, Knoxville, TN, USA

© Springer International Publishing Switzerland 2016
J. I. Mechanick, R. F. Kushner (eds.), *Lifestyle Medicine,* DOI 10.1007/978-3-319-24687-1_8

controlled trial comparing three groups: two patient education and counseling groups ("assistance" and "counseling") and a control group receiving standard care ("advice"). Although nearly all physicians performed the counseling and most rated the acceptability as high [12], the results showed that neither of the counseling interventions increased physical activity levels more than standard care.

Other studies have examined physician counseling for exercise. Some of these studies showed improvements in physical activity, while others did not [13]. A comprehensive review of these studies by the US Preventative Services Task Force (USPSTF) concluded that there was insufficient evidence that physician counseling increased patients' activity levels [14]. A recent review by Tulloch et al. [13] found that only 50% of interventions delivered by physicians were effective at increasing physical activity, while 71–100% of interventions delivered by other allied health professionals were effective. Despite conflicting results on the effectiveness of physical activity counseling in primary care settings, the importance of active lifestyles for promoting health and wellness is well documented [15]. Thus, various groups have worked to reduce the barriers to physician counseling and to improve the effectiveness of these programs.

Exercise Is Medicine

In 2007, the "Exercise is Medicine" program was launched by the American Medical Association and American College of Sports Medicine (ACSM). It was designed to encourage physicians to record physical activity as a vital sign during each office visit. Patients who were able to exercise were encouraged to perform at least 30 min of aerobic activity and 10 min of stretching and muscle strengthening exercise per day. The program increased awareness of tools that physicians can use in counseling their patients about exercise, as well as assessing physical activity and fitness. The *Physical Activity as a Vital Sign* survey is a validated instrument that has been shown to increase the number of patients who have their physical activity assessed [16] (Table 8.1). Furthermore, the use of an exercise vital sign (EVS) results in more patients receiving counseling from their physicians [17] (Table 8.2). The *Stages of Exercise Behavior Change* survey [18] allows respondents to select one of five possible choices that reflect attitudes toward exercise. They

Table 8.1 Physical activity as a vital sign. (From: Greenwood JL, Joy EA, and Stanford JB. The physical activity vital sign: a primary care tool to guide counseling for obesity. *Journal of Physical Activity and Health*. 2010: 7(5):571–576)

How many *days during the past week* have you performed physical activity where your heart beats faster and your breathing is harder than normal for 30 min or more?
How many *days in a typical week* do you perform activity such as this?

are then classified into one of the following categories: (1) precontemplation, (2) contemplation, (3) initiation, (4) action, and (5) maintenance. The *Physical Activity Readiness Questionnaire (PAR-Q)* can be used to gauge the safety of exercise prior to starting a program. Exercise is Medicine also includes tools that simplify the process of prescribing exercise to patients; otherwise, doctors can refer patients to an exercise physiologist.

The barriers to physician and other HCP counseling include time constraints, lack of incentives and reimbursement, lack of standard protocols, inadequate training in behavioral counseling, lack of success in the counseling role, and the absence of a coordinated and systematic approach in practice [19]. In addition, general practitioners who are inactive themselves are about one third as likely to promote exercise to their patients compared to those who are active [19]. Tools have been developed to assist doctors in overcoming barriers, but the time demands on busy primary care doctors are still a barrier.

While exercise advice can be dispensed in a few minutes, behavioral counseling is a more complicated process requiring multiple office visits. The 5 As (assess, advise, agree, assist, and arrange) model has been shown to be effective for smoking cessation and can also be applied to physical activity promotion [20, 21]. However, many physicians and other HCPs do not always have time to do this during routine office visits. This has led researchers to ask if a less intensive approach (i.e., a pedometer + daily step goal + activity log + subsequent follow-up) can succeed in getting inactive patients to increase their steps per day.

Table 8.2 Exercise vital sign survey. (From: Sallis R. Exercise is medicine: a call to action for physicians to assess and prescribe exercise. *Physician and Sportsmedicine*. 2014; 43(1):23–26)

On average, how many days per week do you engage in moderate-to-vigorous physical activity like a brisk walk?
On those days, how many minutes do you engage in physical activity at this level?

Using Pedometers to Encourage Physical Activity in Patients

Recent studies conducted in primary care settings over the past 5–10 years have shown that pedometers are effective in motivating sedentary patients to be more physically active. These pedometer interventions fall into one of the two categories: randomized clinical trials (including one or more control groups of some type) or quasi-experimental studies lacking a control group. Randomized clinical trials are generally considered to provide stronger evidence of health outcomes. However, in these studies, since the control group lacked pedometer-determined steps per day, the studies had to rely on self-reported physical activity based on questionnaires. One study, however, did use an objective monitor capable of recording steps, in addition to the pedometer, and found that the intervention group had significantly greater improvements (2100 steps per day) as compared to controls [22]. Other studies examining pedometer use in primary care settings have not included a control group or did not perform between-group comparisons on steps. In general, those studies find that the use of a pedometer + daily step goal + activity log (with subsequent follow-up by the physician or other HCPs) resulted in an increase of approximately 2500 steps per day [23–25]. These findings are generally consistent with other studies that have examined pedometer programs, conducted in different settings [26].

Physical Activity Monitors

In the next section, we will discuss some devices that are used to track physical activity in patients. In many cases, pedometers can provide accurate enough data to be used in clinical practice, and the preferred metric is "steps." For more detailed information, researchers and practitioners may select a more expensive, research-grade physical activity monitor that stores second-by-second data on physical activity over several weeks. Such high-tech devices can be used to track the pattern of activity throughout the day (i.e., the frequency, intensity, and duration of exercise bouts), physical activity energy expenditure (PAEE), and other variables.

Spring-Levered Pedometers

The simplest device for assessing physical activity is the pedometer. Worn on the belt or waistband, a pedometer counts the number of steps taken throughout the day. Most pedometers use a spring-suspended horizontal lever arm that moves up and down in response to vertical accelerations of the body that occur when walking or running. The most accurate and reliable spring-levered pedometer is the Yamax Digi-Walker SW-200 (Yamasa Corp., Tokyo, Japan) (Fig. 8.1). This model only displays steps and has a reset button to re-zero the steps at the end of the day. The retail cost is approximately $20.

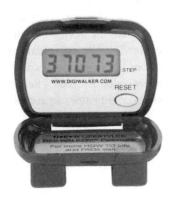

Fig. 8.1 Yamax SW-200 spring-levered pedometer. (Figure courtesy of Dr. Teresa Vollenweider)

The Yamax Digi-Walker is accurate to within +3% for walking speeds of 3 mph and faster with high reliability [27, 28]. This pedometer is designed to avoid double counting of steps during brisk walking or running. For these reasons, the Yamax Digi-Walker is the most widely used pedometer in research and clinical settings. However, two limitations of the device are that it undercounts steps in obese individuals since it does not work as well when tilted on the belt, and it undercounts steps at slow walking speeds, recording about 75% of steps at 2 mph and 50% of steps at 1 mph [29].

When using pedometers to prescribe exercise, it important to use an accurate pedometer. To perform a quick check on accuracy, have the patient put on the pedometer, re-zero it, and take 20 steps in a hallway. The pedometer should record within 1–2 steps of the 20. Written instructions should be given [30]:

- The pedometer should be worn at all times except when bathing or in bed.
- We want you to record the total number of steps you take each day.
- As soon as you wake up each morning, put the step counter on your clothing and wear it all day.
- Just before you go to bed at night, please remove the pedometer, write down the number of steps for that day (in your activity log), and then re-zero the pedometer.
- Repeat the procedure the next day.

The following categories can be used to classify pedometer-determined steps per day in healthy adults: sedentary lifestyle (5000 steps per day), 5000–7499 steps per day (low active), 7500–9999 steps per day (somewhat active), 10,000–12,499 steps per day (active), 12,500 or more steps per day (highly active) [31]. The ACSM advises that patients who take at least 8000 steps per day are likely to meet the national recommendation of 30 min of physical activity per day.

Since there is day-to-day variability in step counts, it takes about 1 week to get a reliable measure of a person's steps per day. Thus, patients should be instructed to wear the pedometer for a week as they go about their daily activities in order to determine their baseline value. Then, they should be given a goal for increasing daily step counts. The goal can either be to increase their daily steps by a certain amount above baseline (e.g., 3000 steps, which is roughly equivalent to 30 min of walking and 1.5 miles) or to achieve a total daily step count that is known to have health benefits (e.g., 10,000 steps). Alternatively, patients can be allowed to self-select goals that they feel are achievable given their medical conditions. Since a cadence of 100 steps per minute is roughly equivalent to 3 metabolic equivalent (METs), this can be helpful in ensuring that the intensity is in the moderate-to-vigorous range. In addition to the pedometer and daily step goal, it is important for participants to log their steps so that they can see their improvement, referred to as

Fig. 8.2 Omron HJ-720 ITC, a pedometer with piezoelectric accelerometer internal mechanism. (Figure courtesy of Omron Healthcare, Inc.)

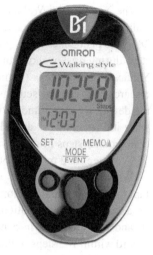

Fig. 8.3 ActiGraph Link physical activity monitor. An example of an accelerometer-based wearable monitor used in research. (Figure courtesy of ActiGraph, LLC)

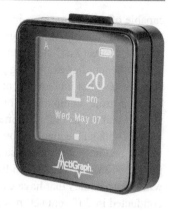

self-monitoring. Asking patients to show their activity logs to the HCP provides a level of accountability and an opportunity to discuss it at the next office visit.

Piezoelectric Data-Storing Pedometers

A new type of pedometer uses an accelerometer for step counting, rather than a mechanical device. The internal mechanism uses a piezoelectric material that responds to acceleration; steps are registered by counting the number of acceleration peaks or zero-crossings. These devices are far more accurate than spring-levered pedometers in individuals with obesity. Thus, they are a good choice for patients who carry excess weight. Piezoelectric pedometers still have the problem of not detecting all steps at slow walking speeds; however, the errors are not as great as with the previous generation of pedometers.

The New-Lifestyles NL-1000 (New-Lifestyles, Lees Summit, MO; $55), Omron HJ-720ITC (Omron Healthcare, Lake Forest, IL; $40), and FitBit Zip (FitBit, Inc., San Francisco, CA; $59) are examples of accelerometer-based pedometers. These devices have good validity for step counting. Another advantage is that they can store data in memory. The New-Lifestyles pedometer can store 8 days in 1-day epochs; the Omron can store 41 days in 1-hour epochs (Fig. 8.2). With the New-Lifestyles pedometer, the data must be retrieved manually by scrolling back through the days; however, the Omron and FitBit allow data to be downloaded to a computer in the home or clinic, or they can be transferred to the patient's laptop or smartphone and uploaded to a website. An advantage of these two data-storing pedometers is that they do not rely on patients to log their steps, and besides, clinicians can obtain a more accurate picture of the patient's activity. In addition, both Omron Healthcare, Inc. (www.Omronfitness.com) and FitBit (www.Fitabase.com) have developed web-based platforms to simplify data management for tracking large numbers of individuals.

Accelerometers

The ActiGraph GT3X+ (ActiGraph, LLC, Pensacola, FL) is the most widely used triaxial accelerometer-based activity monitor in research; the newest generation is called the ActiGraph Link (Fig. 8.3). Other similar devices include the Actiwatch (Phillips Healthcare, Andover, MA), GENEActiv (ActivInsights, Kimbolton, UK), and RT3 (Stayhealthy, Inc., London, UK). The ActiGraph was introduced more than 20 years ago, and although successive generations have become smaller/lighter and the memory capacity has been expanded, the device output has remained relatively stable over time. The ActiGraph has good reliability [32] and technical validity [33]. The ActiGraph measures body acceleration, filters the raw data, and integrates it to yield a metric called "activity counts per minute." The researcher then applies activity count cut points that categorize each minute of the day into sedentary, light, moderate, or vigorous activity. Barriers to the use of this device in clinical practice include high cost ($225 each + $1495 for ActiLife research software) and labor-intensive procedures for processing the data after they are collected.

The ActiGraph Study Admin Portal was developed in 2014 to facilitate the use of the ActiGraph GT3X+ in clinical trials. This was introduced in 2014 to simplify data management for medical researchers who wish to conduct single or multicenter trials while standardizing the data and making the data postprocessing invisible to the user. An overall study coordinator works with the company to design the study protocol, then site coordinators are trained in the protocol (e.g., initialization of the devices, placement site on the patient, and length of the observation period). After the data are collected, the device is connected to a computer by a USB cable. The site coordinator uploads data to a cloud-based server where postprocessing occurs automatically. Each site coordinator can access the data collected at their site and the study coordinator can access all of the data.

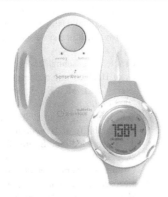

Fig. 8.4 SenseWear Armband Pro 3 activity monitor; it uses acceleration, skin temperature, heat flux, and galvanic skin response to estimate energy expenditure (kcal/day). (© Image courtesy of BodyMedia, Inc.)

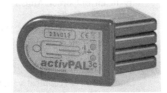

Fig. 8.5 activPAL wearable monitor, designed for detecting posture and physical activity. (Figure courtesy of PAL Technologies Ltd.)

SenseWear Armband

The SenseWear Pro3 Armband (BodyMedia, Inc., Pittsburgh, PA) is a new physical activity monitor that provides data on steps and caloric expenditure (Fig. 8.4). This multisensor device is worn on the upper arm, over the triceps muscle, and measures acceleration, skin temperature, heat flux, and galvanic skin response. The cost of the device is $500, display $100, and software $2500.

A unique feature of the SenseWear Armband is the use of "machine learning" algorithms to estimate energy expenditure [34]. As a result, the SenseWear Armband is currently one of the most accurate devices on the market for estimating the rate of caloric burn in various activities [35, 36]. It has been validated for total daily energy expenditure (TDEE) and PAEE over 2 weeks, with favorable comparisons to the doubly labeled water technique [37]. The SenseWear Armband has been used in a study of energy balance: When combined with a group weight loss program, armband use is associated with significant weight loss over 9 months [38].

activPAL

The activPAL (PAL Technologies Ltd., Glasgow, Scotland) is a device worn on the thigh that detects the amount of time that is spent lying/sitting, standing, and ambulating (Fig. 8.5). The mechanism is a triaxial accelerometer that senses not only dynamic acceleration due to body movements but also static acceleration due to gravity. From the latter, it can detect the angle of inclination of the thigh, allowing it to discriminate between sitting/lying and standing. The cost of the device is $519 + $770 for the docking station

and software. The activPAL is very accurate for detecting the amount of time spent in various body positions [39].

Conclusions

Primary care HCPs can provide advice or counseling to their patients regarding physical activity. Unfortunately, there is still a lack of consensus on the efficacy of physical activity counseling, in part, due to differences in study designs, implementation, and patient populations. Simple, brief questionnaires can be used to assess where a patient stands regarding exercise. These include *Physical Activity as a Vital Sign, PAR-Q,* and *Stages of Exercise Behavior Change.* Recent studies conducted in primary care settings indicate that using pedometers (in conjunction with a daily step goal, activity log, and follow-up) may be helpful in encouraging patients to increase their levels of physical activity, leading to more active and healthier lifestyles. Other types of more sophisticated activity monitors can provide further data in research settings. Time constraints are a significant barrier to the implementation of physical activity counseling in primary care, although pedometer-based programs focused on daily step goals may help motivate patients and increase adherence.

References

1. Hallal PC, Andersen LB, Bull FC, Guthold R, Haskell W, Ekelund U. Global physical activity levels: surveillance progress, pitfalls, and prospects. Lancet. 2012;380(9838):247–57. Epub 2012/07/24.

2. Lee IM, Shiroma EJ, Lobelo F, Puska P, Blair SN, Katzmarzyk PT. Effect of physical inactivity on major non-communicable diseases worldwide: an analysis of burden of disease and life expectancy. Lancet. 2012;380(9838):219–29. Epub 2012/07/24.

3. Carlson SA, Fulton JE, Schoenborn CA, Loustalot F. Trend and prevalence estimates based on the 2008 physical activity guidelines for Americans. Am J Prev Med. 2010;39(4):305–13. Epub 2010/09/15.

4. Song M, Carroll DD, Fulton JE. Meeting the 2008 physical activity guidelines for Americans among U.S. youth. Am J Prev Med. 2013;44(3):216–22. Epub 2013/02/19.

5. Physical Activity Guidelines Advisory Committee. Physical activity guidelines advisory committee report 2008. Washington, DC: U.S. Department of Health and Human Services; 2008.

6. U.S. Department of Health and Human Services. 2008 physical activity guidelines for Americans. 2008. http://www.health.gov/PAGuidelines/Report/Default.aspx. Accessed 7 Nov 2010. (61)

7. U.S. Department of Health and Human Services. Health, United States. 2013. With special feature on death and dying. http://www.cdc.gov/nchs/hus.htm. Accessed 24 June 2014.

8. Wee CC, McCarthy EP, Davis RB, Phillips RS. Physician counseling about exercise. JAMA. 1999;282(16):1583–8. Epub 1999/11/05.

9. Long BJ, Calfas KJ, Wooten W, Sallis JF, Patrick K, Goldstein M, et al. A multisite field test of the acceptability of physical activity

counseling in primary care: project PACE. Am J Prev Med. 1996;12(2):73–81. Epub 1996/03/01.

10. Calfas KJ, Long BJ, Sallis JF, Wooten WJ, Pratt M, Patrick K. A controlled trial of physician counseling to promote the adoption of physical activity. Prev Med. 1996;25(3):225–33. Epub 1996/05/01.

11. Writing Group for the Activity Counseling Trial Research Group. Effects of physical activity counseling in primary care: The Activity Counseling Trial: a randomized controlled trial. JAMA. 2001;286(6):677–87. Epub 2001/08/10.

12. Albright CL, Cohen S, Gibbons L, Miller S, Marcus B, Sallis J, et al. Incorporating physical activity advice into primary care: physician-delivered advice within the activity counseling trial. Am J Prev Med. 2000;18(3):225–34. Epub 2000/03/21.

13. Tulloch H, Fortier M, Hogg W. Physical activity counseling in primary care: who has and who should be counseling? Patient Educ Couns. 2006;64(1–3):6–20. Epub 2006/02/14.

14. Eden KB, Orleans CT, Mulrow CD, Pender NJ, Teutsch SM. Does counseling by clinicians improve physical activity? A summary of the evidence for the U.S. Preventive Services Task Force. Ann Intern Med. 2002;137(3):208–15. Epub 2002/08/06.

15. Peterson JA. Get moving! Physical activity counseling in primary care. J Am Acad Nurse Pract. 2007;19(7):349–57. Epub 2007/08/08.

16. Sallis RE, Coleman KJ. Self-reported exercise in patients using an exercise vital sign (abstract). Med Sci Sports Exerc. 2011;43(5):376.

17. Grant RW, Schmittdiel JA, Neugebauer RS, Uratsu CS, Sternfeld B. Exercise as a vital sign: a quasi-experimental analysis of a health system intervention to collect patient-reported exercise levels. J Gen Intern Med. 2014;29(2):341–8. Epub 2013/12/07.

18. Marcus BH, Simkin LR. The stages of exercise behavior. J Sports Med Phys Fitness. 1993;33:83–8.

19. McKenna J, Naylor PJ, McDowell N. Barriers to physical activity promotion by general practitioners and practice nurses. Br J Sports Med. 1998;32(3):242–7. Epub 1998/10/17.

20. Meriwether RA, Lee JA, LaFleur AS, Wiseman P. Physical activity counseling. Am Fam Physician. 2008;77(8):1129–36.

21. Whitlock EP, Orleans CT, Pender N, Allan J. Evaluating primary care behavioral counseling interventions: an evidence-based approach. Am J Prev Med. 2002;22(4):267–84. Epub 2002/05/04.

22. Mutrie N, Doolin O, Fitzsimons CF, Grant PM, Granat M, Grealy M, et al. Increasing older adults' walking through primary care: results of a pilot randomized controlled trial. Fam Pract. 2012;29(6):633–42. Epub 2012/07/31.

23. McKay J, Wright A, Lowry R, Steele K, Ryde G, Mutrie N. Walking on prescription: the utility of a pedometer pack for increasing physical activity in primary care. Patient Educ Couns. 2009;76(1):71–6. Epub 2008/12/23.

24. Sherman BJ, Gilliland G, Speckman JL, Freund KM. The effect of a primary care exercise intervention for rural women. Prev Med. 2007;44(3):198–201. Epub 2006/12/23.

25. Stovitz SD, VanWormer JJ, Center BA, Bremer KL. Pedometers as a means to increase ambulatory activity for patients seen at a family medicine clinic. J Am Board Fam Pract. 2005;18(5):335–43. Epub 2005/09/09.

26. Bravata DM, Smith-Spangler C, Sundaram V, Gienger AL, Lin N, Lewis R, et al. Using pedometers to increase physical activity and improve health: a systematic review. JAMA. 2007;298(19):2296–304.

27. Crouter SE, Schneider PL, Karabulut M, Bassett DR Jr. Validity of 10 electronic pedometers for measuring steps, distance, and energy cost. Med Sci Sports Exerc. 2003;35(8):1455–60. Epub 2003/08/06.

28. Schneider PL, Crouter SE, Lukajic O, Bassett DR Jr. Accuracy and reliability of 10 pedometers for measuring steps over a 400-m walk. Med Sci Sports Exerc. 2003;35(10):1779–84. Epub 2003/10/03.

29. Crouter SE, Schneider PL, Bassett DR Jr. Spring-levered versus piezo-electric pedometer accuracy in overweight and obese adults. Med Sci Sports Exerc. 2005;37(10):1673–9. Epub 2005/11/02.

30. Bassett DR, Schneider PL, Huntington GE. Physical activity in an old order Amish community. Med Sci Sports Exerc. 2004;36(1):79–85.

31. Tudor-Locke CE, Bassett DR. How many steps are enough? Pedometer-determined physical activity indices. Sports Med. 2004;34(1):1–8.

32. Santos-Lozano A, Marin PJ, Torres-Luque G, Ruiz JR, Lucia A, Garatachea N. Technical variability of the GT3X accelerometer. Med Eng Phys. 2012;34(6):787–90. Epub 2012/03/16.

33. John D, Sasaki J, Staudenmayer J, Mavilia M, Freedson PS. Comparison of raw acceleration from the GENEA and ActiGraph GT3X + activity monitors. Sens Basel Sens. 2013;13(11):14754–63. Epub 2013/11/02.

34. Ball TJ, Joy EA, Goh TL, Hannon JC, Gren LH, Shaw JM. Validity of two brief primary care physical activity questionnaires with accelerometry in clinic staff. Prim Health Care Res Dev. 2015;16:100–8. Epub 2014/01/30.

35. Crouter SE, Churilla JR, Bassett DR Jr. Estimating energy expenditure using accelerometers. Eur J Appl Physiol. 2006;98(6):601–12. Epub 2006/10/24.

36. Dudley P, Bassett DR, John D, Crouter SE. Validity of an armband physical activity monitor in measuring energy expenditure during eighteen different activities. J Obes Wt Loss Ther. 2012; 2(7):146. [Internet]

37. Johannsen DL, Calabro MA, Stewart J, Franke W, Rood JC, Welk GJ. Accuracy of armband monitors for measuring daily energy expenditure in healthy adults. Med Sci Sports Exerc. 2010;42(11):2134–40.

38. Shuger SL, Barry VW, Sui X, McClain A, Hand GA, Wilcox S, et al. Electronic feedback in a diet- and physical activity-based lifestyle intervention for weight loss: a randomized controlled trial. Int J Behav Nutr Phys Act. 2011;8:41. Epub 2011/05/20.

39. Kozey-Keadle S, Libertine A, Lyden K, Staudenmayer J, Freedson P. Validation of wearable monitors for assessing sedentary behavior. Med Sci Sports Exerc. 2011;43(8):1561–7.

Metabolic Profiles—Based on the 2013 Prevention Guidelines

9

Neil J. Stone, John Wilkins and Sakina Kazmi

Abbreviations

ABI	Ankle Brachial Index
ACC-AHA	American College of Cardiology-American Heart Association
ASCVD	Atherosclerotic cardiovascular disease
CAC	Coronary artery calcium
CI	Confidence interval
cIMT	Carotid intima-media thickness
CHD	Coronary heart disease
CKD	Chronic kidney disease
CVD	Cardiovascular disease
DPP	Diabetes Prevention Program
GFR	Glomerular filtration rate
HDL-C	High-density lipoprotein cholesterol
IDL	Intermediate-density lipoprotein
LDL-C	Low-density lipoprotein cholesterol
MetS	Metabolic syndrome
MESA	Multi-Ethnic Study of Atherosclerosis
NHANES	National Health and Nutrition Examination Surveys
NMR	Nuclear magnetic resonance
PAD	Peripheral artery disease
RR	Relative risk
T2D	Type-2 diabetes
TG	Triglycerides
TOS	The Obesity Society
VLDL	Very low-density lipoprotein

Introduction

This chapter reviews the utility of measuring biometric parameters as they relate to the practice of lifestyle medicine and estimating risk for type-2 diabetes (T2D) and atherosclerotic cardiovascular disease (ASCVD). All of the new 2013 American College of Cardiology-American Heart Association (ACC-AHA) Prevention Guidelines emphasize the key role of lifestyle in the prevention of ASCVD [1–3]. The 2013 AHA/ACC Guideline on Lifestyle Management to Reduce Cardiovascular Risk, as the title implies, provides evidence-based lifestyle recommendations for those who need to lower low-density lipoprotein cholesterol (LDL-C) and/or elevated blood pressure [1]. The 2013 AHA/ACC/The Obesity Society (TOS) Guideline for the Management of Overweight and Obesity in Adults addresses lifestyle issues related to those with excess weight and obesity [2]. The 2013 ACC/AHA Guideline on the Assessment of Cardiovascular Risk presented a 30-year or lifetime ASCVD risk estimation on the basis of traditional risk factors for adults aged 20–59 years who are free from ASCVD and not at high short-term risk [3]. This guideline noted that this long-term and lifetime risk information was most appropriate to motivate improved lifestyle change in younger individuals aged 20–59 years. Finally, the 2013 ACC/AHA Guideline on the Treatment of Blood Cholesterol to Reduce Atherosclerotic Cardiovascular Risk in Adults specifically noted: "It must be emphasized that lifestyle modification (i.e., adhering to a heart-healthy diet, regular exercise habits, avoidance of tobacco products, and maintenance of a healthy weight) remains a crucial component of health promotion and ASCVD risk reduction, both

N. J. Stone (✉)
Feinberg School of Medicine, Northwestern University, 676 N. St. Clair, Suite 600, Chicago, IL 60611, USA
e-mail: n-stone@northwestern.edu

J. Wilkins
Department of Preventive Medicine, Feinberg School of Medicine, Northwestern University, Chicago, IL, USA

J. Wilkins · S. Kazmi
Department of Cardiology, Feinberg School of Medicine, Northwestern University, Chicago, IL, USA

© Springer International Publishing Switzerland 2016
J. I. Mechanick, R. F. Kushner (eds.), *Lifestyle Medicine,* DOI 10.1007/978-3-319-24687-1_9

Table 9.1 Metabolic syndrome factors in 2013 Guidelines

Metabolic factors	2013 AHA/ACC Guideline on Lifestyle Management to Reduce Cardiovascular Risk	2013 AHA/ACC/TOS Guideline for the Management of Over-weight and Obesity in Adults	2013 ACC/AHA Guideline on the Assessment of Cardiovascular Risk
Waist circumference[a]	N/A	Advised measuring waist circumference (expert opinion)	Not a variable in ASCVD risk estimator
Elevated TG	TG decreased when *trans* fats were replaced by MUFA/PUFA; TG also reduced by resistive exercise	Sustained weight loss of 3–5% is likely to result in clinically meaningful reductions in TG	Not a variable in ASCVD risk estimator
Low HDL-C	HDL-C raised when *trans* fatty acids were replaced by MUFA/PUFA/SF; also raised by aerobic exercise	Greater amounts of weight loss will improve HDL-C	Variable in ASCVD risk estimator
Systolic blood pressure (BP)	Recommends lifestyle changes to lower BP	Greater amounts of weight loss will improve BP	Variable in ASCVD risk estimator
Elevated blood glucose	N/A	Sustained weight loss of 3–5% is likely to result in clinically meaningful reductions in glucose, A1C, and risk of diabetes	Variable in ASCVD risk estimator

AHA American Heart Association, *ACC* American College of Cardiology, *TOS* The Obesity Society, *N/A* not applicable, *ASCVD* atherosclerotic cardiovascular disease, *TG* triglycerides, *MUFA* monounsaturated fatty acids, *PUFA* polyunsaturated fatty acids, *HDL-C* high-density lipoprotein cholesterol, *SF* saturated fatty acids
[a] Cutoff points are population specific and country specific

prior to and in concert with the use of cholesterol-lowering drug therapies." [4].

Metabolic Syndrome

Some critics of the new guidelines noted that metabolic syndrome (MetS) and other biomarkers of use in clinical practice were not recommended for the basic treatment algorithm. Adult Treatment Panel III put the concept of the "metabolic syndrome" in sharp focus as a crucial consideration for those in need of therapeutic lifestyle change [5]. Three or more of the following clinical metabolic parameters are required for diagnosis: waist circumference, elevated triglycerides (TG), low high-density lipoprotein cholesterol (HDL-C), elevated blood sugar, or elevated blood pressure. One strong advantage of MetS was its ability to identify metabolic factors that improve with lifestyle change [6]. Although the MetS construct predicts T2D and coronary heart disease (CHD), there have been calls for definitive trials to see if MetS independently predicts CHD [7]. The obesity guideline provides an evidence base to understand improvements in MetS risk factors that occur with lifestyle changes [2]. Table 9.1 lists some of the traditional risk variables included in the pooled cohort equations and the overlap with variables of the MetS. Furthermore, both lifestyle and obesity/overweight recommendations discuss exercise, diet, and weight management strategies that improve MetS variables.

Biomarkers to Inform ASCVD Clinician–Patient Risk Discussion

The 2013 ACC/AHA Guideline on the Assessment of Cardiovascular Risk noted four variables that could inform a risk decision when a quantitative risk decision was uncertain. These variables were chosen to improve discrimination, calibration, and net reclassification criteria; in other words, they can serve as "tie-breakers" when a risk decision is uncertain based on traditional risk factors. These variables included:

- Family history of premature ASCVD
- Coronary artery calcium (CAC) score ≥300 Agatston units or ≥75th percentile (from Multi-Ethnic Study of Atherosclerosis (MESA) based on age, race, and sex; see http://www.mesa-nhlbi.org/CACReference.aspx)
- High-sensitivity C-reactive protein (hs-CRP) ≥2.0 mg/L
- Ankle brachial index (ABI; Table 9.2)

Premature parental onset of cardiovascular disease (CVD) is defined as the incidence of a CVD event before the age of 55 years among first-degree male relatives and before the age of 65 years among first-degree female relatives [3]. Family history of premature CVD is observed to be an independent predictor of CVD risk, partially due to the fact that several risk factors of CVD, including dyslipidemia, T2D obesity, and hypertension, are genetically linked [8]. However, the link between family history of premature CVD and CVD risk is still present even after adjusting for traditional risk factors [8, 9]. The link is substantial; approximately 75% of patients with a premature CVD event have a family history of premature CVD [10, 11]. Yet, in a study including data from the

Table 9.2 Variables chosen by the Risk Assessment Guideline to improve discrimination, calibration, and net reclassification criteria

Measured variable	Criteria
Family history of premature ASCVD	First-degree relatives with premature CVD: male <55; female <65
hs-CRP	≥2.0 mg/L
CAC score	≥300 Agatston units or ≥75th percentile based on age, sex, and ethnicity (MESA calculator)
ABI	<0.9

For additional information, see http://www.mesa-nhlbi.org/CACReference.aspx

ABI ankle brachial index, *ASCVD* atherosclerotic cardiovascular disease, *CAC* coronary artery calcium, *CVD* cardiovascular disease, *hs-CRP* high-sensitivity C-reactive protein, *MESA* Multi-Ethnic Study of Atherosclerosis

Framingham parental and offspring cohorts, researchers observed that inclusion of family history with the traditional risk assessment increased risk among offspring who were at intermediate risk owing to borderline cholesterol and blood pressure levels [9]. Consideration of family history of premature CVD added little value for those at very low or very high risk.

High CAC scores are associated with CVD, and the addition of CAC scores to existing risk assessment models has shown to predict increased CVD risk beyond the traditional risk factors. MESA indicated improvement of the "c-statistic," an index of the ability of the prediction model to discriminate future cases from non-cases, from 0.79 to 0.83 with inclusion of CAC to the Framingham risk assessment model [8]. The Framingham risk score utilized age, sex, blood pressure, blood pressure treatment status, tobacco usage, cholesterol, and HDL-C. In this sense, it differed from the pooled cohort equations used by the 2013 ACC-AHA Prevention Guidelines. They used CVD (heart attack and stroke) as endpoints and also utilized diabetes in the model. Relative risk (RR) for CVD events increases with higher CAC burden [8], even among patients at low ASCVD risk [12]. However, the addition of CAC to traditional risk factors has conferred the most improvement to risk prediction among asymptomatic individuals with intermediate risk [12]. Patients at intermediate risk of ASCVD have also been viewed as the target population for which CAC scores may be considered by the 2013 Risk Assessment Guideline [3].

ABI involves a simple clinical assessment to diagnose peripheral artery disease (PAD) and has been linked to future CVD events [8]. ABI has shown limited added value to traditional risk models of ASCVD for asymptomatic patients. However, the net reclassification improvement of adding ABI might be more pertinent to and higher for patients of older age and/or patients with intermediate ASCVD risk [13].

hs-CRP is an extensively studied serum biomarker of CHD risk. Although currently available data do not support that hs-CRP is in the causal pathway of CHD events [14], elevated levels of hs-CRP have a robust, independent association with CHD risk. Using meta-analytic techniques, Buckely et al. [15] reported an RR of 1.58 (95% confidence interval (CI) 1.37–1.85) for the highest quartile to the lowest quartiles of hs-CRP. Although these associations are robust, adding hs-CRP as another variable in the traditional Framingham risk equations results in a modest, at best, increase in the c-statistic, indicating that hs-CRP value in the population-wide

assessment of CHD risk in asymptomatic patients may be limited [16–18]. However, in patients at clinical thresholds for treatment, hs-CRP may be helpful at reclassifying people to a treatment or nontreatment group [19]. Furthermore, in the Justification for the Use of Statins in Prevention: an Intervention Trial Evaluating Rosuvastatin (JUPITER) study [20], individuals with hs-CRP ≥2.0 mg/L who were overweight, prehypertensive, with modest dyslipidemia (41% had MetS), and were treated with 20 mg rosuvastatin per day had a nearly 50% reduction in the risk for CHD, stroke, and revascularization compared to individuals who were on placebo. It should be noted, however, that this trial was a primary prevention trial of rosuvastatin, not a trial designed to test the clinical utility of checking hs-CRP, as there was no "normal" CRP arm. In light of these data, hs-CRP may be a useful marker when an individual's risk assessment is deemed insufficient to make a risk decision about statin treatment.

Additional Biomarkers Considered for ASCVD Risk Estimator

The 2013 ACC/AHA Guideline on the Assessment of Cardiovascular Risk carefully discussed evidence for not recommending variables such as apolipoprotein B100 (ApoB), glomerular filtration rate (GFR), microalbuminuria, carotid intima-media thickness (cIMT), and cardiorespiratory fitness. However, there exists concern over the exclusion of these variables. The Risk Assessment Guideline specifically asked a critical question: "What is the evidence with regard to reclassification or contribution to risk assessment when hs-CRP, ApoB, GFR, microalbuminuria, family history, cardiorespiratory fitness, ABI, CAC, or cIMT are considered in addition to the variables that are in the traditional risk scores?" To determine if these risk factors should be added to the traditional assessment when a quantitative assessment of ASCVD risk is uncertain, the risk assessment working group considered availability, cost, assay reliability, and direct and indirect (downstream) adverse effects of testing [21]. It should be noted that risk markers such as ApoB, microalbuminuria, cardiorespiratory fitness, and cIMT could not be evaluated in creating the pooled cohort equations due to the absence of data or lack of inclusion in the appropriate examination cycle of one or more of the cohorts studied. Moreover, unlike the other risk factors listed above, the above risk markers were not recommended as potential adjuncts to quantitative risk estimation. This was not arbitrary. The panel evaluated the degree to which each of these variables added to risk assessment in terms of improved discrimination, calibration, reclassification, and cost-effectiveness. Nonetheless, each of the variables has a place in clinical evaluation. For example, an assessment of cardiorespiratory fitness is an important risk factor to discuss with patients when lifestyle changes are considered; this highlights the point that clinicians are remiss not to address sedentary behaviors [22].

Measurement of ApoB concentrations may also offer improved diagnosis in genetic lipid disorders and may indicate high-risk patients with seemingly normal or low-risk lipid patterns [23, 24]. Since ApoB is in a 1:1 ratio with atherogenic lipoprotein particles (LDL, very low-density lipoprotein (VLDL), and intermediate-density lipoprotein (IDL)), measurement of ApoB yields an estimate of atherogenic particle number [25]. This measure may be helpful in individuals with characteristics of MetS (e.g., insulin resistance and central obesity) who have low to normal levels of LDL-C, because some of these individuals may have a high number of cholesterol-depleted ApoB lipoproteins [26]. Thus, their ASCVD risk may be higher than the level of LDL-C would suggest. In fact, in several community-based cohort studies, individuals with low to normal levels of LDL-C, but high levels of ApoB, had significantly greater CHD risk than individuals who had low LDL-C and low ApoB [27, 28]. When studied in the asymptomatic population at large, however, addition of ApoB to traditional risk prediction models did not substantially improve the discrimination capacity (c-statistic) of the Framingham risk prediction model [29].

Those with T2D and hypertension benefit from assessment of microalbuminuria [30]. When albumin in the urine is elevated in the 30–300 mg range (above this it can be detected simply with a urine dipstick test), it can predict complications in those with T2D as well as be a marker for atherosclerotic events [31]. Furthermore, the presence of chronic kidney disease (CKD), indicated by decreased GFR, did not merit a separate "statin benefit" category. Indeed, most patients with CKD over age 40, with the exception of those on chronic hemodialysis, qualify for statin treatment when quantitative risk assessment is performed as recommended by the 2013 ACC-AHA Guidelines [3].

cIMT is linked to coronary artery disease and stroke events [32]. However, the new Risk Assessment Guideline noted limited added significance of this variable to the traditional risk factors for a first ASCVD event [3].

Role of LDL-C, LDL Particles, and Non-HDL-C to Predict ASCVD Risk

There are additional biomarkers such as LDL-C, LDL particles, and non-HDL-C (total cholesterol minus HDL) that play a role in ASCVD risk estimation. Nuclear magnetic resonance

(NMR) can be used to determine quantitation of lipoprotein particles and their sizes. NMR quantifies lipoproteins according to the amplitudes of spectral signals emitted by lipoprotein subclasses rather than provides quantitation of cholesterol content [33]. Thus, NMR yields unique information about lipoprotein subclasses and incident T2D [34]. Indeed, a simple means of determining insulin resistance may be predicted by an NMR-derived score [35]. On the contrary, in a prospective study of healthy women, cardiovascular disease risk prediction by NMR was comparable but not superior to that of standard lipids or apolipoproteins [36]. Table 9.3 lists various lipid variables along with their adjusted hazard ratios for incident CVD observed in the Women's Health Study. LDL particle size can confirm a small, dense LDL phenotype. Moreover, LDL particles predict LDL-associated atherosclerotic risk better than LDL-C levels when the two markers are discordant [37]. On the other hand, LDL particles correlate closely with non-HDL-C. The new guidelines use total and HDL-C (which can be non-fasting) for the pooled cohort equations in the ASCVD risk estimator to determine estimated the 10-year ASCVD risk. Thus, the new guidelines are essentially using non-HDL, not LDL to determine estimated short- and long-term ASCVD risk. This is important because the patients most in need of lifestyle counseling, those with MetS variables, often have an elevated non-HDL more prominently than an elevated LDL, as shown using lipid data[1] from the National Health and Nutrition Examination Surveys (NHANES) 2005–2010 [38]. For most patients, non-HDL-C will provide a useful barometer of how patients are doing with lifestyle change if they have MetS. As a guidepost (not a fixed target), getting

Table 9.3 Lipids, NMR lipoproteins, and immunoassay apoproteins along with incident CVD in 27,673 initially healthy women in the Women's Health Study [37]

Variable	Adjusted hazard ratio (95% CI) for incident CVD (log scale)
LDL NMR size (lowest quintile)	1.06 (adjusted only for non-lipid risk factor)
LDL cholesterol	1.74
HDL cholesterol (lowest quintile)	2.08
Total LDL 100 particles	2.51
Non-HDL cholesterol	2.52
Apolipoprotein B 100	2.57
Triglycerides	2.58
Apolipoprotein B100/A-1	2.79
Total/HDL cholesterol	2.82

CI confidence interval, *CVD* cardiovascular disease, *HDL* high-density lipoprotein, *LDL* low-density lipoprotein, *NMR* nuclear magnetic resonance

---

[1] Lipid data from NHANES surveys 2005–2010 showed participants with high non-HDL-C and normal LDL-C values were older and more likely to be men, Hispanic and have impaired fasting glucose, T2D, and MetS.

non-HDL-C under 130 mg/dl indicates a low-risk range for primary prevention.

Markers of Risk Versus Fixed Risk Targets

There is some confusion over biomarkers as markers of risk versus fixed risk targets—not all biomarkers that offer utility as markers of risk warrant usefulness as risk targets of treatment. There are examples where biomarkers can serve as both markers of risk and as risk targets. For example, LDL-C, non-HDL-C, and LDL particles are all markers of risk for ASCVD. LDL-C, for example, is an important causal factor for atherosclerosis, but is a relatively poor biomarker in that it does not easily separate those at risk from those not at risk. The 2013 ACC-AHA Guidelines believe that utilizing arbitrary fixed targets can lead to unproven additional drug therapy. The 2013 ACC-AHA Guidelines advocate a comprehensive program for lifestyle in addition to medications proven to be safe and effective in randomized controlled trials, such as statins, ezetimibe, bile acid sequestrants, and fibrates. Niacin can aggravate the MetS by increasing insulin resistance and should not be used simply because it raises HDL-C [39]. Similarly, MetS is a marker for T2D and ASCVD risks [5], and due to lack of any drugs to specifically treat MetS, lifestyle change is the recommended treatment, as successfully adapted by interventions such as the Diabetes Prevention Program (DPP) [40].

Finally, we would like to stress the importance of lifestyle change in secondary prevention patients. The Treat to New Targets Study compared high-intensity statin therapy (atorvastatin 80 mg/day) with moderate-intensity statin therapy (10 mg/day) in those with chronic coronary artery disease [41]. They found that factors such as increased body mass index, smoking, hypertension, and diabetes mellitus predicted residual risk. Thus, we endorse, as do the 2013 Guidelines, the implementation of a multifaceted prevention approach that has a strong lifestyle component to address more completely the causes of residual risk.

Conclusion

Risk factor assessment panels incorporating large numbers of biometric parameters can estimate ASCVD risks and serve as quantitative tools in lifestyle medicine. The 2013 ACC-AHA Guidelines recommend using the pooled cohort equations for estimating lifetime risk in adults 20–59 years as well as for estimating 10-year risk in adults between 40–75 years [3]. An estimation of lifetime risk can be used to aid lifestyle discussions with the patient while the latter 10-year risk equations can be used to begin a risk discussion to explore the merits of statin therapy in those primary prevention patients without T2D but with a 10-year estimated risk of 7.5% of more. These can be easily accessed by the ACC-AHA risk estimator available online [42]. The assessment of the MetS continues to be of clinical value to the clinician as it identifies metabolic parameters that are easily measurable, understood by the patient as markers of a poor cardio-metabolic prognosis, and importantly, markers that all improve with lifestyle changes.

References

1. Eckel RH, Jakicic JM, Ard JD, de Jesus JM, Houston Miller N, Hubbard VS, Lee IM, Lichtenstein AH, Loria CM, Millen BE, Nonas CA, Sacks FM, Smith SC Jr, Svetkey LP, Wadden TA, Yanovski SZ. 2013 AHA/ACC Guideline on lifestyle management to reduce cardiovascular risk: a report of the American College of Cardiology/American Heart Association Task Force on Practice Guidelines. J Am Coll Cardiol. 2014;63(25 Pt B):2960–84.
2. Jensen MD, Ryan DH, Apovian CM, Ard JD, Comuzzie AG, Donato KA, Hu FB, Hubbard VS, Jakicic JM, Kushner RF, Loria CM, Millen BE, Nonas CA, Pi-Sunyer FX, Stevens J, Stevens VJ, Wadden TA, Wolfe BM, Yanovski SZ. 2013 AHA/ACC/TOS Guideline for the management of overweight and obesity in adults: a report of the American College of Cardiology/American Heart Association Task Force on Practice Guidelines and The Obesity Society. J Am Coll Cardiol. 2014;63(25 Pt B):2985–3023.
3. Goff DC Jr, Lloyd-Jones DM, Bennett G, Coady S, D'Agostino RB Sr, Gibbons R, Greenland P, Lackland DT, Levy D, O'Donnell CJ, Robinson JG, Schwartz JS, Shero ST, Smith SC Jr, Sorlie P, Stone NJ, Wilson PW. 2013 ACC/AHA Guideline on the assessment of cardiovascular risk: a report of the American College of Cardiology/American Heart Association Task Force on Practice Guidelines. J Am Coll Cardiol. 2014;63(25 Pt B):2935–59.
4. Stone NJ, Robinson JG, Lichtenstein AH, Bairey Merz CN, Blum CB, Eckel RH, Goldberg AC, Gordon D, Levy D, Lloyd-Jones DM, McBride P, Schwartz JS, Shero ST, Smith SC Jr, Watson K, Wilson PW. 2013 ACC/AHA Guideline on the treatment of blood cholesterol to reduce atherosclerotic cardiovascular risk in adults: a report of the American College of Cardiology/American Heart Association Task Force on Practice Guidelines. J Am Coll Cardiol. 2014;63(25 Pt B):2889–934.
5. Grundy S. Approach to lipoprotein management in 2001 National Cholesterol Guidelines. Am J Cardiology. 2002;90(8A), 11i–21i.
6. Ferland A, Eckel RH. Does sustained weight loss reverse the metabolic syndrome? Curr Hypertens Rep. 2011;13(6):456–64.
7. Motillo S, Filion KB, Genest J, Joseph L, Pilote L, Poirier P, Rinfret S, Schiffrin EL, Eisenberg MJ. The metabolic syndrome and cardiovascular risk: a systematic review and meta-analysis. J Am Coll Cardiol. 2010;56:1113–32.
8. Greenland P et al. ACCF/AHA Guideline for assessment of cardiovascular risk in asymptomatic adults: a report of the American College of Cardiology Foundation/American Heart Association Task Force on Practice Guidelines. J Am Coll Cardiol. 2010;56(25):e50–103.
9. Lloyd-Jones DM, Nam B, D'Agotino RB, Murabito JM, Wang TJ, Wilson PWF, O'Donnell CJ. Parental cardiovascular disease as a risk factor for cardiovascular disease in middle-aged adults—a prospective study of parents and offspring. JAMA. 2004;291(18):2204–11.

10. Williams RR, Hunt SC, Heiss G. Usefulnes of cardiovascular family history data for population-based preventive medicine and medical research (the Healthy Family Tree Study and the NHLBI Family Heart Study). Am J Cardiol. 2001;87:129–35.

11. Hawe E, Talmud PJ, Miller GJ, Humphries SE. Family history is a coronary heart disease risk factor in the Second Northwick Park Heart Study. Ann Hum Genet. 2003;87:97–106.

12. Okwuosa TM, Greenland P, Lakoski SG, Ning H, Kang J, Blumenthal RS, Szklo M, Crouse JR 3rd, Lima JA, Liu K, Lloyd-Jones DM. Factors associated with presence and extent of coronary calcium in those predicted to be at low risk according to Framingham risk score (from the Multi-ethnic Study of Atherosclerosis). Am J Cardiol. 2011;107:879–85.

13. Lin JS, Olson CM, Johnson ES, Whitlock EP. The ankle-brachial index for peripheral artery disease screening and cardiovascular disease prediction among asymptomatic adults: a systematic evidence review for the U.S. Preventive Services Task Force. Ann Intern Med. 2013;159:333–41.

14. Elliott P, Chambers JC, Zhang W. Genetic loci associated with C-reactive protein levels and risk of coronary heart disease. JAMA. 2009;302:37–48.

15. Buckley DI, Fu R, Freeman M, Rogers K, Helfand M. C-reactive protein as a risk factor for coronary heart disease: a systematic review and meta-analyses for the U.S. Preventive Services Task Force. Ann Intern Med. 2009;151:483–95.

16. Wilson PW, Nam BH, Pencina M, et al. C-reactive protein and risk of cardiovascular disease in men and women from the Framingham Heart Study. Arch Intern Med. 2005;165:2473–8.

17. Cook NR, Buring JE, Ridker PM. The effect of including C-reactive protein in cardiovascular risk prediction models for women. Ann Intern Med. 2006;145:21–9.

18. Van der Meer IM, de Maat MP, Kiliaan AJ, et al. The value of C-reactive protein in cardiovascular risk prediction: the Rotterdam Study. Arch Intern Med. 2003;163:1323–8.

19. Wilson PW, Pencina M, Jacques P, et al. C-reactive protein and reclassification of cardiovascular risk in the Framingham Heart Study. Circ Cardiovasc Qual Outcomes. 2008;1:92–7.

20. Ridker PM, Danielson E, Fonseca FA. Rosuvastatin to prevent vascular events in men and women with elevated C-reactive protein. N Engl J Med. 2008;359:2195–207.

21. Hlatky MA, Greenland P, Arnett DK, Ballantyne CM, Criqui MH, Elkind MS, Go AS, Harrell FE Jr, Hong Y, Howard BV, Howard VJ, Hsue PY, Kramer CM, McConnell JP, Normand SL, O'Donnell CJ, Smith SC Jr, Wilson PW, American Heart Association Expert Panel on Subclinical Atherosclerotic Diseases and Emerging Risk Factors and the Stroke Council. Criteria for evaluation of novel markers of cardiovascular risk: a scientific statement from the American Heart Association. Circulation. 2009;119(17):2408–16.

22. Khan KM, Weiler R, Blair SN. Prescribing exercise in primary care—ten practical steps on how to do it. BMJ. 2011;343:d4141.

23. Sniderman A, Couture P, de Graaf J. Diagnosis and treatment of apolipoprotein B dyslipoproteinemias. Nat Rev Endocrinol. 2010;6(6):335–46.

24. Ford ES, Li C, Sniderman A. Temporal changes in concentrations of lipids and apolipoprotein B among adults with diagnosed and undiagnosed diabetes, prediabetes, and normoglycemia: findings from the National Health and Nutrition Examination Survey 1988–1991 to 2005–2008. Cardiovasc Diabetol. 2013;30(12):26.

25. Barter PJ et al. Apo B versus cholesterol in estimating cardiovascular risk and in guiding therapy: report of the thirty-person/ten-country panel. J Intern Med. 2006;259(3):247–58.

26. Sniderman AD, Williams K, Contois JH, et al. A meta-analysis of low-density lipoprotein cholesterol, non-high-density lipoprotein cholesterol, and apolipoprotein B as markers of cardiovascular risk. Circ Cardiovasc Qual Outcomes. 2011;4(3):337–45.

27. Sniderman AD, De Graaf J, Couture P. Low-density lipoprotein-lowering strategies: target versus maximalist versus population percentile. Curr Opin Cardiol. 2012;27(4):405–11.

28. AD1 S, St-Pierre AC, Cantin B, et al. Concordance/discordance between plasma apolipoprotein B levels and the cholesterol indexes of atherosclerotic risk. Am J Cardiol. 2003;91(10):1173–7.

29. Ingelsson E, Schaefer EJ, Contois JH, et al. Clinical utility of different lipid measures for prediction of coronary heart disease in men and women. JAMA. 2007;298(7):776–85.

30. Bakris GL, Molitch M. Microalbuminuria as a risk predictor in diabetes: the continuing saga. Diabetes Care. 2014;37(3):867–75.

31. Tagle R, Acevedo M, Vidt D. Microalbuminuria: is it a valid predictor of cardiovascular risk? Cleve Clin J Med. 2003;70(3):255–61.

32. Zhang Y, Guallar E, Qiao Y, Wasserman BA. Is carotid intima-media thickness as predictive as other noninvasive techniques for the detection of coronary artery disease? Arterioscler Thromb Vasc Biol. 2014;34(7):1341–5.

33. Mora S, Szklo M, Otvos JD, et al. LDL particle subclasses, LDL particle size, and carotid atherosclerosis in the Multi-Ethnic Study of Atherosclerosis (MESA). Atherosclerosis. 2007;192:211–7.

34. Mora S, Otvos JD, Rosenson RS, Pradhan A, Buring JE, Ridker PM. Lipoprotein particle size and concentration by nuclear magnetic resonance and incident type 2 diabetes in women. Diabetes. 2010;59(5):1153–60 (2010 Feb 25).

35. Shalaurova I, Connelly MA, Garvey WT, Otvos JD. Lipoprotein insulin resistance index: a lipoprotein particle-derived measure of insulin resistance. Metab Syndr Relat Disord. 2014;12(8):422–9.

36. Mora S, Otvos JD, Rifai N, Rosenson RS, Buring JE, Ridker PM. Lipoprotein particle profiles by nuclear magnetic resonance compared with standard lipids and apolipoproteins in predicting incident cardiovascular disease in women. Circulation. 2009;119(7):931–9.

37. Otvos JD, Mora S, Shalaurova I, Greenland P, Mackey RH, Goff DC Jr. Clinical implications of discordance between low-density lipoprotein cholesterol and particle number. J Clin Lipidol. 2011;5(2):105–13.

38. Kilgore M, Muntner P, Woolley JM, Sharma P, Bittner V, Rosenson RS. Discordance between high non-HDL cholesterol and high LDL-cholesterol among US adults. J Clin Lipidol. 2014;8(1):86–93.

39. Tuteja S, Rader DJ. Dyslipidaemia: cardiovascular prevention–end of the road for niacin? Nat Rev Endocrinol. 2014;10:646–47.

40. Orchard TJ, Temprosa M, Goldberg R, Haffner S, Ratner R, Marcovina S, Fowler S. The effect of metformin and intensive lifestyle intervention on the metabolic syndrome: the diabetes prevention program randomized trial. Ann Intern Med. 2005;142:611–9.

41. Mora S, Wenger NK, DeMicco DA, Breazna A, Boekholdt SM, Arsenault BJ, Deedwania P, Kastelein JJP, Waters DD. Determinants of residual risk in secondary prevention patients treated with high- versus low-dose statin therapy: the Treating to New Targets (TNT) study. 125(16):1979–87.

42. 2013 Prevention Guidelines ASCVD Risk Estimator. http://www.acc.org/tools-and-practice-support/mobile-resources/features/2013-prevention-guidelines-ascvd-risk-estimator. Accessed 15 March 2015.

The Chronic Care Model and the Transformation of Primary Care

10

Thomas Bodenheimer and Rachel Willard-Grace

Abbreviations

CCM	Chronic care model
EMR	Electronic medical record
A1C	Hemoglobin A1c
NCQA	National Committee on Quality Assurance
PCMH	Patient-centered medical home
RN	Registered nurse
T2D	Type-2 diabetes

Introduction

In the late 1990s, Ed Wagner and associates at the MacColl Institute for Health Care Innovation formulated a new model for the care of patients with chronic illness [1]. Since then, the chronic care model (CCM) has been universally embraced as the guide for improving chronic care.

Performance data reveal that chronic care needs a great deal of improvement. For example, 54% of people with hypertension are poorly controlled [2], 67% with elevated cholesterol have not reached lipid-lowering goals [3], and 48% of people with diabetes have not achieved glycemic control [4].

Because the majority of chronic illness care is performed within the primary care setting, the CCM constitutes a major rethinking of primary care practice. This chapter will describe the six components of the CCM, review some of the evidence linking CCM components to improved clinical outcomes, highlight the self-management support component as the foundation of chronic illness care, and finally explore the relationship between the CCM and the overall transformation of primary care.

Describing the Chronic Care Model

Chronic care takes place within three overlapping galaxies: (1) the entire community, with its myriad resources and numerous public and private policies; (2) the health-care system, including its payment structures; and (3) the provider organization, most importantly the primary care practice, whether a community health center, a small physician practice, or an integrated delivery system. One component—community resources and policies—subsumes the entire community galaxy and a second component—the health-care system—resides in the second galaxy. The four other components—decision support, delivery system design, clinical information systems, and self-management support—are features of the primary care practice itself. Efforts to implement these four primary care-centered components of the CCM have been central to the vibrant campaign to transform primary care practice in the USA and in other nations.

Component 1. Community Resources and Policies

To improve chronic care, provider organizations need linkages with community-based resources, for example, exercise programs, parks and recreation facilities, safe neighborhoods, senior centers, public health laws and regulations, and self-help groups. Community linkages—for example, with hospitals offering patient education classes or home care agencies—are especially helpful for small physician offices with limited resources.

Component 2. Health-Care Organization

The structure, goals, and values of the larger system in which primary care practices exist have a profound influence on chronic care. If the entire health-care system, or the larger provider organization of which a primary care practice is a part, does not view chronic care as a priority, improvement

T. Bodenheimer (✉) · R. Willard-Grace
Department of Family and Community Medicine, University of California, San Francisco, San Francisco CA, USA
e-mail: TBodenheimer@fcm.ucsf.edu, tbodie@earthlink.net

© Springer International Publishing Switzerland 2016
J. I. Mechanick, R. F. Kushner (eds.), *Lifestyle Medicine*, DOI 10.1007/978-3-319-24687-1_10

will not take place. If primary care practices are reimbursed only for clinician visits, the practices will have a difficult time implementing other CCM components which require the participation of team members whose work is not paid for. If millions of people have no health insurance, they cannot afford the care that is essential for controlling their chronic conditions. If low- or medium-income families with health insurance face large deductibles and co-payments, they will also have difficulty accessing primary care services.

Component 3. Decision Support

Evidence-based clinical practice guidelines provide standards for optimal chronic care and should be integrated into daily practice through reminders. Guidelines are reinforced by physician "champions" who lead educational sessions for practice teams. Ideally, specialist expertise is a mere telephone call or e-consultation away. Practices that have fully implemented decision support have embedded practice guidelines into the electronic medical record, available for clinicians to consult with one click of the mouse.

Component 4. Delivery System Design

The "tyranny of the urgent" refers to the prioritization of acute problems over chronic and preventive care. To combat this phenomenon, planned visits whose only agenda is the management of the patient's chronic conditions are required. This usually means having non-clinician ("clinician" refers to physicians, nurse practitioners, and physician assistants, the personnel with the most training) team members—nurses, pharmacists, health educators, or health coaches—leading the planned visits. This change in practice design requires that primary care practices develop well-functioning teams in place of clinician-only care. The clinician role becomes the treatment of patients with acute problems, management of stubbornly difficult and complex chronic care patients, and the training and mentoring of non-clinician team members. Non-clinician personnel are trained to support patient self-management, arrange for routine periodic tasks (e.g., laboratory tests for diabetic patients, eye examinations, and foot examinations), and ensure appropriate follow-up.

Component 5. Clinical Information Systems

Computerized information has three important roles: (1) reminder systems that help primary care teams adhere to practice guidelines; (2) feedback to clinicians and teams, showing how each is performing on chronic illness measures such as hemoglobin A1c (A1C) and lipid levels; and (3) registries for conducting population-based care. Registries, a central feature of the CCM, are lists of all patients with a particular chronic condition in a practice's or clinician's panel. The registry feeds into a reminder pop-up message on the electronic medical record, which flags laboratory work or examinations not performed according to schedules recommended by clinical practice guidelines. Non-clinician practice personnel, panel managers, periodically review the registry to identify and contact patients overdue for routine studies or with poor disease control in order to bring those patients into care.

Component 6. Self-Management Support

For chronic conditions, patients themselves become the principal caregivers [5]. Management of these illnesses can be taught to most patients, and substantial segments of that management—healthy eating, exercise, and medication use—are under the direct control of the patient. Self-management support involves collaboratively helping patients and their families acquire the knowledge, skills, and confidence to manage their chronic illness. Self-management is particularly important for the successful implementation of lifestyle medicine.

Interdependence of the Components

The six components of the CCM build upon one another. Delivery system redesign and the formation of primary care teams with a division of labor are essential to teach self-management because physicians do not have time for this activity. For registries to be successful, redesigning delivery systems is necessary so that one member of a primary care team is responsible for working the registry. Clinical practice guidelines, a key decision-support tool, provide the evidence upon which the physician feedback data and reminder systems are based.

As its ultimate goal, the CCM envisions an informed, activated patient interacting with a prepared, proactive practice team, resulting in satisfying encounters and improved outcomes [1]. Is the model a utopian concept, impossible to implement in the rough-and-tumble world of primary care? A number of organizations have attempted to introduce the model. Some have enjoyed success, while others were unable to sustain the improvements. For practices across the country, the CCM remains an ideal toward which to aspire.

Evidence Supporting Chronic Care Model Components

Since the CCM was introduced in the late 1990s, considerable evidence has accumulated to support the four primary care-based components of the model.

Decision Support

Creating practice guidelines for the care of chronic illness has only a minimal impact on quality unless the guidelines are woven into the daily fabric of patient care, most effectively by integrating them into the electronic medical record (EMR) [6]. In a randomized trial, patients with diabetes whose physicians used an EMR-based decision support system had significantly better levels of A1C and systolic blood pressure than patients of physicians without such decision support [7]. Electronic decision support improves safety and reduces costs as well. A review of 20 studies of computerized decision support found evidence that they reduced prescribing error rates on the order of 50% [8]. Electronic decision support evaluations confirm their usefulness but add a cautionary note. Studies find that clinicians override 49–96% of the decision support alerts. Higher specificity of alerts coupled with clear explanations may help improve the utility of decision aids and their ability to prevent error [9].

Delivery System Design

Growing evidence demonstrates that redesign of the delivery system can improve chronic care. Effective self-management support requires proactive, planned care in which the proper team member has dedicated time to focus on self-management support [10]. Planned group visits for patients with diabetes significantly reduced A1C levels and hospital use for these patients in the Kaiser Permanente system [11].

In one study, patients with diabetes participated in a 20-min planned pre-visit with a clinic assistant to set the agenda and prepare questions for the ensuing physician visit. The engaged patients achieved an average A1C reduction from 10.6 to 9.1%, while A1C levels for a control group increased from 10.3 to 10.6%. Audiotapes of the physician visits showed that the engaged patients were twice as effective as controls in eliciting information from the physician [12].

Longer, more structured planned visits create an opportunity for primary care team members, often nurses, to provide care management for patients with chronic conditions. Care management refers to more intensive engagement with patients, generally taking place during planned visits and phone calls by a non-physician member of the care team [13]. In a systematic review of 41 studies of patients with diabetes, the involvement of a nurse care manager—providing patient education, self-management support, and in some cases medication management using protocols—was associated with improved glycemic and lipid control. When nurse care managers are closely integrated with or embedded in primary care, they have been shown to improve outcomes and reduce costs for elderly and complex, chronically ill populations. A period of more intensive surveillance and involvement by a nurse or other clinical care managers has been shown to improve outcomes for more complex patients with chronic illness [14].

An important feature of planned chronic illness care is regular follow-up. The benefits of self-management support for patients with diabetes diminish over time without scheduled follow-up, and the total time caregivers spend with patients correlates with glycemic control. Similarly, regular follow-up is necessary for hypertension management; moreover, reviews of trials of patients with heart failure discharged from the hospital find that nurse-led follow-up is associated with large reductions in heart failure readmissions. Patients with consistent follow-up have better adherence to medications and lifestyle behaviors [15].

Clinical Information Systems

A systematic review found that registries identifying and bringing at-risk patients with diabetes into care result in improved glycemic control compared with usual care [16]. A randomized trial found that primary practices that utilized disease registries improved A1C and LDL-cholesterol levels for patients with diabetes, if the registries were used to generate reminders to patients to come in for care [17].

Self-Management Support

Considerable evidence reveals that individual and group interventions emphasizing patient empowerment and the acquisition of self-management skills are effective in improving care for diabetes, asthma, and other chronic conditions [18]. Self-management support is associated with improved glycemic control [10]. In a review of 39 chronic care improvement interventions, self-management support was the CCM intervention most commonly associated with improved processes or outcomes of care [1]. In a systematic review of 72 studies of patients with diabetes, self-management training was positively associated with patient knowledge, frequency, and accuracy of blood glucose self-monitoring, self-reported dietary habits, and glycemic control in studies with short follow-up (less than 6 months) [19]. In a randomized controlled trial of low-income patients with poorly controlled diabetes, patients who were provided with self-management support by peer health coaches (other patients with diabetes) had significantly improved A1C levels compared with controls [20]. Most experts now recommend that self-management support be an integral component of all clinical interactions with patients with chronic health problems.

Multiple Chronic Care Model Components

The CCM was designed to build on the interrelationships among the six components. Several studies have found that the presence of multiple CCM components is associated with better quality of care [18]. In a meta-analysis of CCM components used for patients with asthma, congestive heart failure, depression, and diabetes, four elements of the model (delivery system design, self-management support, decision support, and clinical information systems) were associated with better outcomes and processes. Delivery system design and self-management support appeared to be the most effective CCM components [21]. In a study of 20 primary care practices, patients with diabetes cared for in practices that had implemented more CCM components had a lower risk of developing coronary heart disease than patients cared for in practices with fewer CCM components [22].

Implementing the Chronic Care Model in Primary Care

Implementing CCM components into primary care requires transforming primary care practices. While humane, empathetic, and competent clinicians can provide excellent chronic care, they cannot sustain such efforts indefinitely. Ensuring that all clinicians provide high-quality chronic care to every patient requires systems that incorporate CCM components.

In 2007, four primary care professional societies coalesced around a vision for primary care—the Joint Principles of the Patient-Centered Medical Home. The patient-centered medical home (PCMH) has been adopted as a designation of practices with the capacity to implement the entire CCM. This vision was based on four pillars of primary care practice elaborated by Barbara Starfield in 1992: first-contact care, continuity of care, comprehensive care, and coordination of care. The publication of the Joint Principles stimulated efforts to define the PCMH, for example, the National Committee on Quality Assurance (NCQA) PCMH recognition standards. While such standards can be a useful tool, they do not go far enough. A more transformative approach is provided by the 10 Building Blocks of High-Performing Primary Care. The building blocks represent a system-level change in how primary care practices are organized [23].

The building blocks were derived from case studies of, and site visits to, exemplar primary care practices. The PCMH has been adopted as a designation of practices with the capacity to implement the entire CCM. A surprising observation about these practices is that they tended to share several unifying characteristics that were categorized as the 10 Building Blocks. The building blocks have become a model that primary care practices can adopt to become patient-centered medical homes with the capacity to operationalize CCM components. The 10 Building Blocks are shown in Fig. 10.1a, b and reviewed in the following section in relation to the CCM.

These building blocks were derived from site visits to high-performing primary care practices and clinics. The unanimity with which these principles are put into practice suggests that there is one basic model—with individual variation—for primary care excellence.

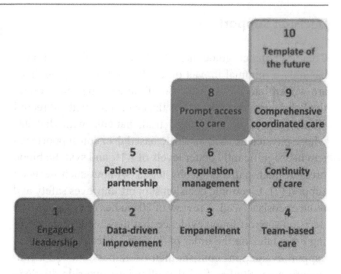

Fig. 10.1 Building blocks of high-performing primary care: the Share The Care model. (Courtesy of Center for Excellence in Primary Care, University of California, San Francisco)

1. Engaged leadership, including patients, creating a practice-wide vision with concrete objectives and goals
2. Data-driven improvement using computer-based technology
3. Empanelment
4. Team-based care
   (a) Culture shift: share the care
   (b) Stable teamlets
   (c) Co-location
   (d) Staffing ratios adequate to facilitate new roles
   (e) Standing orders/protocols
   (f) Defined workflows and workflow mapping
   (g) Defined roles with training and skills checks to reinforce those roles
   (h) Ground rules
   (i) Communication: team meetings, huddles, and minute-to-minute interaction
5. Patient–team partnership
   (a) Evidence-based care
   (b) Health coaching
   (c) Informed, activated patients
   (d) Shared decision-making
6. Population management
   (a) Panel management
   (b) Self-management support (health coaching)
   (c) Complex care management
7. Continuity of care
8. Prompt access to care
   (a) Weekday hours
   (b) Nights/weekends
   (c) Phone access
9. Comprehensiveness and care coordination
   (a) Within the medical neighborhood
   (b) With community partners
   (c) With family and caregivers

10. Template of the future: escape from the 15-min visit
    (a) E-visits
    (b) Phone visits
    (c) Group visits
    (d) Visits with nurses and other team members
    (e) Requires payment reform

For detailed descriptions of six of these building blocks, see the California HealthCare Foundation report, The Building Blocks of High-Performing Primary Care: Lessons from the Field, April 2012 (www.chcf.org).

Building Block 1. Engaged Leadership

High-performing practices have leaders fully engaged in the process of change, such as reforming teams and empowering staff to take on new roles in self-management support or redesigning the workflow to facilitate planned visits. Leaders work with frontline staff and patients to develop strategic goals and to create concrete, measurable objectives, some of which are chronic care performance goals. Examples of these goals include: the percent of patients with diabetes who have A1C greater than 9 % will drop from 20 to 10 % by December 31, 2014; or the percent of patients with asthma who have attended planned visits to learn inhaler skills and to adopt asthma action plans will increase from 20 to 60 % by June 30, 2015. The visible support and promotion of practice improvement by organization leaders is a major predictor of success. Conversely, lack of leadership support predicts failure [6].

Building Block 2. Data-driven Improvement

Monitoring progress toward chronic care objectives requires data systems that track clinical metrics for conditions such as diabetes, obesity, hypertension, depression, congestive heart failure, and chronic obstructive pulmonary disease. To ensure that all patients with chronic conditions receive the periodic tasks known to improve care (e.g., regular A1C and LDL-cholesterol laboratory tests), practices need registries that list all patients with chronic conditions together with the dates and results of studies, and furthermore, practices need personnel with training and time to review the registries and contact patients with gaps in their care. Registries are part of the CCM clinical information systems component and the personnel—called population managers—are part of delivery system design.

Building Block 3. Empanelment

Empanelment means linking each patient to a care team and a primary care clinician. Empanelment is the basis for the therapeutic relationship that is essential for good patient outcomes. Empanelment interacts closely with data-driven improvement because defined panels provide a denominator for performance measures. For example, within a particular practice, how do the clinicians know the percent of their patients with diabetes that have A1C levels above 9 %? First, the clinicians need to know the denominator: how many patients with type-2 diabetes (T2D) are in their panel.

Building Block 4. Team-based Care

Exemplar practices have created teams with well-trained non-clinicians who share the care with clinicians [24]. Team formation is the essence of delivery system design. While team composition varies widely among practices, a common team structure features two-person teamlets working within a larger team. Patients are empaneled to a teamlet, which often consists of a clinician and a medical assistant who always work together. Supporting several teamlets might be a behavioral health provider, a registered nurse (RN) complex care manager, pharmacist, or a social worker who sees patients with more complex needs.

In an analysis of 66 studies, the two most effective strategies to improve glycemic control for patients with diabetes were team formation and care management. These strategies are interlocked because care management is generally performed by non-clinician team members (nurses or pharmacists) in planned visits. Diabetes outcomes were best when the team members had standing orders to make medication adjustments without awaiting physician authorization [25].

Building Block 5. Patient–Team Partnership

Patient–team partnerships are achieved when the patient is empowered as an expert in her life to share decision-making with a team using evidence-based care guidelines. Patient–team partnerships rely on a relationship of trust. Patients with chronic disease have better outcomes when they enjoy a trusting relationship with a clinician and team. This partnership is the intersection of the informed, activated patient and the proactive practice team, as described in the CCM, which leads to productive interactions.

Building Block 6. Population Management

The CCM is a population-centered concept, aiming to improve chronic care for entire populations. Practices are tasked to move from the traditional model of caring for those patients who happen to come for appointments to a new paradigm with the goal that all patients empaneled to the practice are as healthy as possible. Population management requires both clinical information systems to risk-adjust a practice's panel of patients in order to determine who needs which services and delivery system redesign to create teams with personnel who are responsible for population management.

All patients need routine preventive services, a function often called panel management. Studies have shown that panel management is best performed by a non-clinician such as a medical assistant because clinicians lack the time to ensure that all gaps in care are addressed [26]. Standing orders enable panel managers to address care gaps without involving the clinician. Routine care is ideally complete before the clinician enters the exam room, so that visits can focus on addressing patient concerns and strengthening the clinician–patient relationship.

For patients with chronic conditions, population management entails the care team providing self-management support—also called health coaching—at every visit. All team members—clinicians, medical assistants, RNs, registered dietitians, and pharmacists—should view self-management support as part of what they do every time they see a patient. Patients with poorly controlled chronic conditions often require longer planned visits with a team member trained in health coaching. Health coaching assesses patients' knowledge and motivation, provides information and skills, and engages patients in behavior-changing action plans known to improve outcomes [27]. Patients with diabetes who are working with health coaches have better outcomes than those without health coaches [20].

For the 5–10% of patients in a population who have complex health-care needs and are high utilizers of expensive services, a population management approach provides intensive care management from a specialized team led by RNs and/or social workers. These intensive teams have been shown to improve care and reduce costs for complex patients [28].

Building Block 7. Continuity of Care

Continuity of care is the operational substrate upon which trusting relationships between patients and care teams are established. Continuity over time is associated with improved preventive and chronic care, greater patient and clinician experience, and lower costs [29]. Achieving continuity requires empanelment, which links each patient to a clinician and teamlet. High-performing practices measure continuity for each clinician/teamlet, with the metric being the number of visits by a patient panel to the teamlet to which the patients are empaneled divided by the total number of primary care visits by that patient panel. Failing to optimize continuity of care seriously undermines good chronic care.

Building Block 8. Enhanced Access

All CCM components depend on the ability of patients to gain timely access to appointments with their care team, access during nights and weekends, and access by phone or e-mail. Practices are more successful at improving access if they empanel all patients to a provider and team, as well as build teams that empower non-clinicians to independently provide care for appropriate patients. This process adds capacity to meet patient demand.

Building Block 9. Comprehensiveness and Care Coordination

Comprehensiveness means that primary care addresses a wide range of patient needs, while care coordination is the linking of primary care with services that primary care is unable to provide. The care coordination model [http://www.improvingchroniccare.org] proposes four key changes that must be implemented to foster excellent care coordination:

1. The primary care practice assumes accountability for care coordination.
2. Primary care provides support to patients needing specialty, hospital, or long-term care services, helping patients identify high-quality referral sites, assisting them to make appointments, tracking referrals to ensure that patients attend their appointments, and sometimes offering patient navigators to provide transportation, interpretation, and comfort to patients.
3. Primary care initiates agreements with specialists and hospitals that facilitate access and information sharing.
4. Primary care develops electronic connectivity with as many referral partners as possible to facilitate rapid information exchange; these changes fall under the delivery system design CCM component.

Building Block 10. Alternative Encounter Types

Traditional primary care has celebrated the patient–clinician relationship through face-to-face visits. In contrast, innovative practices are redesigning their delivery system through alternative encounters: phone visits, interactions via electronic patient portals, group visits, and visits with non-clinician care team members. Full implementation of this future vision requires payment reform that does not reward primary care only for in-person clinician visits. The alternative encounter types should preserve continuity of care and long-term trusting relationships between patients and their care team.

Self-Management Support: The Heart of the Chronic Care Model and the Building Blocks

Of the 8760 h in a year, people living with chronic illness spend approximately 1 h with their primary care provider. The other 8759 h are spent at home, at work, and in the community. The choices that most impact health are self-care decisions: whether to eat chips or vegetables on break, whether to walk or watch television after work, or whether to pick up medications today or go without for a few days. If primary care is to make a significant impact on health, it must help patients acquire the knowledge, skills, and confidence to make healthy choices.

Thus, self-management support is at the heart of the CCM and primary care's building blocks. Self-management support (health coaching) is not didactic education—telling people what they should and should not do—which does not improve clinical outcomes [15]. Self-management support empowers patients to identify and work toward their own health goals and to more actively manage their conditions. Improved clinical outcomes and patient experience have been reported in self-management support programs relying on RNs, medical assistants, volunteers, and other patients with the same condition.

Several key components of self-management support (health coaching) are given below.

- Making sure patients, for example those with diabetes, know their laboratory numbers (A1C and LDL-cholesterol), know the evidence-based goals for these numbers, and know how to bring their number to the goal
- Asking patients to "close the loop"—to teach back the specifics of their care plan. This practice addresses the reality that 50% of patients do not remember their physician's recommendations
- Engaging patients in setting goals and making short-term, achievable action plans to reach these goals. In a randomized trial, patients with diabetes who are making action plans had significantly improved A1C levels compared with patients with diabetes receiving traditional patient education [30]
- Because medication adherence is critical for improving chronic illness outcomes, patients deserve collaborative discussions to increase their knowledge of their medications and to address barriers to taking their medications

Moving Upstream: Implications for Lifestyle Medicine

For people with chronic disease, primary care tends to emphasize medication management. The CCM, with its most important component being self-management support,

places equal importance on lifestyle medicine—engaging people in setting healthy goals that change how they live their day-to-day lives.

Most health-care-related dollars are dedicated to caring for people who are already sick, a decidedly downstream approach. The CCM challenges us to consider what happens within the broader community—outside the walls of the health center—to impact the upstream causes of poor health. An upstream approach has a far greater influence on health. While excellent management of diabetes adds an average of 3 months to a patient's life, preventing diabetes adds 6 years. Yet, seeking upstream solutions is challenging. The root causes of poor health stem from complex issues such as lack of economic opportunity or unsafe environments. The community resources component of the CCM is the upstream element, which is often beyond the capacity of primary care practices.

What is the role of primary care in working upstream? The engagement of primary care in the community may be seen along the continuum of the river's course. At the river's end is medical care for complications of poor health. A little way up the river, we might find proactive care such as routine labs to monitor control of chronic conditions and self-management support designed to help patients take greater control over their health. Higher upriver, we see primary care emerging from the clinic to engage in the outside community, perhaps through community health workers and partnerships with community organizations to help people lose weight, become more active, and stop smoking. Further upstream, primary care practices are support of public health policy initiatives or become focal points for community activation. For example, the Mound Bayou Health Center in rural Mississippi became the catalyst for job training programs, a farm cooperative, and small businesses that began creating jobs [31].

Along the riverbanks, patients are an untapped resource. Initiatives designed to improve health by empowering and employing community members as promoters or community health workers create ripple effects, as newly empowered community members identify and tackle other barriers to their health and well-being [32].

Where along the river path a primary care practice chooses to invest its energy may depend on the resources it brings to bear, the needs of the community it serves, and whether there are other leaders within the community to drive forward change. Certainly, primary care has a unique opportunity to provide targeted self-management support and medical care that cannot be provided in other environments. At the same time, primary care practices are part of the communities they serve, and they may be catalysts for change that echoes beyond their walls.

References

1. Bodenheimer T, Wagner EH, Grumbach K. Improving primary care for patients with chronic illness, parts 1 and 2. JAMA. 2002;288:1775–9, 1909–14.
2. Centers for Disease Control and Prevention (CDC). Vital signs: prevalence, treatment, and control of hypertension—United States, 1999–2002 and 2005–2008. MMWR Morb Mortal Wkly Rep. 2011;60(4):103–8.
3. Centers for Disease Control and Prevention (CDC). Vital signs: prevalence, treatment, and control of high levels of low-density lipoprotein cholesterol—United States, 1999–2002 and 2005–2008. MMWR Morb Mortal Wkly Rep. 2011;60(4):109–14.
4. Casagrande SS, Fradkin JE, Saydah SH, Rust KF, Cowie CC. The prevalence of meeting A1C, blood pressure, and LDL goals among people with diabetes, 1988–2010. Diabetes Care. 2013;36:2271–9.
5. Bodenheimer T, Lorig K, Holman H, Grumbach K. Patient self-management of chronic disease in primary care. JAMA. 2002;288:2469–75.
6. Wagner EH, Austin BT, Davis C, Hindmarsh M, Schaefer J, Bonomi A. Improving chronic illness care: translating evidence into action. Health Aff. 2001;20:64–78.
7. O'Connor PJ, Sperl-Hillen JM, Rush WA, et al. Impact of electronic health record clinical decision support on diabetes care: a randomized trial. Ann Fam Med. 2011;9:12–21.
8. Schedlbauer A, Prasad V, Mulvaney C, Phansalkar S, Stanton W, Lip B, et al. What evidence supports the use of computerized alerts and prompts to impove clinicians' prescribing behavior? J Am Med Inform Assoc. 2009;16:531–8.
9. van der Sijs H, Aarts J, Vulto A, Berg M. Overriding of drug safety alerts in computerized physician order entry. J Am Med Inform Assoc. 2006;13:138–47.
10. Stellefson M, Dipnarine K, Stopka C. The chronic care model and diabetes management in US primary care settings: a systematic review. Prev Chronic Dis. 2013;10:E26.
11. Sadur CN, Moline N, Costa M, Michalik D, Mendlowitz D, Roller S, et al. Diabetes management in a health maintenance organization. Efficacy of care management using cluster visits. Diabetes Care. 1999;22:2011–7.
12. Greenfield S, Kaplan SH, Ware JE, Yano EM, Frank HJL. Patients' participation in medical care: effects on blood sugar control and quality of life in diabetes. J Gen Intern Med. 1988;3:448–57.
13. Wagner EH, Bennett SM, Austin BT, Greene SM, Schaefer JK, vonKorff M. Finding common ground: patient-centeredness and evidence-based chronic illness care. J Altern Complement Med. 2005;11(Suppl 1):s7–15.
14. Renders CM, Valk GD, Griffin SJ, Wagner EH, van Eijk JTM, Assendelft WJJ. Interventions to improve the management of diabetes in primary care, outpatient, and community settings. Diabetes Care. 2001;24:1821–33.
15. Bodenheimer T. A 63-year-old man with multiple cardiovascular risk factors and poor adherence to treatment plans. JAMA. 2007;298:2048–55.

16. Griffin S, Kinmonth AL. Diabetes care: the effectiveness of systems for routine surveillance for people with diabetes. Cochrane Database Syst Rev. 2000;(2):CD000541.
17. Stroebel RJ, Scheitel SM, Fitz JS, et al. A randomized trial of three diabetes registry implementation strategies in a community internal medicine practice. Jt Comm J Qual Improv. 2002;28:441–50.
18. Coleman K, Austin BT, Brach C, Wagner EH. Evidence on the Chronic Care Model in the new millennium. Health Aff. 2009;28:75–85.
19. Norris SL, Engelgau MM, Narayan KMV. Effectiveness of self-management training in type 2 diabetes. Diabetes Care. 2001;24:561–87.
20. Thom DH, Ghorob A, Hessler D, De Vore D, Chen E, Bodenheimer T. Impact of peer health coaching on glycemic control in low-income patients with diabetes: a randomized controlled trial. Ann Fam Med. 2013;11:137–44.
21. Tsai AC, Morton SC, Mangione CM, Keeler EB. A meta-analysis of interventions to improve care for chronic illness. Am J Manag Care. 2005;11:478–88.
22. Parchman ML, Zeber JE, Romero RR, Pugh JA. Risk of coronary artery disease in type 2 diabetes and the delivery of care consistent with the chronic care model in primary care settings: a STARNet study. Med Care. 2007;45:1129–34.
23. Bodenheimer T, Ghorob A, Willard-Grace R, Grumbach K. The 10 building blocks of high-performing primary care. Ann Fam Med. 2014;12:166–71.
24. Willard R, Bodenheimer T. The building blocks of high-performing primary care: lessons from the field. California HealthCare Foundation, 2012.
25. Shojania KG, Ranji SR, McDonald KM, Grimshaw JM, Sundaram V, Rushakoff RJ, Owens DK. Effects of quality improvement strategies for type 2 diabetes on glycemic control. JAMA. 2006;296:427–40.
26. Chen EH, Bodenheimer T. Improving population health through team-based panel management. Arch Intern Med. 2011;171:1558–9.
27. Bennett HD, Coleman EA, Parry C, Bodenheimer T, Chen EH. Health coaching for patients. Fam Pract Manag. 2010;17:24–9.
28. Bodenheimer T, Berry-Millett R. Care management for patients with complex healthcare needs. Robert Wood Johnson Foundation, 2009.
29. Saultz JW, Lochner J. Interpersonal continuity of care and care outcomes: a critical review. Ann Fam Med. 2005;3:159–66.
30. Naik AD, Palmer N, Petersen NJ, Street RL Jr, Rao R, Suarez-Almazor M, Haidet P. Comparative effectiveness of goal setting in diabetes mellitus group clinics: randomized clinical trial. Arch Intern Med. 2011;171:453–9.
31. Geiger HJ. The first community health centers: a model of enduring value. J Ambul Care Manage. 2005;28:313–20.
32. Wiggins N. Popular education for health promotion and community empowerment: a review of the literature. Health Promot Int. 2011;27:356–71.

Guidelines for Healthy Eating

11

Linda Van Horn

Abbreviations	
ACC/AHA	American College of Cardiology/American Heart Association
AHA	American Heart Association
AHEI	Alternative Healthy Eating Index
AI	Adequate intake
BP	Blood pressure
CDC	Centers for Disease Control
DASH	Dietary approaches for stopping hypertension
DGAC	Dietary Guidelines Advisory Committee Report
DHHS	Department of Health and Human Services
DRIs	Dietary reference intakes
EAR	Estimated average requirement
FFQ	Food-frequency questionnaire
FNB	Food and Nutrition Board
HEI	Healthy Eating Index
HDL–C	High-density lipoprotein–cholesterol
IOM	Institute of Medicine
LDL-C	Low-density lipoprotein cholesterol
NEL	Nutrition Evidence Library
NHANES	National Health and Nutrition Examination Survey
RDAs	Recommended dietary allowances
T2D	Type-2 diabetes
UL	Upper intake level
USDA	US Department of Agriculture
USDGs	US Dietary Guidelines
WCRF/AICR	World Cancer Research Fund/American Institute for Cancer Research

L. Van Horn (✉)
Department of Preventive Medicine, Northwestern University Feinberg School of Medicine, 680 North Lake Shore Drive, Suite 1400, Chicago, IL 60611, USA
e-mail: lvanhorn@northwestern.edu

© Springer International Publishing Switzerland 2016
J. I. Mechanick, R. F. Kushner (eds.), *Lifestyle Medicine*, DOI 10.1007/978-3-319-24687-1_11

Introduction and Historical Perspective

"Let food be thy medicine and medicine be thy food"—Hippocrates, 400 BC.

Diet and food intake have long been recognized as major contributors to health. It is exciting to consider how far we have come from the earliest days of nutrition research when mysteries prompted questions like how could plant-based foods, like grass, nourish animals, like cows, even though animals, like people, were composed of blood and tissue? When the elements were identified in the eighteenth century, the discovery of nitrogen led to further identification of compounds like albumin, then protein, and the recognition that it provided energy for the body to do work. Not until the late nineteenth century did the study of body heat or *calorimetry* progress along with the identification of inorganic elements, like minerals. Fatty acids were also identified and differentiated. Stunning discoveries such as ascorbate could cure scurvy and "something," other than a mineral, in rice polishings could cure beriberi all evolved during the late 1880s and early 1900s. Thiamine was eventually identified as the anti-beriberi factor, along with other "vital amines" that became known as "vitamins" [1]. Subsequently, nutritional biochemists like E.V. McCollum, Marguerite Davis, George and Mildred Burr, and countless others contributed to the fundamental understanding of food and diet essentials for health and generated nutrition classification systems that underlie the basics of nutrition research to this day.

Fast-forward to the twentieth century. Animal studies testing various nutrients and dietary factors yielded further evidence confirming the essential nature of certain vitamins, minerals, and macro/micronutrients, but this also yielded recognition of an important concept called "conditional essentiality." This reflects awareness that essential nutrients can in some cases be accommodated by the presence and sufficient quantities of other nutrients. For example, in the 1920s, scientists found that rats fed 10–12 % casein as their source of protein grew faster when 0.5 % cystine (or the reduced form, cysteine) was included in the diet. This amino acid became an essential nutrient as well, but after methionine, another sulfur-containing amino acid, was discovered, it too was found to be essential; when methionine was consumed in sufficient amounts, it eliminated the requirement for cysteine. These and other synergistic nutrient relationships surely represent the origins of preventive medical nutrition and are likely attributable to this notion of "conditional essentiality" or compensatory nutrition. As a further example, studies on premature infants revealed that certain enzymes required for amino acid metabolism developed later in gestation, rendering these preemies incapable of synthesizing taurine, tyrosine, or other essential amino acids. Similarly, the discovery of genetic defects that required enzymes not inherently available but remediable through higher than normal intake of the vitamin component of corresponding coenzymes further demonstrated the ability to modify a person's diet to meet specific nutritional needs. These conceptual breakthroughs constitute the roots of preventive and therapeutic diets that have become increasingly relevant to the teaching and practice of lifestyle medicine.

This chapter addresses the importance of diet and nutrition in the promotion of good health and prevention of disease by applying twenty-first-century evidence, technology, and biostatistical advances to the modern practice of lifestyle medicine. Evolutionary research on diet and health from observational population studies to diet intervention studies documenting adherence to certain eating patterns and therapeutic diets associated with reduced risks for chronic diseases provide the evidence associated with better versus worsening health outcomes. These data constitute the rationale for the national dietary guidelines summarized and compared here. Assessment methodologies that have contributed to these findings and new and emerging research approaches involving biomarkers and objective measures are further highlighted. Finally, consumer-friendly approaches for helping patients eat healthier are provided.

Diet in the Promotion of Health: US Dietary Guidance

Since the 1940s, the Food and Nutrition Board (FNB) of the Institute of Medicine (IOM) has provided guidance regarding the recommended dietary allowances (RDAs) and later, in 1993, the dietary reference intakes (DRIs). While the RDAs were intended to prevent deficiency diseases in healthy populations, the DRIs incorporated advancing science that differentiated adequate intake (AI), from the estimated average requirement (EAR), from the tolerable upper intake level (UL) as well as designations not only for healthy populations but also for individuals and subgroups. These values are available at: http://www.iom.edu/Activities/Nutrition/SummaryDRIs/~/media/Files/Activity%20Files/Nutrition/DRIs/5_Summary%20Table%20Tables%201-4.pdf.

Initial development of national guidelines for diet planning was intended to help reduce hunger and malnutrition that were prevalent in the 1950s–1960s. Over time, and as assessment of population-wide dietary intake has advanced, the prevalence of overnutrition and excess energy intake, especially from non-nutrient-dense sources, has escalated in tandem with the growing obesity epidemic common across all segments of modern society.

The National Health and Nutrition Examination Survey (NHANES) data are used to monitor the health status of the nation. Launched in the early 1960s by the National Center for Health Statistics, part of the Centers for Disease Control (CDC), and periodically repeated thereafter from 1971 to 1994, NHANES data have been collected continuously since 1999, every 2 years on a population-based sample of approximately 5000 individuals with an accompanying health examination. Two 24-h recalls are currently included in this assessment, and these population-based data are used to represent the dietary intake of the healthy US population ages 2 years and older.

Beginning in 1980, the US Department of Agriculture (USDA) and the US Department of Health and Human Services (DHHS) released, for the first time, "Nutrition and Your Health: Dietary Guidelines for Americans" [2] that were based on emerging science of that era as related to diet and its impact on health and disease. They examined both ends of the caloric spectrum and compared current intake with recommendations for health promotion. The guidelines have been revised and updated approximately every 5 years since then. The most recent 2010 US Dietary Guidelines (USDGs) represented a strategic shift from previous guidelines for several reasons [3].

First, all previous guidelines addressed a generally healthy US population, but in 2010, the majority of the population, 72% of men, 64% of women, and a growing number of children and adolescents, were overweight or obese [3]. This alarming factor influenced development of the entire report. Beginning with the review of evidence related to prevention and treatment of overweight as well as the practical application of dietary guidance intended to maximize nutrient density, minimize excessive calorie intake from energy-dense sources, and increase physical energy expenditure, the 2010 USDGs were focused on prevention and treatment of obesity.

Unfortunately, the US dietary intake falls far short of meeting many recommended nutrient and dietary goals. Imbalances in observed versus recommended diet and eating behaviors are common. Population intakes of whole grains, fruits, vegetables, dairy products, fish, and unsaturated oils are far below the goals, whereas intakes of calories, sugar, solid fats, salt, and refined grains far exceed the recommended limits. Indeed, the leading contributor of calories to the US diet is "grain-based desserts," including cake, cookies, doughnuts, and other sweet foods that are high in sugar, salt, saturated fats, *trans* fats, and non-nutrient-dense calories. Figure 11.1 from the 2010 US Dietary Guidelines Advisory Committee Report (DGAC) illustrates the deficiencies and imbalances in nutrient-dense versus energy-dense foods [4].

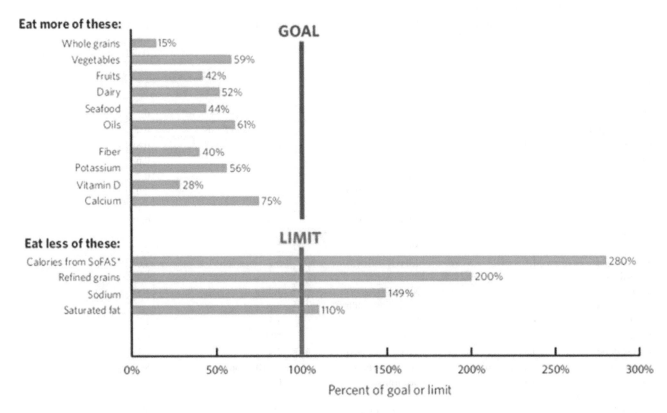

Fig. 11.1 Based on data from: US Department of Agriculture, Agricultural Research Service, and US Department of Health and Human Services, Centers for Disease Control and Prevention. What We Eat in America, NHANES 2001–2004 or 2005–2006. *SoFAS* Solid Fats and Added Sugars

Table 11.1 2010 US Dietary Guidelines recommendations. (Based on data from: US Department of Agriculture, Agricultural Research Service, and US Department of Health and Human Services, Centers for Disease Control and Prevention. What we eat in America, NHANES 2001–2004, 2005–2006)

Limit calorie intake to the amount needed to attain or maintain a healthy weight for adults and for appropriate weight gain in children and adolescents
Consume foods from all food groups in nutrient-dense forms and in recommended amounts
Reduce intakes of solid fats with oils (major sources of saturated and *trans*-fatty acids)
Replace solid fats with oils (major sources of polyunsaturated and monounsaturated fatty acids) when possible
Reduce intake of added sugars
Reduce intake of refined grains and replace some refined grains with whole grains
Reduce intake of sodium (major component of salt)
If consumed, limit alcohol intake to moderate levels
Increase intake of vegetables and fruits
Increase intake of whole grains
Increase intake of milk and milk products and replace whole milk and full-fat milk products with fat-free or low-fat choices to reduce solid fat intake
Increase seafood intake by replacing some meat or poultry with seafood

This is especially troubling from a health promotion and lifestyle medicine perspective. The absence of essential nutrients inherent in these under-consumed foods and the lost opportunity to achieve calorie balance from satiety-producing increased servings of high-fiber, unsaturated fatty acid-containing foods contribute to the risk of chronic diseases.

The 2010 USDGs were also first to utilize the newly developed Nutrition Evidence Library (NEL) and embarked on an entirely systematic, evidence-based review of the a priori diet questions, considered most essential to health and disease. Carefully developed eligibility criteria related to study design, sample size, assessment methodology, and validity of results directed selection of the relevant studies reviewed and ranked them according to the quality, consistency, quantity, impact, and generalizability of the findings. On this basis, the 2010 USDGs were developed and ultimately produced the following recommendations (see Table 11.1).

Table 11.2 Comparison of Mediterranean, DASH, and 2010 USDA recommended food pattern with current dietary intake. (Adapted from Dietary Guidelines for Americans 2010[a])

Pattern	Usual US intake in adults[b]	Mediterranean patterns[a] Greece (G) Spain (S)	DASH[a]	USDA food pattern (US Dietary Guidelines)
Food Groups				
Vegetables: Total (all cups/day)	1.6	1.2 (S)—4.1 (G)	2.1	2.5
Dark green	0.1	ND[c]	ND	0.2
Beans and peas	0.1	<0.1(G)—0.4 (S)	See protein foods	0.2
Red and orange	0.4	ND	ND	0.8
Other	0.5	ND	ND	0.6
Starchy	0.5	ND—0.6 (G)	ND	0.7
Fruits and juices (cups/day)	1.0	1.4 (S)—2.5 (G) (includes nuts)	2.5	2.0
Grains: total (oz)	6.4	2.0 (S)—5.4 (G)	7.3	6.0
Whole grains (oz)	0.6	ND	3.9	≥3.0
Milk and dairy products (cups/day)	1.5	1.0 (G)—2.1 (S)	2.6	3.0
Meat (all in oz/day)	2.5	3.5 (G)—3.6 (S) (including poultry)	1.4	1.8
Poultry	1.2	ND	1.7	1.5
Eggs	0.4	ND—1.9 (S)	ND	0.4
Fish/seafood	0.5	0.8 (G)—2.4 (S)	1.4	1.2
Beans and peas	See vegetables	See vegetables	0.4 (0.1 cup)	See vegetables
Nuts, seeds, and soy products (oz)	0.5	See fruits	0.9	0.6
Oils (g/day)	18	19 (S)—40 (G)	25	27
Solid fats (g)	43	ND	ND	16[d]
Added sugars (g)	79	ND—24 (G)	12	32[d]
Alcohol (g)	9.9	7.1 (S)—7.9 (G)	ND	ND[e]

[a] US Department of Agriculture and US Department of Health and Human Services. Dietary Guidelines for Americans 2010, 7th Edition, Washington, DC: US Government Printing Office, December 2010

[b] Source: US Department of Agriculture, Agricultural Research Service, and US Department of Health and Human Services, Centers for Disease Control and Prevention. What We Eat In America, NHANES 2001–2004, 1 day mean intakes for adult males and females, adjusted to 2000 calories and averaged

[c] *ND* not determined

[d] Amounts of solid fats and added sugars are examples only of how calories from solid fats and added sugars in the USDA Food Patterns could be divided

[e] In the USDA Food Patterns, some of the calories assigned to limits for solid fats and added sugars may be used for alcohol consumption instead

Current US dietary intake does not meet these recommendations (Fig. 11.1). Accumulating data further document compelling reasons why the observed dietary intake poses a major risk factor for developing chronic diseases, especially cardio-metabolic, including type-2 diabetes (T2D), and cancer. The 2010 USDGs' Advisory Committee [3] reviewed the growing, but relatively limited, database at that time, reflecting more than a single nutrient- or food-associated risk for disease. Beyond the well-known evidence surrounding saturated/*trans*-fatty acid intake and low-density lipoprotein cholesterol (LDL-C), or sodium and blood pressure (BP), or sugar and obesity was new evidence from studies that reported outcomes based on total eating patterns. The Dietary Approaches for Stopping Hypertension (DASH) and the Mediterranean style-eating pattern are not singular, structured diets. Rather, these are eating patterns representing a mixture of vegetables, legumes, unsalted nuts, fruits, whole grains, fish, and unsaturated (DASH) or olive (Mediterranean) oils, with moderate alcohol (Mediterranean) or low-fat dairy (DASH) and very little red/processed meat, sweets, or refined grains [5–7].

Table 11.2 compares the Mediterranean dietary patterns, DASH, and the 2010 USDA-recommended food pattern with current dietary intake on the basis of a 2000-calorie intake. Intakes of vegetables, fruit, dairy, fish, and oils are noticeably lower in the usual US intakes. Conversely, alcohol, solid fats, and added sugars exceed the limits reflected in the Mediterranean, DASH, and USDA food patterns.

Table 11.3 World Cancer Research Fund/American Institute for Cancer Research 2007 Recommendations for Cancer Prevention. [8]

1. Be as lean as possible without becoming underweight
2. Be physically active for at least 30 min every day
3. Avoid sugary drinks. Limit consumption of energy-dense foods
4. Eat more of a variety of vegetables, fruits, whole grains, and legumes such as beans
5. Limit consumption of red meats (such as beef, pork, and lamb) and avoid processed meats
6. If consumed at all, limit alcoholic drinks to 2 for men and 1 for women a day
7. Limit consumption of salty foods and foods process with salt (sodium)
8. Don't use supplements to protect against cancer
9. It is best for mothers to breastfeed exclusively for up to 6 months and then add other liquids and foods
10. After treatment, cancer survivors should follow the recommendations for cancer prevention

Other National Dietary Guidelines: Prevention of Cancer, Cardiovascular Disease, and Obesity

In addition to the USDA's evidence-based dietary guidelines, other disease-specific national organizations have likewise conducted evidence-based reviews underlying their own guidelines as well. Most notable among these are dietary guidelines specifically focused on prevention of cancer and cardiovascular diseases.

In 2007, the World Cancer Research Fund/American Institute for Cancer Research (WCRF/AICR) published "Food, Nutrition, Physical Activity, and the Prevention of Cancer: A Global Perspective" [8]. Considered the most comprehensive report on diet and cancer ever produced, the reviewers included over 7000 studies that met the a priori established eligibility criteria. Now designated as a continuous process of review, the WCRF/AICR has published ten recommendations for cancer prevention as derived from the Second Expert Panel Report [8]. After intensive and comprehensive comparisons regarding nutrients, foods, food groups, and eating patterns, the recommendations are more behavioral than nutrient-based, as listed in Table 11.3.

There is an emphasis on plant-based foods; an avoidance of solid fats, sugars, salt, and processed meats; and a strong endorsement of daily physical activity to promote leanness and avoidance of weight gain. Rather than specific nutrient recommendations, the above guidelines are more general and lifestyle-oriented with an overarching goal of prevention of obesity. Encouragement of regular activity and a focus on nutrient-dense foods illustrates the preferred approach achieving and maintaining weight control.

More recently, in 2013, the American Heart Association (AHA) published the "American College of Cardiology/American Heart Association (ACC/AHA) Guidelines on Lifestyle Management to Reduce Cardiovascular Risk" [9]. A specific focus was placed on reducing the LDL-C and BP, both considered major risk factors. Based on a comprehensive, systematic review of the literature, the expert panel specifically recommended that saturated fat be limited to no more than 6% of total calories/day and that sodium intake be reduced, but just as was recommended by the USDGs, a

DASH-type diet reduced in sodium was advocated as a model eating pattern for implementing these nutrient-specific recommendations, along with increased physical activity. The diet recommendations for LDL-C lowering and BP lowering were based on strong evidence statements addressing key critical questions posed in developing the lifestyle guideline. The rationale and approach for these two cardiovascular targets are detailed below. Recommendations for the practical implementation of the ACC/AHA diet recommendations are provided in Table 11.4.

ACC/AHA Diet Recommendations for LDL-C Lowering

Advise adults who would benefit from LDL-C lowering to:

1. Consume a dietary pattern that emphasizes intake of vegetables, fruits, and whole grains; includes low-fat dairy products, poultry, fish, legumes, nontropical vegetable oils, and nuts; and limits intake of sweets, sugar-sweetened beverages, and red meats. Adapt this dietary pattern to appropriate calorie requirements, personal and cultural food preferences, and nutrition therapy for other medical conditions (including diabetes). Achieve this pattern by following plans such as the DASH dietary pattern, the USDA Food Pattern, or the AHA diet.
2. Aim for a dietary pattern that achieves 5–6% of calories from saturated fat.
3. Reduce percent of calories from saturated fat.

Reducing saturated fat intake lowers both LDL-C and high-density lipoprotein–cholesterol (HDL–C). Since the absolute effect tends to be greater for LDL-C than HDL–C, reducing saturated fat intake has a beneficial effect on the lipid profile. Given that reducing saturated fat intake lowers LDL-C regardless of whether the saturated fat is replaced by carbohydrate, monounsaturated fatty acids, or polyunsaturated fatty acids, the work group does not specify which of these 3 macronutrients should be substituted in place of saturated fat. However, favorable effects on lipid profiles are greater

Table 11.4 The American Heart Association's Heart Healthy Diet Recommendations. (American Heart Association Healthy Diet Guidelines. 2014: http://www.heart.org/HEARTORG/GettingHealthy/NutritionCenter/HealthyCooking/Healthy-Diet-Guidelines_UCM_430092_Article.jsp)

Balance the number of calories you eat and physical activity to maintain a healthy body weight (this means not eating more calories than you need)
Make your diet rich in fruits and vegetables. A typical adult should try for 9–10 servings (4.5 cups) of fruits and vegetables every day
Choose whole grains and high-fiber foods (three 1-oz. servings per day). A diet rich in fiber can help manage your weight because fiber keeps you feeling fuller longer, so you eat less
Eat fish, especially oily fish like salmon or albacore tuna, twice a week to get omega-3 fatty acids
Limit saturated and *trans* fat and cholesterol by choosing lean meats, selecting fat-free (skim), 1% and low-fat dairy products, and avoiding hydrogenated fats (margarine, shortening, cooking oils, and the foods made from them). A person needing 2000 calories each day should consume less than 16 g saturated fat, less than 2 g *trans* fat, and between 50 and 70 g of total fat and limit cholesterol to no more than 300 mg each day
Limit the amount of added sugars you consume to no more than half of your daily discretionary calorie allowance. For most American women, this is no more than 100 calories/day and no more than 150 calories/day for men (or approximately 6 teaspoons/day for women and 9 teaspoons/day for men). Limit sugar-sweetened beverages to no more than 450 calories (36 oz.) per week
Choose and prepare foods with little or no salt (sodium) to maintain a healthy blood pressure. Keep sodium intake to 1500 mg/day or less. Limit processed meat (such as sandwich meat, sausages, and hot dogs) to fewer than two servings per week
Try to eat four servings per week of nuts, seeds, or legumes (beans)
If you choose to consume alcohol, do so in moderation. This means an average of one to two drinks per day for men and one drink per day for women
If you eat out, pay attention to portion size and the number of calories in your meal

when saturated fat is replaced by polyunsaturated fatty acids, followed by monounsaturated fatty acids, and then carbohydrates. It is important to note that there are various types and degrees of refinement of carbohydrates. Substitution of saturated fat with whole grains is preferable to refined carbohydrates.

ACC/AHA Diet Recommendations for BP Lowering

Advise adults who would benefit from BP lowering to:

1. Consume a dietary pattern that emphasizes intake of vegetables, fruits, and whole grains; includes low-fat dairy products, poultry, fish, legumes, nontropical vegetable oils, and nuts; and limits intake of sweets, sugar-sweetened beverages, and red meats. Adapt this dietary pattern to appropriate calorie requirements, personal and cultural food preferences, and nutrition therapy for other medical conditions (including diabetes mellitus). Achieve this pattern by following plans such as the DASH dietary pattern, the USDA Food Pattern, or the AHA diet. Rationale: This recommendation is based largely on studies of the DASH dietary pattern (DASH and DASH Sodium), which provided the highest-quality evidence for this food-based dietary pattern, causing improvements in lipid profiles and BP.

2. Consume no more than 2400 mg/day of sodium; further reduction of sodium intake to 1500 mg/day is desirable since it is associated with an even greater reduction in BP; reduce sodium intake by at least 1000 mg/day even if the desired daily sodium intake is not yet achieved.

3. Combine the DASH dietary pattern with lower sodium intake. One well-conducted trial demonstrated clinically meaningful lowering of BP when sodium was reduced to 2400 mg/day, with lower BPs achieved when sodium intake was reduced to 1500 mg/day [10]. A healthy dietary pattern, as exemplified by DASH, and reduced sodium intake independently reduce BP [11]. However, the BP-lowering effect is greater when these dietary changes are combined. In the 60% of US adults with hypertension (HTN) or pre-HTN, simultaneously implementing dietary recommendations number 1 and number 2 for BP lowering can prevent and control HTN more than either intervention alone [12, 13].

Assessment of Diet Quality and Adherence

Major advances have been made not only in reporting the research outcomes documenting diet–disease associations but also the research validating the assessment methodology itself. Research-quality diet assessment relies on the use of validated methodology. This ranges from interviewer-administered multiple 24-h recalls (24 HR) linked to a credible, current, and detailed nutrient data base to a standardized food-frequency questionnaire (FFQ) that can vary in length from a "screener" regarding a specific food or food group, such as vegetables, to a detailed list of foods intended to capture the majority of the diet [14]. Multiple 24 HR have been recognized as the preferred method for estimating population level or group dietary intakes [15], but due to the labor and expense involved, the FFQ is much more commonly used in epidemiologic research, thereby raising questions about underreporting in these data [16].

With advances in technology and metabolomics research, objective biomarkers are being identified that can potentially improve the accuracy of self-reported dietary data [17]. Calibration of self-reported dietary assessment methods including 24 HR and FFQs based on measures of biomarkers from metabolomic or clinical measures are emerging as enhanced approaches to nutritional assessment [18]. For example, a recent case–control study among the Framingham offspring reported that five branched-chain and aromatic amino acids were significantly associated with future risk of developing diabetes among individuals who were normoglycemic at baseline [19]. Ultimately, establishing a nutritional assessment method that does not solely rely on self-reported diet intake data but also includes objective measures of food, nutrient, and even phytochemical intake will provide a more realistic and reliable measure of diet intake that can foster generation of hypotheses related to potential mechanisms.

Diet quality scoring systems have been developed to help evaluate overall nutrient density of a diet compared with recommended intake. The 2010 Healthy Eating Index (HEI) reinforces the validity and reliability of this scoring system developed to measure overall diet quality compared with the USDGs [20] and has been shown to be associated with decreased risk of cardiovascular diseases, cancer, and all-cause mortality [21]. Unfortunately, as illustrated in Fig. 11.1, the overall quality of the American diet remains woefully low with an overall score that is approximately 50 % of the maximum total and an empty calorie score that is more than double the maximum score. Other scoring systems have been developed and validated to evaluate adherence to the DASH and Mediterranean Diets [22, 23]. The Alternative Healthy Eating Index (AHEI) also strongly predicts chronic disease [24].

From a consumer/patient perspective, there are many user-friendly diet assessment tools that are now available. The USDA has developed a free online tool called Super-Tracker (https://www.supertracker.usda.gov/) for use in assessing adherence to the My Plate recommendations or any other dietary guidelines. Other assessment tools are available as smartphone applications, both commercially and for free, that can help patients assess their own level of adherence to these recommendations.

Healthy Eating: Start at the Beginning

Before concluding this chapter on healthy eating that is largely focused on adults, it is increasingly reported that a healthy lifestyle begins in utero, and the benefits of exclusive breast feeding at birth and for several months postpartum are tremendous [25, 26]. As indicated in the WCRF/AICR guidelines, human milk is highly recommended as the only source of nourishment in newborns and preferably for the first 6 months of life. This has been recommended by the USDGs as well, based on rapidly growing evidence that breastfeeding provides long-term benefits for mother and baby alike in regard to prevention of chronic disease. Delay of solid foods to no sooner than 4 months of age and preferably 6 months is further recommended for both weight control and diet quality purposes.

Summary and Conclusions

Taken together, the dietary guidelines from various national organizations have provided an overview of the evidence associated with healthy eating. The 2010 USDGs have reviewed the data on diet and disease that have resulted in the above recommendations.

Likewise, guidelines from the ACC/AHA have provided an even more focused view of diet as it may help prevent cardiovascular disease, and the (WCRF/AICR) have similarly addressed prevention of cancer. Table 11.2 summarizes and compares the USDA Dietary Guidelines with the DASH and Mediterranean Diets based on the specific foods and recommended amounts. Some differences across these eating patterns include the amount and choice of dietary fatty acids (e.g., olive oil vs. other polyunsaturated oils), the inclusion of low-fat dairy products, type and amount of red meat, inclusion and amount of wine intake, and tolerance for greater (USDA) versus lower sugar intake. These are decisions that can be made based on taste and cultural preferences but also the high priority to maintain weight control. The goal is a nutrient-dense, calorie-controlled diet combined with a physically active lifestyle. Helping patients select the approach that is most likely to achieve long-term adherence may be the most important contribution that the lifestyle medicine provider can make.

References

1. Murray D, Holben D, Raymond J. Food and nutrient delivery: planning the diet with cultural competency. In: Mahan K, Escott-Stump S, Raymond J, editors. Krause's food and the nutrition care process. 13 ed. USA: Elsevier/Saunders; 2012. p. 274–90.
2. U.S. Senate Appropriations Subcommittee on Agriculture, Rural Development, Food and Drug Administration, and Related Agencies. Dietary guidelines for Americans: hearing before a subcommittee of the Committee on Appropriations, United States Senate, Ninety-sixth Congress, second session: special hearing, Department of Agriculture, Department of Health and Human Services, nondepartmental witnesses. Washington: U.S. Govt. Print. Off.: for sale by the Supt. of Docs., U.S. Govt. Print. Off.; 1980. iv, 306 p.
3. United States Department of Health and Human Services., United States Department of Agriculture., United States. Dietary Guidelines Advisory Committee. Dietary guidelines for Americans, 2010. 7th ed. Washington, DC: G.P.O.; 2010. xi, 95 p.
4. Van Horn L, Dietary Guidelines Advisory C. Development of the 2010 US Dietary Guidelines Advisory Committee Report: perspectives from a registered dietitian. J Am Diet Assoc. 2010;110(11):1638–45.

5. Appel LJ, Moore TJ, Obarzanek E, Vollmer WM, Svetkey LP, Sacks FM, et al. A clinical trial of the effects of dietary patterns on blood pressure. DASH Collaborative Research Group. N Engl J Med. 1997;336(16):1117–24.

6. Willett WC, Sacks F, Trichopoulou A, Drescher G, Ferro-Luzzi A, Helsing E, et al. Mediterranean diet pyramid: a cultural model for healthy eating. Am J Clin Nutr. 1995;61(6 Suppl):1402S–6S.

7. Stamler J. Toward a modern Mediterranean diet for the 21st century. Nutr Metab Cardiovasc Dis: NMCD. 2013;23(12):1159–62.

8. American Institute for Cancer Research, World Cancer Research Fund. Food, nutrition, physical activity and the prevention of cancer: a global perspective: a project of World Cancer Research Fund International. Washington, DC: American Institute for Cancer Research; 2007. xxv, 517 p.

9. Eckel RH, Jakicic JM, Ard JD, Hubbard VS, de Jesus JM, Lee IM, et al. 2013 AHA/ACC guideline on lifestyle management to reduce cardiovascular risk: a report of the American College of Cardiology/American Heart Association Task Force on practice guidelines. Circulation. 2014;129(25 Suppl 2):S76–99.

10. Sacks FM, Svetkey LP, Vollmer WM, Appel LJ, Bray GA, Harsha D, et al. Effects on blood pressure of reduced dietary sodium and the dietary approaches to stop hypertension (DASH) diet. DASH-Sodium Collaborative Research Group. N Engl J Med. 2001;344(1):3–10.

11. Vollmer WM, Sacks FM, Ard J, Appel LJ, Bray GA, Simons-Morton DG, et al. Effects of diet and sodium intake on blood pressure: subgroup analysis of the DASH-sodium trial. Ann Intern Med. 2001;135(12):1019–28.

12. Bray GA, Vollmer WM, Sacks FM, Obarzanek E, Svetkey LP, Appel LJ, et al. A further subgroup analysis of the effects of the DASH diet and three dietary sodium levels on blood pressure: results of the DASH-sodium trial. Am J Cardiol. 2004;94(2):222–7.

13. Sacks FM, Campos H. Dietary therapy in hypertension. N Engl J Med. 2010;362(22):2102–12.

14. Block G, Gillespie C, Rosenbaum EH, Jenson C. A rapid food screener to assess fat and fruit and vegetable intake. Am J Prev Med. 2000;18(4):284–8.

15. Institute of Medicine. Dietary reference intakes: applications in dietary assessment. Washington, DC: National Academy Press; 2000.

16. Rhodes DG, Murayi T, Clemens JC, Baer DJ, Sebastian RS, Moshfegh AJ. The USDA automated multiple-pass method accurately assesses population sodium intakes. Am J Clin Nutr. 2013;97(5):958–64.

17. Scalbert A, Brennan L, Manach C, Andres-Lacueva C, Dragsted LO, Draper J, et al. The food metabolome: a window over dietary exposure. Am J Clin Nutr. 2014;99(6):1286–308.

18. Prentice RL, Huang Y, Kuller LH, Tinker LF, Horn LV, Stefanick ML, et al. Biomarker-calibrated energy and protein consumption and cardiovascular disease risk among postmenopausal women. Epidemiology. 2011;22(2):170–9.

19. Wang TJ, Larson MG, Vasan RS, Cheng S, Rhee EP, McCabe E, et al. Metabolite profiles and the risk of developing diabetes. Nat Med. 2011;17(4):448–53.

20. Guenther PM, Kirkpatrick SI, Reedy J, Krebs-Smith SM, Buckman DW, Dodd KW, et al. The healthy eating index-2010 is a valid and reliable measure of diet quality according to the 2010 Dietary Guidelines for Americans. J Nutr. 2014;144(3):399–407.

21. Reedy J, Krebs-Smith SM, Miller PE, Liese AD, Kahle LL, Park Y, et al. Higher diet quality is associated with decreased risk of all-cause, cardiovascular disease, and cancer mortality among older adults. J Nutr. 2014;144(6):881–9.

22. Fung TT, Hu FB, Wu K, Chiuve SE, Fuchs CS, Giovannucci E. The Mediterranean and dietary approaches to stop hypertension (DASH) diets and colorectal cancer. Am J Clin Nutr. 2010;92(6):1429–35.

23. Bertoia ML, Triche EW, Michaud DS, Baylin A, Hogan JW, Neuhouser ML, et al. Mediterranean and dietary approaches to stop hypertension dietary patterns and risk of sudden cardiac death in postmenopausal women. Am J Clin Nutr. 2014;99(2):344–51.

24. Chiuve SE, Fung TT, Rimm EB, Hu FB, McCullough ML, Wang M, et al. Alternative dietary indices both strongly predict risk of chronic disease. J Nutr. 2012;142(6):1009–18.

25. Fields DA, Demerath EW. Relationship of insulin, glucose, leptin, IL-6 and TNF-alpha in human breast milk with infant growth and body composition. Pediatr Obes. 2012;7(4):304–12.

26. Owen CG, Martin RM, Whincup PH, Davey-Smith G, Gillman MW, Cook DG. The effect of breastfeeding on mean body mass index throughout life: a quantitative review of published and unpublished observational evidence. Am J Clin Nutr. 2005;82(6):1298–307.

A Review of Commercial and Proprietary Weight Loss Programs

Nasreen Alfaris, Alyssa Minnick, Patricia Hong and Thomas A. Wadden

Abbreviations

ADA	American Diabetes Association
BDD	Balanced deficit diet
BMI	Body Mass Index
DSE	Diabetes support and education
DSME	Diabetes self-management education
HCP	Health-care professionals
HMR	Health Management Resources
LCDs	Low-calorie diets
NHLBI	National Heart, Lung, and Blood Institute
NIH	National Institutes of Health
POWER	Practice-based opportunities for weight reduction
RCTs	Randomized controlled trials
T2D	Type-2 diabetes
VLCD	Very low-calorie diet

The 2013 Guidelines for the Management of Overweight and Obesity in Adults [1] included an assessment of the efficacy of commercial weight loss programs and whether primary care health-care professionals (HCP) could recommend their use to patients. The expert panel noted the limited number of high quality studies conducted in this area but concluded that, "Some commercial-based programs that provide a comprehensive lifestyle intervention can be prescribed as an option for weight loss, provided there is peer-reviewed published evidence of their safety and efficacy."

This chapter examines the efficacy of the major commercial and proprietary weight loss programs (in the USA) as assessed in randomized controlled trials (RCTs). Additional sources, including web sites and telephone inquiries, were used to obtain information about programs' costs and principal treatment components, as well as the training of interventionists. We review three general types of programs: (1) traditional nonmedical programs, such as Weight Watchers® and Jenny Craig®, that offer diet and physical activity recommendations, accompanied by person-to-person individual or group lifestyle counseling; (2) medically supervised programs, such as HMR® and OPTIFAST®, which offer low- or very-low-calorie, portion-controlled diets, combined with person-to-person lifestyle counseling; and (3) remotely delivered programs that offer lifestyle interventions using e-mail, text messaging, the web, or similar methods. This last category is the fastest growing but the one that has been least evaluated because of its very recent emergence. Programs in the first category (e.g., Weight Watchers®) are increasing their online presence and use of apps, but these components have not been widely evaluated to date. We excluded commercial self-help approaches based solely on written materials (e.g., diet books) , over-the-counter meal replacement plans, or similar products.

Plan of the Review

We searched the Pubmed database for articles published between January 1, 1998 and July 14, 2014 using the terms *obesity*; *weight loss,* and *commercial*; combined with each of the following text terms: *diet, reducing, nutrition, behavior therapy, low calorie, cognitive therapy, physical activity,* and *technology*. The search was limited to RCTs. Studies were excluded if they included fewer than ten participants per treatment group, treated children and adolescents, did not state the duration of the intervention, or lasted fewer than 12 weeks. In addition, we only included studies in which programs were assessed under conditions relatively similar to those in which the programs are offered to the public.

N. Alfaris (✉)
Center for Weight and Eating Disorders, University of Pennsylvania Perelman School of Medicine, 3535 Market Street, Suite 3021, Philadelphia, PA 19104, USA
e-mail: nasreen.alfaris@UPHS.upenn.edu

A. Minnick · P. Hong · T. A. Wadden
Departments of Medicine and Psychiatry, University of Pennsylvania Perelman School of Medicine, Philadelphia, PA, USA

© Springer International Publishing Switzerland 2016
J. I. Mechanick, R. F. Kushner (eds.), *Lifestyle Medicine,* DOI 10.1007/978-3-319-24687-1_12

Nonmedical Commercial Weight Loss Programs

Nonmedical commercial programs are staffed by HCP, former clients, or laypersons trained by the parent company (Table 12.1). These programs do not provide medical supervision. Therefore, persons with weight-related medical complications must be monitored by their own primary care practitioners when participating in such interventions. Nonmedical commercial programs typically aim to induce weight loss of 0.5–0.9 kg/week (1–2 lb/week), which is considered a safe rate [1]. Three nonmedical commercial weight loss programs are included in this review—Weight Watchers®, Jenny Craig®, and Nutrisystem®. An overview of the programs' components can be found in Table 12.1.

Weight Watchers®

The Weight Watchers® program prescribes a balanced, moderate-calorie-deficit diet. Clients are offered a food plan (e.g., PointsPlus®), a physical activity plan based on current National Institutes of Health (NIH) guidelines, and behavior modification principles and techniques [2]. Clients can access resources through in-person group meetings or online. One-hour, face-to-face group meetings are held weekly and are led by successful program completers who offer support and guidance, as well as written materials and weigh-ins [2]. At the time of this writing, the estimated cost of participating in Weight Watchers® for 3 months (i.e., meetings and online tools) was US$128.85 (Table 12.2).

Outcome Data Weight Watchers® has sponsored at least seven RCTs of its program (the five largest and longest of which are reviewed here). In a multicenter study, Heshka et al. [3, 4] randomly assigned 423 participants to Weight Watchers® or a self-help intervention that included two visits with a dietitian (Table 12.3). Participants in Weight Watchers®, who were provided weekly group meetings, lost an average of 4.8 kg of initial weight at week 26 and maintained a loss of 2.9 kg at year 2, compared with significantly smaller values of 2.9 and 0.2 kg, respectively, for those who received the self-help intervention. (Statistical comparisons between groups, when available, are shown in Table 12.3.) Participants who attended the most meetings over the 2 years achieved the greatest weight losses. As shown in Table 12.3, 34% of Weight Watchers® participants maintained a loss ≥5% of initial weight at year 2, compared with 21% of those in self-help. Weight loss of this amount is considered clinically meaningful [1, 5].

In a multinational study, Jebb et al. [6] assigned 772 participants from primary care practices in Australia, Germany, and the UK to 12 months of weekly Weight Watchers® meetings or to a usual care program provided by participants' own

practitioners. Weight Watchers® participants lost an average of 4.1 kg at month 12 compared with 1.8 kg for usual care. Weight losses were similar in all countries. Attrition, however, was high in both interventions, with rates of 39 and 45.8%, respectively.

In another multisite study, Jolly et al. [7] assigned 740 men and women to 1 of 8 intervention arms for 12 weeks. At year 1, Weight Watchers® participants lost 3.5 kg, compared to a smaller 0.8 kg for those assigned to a usual care comparator group provided by participants' primary care HCP. Weight losses of other interventions fell in between these two groups.

In a single-site study, Johnston et al. [8] assigned 292 men and women to Weight Watchers® or a self-help program (consisting of informational materials on diet and exercise). At month 6, Weight Watchers® participants lost an average of 4.6 kg, compared with 0.6 kg for self-help. Attrition in both groups was low (i.e., 11.6 and 12.4%, respectively). Participants in Weight Watchers® who used all modes of participation (including face-to-face meetings, web site, and mobile applications) lost the most weight.

In another single-site study, [9] 141 men and women were assigned to Weight Watchers® alone, a group behavioral weight loss alone, or a group behavioral weight loss treatment combined with Weight Watchers®. At week 48, average weight losses in the three groups were 6.0, 5.5, and 3.6 kg, respectively (p=0.03 for the comparison of groups 1 and 3). Adding brief behavioral weight loss treatment to the Weight Watchers® program did not improve outcomes.

Examining these five trials together, at 12 to 24 months, 31–51% of participants who received the Weight Watchers® program achieved a loss ≥5% of initial weight. These findings suggest that primary care HCP can consider Weight Watchers® as a behavioral weight loss option with appropriate patients, as indicated by the recent 2013 Obesity Guidelines published by The Obesity Society and American College of Cardiology/American Heart Association Task Force (Obesity Guidelines) [1].

Jenny Craig®

Jenny Craig® provides a lifestyle intervention combined with low-calorie meal replacements that provide 1200–2300 calories per day, as combined with some fresh foods [10]. Clients are offered face-to-face individual counseling or telephone-based counseling by trained interventionists, both in conjunction with online resources. The estimated cost of Jenny Craig® for 3 months of intervention and meal replacements is US$1984.00.

Outcome Data In a single-site randomized trial, Rock et al. [11] assigned 70 participants to Jenny Craig® or usual care.

Table 12.1 Key components of selected commercial and organized self-help weight loss programs

Program	Staff qualifications	Diet	Physical activity	Behavior modification	Face-to-face contact	Electronically delivered contact
Nonmedical programs						
Weight Watchers®	Successful lifetime member (successful program completer)	Low-calorie, exchange diet; clients prepare own meals	Recommends increasing exercise over time	Behavioral weight control methods	Weekly group meetings	Food and activity tracker, newsletter, forum, mobile app
Jenny Craig®	Company-trained counselor	Low-calorie diet of prepackaged Jenny Craig meals only	Increased PA with goal setting and follow through; 30 min of PA ≥5 days/week	Manual on weight loss strategies provided	Individual sessions, weekly contact	Jenny at home offers contact via phone and Internet
Nutrisystem®	Health-care professional with behavioral weight control experience	Low-calorie diet provided through meal replacement products	Personalized "My Daily 3" activity plan	Behavioral weight control methods	Access to counselors, dietitians, community, and tracking tools	Online forum, tracking tools, blog, dining out guide
Medically supervised						
Health Management Resources®	Licensed physician and other health-care providers	Low-calorie or very-low-calorie diet provided through meal replacement products	Walking and calorie charts provided in lifestyle classes	Included in lifestyle classes; accountability and skill acquisition emphasized	Group sessions and weekly classes; some telephone support	None
OPTIFAST®	Licensed physician and other health-care providers	Low-calorie diet provided through meal replacement products	PA modules taught in lifestyle classes	Included in lifestyle classes; stress management and social support emphasized	Group sessions and weekly classes; some telephone support	None
Medifast®/Take Shape for Life	Not applicable	Low-calorie or very-low-calorie diet provided through meal replacement products	May be included in Take Shape for Life	May be included in Take Shape for Life	Included in Take Shape for Life	24 h online support through the Medifast community
Remotely delivered						
eDiets.com	Company-trained counselors and company dietitians	Low-calorie diet provided through "virtual dietitian" program; clients prepare own meals	PA seminar as part of eDiets.com University	Included in eDiets.com University; stress management emphasized	None	Individual and group Internet support
VTrim®	Company-trained counselors and company dieticians	Low-calorie diet plan; clients prepare own meals	PA goals and planning	Included in the two consecutive 12-week online courses	None	Individual and group Internet support
Innergy™	Johns Hopkins-trained coaches	Low calorie diet plan; clients prepare own meals	PA goals and planning	Included in phone calls and online account resources	None	Individual and group Internet support
The Biggest Loser® Club	Company-trained counselors and company dieticians	Low-calorie diet plan through "virtual dietitian" program; clients prepare own meals	PA goals and planning; 8-week online exercise bootcamp for extra cost	Included in the online account resources	None	Individual and group Internet support

Low-calorie diets typically provide 1200–1500 kcal/day for women and 1500–1800 kcal/day for men. Alternatively, the goal is to induce an energy deficit of 500–1000 kcal/day; *PA* physical activity

Table 12.2 Estimated program costs for commercial and organized self-help weight loss programs

Program	Membership fee or initial cost	Periodic fees	Meal plan	Other	Estimated cost of 3-month program
Nonmedical programs					
Weight Watchers®	Meetings and online tools	US$42.95/month	None	None	US$128.85
	Online standard monthly US$29.95	Monthly fee US$18.95	None	None	US$86.80
	Meetings only US$20.00	US$12–14/meeting	None	None	US$188.00
Jenny Craig®	US$49	US$29/month[a]	US$105–154/week[b]	None	US$1984.00
Nutrisystem®	Basic- 28 day; three meals and dessert daily US$244.99	None	US$244.99 per month	None	US$734.97
	Core program—28 day; three meals and dessert daily. Customized menu options, weight loss counselor. US$284.99	None	US$284.99/month	None	US$854.97
	Select Program—28 day; three meals and dessert daily. Customized menu options, weight loss coaches. Eighteen days of ready-to-go and frozen menu options. US$329.99	None	US$329.99/month	None	US$989.97
Medically supervised					
Health Management Resources®	None	US$600–700/13 weeks	Powder US$3/envelope ready to drink US$3.50/can	Maintenance visits at extra cost	US$600–700 + cost of food (~US$1350)
OPTIFAST®	US$150–300 for medical evaluation	US$35/week for medical visits; US$10/week for behavior modification classes; US$210 for lab test[d]	~US$200 for 84 packs	Maintenance visits at extra cost	US$1200 for shakes + cost of visits and initial evaluation
Medifast®/Take Shape For Life	None	Not required[d]	US$339 for 4-week package	Physicians visit at extra cost	US$1017 for food + cost of visits
Remotely delivered					
eDiets.com	None	US$9.95/month	None	Dietary supplements, prepared meals, meal replacements, nutrition books, and exercise equipment at extra cost	US$29.85
VTrim®	None	US$395/12-week course	None	Monthly online maintenance course at extra cost	US$395 (US$790 for two consecutive 12-week courses)
Innergy™	None	US$27.74/month for 12-month weight loss[c]	None	None	US$82.41 for 3 months of weight loss[c]
		US$13.73/month for 12-month maintenance[c]			US$41.19 for 3 months of maintenance[c]
The Biggest Loser® Club	None	US$39.99	None	8-week online exercise bootcamp for extra cost	US$39.99

All costs are presented in US dollars (US$) and were estimated from discussions with company representatives and calls to programs in New Jersey, to limit geographic variations in cost. The information for Jenny Craig® was provided through their corporate site because information could not be obtained through company representatives
[a] Plus the cost of shipping if applicable. Recurring billing required via credit card
[b] Does not include fruits, vegetables and other grocery items
[c] Costs for Johns Hopkins University employees. Costs may vary for other employers and health systems
[d] Costs estimated in 2005, Contacted centers but unable to obtain updated cost

Table 12.3 Summary of results for commercial and organized self-help weight loss programs

Nonmedical programs

Program (Reference)	Study design	Subjects, N; Mean initial BMI or weight	Women %	Duration	Treatment regimen	Short-term weight loss	Long-term weight loss	Long-term attrition
Weight Watchers® [3, 4]	Multisite randomized trial	423; 33.7 kg/m²	85	2 year	Weight Watchers group	−4.8 kg at week 26[a]; 53% lost ≥5%[a]	−2.9 kg at year 2[a]; 34% lost >5%[a]	28.9% at year 2
					Self-help (two visits with a dietitian)	−1.4 kg at week 26[b]; 16% lost ≥5%[b]	−0.2 kg at year 2[b]; 21% lost >5%[b]	25.0% at year 2
Weight Watchers® [6]	Multisite randomized trial	772; 31.4 kg/m²[c]	86.5	1 year	Weight Watchers		−4.1 kg at year 1[a]; 45% lost ≥5%	39.0% at year 1
					Standard Care		−1.8 kg at year 1[b]; 22% lost ≥5%	45.8% at year 1
Weight Watchers® [7]	Multisite randomized trial	740; 33.6 kg/m²[c]	69.3	1 year	Weight Watchers	−4.4 kg at week 12; 46% lost ≥5%	−3.5 kg at year 1; 31% lost ≥5%	18.0% at year 1
					General practice one-to-one support	−1.4 kg at week 12; 16% lost ≥5%	−0.8 kg at year 1; 16% lost ≥5%	34.3% at year 1
Weight Watchers® [8]	Single site randomized trial	292; 33.0 kg/m²	89.8	6 month	Weight Watchers		−4.6 kg at month 6[a]	11.6% at month 6
					Self-help		−0.6 kg at month 6[b]	12.4% at month 6
Weight Watchers® [9]	Single site randomized trial	141; 36.2 kg/m²	90	48 week	Behavioral Weight Loss Treatment	−6.0 kg at week 24[a]; 47.8% lost ≥5%[a]	−5.4 kg at week 48[a]; 41.3% lost ≥5%[a]	29.2% at week 48
					Weight Watchers	−5.1 kg at week 24[a]; 40.8% lost ≥5%[a]	−6.0 kg at week 48[b]; 51.0% lost ≥5%[a]	16.3% at week 48
					Combined Treatment	−4.9 kg at week 24[a]; 41.3% lost ≥5%[a]	−3.6 kg at week 48[a]; 32.6% lost ≥5%[a]	19.1%at week 48
Jenny Craig® [11]	Single site randomized trial	70; 34.0 kg/m²	100	1 year	Jenny Craig Intervention	−7.2 kg at month 6[a]	−6.6 kg at year 1[a]	8.6% at year 1
					Usual Care Control Group	−0.3 kg at month 6[b]	−0.7 kg at year 1[b]	5.7% at year 1
Jenny Craig® [12]	Multisite randomized trial	446; 442; 33.9 kg/m²[c]	100	2 year	Center-based intervention	−10.1 kg at year 1[a]	−7.4 kg at year 2[a]; 62% lost ≥5%[a]	10.7% at year 2
					Telephone-based intervention	−8.5 kg at year 1[a]	−6.2 kg at year 2[a]; 56% lost ≥5%[a]	6.7% at year 2
					Usual Care	−2.9 kg at year 1[b]	−2.0 kg at year 2[b]; 29% lost ≥5%[b]	8.8% at year 2
Nutrisystem® [17]	Single site randomized trial	69; 39.0 kg/m²	71.0	6 month	Portion-Controlled Diet	−8.2 kg at month 3[a]		2.9% at month 6
					Diabetes Support and Education	−0.6 kg at month 3[b]		0.0% at month 6
Nutrisystem® [18]	Multisite randomized trial	100; 35.8 kg/m²	59.0	6 month	Portion-Controlled Diet	−5.6 kg at month 3	−7.3 kg at month 6[a]; 54% lost ≥5%[a]	2.0% at month 6
					Diabetes Support and Education	−1.8 kg at month 3	−2.2 kg at month 6[b]; 14% lost ≥5%[b]	0.0% at month 6

Table 12.3 (continued)

Program (Reference)	Study design	Subjects, N; Mean initial BMI or weight	Women %	Duration	Treatment regimen	Short-term weight loss	Long-term weight loss	Long-term attrition
Medically supervised								
HMR® [24]	Single site randomized trial	69; 38 kg/m²	100.0	90 day	HMR		−20.4 kg at day 90	Not given
					HMR + Endurance Exercise		−21.4 kg at day 90	Not given
					HMR + Weight Training		−20.9 kg at day 90	Not given
					HMR + Endurance Exercise and Weight Training		−22.9 kg at day 90	Not given
HMR® [25]	Single site randomized trial	40; 30–40 kg/m²	47.5	12 week	HMR + food	−15.5 kg at week 12	−8.8 kg year 1[c]	7.5 % at year 1[c]
					HMR + food	−14.9 kg at week 12		
HMR® [26]	Single site randomized trial	45; 35 kg/m²	76	24 week	HMR		−13.9 kg at week 24[a]	21.7 % at week 24
					Usual Care		−0.7 kg at week 24[b]	40.9 % at week 24
HMR® [27]	Single site randomized trial	295; 35.1 kg/m²	~70%	18 month	HMR + face-to-face weight management clinic	−13.5 kg at month 6; 86 % lost ≥5 %[a]	−8.4 kg at month 18; 61.7 % lost ≥5 %[a]	26 % at month 18
					HMR + group conference calls	−12.6 kg at month 6; 91 % lost ≥5 %[a]	−7.5 kg at month 18; 59.7 % lost ≥5 %[a]	28 % at month 18
OPTIFAST® [29]	Single site randomized trial	49; 39.5 kg/m²	100.0	1 year	OPTIFAST	−20.5 kg at week 17[a]	−17.3 kg at year 1[a]	17.9 % at year 1
					Balanced-Deficit Diet	−9.1 kg at week 17[b]	−14.4 kg at year 1[b]	19.0 % at year 1
OPTIFAST® [30]	Single site randomized trial	201; 36.6 kg/m²	100.0	18 month	OPTIFAST + regular food (time-dependent)	−15.2 kg at randomization	−8.2 kg at month 18	6.0 % at month 18
					OPTIFAST + regular food (weight dependent)	−15.0 kg at randomization	−8.6 kg at month 18	4.3 % at month 18
					OPTIFAST + stimulus narrowing (time-dependent)	−14.9 kg at randomization	−6.0 kg at month 18	15.6 % at month 18
					OPTIFAST + stimulus narrowing (weight dependent)	−14.2 kg at randomization	−2.8 kg at month 18	10.2 % at month 18
Medifast® [32]	Single site randomized trial	119; 35.3 kg/m²	53.7	86 week	Medifast Plus	−4.8 kg at week 34[b], 61.3 % lost ≥5 %	−1.3 kg at week 86[b], 43.8 % lost ≥5 %[a]	70.4 % at week 86
					Standard Diet	−1.5 kg at week 34[a], 23.5 % lost ≥5 %[b]	−0.5 kg at week 86[a], 25.0 % lost ≥5 %[a]	86.2 % at week 86
Medifast® [33]	Single site randomized trial	90; 38.5 kg/m²	58.0	40 week	Medifast 5&1 plan	−13.5 kg at week 16[a], 92.9 % lost ≥5 %	−8.9 kg at week 40[a], 61.5 % lost ≥5 %[a]	42.2 % at week 40
					Food-based plan	−6.5 kg at week 16[b], 55.0 % lost ≥5 %[b]	−5.7 kg at week 40[b], 30.0 % lost ≥5 %[b]	55.6 % at week 40

Table 12.3 (continued)

Program (Reference)	Study design	Subjects, N; Mean initial BMI or weight	Women %	Duration	Treatment regimen	Short-term weight loss	Long-term weight loss	Long-term attrition
Medifast® [34]	Single site randomized trial	120; 40.4 kg/m²	50.0	1 year	Medifast 5&1 plan	−7.5 kg at month 6 [a]	−4.7 kg at year 1 [a]	16.7% at year 1
					Food-based plan	−3.8 kg at month 6 [b]	−1.9 kg at year 1	25.0% at year 1
Remotely delivered								
eDiets.com [37]	Single-site randomized trial	46; 33.5 kg/m²	100	1 year	eDiets.com	−0.7 kg at week 16 [a]	−0.8 kg at year 1 [a]	34.8% at year 1
					LEARN Program for Weight Management 2000	−3.0 kg at week 16 [b]	−3.3 kg at year 1 [b]	33.3% at year 1
VTrim® vs. eDiets.com [40]	Single-site randomized trial	124; 32.4 kg/m²	81.5	1 year	eDiets.com	−3.3 kg at month 6 [a]	−2.6 kg at year 1 [a]; 37.5% lost ≥5%[a]	23% at year 1
					VTrim	−6.8 kg at month 6 [b]	−5.1 kg at year 1 [b]; 65% lost ≥5%	35% at year 1
Innergy™ [43]	Single-site randomized trial	415; 36.6 kg/m²	63.6	2 year	In-person support	−5.8 kg at month 6 [a]; 46.0% lost ≥5%[a]	−5.1 kg at year 2 [a]; 41.4% lost ≥5%[a]	5% at year 2
					Remote-only support	−6.1 kg at month 6 [a]; 52.7% lost ≥5%[a]	−4.6 kg at year 2 [a]; 38.2% lost ≥5%[a]	13% at year 2
					Control/Waitlist	−1.4 kg at month 6 [b]; 14.2% lost ≥5%[b]	−0.8 kg at year 2 [b]; 18.8% lost ≥5%[b]	Not given
The Biggest Loser® Club [45, 46, 47]	Single-site randomized trail	309; 32.3 kg/m²	58.3	24 week	Basic version	−2.3 kg at week 12 [a]	−3.0 kg at week 24 [a]; 28.7% lost ≥5%[a]	31.5% at week 24
					Enhanced version	−3.1 kg at week 12 [a]	−3.9 kg at week 24 [a]; 36.7% lost ≥5%[a]	19% at week 24
					Control/Waitlist	0.5 kg at week 12 [b]	N/A[f]	N/A[f]

Values shown for BMI are means. Values shown for weight change are mean changes. For each study, under "weight change" values within columns labeled with different letters (a, b) are significantly different from each other at $P<0.05$. Values with the same letter (a) are not significantly different.

c Calculated value from data provided

d The study does not report p-values for the difference between Weight Watchers® and Usual Care

e 1-year follow-up data provided for all participants in the study. Follow-up data was not reported for each group separately

f Participants in the control condition were re-randomized into the basic and enhanced groups after week 12

Participants in Jenny Craig® received weekly face-to-face meetings with a trained interventionist, plus meal replacements, while those in usual care received diet and exercise information from a dietitian at baseline and week 16. At month 12, those in Jenny Craig® lost an average of 6.6 kg of initial weight, compared with 0.7 kg for participants in usual care. Attrition was low in both groups, as shown in Table 12.3.

In a multisite randomized trial, Rock et al. [12] allocated 446 participants to a center-based (face-to-face) intervention, telephone-based program, or usual care. Participants in the two interventions received weekly contact (in-person or by phone) for the entire 2-year study (although not all participants used this benefit). Those in usual care received diet and exercise information from a dietitian at baseline and month 6. At month 24, participants in the center-based intervention lost 7.4 kg, those treated by telephone lost 6.2 kg, and those in usual care lost 2.0 kg. As shown in Table 12.3, 62% of those in the first group and 56% in the second lost ≥5% of initial weight, compared with 29% in the third. Attrition was low in all groups.

Short- and long-term weight losses produced by Jenny Craig® generally were larger than those achieved in Weight Watchers® trials, likely because of the provision of portion-controlled meals in the former program. Portion-controlled meals, served as shakes or prepared foods, increase mean weight loss by approximately 3–4 kg (in 3 months) as compared with the prescription of an equivalent calorie diet of self-selected conventional foods [13, 14]. The greater weight loss with Jenny Craig®, compared with Weight Watchers®, comes at a higher cost, some of which, however, would be accounted for by the need for Weight Watchers® participants to buy conventional foods. The success of the telephone-delivered program in the Jenny Craig® trial, which nearly matched the efficacy of face-to-face counseling, is particularly noteworthy. Telephone-delivered counseling potentially is more convenient to patients, eliminates travel costs, and can be provided to individuals in remote areas [15]. The Obesity Guidelines [1] included Jenny Craig® as one of the commercial programs that primary care HCP could consider recommending.

Nutrisystem®

The Nutrisystem® program offers low-calorie meal replacements, telephone support for consumers who seek it (provided by dietitians and trained interventionists) and online tracking tools [16]. Estimated 3-month costs for Nutrisystem® range from US$734.97 for the Basic Plan, which includes a set menu, to US$1259.97 for the Uniquely Yours plan, which offers flexible menu customization and greater access to weight loss coaches. The high cost of this program,

relative to Weight Watchers®, results from the cost of the prepackaged foods provided by Nutrisystem®.

Outcome Data In a single site trial, Foster et al. [17] assigned 69 overweight/obese individuals with type-2 diabetes (T2D) to Nutrisystem® or a control program of diabetes support and education (DSE). Participants in the former group attended 12 group behavioral sessions over 3 months and received Nutrisystem® portion-controlled meals, while those in DSE had 3 group meetings. At month 3, participants assigned to Nutrisystem® lost 8.2 kg of initial weight, compared to 0.6 kg for DSE. The two groups achieved reductions in hemoglobin A1c (A1C) of −0.9 and −0.03%, respectively. This study was extended for 3 months as an open-label trial with the DSE participants receiving the Nutrisystem® meal plan. Mean weight losses at month 6 were 9.7 and 5.3% for the original Nutrisystem® and DSE arms, respectively.

In a two-center trial, Foster et al. [18] assigned 100 overweight/obese participants with T2D to Nutrisystem® or diabetes self-management education (DSME). Participants in the first condition received 9 group behavioral treatment sessions, while those in DSME had 9 group meetings that provided recommendations for diet, physical activity, and diabetes management. Participants, however, were not given specific instructions for behavior change. At month 6, Nutrisystem® participants lost 7.3 kg of initial weight, compared with 2.2 kg in DSME. Changes in A1C were −0.7 and −0.4%, respectively. Attrition was low in both treatment arms in both studies.

Approximately 54% of participants in the second Nutrisystem® trial lost ≥5% of initial weight, suggesting the potential clinical benefits of this program (as does the reduction in A1C). The results, however, from those two trials may not be representative of those typically achieved by consumers. This is because Nutrisystem® does not offer face-to-face behavioral counseling, as provided in these two research trials. It is possible that Nutrisystem®'s telephone-based counseling would produce weight losses comparable to those achieved with the face-to-face meetings provided in the research studies, a hypothesis worth testing. Long-term trials (i.e., 12–24 months) of Nutrisystem® also are needed.

Limitations

We note that our cost estimates (Table 12.2) for these three programs did not consider promotional discounts offered by the companies. In addition, some programs require the purchase of fresh foods in addition to those provided by the program, expenditures that were not incorporated in our cost estimates. Other factors, such as the user friendliness of a program's web sites or consumers' ratings of the foods provided, were not evaluated. All of these factors may play a role in a dieter's decision to participate in a program. The Weight Watchers® program would appear to induce weight loss at a lower cost than Jenny Craig® or Nutrisystem®. However, potential participants should attempt to estimate their weekly food costs while participating in Weight Watchers® to determine the ultimate difference in costs between the three programs.

Medically Supervised Proprietary Programs

Medically supervised very low-calorie diet (VLCD) programs were very popular in the 1980s, perhaps reaching their zenith in 1989 when Oprah Winfrey announced to her television audience that she had lost 67 lb on the OPTIFAST® Program [14]. VLCDs provide ≤ 800 kcal/day (typically 400–800 kcal) with large amounts of dietary protein (70–100 g/day) to preserve lean body mass [19, 20]. These diets usually are served as a powdered protein that is mixed with water, yielding a "shake." Protein, however, also may be obtained from lean meat, fish, and fowl, served as conventional foods [14, 19]. In either case, the diets are supplemented with vitamins and minerals (particularly potassium).

Patients must complete a history, physical examination, and laboratory tests prior to receiving a VLCD to ensure they have no contraindications (e.g., cardiovascular, renal, or hepatic) to severe caloric restriction [14, 19]. Thereafter, they meet with a physician, or other primary care HCP, approximately every 2–4 weeks to review their rate of weight loss, vital signs, and any adverse events (including dry skin, constipation, headache, and postural hypotension). Patients typically are provided weekly individual or group behavioral counseling, designed to facilitate their adherence to the VLCD and increase their physical activity. After approximately 12–16 weeks of the VLCD (and an average weight loss of 15–20 kg), conventional foods are gradually reintroduced during a 3–6 week refeeding period, with continued behavioral instruction in adopting healthy eating habits [14, 19]. The cost of such treatment, including expenses for medical care, counseling, and the diet, is often US$2500–3500 for approximately 6 months [21]. Patients usually must pay most of the expenses out of pocket, because medical weight management is not covered by their insurance plans.

Weight management guidelines issued in 1998 by the National Heart, Lung, and Blood Institute did not recommend the use of VLCDs because of findings of rapid weight regain following the termination of these diets [20]. Long-term weight losses (i.e., 1-year follow-up or more) achieved with VLCDs were not significantly greater than those achieved with low-calorie diets (LCDs), comprised of conventional foods that provided 1000–1200 kcal/day, and induced weight loss at a lower cost than VLCDs [14, 20]. The Obesity Guidelines [1] similarly concluded that VLCDs were effective short-term but should only be recommended in limited circumstances, such as inducing weight loss before bariatric surgery or other medical procedures.

Today, most companies that manufacture VLCDs also offer LCDs, typically providing more than 1000 kcal/day. Liquid shakes remain a component of the diet but have been complemented by high protein meal bars and soups, as well as shelf-stable prepared entrees. The increased calories in LCDs have led some companies to reduce (or eliminate) their medical screening and monitoring [22, 23]. These companies sell shakes and other foods online or by phone to consumers who are instructed to see their own primary care HCP prior to weight loss. Behavioral counseling may be provided on a web site or by phone, thus, eliminating any face-to-face contact with program staff. The decreased medical and behavioral care has substantially reduced the cost of treatment as compared with VLCDs, although apparently with reductions in the amount of weight loss.

The largest medically supervised programs are Health Management Resources® (Boston, MA), OPTIFAST® (Nestle Health Care Nutrition, Fremont, MI), and Medifast® (Jason Pharmacuticals, Inc., Owings Mills, MD).

Health Management Resources (HMR)®

HMR® has offered a medically supervised VLCD intervention since 1983 [22]. Today, the program incorporates meal replacements using HMR® shakes, entrees, multigrain hot cereal, and meal bars. All participants who enroll at an HMR® clinical site undergo medical screening. Based on the amount of weight loss desired, as well as body mass index (BMI) and medical history, participants can choose between the *Decision-Free® Diet* plan and the *Healthy Solutions® Diet* plan [22]. Both plans offer a 3-phase meal replacement program, the initial phase being active weight loss, followed by a transition (refeeding) phase, and finally weight maintenance. Participants in the *Decision-Free® Diet* program usually need to lose ≥ 14 kg (30 lb) and receive a medically supervised VLCD that provides 500–800 kcal/day. Participants attend weekly group behavioral weight loss sessions.

The *Healthy Solutions® Diet* plan is for participants with < 14 kg (30 lb) to lose. It provides a meal replacement diet that ranges from 1200–1600 kcal/day. Participants in this program attend weekly group behavioral meetings at a local clinical center as well, but other than the initial screening, no medical supervision is required [22]. The projected cost of 3 months of this program is US$600–700, plus the cost of food (~US$1350; Table 12.3).

Outcome Data A number of RCTs of the HMR® plan have been conducted over the past 25 years at academic research centers. Donnelly et al. [24] randomly assigned 69 obese females to a VLCD (521 kcal/day) comprised of HMR® shakes or to the same diet combined with three different types or intensities of exercise. All participants attended weekly group behavioral weight loss sessions for 3 months, with additional supervised exercise for some treatment arms. There were no statistically significant differences in weight loss between the four groups, all of which lost 20–23 kg (and ~45% of body fat). A follow-up evaluation was not included.

Anderson et al. [25] randomly allocated 40 participants with T2D (average A1C of about 8.5%) to either HMR® liquid diet alone or to the same diet combined with an evening meal of conventional foods. Both diets provided 800 kcal/day and all participants received behavioral counseling. Both groups lost approximately 15 kg at week 12 and the A1C declined to approximately 6% (with no significant differences between groups on either measure). At year 1, follow-up of 37 participants (in the two groups combined) revealed an average loss of 8.8 kg (from baseline), highlighting the common problem of weight regain following a VLCD.

In a second study, Anderson et al. [26] assigned 45 obese individuals to either a usual care condition that provided three counseling visits with a registered dietitian over 24 weeks or to an HMR® diet of 1200 kcal/day which prescribed 3 shakes, 2 entrees, and 5 servings of fruits or vegetables. Participants attended weekly 90-min weight loss classes the first 16 weeks and 60-min maintenance classes for the remaining 8 weeks. Attrition at week 16 averaged 15.6%, at which time HMR® participants lost significantly more weight than those in usual care (−12.5 kg vs. −0.7 kg) and had larger reductions in waist circumference (−11.6 cm vs. −0.4 cm). Similar weight losses were observed at week 24, after the 8-week weight maintenance program.

Donnelly et al. [27] randomly assigned 295 participants to receive an HMR® diet which was combined with behavioral counseling, delivered either in face-to-face meetings or by group conference calls. Meetings were held weekly during the initial weight loss phase (months 1–6), twice per month during months 7–9, monthly during months 10–12, and every other month through month 18. During the first 6 months, energy intake was reduced to roughly 1200–1500 kcal/day using HMR® foods, consisting of liquid shakes or prepared conventional foods, combined with fruits and vegetables. Participants in the face-to-face and telephone counseling groups lost 13.5 and 12.6 kg, respectively, at month 6. More than 85% of participants in both groups lost ≥5% of initial weight. At month 18, however, both groups regained an average of 5 kg from their 6-month weight loss.

OPTIFAST®

The OPTIFAST® program has provided medically supervised weight management since 1974 [28]. Participants in the program receive meal replacements combined with comprehensive medical supervision and behavioral counseling.

The program typically consists of three phases: a 12-week weight loss phase, followed by a refeeding period in which conventional foods are gradually reintroduced, and finally a long-term weight management phase [28]. A precise estimate of the cost of the program in 2014 is difficult to obtain, but in 2005 the program was estimated to cost US\$1800–2000 for 3 months [21].

Outcome Data Wadden et al. [29] randomly assigned 49 women to behavior therapy combined with a balanced deficit diet (BDD) of 1200 kcal/day or behavior therapy combined with a VLCD comprised of OPTIFAST® (i.e., five servings daily, providing 420 kcal/day). Participants in the latter group consumed the VLCD for 16 weeks, followed by the gradual reintroduction of solid foods so that by week 23, participants consumed 1000 kcal/day of conventional foods. Participants in both groups attended weekly group counseling sessions for the first 52 weeks, followed by every-other-week sessions for an additional 26 weeks. At week 16, VLCD participants lost 20.5 kg, compared with a significantly smaller 9.1 kg for those in the BDD group. The VLCD group, however, regained weight rapidly in the ensuing months, so that by month 18, losses in the two groups were 10.9 and 12.2 kg, respectively.

Agras et al. [30] compared four methods of improving the maintenance of weight loss in 201 women with a mean BMI of 36.6 kg/m^2 who, before randomization, had lost approximately 15 kg by participating in a 12-week group behavioral program that included the use of OPTIFAST® (800 kcal/day). Following this intervention, participants entered a refeeding and weight loss maintenance program in which they received group behavior therapy weekly for the first 12 weeks, then every 2 weeks for 3 months, and finally at monthly intervals for the past 3 months. As part of refeeding, participants were randomly assigned to consume either prepackaged foods (meal replacements) or conventional foods, in either a time-dependent manner (i.e., in which new refeeding foods were introduced on a set schedule at weekly intervals) or a weight-dependent manner, in which participants progressed to the next stage of refeeding only when their weight was stable or declining. By the end of the first 3 months, all participants had discontinued the use of OPTIFAST® and they consumed all of their meals and snacks as conventional foods. After 6 additional months of instruction in weight loss maintenance, participants had another 9 months of non-intervention follow-up, through 18 months post-randomization. At this time, 90% of participants completed the study and both groups that had been assigned to consume conventional foods during the refeeding period maintained a loss of approximately 8 kg (i.e., a regain of about 7 kg from the 15 kg loss during the pre-randomization OPTIFAST® program). Participants assigned to consume pre-packaged foods in a time-dependent manner during the refeeding period maintained a mean loss of 6 kg at month 18, while those who were assigned to the weight dependent refeeding program (and consumed prepackaged foods) maintained a loss of only 2.8 kg. Results of this study, with those of Wadden et al. [29], underscore the difficulty of sustaining the large weight losses achieved with a VLCD, even when participants are provided intensive weight loss maintenance counseling.

Medifast®

Medifast® was established in 1980 to manufacture and distribute Medifast® Meals to doctors, who in turn prescribed them to their patients and provided medical supervision and behavioral counseling [23, 31]. Medifast® was redesigned by Jason Pharmaceuticals in 2000 as a direct-to-consumer program [31].

The Medifast® program provides six weight loss plans using low-calorie, low-fat, and low glycemic-index meal replacements. The company reports that the most popular diet is the Medifast 5&1 Plan® which consists of three phases. The first is the weight loss phase, in which patients eat 5 Medifast® meal replacements per day plus a Lean & Green™ meal, comprised of conventional foods that the individual prepares with the help of a grocery list provided by the program. These latter meals provide principally protein and vegetables. During the second phase of the program patients gradually increase their caloric intake, starting from 850–1050 kcal/day the first week to 1150–1550 kcal/day by weeks 4–6. The third phase of the program focuses on weight loss maintenance, in which individuals are prescribed three lean protein and vegetable meals and 3 Medifast® meal replacements [23]. Patients also have the option to visit a Medifast® Weight Control Center for support and medical supervision [23]. We were unable to obtain a precise estimate of the cost of the program, which we calculate (for 3 months) is approximately US$1017 plus the cost of a potential initial evaluation and any subsequent visits.

Outcome Data   Several studies have examined the efficacy of the Medifast® program. Cheskin et al. [32] randomly assigned 119 participants with T2D and a BMI of 25–40 kg/m² to Medifast® Plus for Diabetics or to a 25% energy-deficit diet in accordance with recommendations of the American Diabetes Association (ADA). The participants were assessed at week 34 for weight loss and then 1 year later for weight maintenance. At week 34, only 48 (40.3%) participants in the two groups completed the program. Participants assigned to Medifast® lost significantly more weight than those on the 25% energy-deficit diet and had greater reductions in their waist circumference measurements (−7.3 kg vs. −3.7 kg and −6.9 cm vs. −4.9 cm, respectively). The Medifast® group also had significantly greater reductions in fasting blood glucose levels than

the energy-deficit diet group (−22.2 mg/dl vs.−11.17 mg/dl). Only 24 participants (21.4%) completed the 1-year follow-up evaluation, severely limiting the validity of the data.

Davis et al. [33] randomly assigned 90 adults with a BMI of 30–50 kg/m² to either a Medifast® meal replacement 5&1 Plan® or a self-selected diet of conventional foods, with both prescribing ∼1000 kcal/day. Participants were treated for 16 weeks, at the end of which time those assigned to Medifast® lost 13.5 kg, compared with 6.5 kg for those prescribed a conventional diet. The Medifast® group had a greater decrease in waist circumference than the self-selected diet group (−13 cm vs. −7.8 cm). At a follow-up assessment at week 40, weight losses for the two groups were 8.9 and 5.7 kg, respectively. Results of this study must be interpreted in the light of attrition of 50% at week 16.

Shikany et al. [34] compared the Medifast® 5&1 plan to a reduced energy, food-based diet (∼1000 kcal/day) in 120 participants with a BMI of 35–50 kg/m². Participants completed a 26-week weight loss phase followed by 26 weeks of weight maintenance. At week 26, the Medifast® group lost significantly more weight than the reduced-energy, food-based diet (−7.5 kg vs.-3.8 kg). At week 52, mean weight loss remained greater in the Medifast® group (−4.7 kg vs. −1.9 kg, respectively) and attrition averaged 21%.

Limitations

The data presented here have several limitations. First, most of the RCTs were conducted in academic medical centers and the weight losses achieved may not be representative of those obtained in community medical practices. Second, some of the randomized trials of HMR® and OPTIFAST® examined the efficacy of VLCDs combined with specific behavioral interventions (e.g., weekly, closed-group behavioral sessions) which are no longer provided by the companies, thus, limiting the relevance of the results [29, 30]. Similarly, some studies were not designed to evaluate the medically supervised program per se but instead included the VLCD as a background therapy on top of which to assess the effects of different types of exercise training or methods of refeeding patients (after the VLCD) [24, 30]. It is not clear how these added interventions may have affected the short- or long-term weight losses compared with those typically achieved. Third, several studies had high attrition rates, which limit the confidence that can be placed in the mean weight losses reported. Fourth, many studies did not provide a thorough report of adverse events, which typically are more frequent with these programs than with nonmedical commercial programs. Fifth, there was difficulty obtaining data on the costs of the VLCD and LCD programs, suggesting that consumers may similarly have such difficulty when trying to determine what a course of treatment will cost. For these reasons, the conclusions of the Obesity Guidelines [1] are reiterated that VLCDs should be used in only limited circumstances, such as inducing weight loss in at-risk patients where bariatric surgery is considered as a last resort. On the other hand, LCD meal replacements would appear appropriate for a greater range of obese individuals, but we believe that they should be administered under the care of a primary care HCP.

Remotely Delivered Commercial Weight Loss Programs

Internet and smartphone-based interventions are the latest development in commercial programs and will continue to grow in popularity because of their convenience and low cost. eDiets.com, VTrim®, The Biggest Loser® Club, and Innergy™, have all been evaluated in RCTs and will be reviewed here. A host of other programs are available to consumers (e.g., Nutrisystem.com, Weight Watchers® Online, Alere™, WebMD®, Dietwatch.com), as well as at least 30 smartphone applications (apps), such as MyNetDiary, Lose it!, MyFitnessPal, and Weight Watchers® Diary [35].

eDiets.com

eDiets.com offers clients a choice of low-calorie reducing plans, based on their dietary preferences [36]. Clients choose from seven diets, for all of which they purchase conventional foods and prepare their meals. All of the meal plans are designed to induce a loss of 0.5–0.9 kg/week (1–2 lb/week), a rate similar to that for nonmedical commercial programs. eDiets. com also offers online support (from other members), physical activity planning, and blog posts about diet and exercise. It also provides access to company experts, including dietitians and psychologists. eDiets.com charges US$9.95 for a 1-month membership (equal to US$29.85 for a 3-month program).

Outcome Data A single-site randomized trial [37] assessed the efficacy of eDiets.com (as available between February 2001 and September 2002) compared to a behavioral weight loss manual (LEARN Program for Weight Management 2000) [38]. After 1 year, participants assigned to eDiets.com lost 0.8 kg, compared to a significantly greater 3.3 kg for LEARN participants. These results most likely represent a best-case scenario given that participants in both groups had 11 on-site assessment visits (i.e., brief weigh-ins), as well as five 15-min consultations with a psychologist to assess progress. Such visits likely increased motivation and adherence to the recommended diet and physical activity modifications. The attrition rates for eDiet.com and LEARN participants were 34.8 and 33.3 %, respectively.

VTrim®

VTrim® offers clients two 12-week structured weight loss programs that run consecutively [39]. The weekly 1-h classes are led by company experts in a private online chat room with 12–20 clients. Each online class focuses on a specific strategy to improve eating and exercise habits, such as eating in social situations. The program prescribes both a low-calorie diet and physical activity regimen with the goal of facilitating weight loss of 0.5–0.9 kg/week (1–2 lb/week). The program also includes access to online food and exercise journaling, recipes, calorie calculators, and weekly feedback from the group leaders via the web site or e-mail. VTrim® charges US$395 per 12-week course (US$790 for two consecutive 12-week courses) and also offers a monthly maintenance course for an additional fee.

Outcome Data A single-site randomized trial [40] (conducted from February 2003 through March 2005) examined the effectiveness of VTrim® compared with eDiets.com (described previously). At month 6, participants assigned to VTrim® lost significantly more weight than those using eDiets.com (−6.8 and −3.3 kg), and VTrim® participants maintained greater weight loss at month 12 (−5.1 and −2.6 kg, respectively). In addition, 65 % of VTrim® participants lost ≥5 % of initial weight at month 12 compared to 37.5 % of eDiets.com participants. One-year attrition rates were 35 and 23 %, respectively.

Innergy™

Innergy™ is a phone and web-based weight loss program developed by Johns Hopkins Medicine and Healthways, Inc. and is currently delivered to the public by Healthways, Inc. It is available exclusively through employers, health plans, health systems, physician networks, and government agencies [41]. The program offers a 12-month weight loss intervention, followed by 12 months of maintenance support [42]. It provides one-to-one counseling, via the telephone or web, with coaches trained by Johns Hopkins staff. The Innergy™ web site offers educational resources, self-monitoring tools, personalized e-mail reminders, and progress tracking, as well as online group chats with a coach or other members. The program also encourages clients to communicate with their primary care practitioners and gives clients a shareable progress report for their routine medical visits. The program prescribes a low-calorie diet (of conventional foods) and physical activity with the goal of achieving and maintaining a loss ≥5 % of initial body weight at month 12. For Johns Hopkins University employees, the cost of this program (which is partially subsidized by their employer) is US$27.47 per month for the 12-month weight loss period (i.e., US$329.64 for the first year) and US$13.73 per month for the subsequent 12-month maintenance period (i.e., US$164.76 for the second year) [42]. However, costs may vary across employers and health systems.

Outcome Data The Innergy™ program was modeled on the results of a single-site randomized controlled trial conducted by investigators at John Hopkins University [43]. The Practice-based Opportunities for Weight Reduction (POWER) trial compared the effectiveness of usual care to a 2-year lifestyle intervention that was delivered remotely by telephone (i.e., 33 brief individual calls) or by in-person group and individual meetings (i.e., up to 57 such visits). Participants in the two latter groups also were provided a web-based program that included a curriculum of behavior change and tools for tracking diet and physical activity. At month 24, participants in the remotely delivered and in-person groups lost 5.1 and 4.6 kg of initial weight, respectively, compared with a significantly smaller 0.8 kg for controls. A total of 38.2, 41.4, and 18.8 % of participants in the three groups lost ≥ 5 % of initial weight at month 24 [43].

Findings for the telephone-delivered intervention in the POWER trial are very encouraging, given that 33 brief phone calls produced a clinically meaningful weight loss (months 12 and 24) which was equivalent to that achieved with a more intensive face-to-face intervention. Additional studies are needed of the Innergy™ program to determine if the commercialized version of the POWER study is as effective as the original intervention, which was delivered in a highly structured research setting.

The Biggest Loser® Club

The Biggest Loser® Club is a web site that offers clients food and exercise monitoring tools, menu and exercise planning, educational resources, community forums, and weekly e-mail newsletters [44]. The program prescribes a low-calorie diet and physical activity with the goal of inducing a loss of 0.5–1 kg/week (1–2 lb/week). In addition, the web site offers clients access to a global database, which includes calorie and nutritional information for 200,000 name and generic brand products. The Biggest Loser® Club charges US$19.99 for a 1-month membership or US$39.99 for 3 months.

Outcome Data A single-site randomized controlled trial compared basic and enhanced versions of The Biggest Loser® Club web site to a waitlist control group [45–47]. The enhanced version included all features of the basic version described previously, plus personalized, system-generated weight loss goals, weekly personalized automated feedback for participants, and escalating reminders (e-mail, text message, and phone call) to use the online weight diary.

(We note that the basic version is commercially available, but the enhanced version was delivered by researchers in a "closed test environment.") At week 12, both the basic and enhanced versions produced significantly more weight loss than the control group, with no difference between the first two groups (−2.3, −3.1, and +0.5 kg, respectively, as determined by last observation carried forward analysis). After week 12, the control participants were re-randomized to either the basic or enhanced group, and all participants received 12 more weeks of intervention. There were no differences in weight loss between the two intervention groups at week 24 (basic = −3.0 kg and enhanced = −3.9 kg, with attrition of 31.5 and 19 %, respectively).

Limitations

Currently, there is limited research to evaluate the efficacy and effectiveness of remotely delivered commercial weight loss programs, and for the research that is available, findings are mixed. For example, the Internet-based eDiets.com program did not produce greater weight loss than the LEARN manual, which included the use of traditional paper and pencil food diaries. LEARN participants lost more weight than those assigned to eDiets.com, who reduced < 1.0 kg at year 1 [37, 38]. The VTrim® program also performed better than eDiets.com after 12 months, potentially because of the greater attention provided by the weekly online chats in the former program [40]. Participants assigned to use The Biggest Loser® Club web site lost significantly more weight than a waitlist group, but the web site participants did not achieve clinically meaningful weight losses on average [46]. The most promising results reviewed were obtained in the POWER study (i.e., the basis for Innergy™) with the provision of brief telephone calls by a trained interventionist, combined with participants' use of a web-based intervention [43]. The Obesity Guidelines [1] concluded that feedback from a trained interventionist, as provided in this study, is critical to the success of remotely delivered programs.

Given that a majority of Americans have a smartphone and access the Internet daily, [48] interventions delivered via smartphone, the web, and telephone would appear to be more convenient and more accessible to dieters than traditional store-front programs. Individuals may also use these remote devices to access others' personal stories of successful weight loss; reading these crowdsourced materials has been shown to increase ratings of self-efficacy for losing weight [49]. However, additional RCTs are needed to evaluate commercially available remotely delivered programs, and further research is needed on methods of keeping dieters engaged with these interventions, which are easy to start but also to quit. A personal relationship with a trained interventionist, whether in person, over the phone, or by digital contact, may be necessary to facilitate dieters' accountability and adherence to their program.

Implementation into Practice

Primary care physicians are often the first HCP who identify overweight and obese patients [50, 51]. Therefore, intervention should start at the HCP's office with the goal of educating patients about the causes and consequences of obesity, as well as the benefits of losing 5–10% of initial weight. The HCP must first determine whether patients are ready to lose weight. Those who are not, should be encouraged to prevent further weight gain and their readiness for weight loss should be reassessed at subsequent visits. With a patient who wishes to lose weight, the HCP should review previous successful weight loss efforts and determine whether any of the prior approaches appeal to the individual at present. If not, patient and provider can develop a new weight loss intervention that considers the individual's weight-related comorbidities, as well as preferences for diet, physical activity, and behavioral interventions [1]. A key question for the HCP is whether they wish to provide intensive lifestyle counseling to their overweight/obese patients (with the requirement of weekly to twice monthly counseling visits) or instead prefer to refer patients to other HCPs (e.g., registered dietitian, behavioral psychologist, or nurse) or commercial programs that can provide intensive lifestyle counseling [58].

Overweight and obese individuals should be prescribed lifestyle counseling that will assist them in adhering to a LCD. These individuals should be prescribed LCD consisting of 1200–1500 kcal/day for females, or a 1500–1800 kcal/day for males. An alternative to this, could be prescribing an energy deficit of 500–700 kcal/day. This objective could be achieved using many of the commercial weight loss programs described in this chapter [1].

VLCDs can be used in patients with obesity with a BMI ≥30 kg/m², but should be provided under the supervision of a physician (potentially the patient's primary care physician) and a trained lifestyle interventionist. As noted previously, although these diets produce greater weight losses (~15–25% of body weight) than those observed with LCDs, patients regain about 50% of the lost weight 1–2 years after treatment [52, 53]. The National Heart, Lung, and Blood Institute (NHLBI) expert panel did not recommend the use of VLCD over LCD because there is no difference in the long-term weight loss between the two diets after considering the weight regain associated with VLCDs [14, 54–57].

With a patient who is referred to another HCP or to a commercial weight loss program, the primary care physician still plays a critical, on-going role in the individual's weight loss effort. This includes praising the patient, at routine medical visits, for losing weight, as well as monitoring comor-bid conditions (e.g., T2D, hypertension) that may improve with weight loss. Medications may need to be adjusted with weight change, and the physician here can provide important long-term support when the patient completes a weight loss program. This includes encouraging the patient to monitor his or her weight weekly or more often and to respond appropriately to small weight gains by decreasing calorie intake and increasing physical activity [58].

Conclusions

This review of commercial and proprietary weight loss programs has revealed that two nonmedical programs—Weight Watchers® and Jenny Craig®—have provided evidence of their efficacy in two or more RCTs of 1 year's duration or longer. Both programs were found to produce clinically meaningful weight loss on average and, as recommended by the Obesity Guidelines [1], can be considered by primary care HCP as options for behavioral weight control with appropriate individuals. As noted previously, the programs vary markedly in price, a fact that consumers should investigate carefully before signing up for either. Some of the difference in price may be mitigated by the need for dieters to purchase conventional foods when participating in the Weight Watchers® program.

Liquid meal replacement diets, whether served as VLCDs or LCDs (the latter often combined with conventional foods) were generally found to produce larger weight losses than the nonmedical programs reviewed. However, numerous studies revealed that participants regained weight rapidly when they lost more than 12–15 kg on average. Thus, it may not be beneficial to aim for these larger losses (particularly in view of the costs involved with a VLCD), as implicitly noted by the 1998 [20] and 2013 Obesity Guidelines [1]. The provision of liquid meal replacements directly to consumers was popularized by companies such as SlimFast® and now has been followed by some of the original medically supervised VLCD programs, including HMR® and Medifast®. The switch to LCD programs, particularly those providing >1000 kcal/day, has been accompanied by some companies' eliminating (or reducing) their direct medical screening and monitoring of patients, a responsibility they have passed on to consumers' primary care HCP. We strongly believe that individuals who plan to use a meal replacement LCD for a week or more should see their primary care HCP before doing so. Such diets, for example, can cause hypoglycemia in individuals with T2D, if not used properly [14].

Remotely delivered weight loss interventions (including by mobile phone, apps, and social media) will continue to receive the most attention from developers and consumers in the near future. These approaches currently are not as effective as traditional face-to-face interventions or those delivered by telephone. However, remotely delivered interventions are likely to improve as they provide more opportunities to monitor weight, physical activity, and eating behavior in a convenient manner. In addition, the time is quickly coming when data collected on smart phones, smart scales, and accelerometers will be automatically entered in patients' electronic health record, thus, continually updating primary care HCP on their patients' weight management success.

References

1. Jensen MJ, Ryan DH, Donato KA, et al. Executive summary: guidelines (2013) for the management of overweight and obesity in adults: a report of the American College of Cardiology/American Heart Association Task Force on Practice Guidelines and The Obesity Society published by The Obesity Society and American College of Cardiology/American Heart Association Task Force on Practice Guidelines. Based on a systematic review from The Obesity Expert Panel, 2013. Obesity (Silver Spring). 2014;22:S5–39.
2. Weight Watchers Program www.weightwatchers.com. Accessed 11 July 2014.
3. Heshka S, Greenway F, Anderson JW, et al. Self-help weight loss versus a standard commercial program after 26 weeks: a randomized controlled trial. Am J Med. 2000;109:282–7.
4. Heshka S, Anderson JW, Atkinson RL, et al. Weight loss with self-help compared with a structured commercial program. JAMA. 2003;289:1792–98.
5. Wing RR, Lang W, Wadden TA, et al. Benefits of modest weight loss in improving cardiovascular risk factors in overweight and obese individuals with type 2 diabetes. Diabetes Care. 2011;34:1481–6.
6. Jebb SA, Ahern AL, Olson AD, et al. Primary care referral to a commercial provider for weight loss treatment versus standard care: a randomised controlled trial. Lancet. 2011;378:1485–92.
7. Jolly K, Lewis A, Beach J, et al. Comparison of range of commercial or primary care led weight reduction programmes with minimal intervention control for weight loss in obesity: lighten up randomised controlled trial. BMJ 2011:1–16.
8. Johnston CA, Rost S, Miller-Kovach K, Moreno JV, Foreyt JP. A randomized controlled trial of a community-based behavioral counseling program. Am J Med. 2013;126:19–24.
9. Pinto AM, Fava JL, Hoffmann DA, Wing RR. Combining behavioral weight loss treatment and a commercial program: a randomized clinical trial. Obesity. 2013;21:673–80.
10. Jenny Craig Program http://www.jennycraig.com/site/how-it-works/the-program. Accessed on 11 July 2014.
11. Rock CL, Pakiz B, Flatt SW, Quintana EL. Randomized trial of a multifaceted commercial weight loss program. Obesity. 2007;15:939–49.
12. Rock CL, Flatt SW, Sherwood NE, Karanja N, Pakiz B, Thomson CA. Effect of a free prepared meal and incentivized weight loss program on weight loss and weight maintenance in obese and overweight women: a randomized controlled trial. JAMA. 2010;304:1803–10.
13. Heymsfield BS, van Mierlo CA, van der Knaap HC, Heo M, Frier HI. Weight management using a meal replacement strategy: meta and pooling analysis from six studies. Int J Obes Relat Metab Disord. 2003;27:537–49.
14. Tsai AG, Wadden TA. The evolution of very-low-calorie diets: an update and meta-analysis. Obesity (Silver Spring). 2006;14:1283–93.
15. Perri MG, Limacher MC, Durning PE, et al. Extended-care programs for weight management in rural communities: the treatment of obesity in underserved rural setting (TOURS) randomized trial. Arch Intern Med. 2008;168:2347–54.
16. Nutrisystem Program. http://www.nutrisystem.com/jsps_hmr/how_it_works/why_it_works.jsp. Accessed on 11 July 2014.
17. Foster GD, Borradaile KE, Vander Veur S, et al. The effects of a commercially available weight loss program among obese patients with type 2 diabetes: a randomized study. Postgrad Med. 2009;121:113–8.
18. Foster GD, Wadden TA, Lagrotte CA, et al. A randomized comparison of a commercially available portion-controlled weight-loss intervention with a diabetes self-management education program. Nutr Diabetes. 2013;18:e63.
19. Atkinson RL, Dietz WH, Foreyt JP, et al. Very low-calorie diets: National Task Force on the Prevention and Treatment of Obesity, National Institutes of Health. JAMA. 1993;270:967–74.
20. National Institutes of Health Clinical Guidelines on the Identification, Evaluation, and Treatment of Overweight and Obesity in Adults—The Evidence Report. National Institutes of Health. Obes Res. 1998;6(Suppl 3):51S–209S.
21. Tsai AT, Wadden TA. Systematic review: an evaluation of major commercial weight loss programs in the United States. Ann Intern Med. 2005;142:56–66.
22. HMR Program http://www.hmrprogram.com/. Accessed 1 July 2014.
23. Medifast Program http://www.medifast1.com/. Accessed 1 July 2014.
24. Donnelly JE, Pronk NP, Jacobsen DJ, Pronk SJ, Jakicic JM. Effects of a very-low-calorie diet and physical-training regimens on body composition and resting metabolic rate in obese females. Am J Clin Nutr. 1991;54:56–61.
25. Anderson JW, Brinkman-Kaplan V, Hamilton CC, Logan JE, Collins RW, Gustafson NJ. Food-containing hypocaloric diets are as effective as liquid-supplement diets for obese individuals with NIDDM. Diabetes Care. 1994;17:602–4.
26. Anderson JW, Reynolds LR, Bush HM, Rinsky JL, Washnock C. Effect of a behavioral/nutritional intervention program on weight loss in obese adults: a randomized controlled trial. Postgrad Med. 2011;123:205–13.
27. Donnelly JE, Goetz J, Gibson C, et al. Equivalent weight loss for weight management programs delivered by phone and clinic. Obesity (Silver Spring). 2013;21:1951–9.
28. OPTIFAST Program https://www.optifast.com/Pages/about_us.aspx. Accessed 1 July 2014.
29. Wadden TA, Foster GD, Letizia KA. One-year behavioral treatment of obesity: comparison of moderate and severe caloric restriction and the effects of weight maintenance therapy. J Consult Clin Psychol. 1994;62:165–71.
30. Agras WS, Berkowitz RI, Arnow BA, et al. Maintenance following a very-low-calorie diet. J Consult Clin Psychol. 1996;64:610–3.
31. Take Shape For Life Our parent company. http://www.tsfl.com/about_tsfl/our_parent_company.jsp. Accessed 1 July 2014.
32. Cheskin LJ, Mitchell AM, Jhaveri AD, et al. Efficacy of meal replacements versus a standard food-based diet for weight loss in type 2 diabetes: a controlled clinical trial. Diabetes Educ. 2008;34:118–27.
33. Davis LM, Coleman C, Kiel J, et al. Efficacy of a meal replacement diet plan compared to a food-based diet plan after a period of weight loss and weight maintenance: a randomized controlled trial. Nutr J. 2010;9:11.
34. Shikany JM, Thomas AS, Beasley TM, Lewis CE, Allison DB. Randomized controlled trial of the Medifast 5 & 1 Plan for weight loss. Int J Obes (Lond). 2013;37:1571–8.
35. Pagoto S Schnieder K, Jojic M, DeBiasse M, Mann D. Evidence-based strategies in weight-loss mobile apps. Am J Prev Med. 2013;45:576–82.

36. eDiets.com Program www.ediets.com. Accessed 10 June 2014.
37. Womble LG, Wadden TA, McGuckin BG, Sargent SL, Rothman RA, Krauthamer-Ewing ES. A randomized controlled trial of a commercial internet weight loss program. Obes Res. 2004;12:1011–8.
38. Brownell KD. The LEARN Program for Weight Management Dallas, TX. American Heart Publishing; 2000.
39. The VTrim Program. www.vtrimonline.com/the-vtrim-program/. Accessed 10 June 2014.
40. Gold BC, Burke S, Pintauro S, Buzzell P, Harvey-Berino J. Weight loss on the web: a pilot study comparing a structured behavioral intervention to a commercial program. Obesity (Silver Spring). 2007;15:155–64.
41. Healthways Innergy. www.healthways.com/innergy. Accessed 18 June 2014.
42. Innergy FAQ's http://benefits.jhu.edu/documents/Innergy_FAQ.pdf. Accessed 27 June 2014.
43. Appel LJ, Clark JM, Yeh H, et al. Comparative effectiveness of weight-loss interventions in clinical practice. N Engl J Med. 2011;365:1959–68.
44. www.biggestloserclub.com. Accessed 10 June 2014.
45. Collins CE, Morgan P, Jones P, et al. A 12-week commercial web-based weight-loss program for overweight and obese adults: randomized controlled trial comparing basic versus enhanced features. J Med Internet Res. 2012;14:e57.
46. Collins CE, Morgan P, Hutchesson MJ, et al. Efficacy of standard versus enhanced features in a web-based commercial weight-loss program for obese adults, part 2: randomized controlled trial. J Med Internet Res. 2013;15:e140.
47. Hutchesson MJ, Collins CE, Morgan PJ, Watson JF, Guest M, Callister R. Changes to dietary intake during a 12-week commercial web-based weight loss program: a randomized controlled trial. Clin Nutri. 2014;68:64–70.
48. Pew Research Internet Project Mobile technology fact sheet.http://www.pewinternet.org/fact-sheets/mobile-technology-fact-sheet/. Accessed 27 June 2014.
49. Manuvinakurike R, Velicer WF, Bickmore TW. Automated indexing of internet stories of health behavior change: weight loss attitude pilot study. J Med Internet Res. 2014;16:e285.
50. Grima M, Dixon JB. Obesity-recommendations for management in general practice and beyond. Aust Fam Physician. 2013;42:532–41.
51. Wadden TA, Volger S, Sarwer DB, et al. A two-year randomized trial of obesity treatment in primary care practice. N Engl J Med. 2011;365:1969–79.
52. Wadden TA, Foster GD, Letizia KA, Stunkard AJ. A multicenter evaluation of a proprietary weight reduction program for the treatment of marked obesity. Arch Intern Med. 1992;152:961–6.
53. Anderson JW, Brinkman-Kaplan V, Hamilton CC, Logan JE, Collins RW, Gustafson NJ. Food-containing hypocaloric diets are as effective as liquid-supplement diets for obese individuals with NIDDM. Diabetes Care. 1994;17:602–4.
54. Anderson JW, Konz EC, Frederich RC, Wood CL. Long-term weight-loss maintenance: a meta-analysis of US studies. Am J Clin Nutr. 2001;74:579–84.
55. Mustajoki P, Pekkarinen T. Very low energy diets in the treatment of obesity. Obes Rev. 2001;2:61–72.
56. Saris WH. Very-low-calorie diets and sustained weight loss. Obes Res 2001;9(Suppl 4):295s–301s.
57. Finer N. Low-calorie diets and sustained weight loss. Obes Res 2001;9(Suppl 4):290s–4s.
58. Wadden TA, Butryn ML, Hong P, Tsai AG. Behavioral treatment of obesity in patients encountered in primary care settings: A systematic review. JAMA. 2014;312:1779–91.

Physical Activity Programs

Damon Swift, Neil M. Johannsen and Timothy Church

Abbreviations

ACLS	Aerobics Center Longitudinal Study
AT/RT	Aerobic training/resistance training
BMI	Body Mass Index
CARDIA	Coronary artery risk development in young adults
CHD	Coronary heart disease
CRF	Cardiorespiratory fitness
CVD	Cardiovascular disease
DARE	Diabetes aerobic and resistance exercise
DREW	Dose response to exercise in women
FBG	Fasting blood glucose
HDL	High-density lipoproteins
LDL	Low-density lipoprotein
MET	Metabolic equivalents of task
OGTT	Oral glucose tolerance test
PA	Physical activity
STRRIDE	Studies of targeted risk reduction intervention through defined exercise
T2D	Type-2 diabetes
TG	Triglyceride

Introduction

In 2008, the US Department of Health and Human Services released the first set of Federal Physical Activity Guidelines (U.S. Department of Health and Human Services 1–76; http://www.health.gov/paguidelines/). While several iterations of the US dietary guidelines have occurred over the past decades, the 2008 Physical Activity Guidelines represent the first federal physical activity (PA) recommendations to improve the health of Americans. The process of how these guidelines were developed is worth discussing, considering the lack of prospective, longitudinal evidence. An Advisory Committee was commissioned to produce a summary of the PA research categorized according to health status (healthy adults, diabetes, heart disease, disability, etc.). The result was a comprehensive report of over 600 pages with associated references (US Department of Health and Human Services). The Guidelines mirror the findings of this report and are similar to recommendations from other groups such as the Centers for Disease Control and Prevention, American College of Sports Medicine, American Heart Association, American Diabetes Association, and Surgeon General's Report. The new Guidelines represent a tremendous resource for clinicians, researchers, and the lay-public and are referred to frequently in this chapter.

The Guidelines state that in order to attain substantial health benefits from PA or exercise, adults should participate in at least 150 min (2 h and 30 min) a week of moderate-intensity, 75 min (1 h and 15 min) a week of vigorous-intensity aerobic PA, or an equivalent combination of moderate- and vigorous-intensity aerobic activity. The aerobic activity should occur on most days of the week and in bouts of at least 10 min. In addition to aerobic activity, adults should also participate in muscle-strengthening activities (resistance training) that involve all major muscle groups on 2 or more days a week. Two additional, key messages that are reiterated several times in the Guidelines are that (1) participating in some activity is better than no activity and (2) participating in more activity than what is recommended may produce greater health benefits.

The Guidelines address many different health conditions including cardiovascular disease (CVD), type-2 diabetes (T2D), and aging. The research used to make the recommendations stems from published epidemiological and intervention studies along with recommendations that are either inferred from past data or based on the best evidence or guidance from the Advisory Board. As such, the Guidelines for

D. Swift (✉) · T. Church
Preventive Medicine Laboratory, Pennington Biomedical Research Center, Baton Rouge, LA, USA

N. M. Johannsen
School of Kinesiology, LSU College of Human Sciences and Education, Baton Rouge, LA, USA

© Springer International Publishing Switzerland 2016
J. I. Mechanick, R. F. Kushner (eds.), *Lifestyle Medicine*, DOI 10.1007/978-3-319-24687-1_13

Table 13.1 Health benefits associated with regular physical activity

Children and Adolescents
Strong evidence
Improved cardiorespiratory and muscular fitness
Improved bone health
Improved cardiovascular and metabolic health biomarkers
Favorable body composition
Moderate evidence
Reduced symptoms of depression
Adults and Older Adults
Strong evidence
Lower risk of early death
Lower risk of coronary heart disease
Lower risk of stroke
Lower risk of high blood pressure
Lower risk of adverse blood lipid profile
Lower risk of type-2 diabetes
Lower risk of metabolic syndrome
Lower risk of colon cancer
Lower risk of breast cancer
Prevention of weight gain
Weight loss, particularly when combined with reduced calorie intake
Improved cardiorespiratory and muscular fitness
Prevention of falls
Reduced depression
Better cognitive function (for older adults)
Moderate to strong evidence
Better functional health (for older adults)
Reduced abdominal obesity
Moderate evidence
Lower risk of hip fracture
Lower risk of lung cancer·
Lower risk of endometrial cancer
Weight maintenance after weight loss
Increased bone density
Improved sleep quality

specific health outcomes and PA/exercise components are graded as "strong," "moderate," and "weak," based on the available literature (type, number, and quality), consistency of the outcome in the literature, the possibility for *causality* and dose response, and where evidence was limited, the recommendations were at the discretion of the Advisory Board (Table 13.1). Regular PA is important across the age-span to improve fitness (aerobic and muscular), prevent early death, especially from cardiovascular disease, improve metabolic health, and reduce the risk of musculoskeletal disorders including osteoporosis and bone fracture. The sections below will outline the epidemiologic and intervention evidence that support the recommendations for increased PA, especially in sedentary individuals or those with low activity levels, to improve major health outcomes including cardiorespiratory fitness (CRF), metabolic diseases such as T2D, and overweight/obesity.

Importance of Physical Activity and Exercise for Health

As stated previously, the Guidelines recommend that adults obtain 150 min of moderate PA or 75 min (1 h and 15 min) of vigorous-intensity aerobic PA per week to maintain or improve health [1]. In brief, moderate intensity is characterized as a brisk walk whereas a jog is considered the lower boundary of vigorous intensity. This recommendation is based on epidemiological studies which demonstrate a reduction in cardiovascular and all-cause mortality consistent at or above these PA levels [1, 2]. However, only 43.8% of adults participate in recommended levels of aerobic PA, and approximately 30% of adults engage in no leisure time PA (defined as no light to vigorous sessions lasting at least 10 min in duration) [3]. Studies in this area of research typically quantify exercise as either PA (through a validated questionnaire) or evaluate CRF either through an exercise test, where participants are near maximal or maximal levels (e.g., age-predicted maximal heart rate or volitional exhaustion) [4]. CRF is thought to be a more valid measure because it is an objective measure and not prone to the misclassification of PA levels that can occur with subjective questionnaires [5, 6]. Additionally, some studies have observed that CVD mortality is more strongly associated with CRF than with PA [5, 7].

Physical Activity, Cardiorespiratory Fitness, and Heart Disease

According to data from the American Heart Association's Heart Disease and Stroke Statistics [3], heart disease was the leading cause of death in the USA in 2010 accounting for approximately 787,650 deaths, representing 31.9% of all-cause mortality [3]. Low PA or low CRF represent major risk factors for heart disease [8–10] and, moreover, have been shown to be independent of other traditional CVD risk factors, including body mass index (BMI) [11], body fat [11], dyslipidemia [12], and hypertension.

Several major studies have demonstrated PA and CRF as risk factors for heart disease. In addition, studies suggest that PA and CRF may interact with obesity to influence heart disease outcomes. Although PA levels measured through questionnaires have various limitations as mentioned earlier (e.g., self-reported, subjective nature, and misclassification issues) [5–7], many studies report that PA is inversely associated with heart disease risk. For example, in the Harvard Alumni Study, 12,516 middle-aged and older men were followed from 1977 to 1993. PA levels were quantified through the use of a questionnaire asking participants about the amount of daily stairs climbed, distances walked, and recreation sports and activities. The researchers found that an exercise level at or above public health recommendations (~150 min/week)

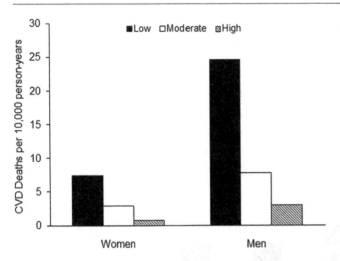

Fig. 13.1 Risk of cardiovascular mortality across levels of cardiorespiratory fitness in women and men. *CVD* cardiovascular disease

was associated with 25–27 % reduction in coronary heart disease (CHD) after adjustment for important confounding variables such as age, BMI, alcohol intake, hypertension, T2D, and smoking status. This study observed that the relationship between PA and CHD displayed an "L"-shaped distribution, meaning that once PA levels were at or above public health definitions, no further reduction in risk of CHD was observed [4]. Similarly, in the Nurses' Health study, Li et al. evaluated the effects of PA on CHD in 88,393 women (ages 34–59 years) between the years of 1980 and 2000. PA was measured using a questionnaire that evaluated the amount of time spent each week in moderate and vigorous activities. The researchers observed that women with less than 3.5 h/week of PA had a 34–43 % increased risk in CHD.

Studies that have evaluated the relationship between CRF and CVD mortality have observed similar relationships. In a classic study by Blair et al. [12] from the Aerobics Center Longitudinal Study (ACLS), CRF was measured using a modified Balke treadmill protocol (where the intensity of exercise was periodically increased in standardized fashion until the participant reached at least 85 % of their age-predicted maximum heart rate) performed during preventive medicine examinations in 25,341 men and 7080 women between 1970 to 1989 (Fig. 13.1). A low CRF (lowest 20 % of sample based on age and gender) was associated with 1.7-fold increased risk for CVD mortality in men and 2.4-fold increase in women, after adjustments for smoking status, high cholesterol, systolic blood pressure, BMI > 27 kg/m², and other confounding variables [12]. Lee et al. [11] further evaluated this relationship with respect to body fat in men and observed elevated risk of CVD mortality in unfit men compared to fit men, regardless of whether they were lean (~3-fold), normal body fat (~1.5-fold), or obese (~2.7-fold). Population level studies have also shown that improvements in CRF are associated with a reduction of CVD mor-

tality, suggesting that public health promotion may have an important role in reducing the risk of heart disease. Lee et al. [13], using data from the ACLS database, showed that men categorized with an initially low CRF, but increased their CRF level at the second examination, had a 42 % reduction in CVD mortality, compared to those that remained unfit. Additionally, these analyses were adjusted for a set of potential confounding variables including changes in BMI between both examinations. While these data are certainly provocative and clinically important, a major limitation of the literature at the present time is the power to investigate the influence of racial descent considering that the majority of the ACLS database is composed of white men.

The data above suggest that baseline levels of PA or CRF, as well as changes in CRF, have a major role in the overall risk of heart disease. In general, PA and CRF reduce the risk of heart disease independent of other traditional CVD risk factors, including BMI.

Physical Activity, Cardiorespiratory Fitness, and Type-2 Diabetes

Approximately 29.1 million Americans have T2D, which represents the seventh leading cause of death in the USA. According to a Scientific Statement released by the American Diabetes Association [14] in 2012, the total estimated medical cost of treating T2D in the USA was US$245 billion, which included US$176 billion in direct medical costs and US$69 billion in reduced productivity. In addition to the health consequences associated with high blood glucose levels, about 70 % of individuals with T2D have concurrent hypertension and 65 % have dyslipidemia, including high low-density lipoprotein (LDL) and high triglyceride (TG) levels. This results in an estimated 1.7-, 1.8-, and 1.5-fold increase in CVD mortality, heart attack, and stroke, respectively, compared with their counterparts without T2D. PA and exercise training is recommended to reduce the overall risk and associated severity of T2D.

Similar to heart disease, research demonstrates an inverse relationship between T2D incidence and PA/CRF levels. In the ACLS, CRF was quantified by a maximal graded exercise test, and T2D risk was determined based on blood glucose values (≥126 mg/dL) at follow-up. In this study, Wei et al. [15] followed 8633 for an average of 6.1 years and found that low CRF levels at baseline were associated with a 2.6-fold increase in risk in the development of T2D. This relationship persisted after statistical adjustments for BMI, age, high blood pressure, high levels of high-density lipoproteins (HDL), total cholesterol, TG, parental T2D, and other confounders [15]. Additionally, Wei et al. [15] found an inverse relationship between CRF at baseline and risk of developing T2D in men who were both overweight and

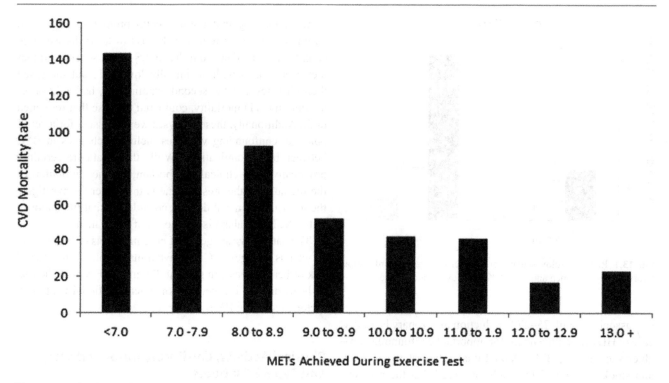

Fig. 13.2 Risk of mortality across cardiorespiratory levels in metabolic equivalents of task *(METs)* in men with diabetes. *CVD* cardiovascular disease

obese. Similar relationships were observed from the ACLS dataset in women, as Sui et al. [16] followed 6249 women for 17 years, and observed a 39% reduction in risk of T2D in those classified as having high CRF, compared to those classified as having low CRF at baseline after statistical adjustments for covariates, including baseline BMI. In overweight women (BMI≥25 kg/m²), the authors observed a 2.6-fold increased risk of T2D incidence in women who were unfit compared to those women who were lean and fit.

Epidemiological studies have also evaluated the effect of CRF change from baseline to follow-up (instead of initial CRF alone) on the risk of developing T2D. In the Coronary Artery Risk Development in Young Adults (CARDIA) study, CRF was quantified using a modified Balke treadmill protocol and T2D was diagnosed through fasting blood glucose (FBG) levels≥126 mg/dll, self-report of diabetes medications, or 2-h post-challenge blood glucose≥200 mg/dL. Carenthon et al. [17] followed 1808 men for 7 years and found that a reduction in CRF (quantified by a 19% reduction in treadmill test duration over 7 years) was associated with a 2-fold and 46% increase in T2D incidence in men and women, respectively, after adjustments for baseline BMI and other potential confounders (age, race, smoking, family history of T2D, and baseline treadmill test duration). In a separate analysis examining change in CRF over the course of 20 years, Carnethon et al. [17] (N=2231) observed that those who were diagnosed with T2D over the course of 20

years had greater reductions in treadmill test duration (men: −37.9%, women: −34.9%; indicating a reduction in CRF) compared to those who did not have T2D (men: −26.5%, women: −27.0%). In the ACLS dataset, Wei et al. [18] observed that men who had an increase in CRF level by just 1 metabolic equivalent of task (or "metabolic equivalent"; MET) between the baseline and follow-up examinations had a 28% reduction in T2D incidence after adjustments for baseline BMI and other covariates.

Fitness is also an important component for survival in individuals with T2D. Church et al. [19] followed 2196 with T2D for an average of 14.6 years and found that men who had low (<8.8 METs) or moderate (8.8 to 10.0 METs) levels of CRF at baseline had a 4.5 and 2.8-fold increased risk of death, respectively, compared to men with high CRF levels (>11.7 METs). Statistical adjustments were made in this analysis for non-modifiable risk factors, modifiable risk factors, and BMI. In another study by Church et al. [20] within the ACLS dataset where 2316 men with T2D were followed for an average of 15.9 years, a 1-MET increase in CRF was associated with a 20% reduction in CVD mortality (Fig. 13.2). Additionally, higher CRF reduced the overall risk of CVD mortality in both normal-weight and obese men with T2D. The relationship of CRF with mortality measures in individuals with T2D has important clinical and public health implications due the high risk of heart disease in individuals with T2D.

In summary, the available evidence suggests that similar to heart disease:

- High CRF reduces the risk of future T2D diagnosis
- Improvements in CRF appear to reduce the risk of T2D diagnosis
- High CRF levels reduce the overall risk of CVD mortality in individuals who have been diagnosed with T2D

Exercise and Physical Activity Programs to Improve Health

The epidemiological data to support the 2008 Federal Physical Activity Guidelines to improve health are abundant [1]. However, the number of intervention studies in which individuals are made to exercise or increase PA levels and are also supported with a large number of participants are few and contain limitations to "real-world" interpretation. However, in order to adequately translate the epidemiological outcomes to the real world, well-designed, adequately powered, randomized controlled lifestyle modification intervention trials must be conducted.

Exercise and Physical Activity Programs to Improve Cardiorespiratory Fitness

Intervention studies typically quantify the adaptations by pre-/post-intervention changes in CRF assessed either by maximal oxygen uptake (VO_{2max} measured by gas exchange), estimated multiple of resting energy expenditure (METs), or simply test duration from a graded exercise test. Unlike epidemiological research, PA levels and exercise doses (volumes) are controlled according to the F.I.T.T. principle (frequency, intensity, time, type; i.e., 30 min of moderate-intensity walking, 3 days/week) or a specific energy expenditure per week (i.e. 1000 kcal/week or 11 kcal/kg body weight per week; KKW). In this way, the changes observed in the outcome data can be directly compared to the dose or intensity of exercise or PA without making inferences about activities as determined by questionnaire data. In appropriately controlled trials, the control group's results—the group that does not do the exercise/PA intervention—represents the general trend for everyone in the study. While many small studies on the effects of exercise/PA on health outcomes exist, it is the larger, clinical trials that merit attention here.

Unlike epidemiological studies examining the effects of CRF on hard outcomes like CVD morbidity and mortality, intervention studies typically examine CRF directly in response to PA or exercise programs. Data to support the effects of aerobic exercise, treadmill walking, cycling, etc., on CRF are plentiful; however, few have the power, and sample diversity, to generalize the results to large sectors of the population. With that said, results from large, randomized controlled trials suggest that CRF increases with total exercise dose (kcal/wk) and intensity (moderate to vigorous) [21, 22]. For example, the Dose Response to Exercise in Women (DREW) study examined the effect of 50, 100, and 150% of the recommended amount of exercise of aerobic exercise at a moderate intensity (~50% peak oxygen uptake; VO_{2peak}) on CRF in 464 postmenopausal women [21]. The DREW study supported the epidemiologically based recommendation that:

1. Some exercise is better than none (50%; 4 KKW).
2. The recommended amount of moderate-intensity aerobic exercise produces significant health benefits (100%; 8 KKW).
3. Greater amounts of exercise may confer additional benefits to health outcomes (150%; 12 KKW) by showing a significant increase in CRF as measured by VO_{2peak} with an average of 72 min and a dose response for increasing CRF up to an average of 192 min/week (Fig. 13.3).

Interestingly, the upper threshold for improving CRF in postmenopausal women was not observed, and the optimal dose of aerobic exercise was not determined.

To date, no studies examining the effect of exercise intensity in a prospective, longitudinal study with at least three separate and distinct exercise intensities have been conducted. However, the available literature suggests that high-intensity exercise confers additional health benefits, in particular, greater gains in CRF [22]. In the Studies of Targeted Risk Reduction Intervention Through Defined Exercise (STRRIDE) study, men and women with mild to moderate dyslipidemia were randomized to one of the following:

1. High amount/high intensity (23 KKW at 65–80% VO_{2peak})
2. Low amount/high intensity (14 KKW at 65–80% VO_{2peak})
3. Low amount/low intensity (14 KKW at 40–55% VO_{2peak})
4. A control group

The higher the amount of exercise and the higher-intensity exercise groups had the largest improvements in fitness suggesting that total exercise dose and exercise intensity have independent effects on fitness. A recent study by Ross et al. [23] found corroborating results to the STRRIDE study using a similar design (with different intensities at high amounts of exercise) in adults with abdominal obesity. It should be noted, however, that standard equations used to estimate caloric expenditure during exercise from the American College of Sports Medicine [24] assume equal biomechanical and muscular efficiency among all people, an assumption that may not be met especially across low- and high-intensity exercise.

The effect of resistance training, alone and in combination with aerobic training, on CRF is minor. However, most stud-

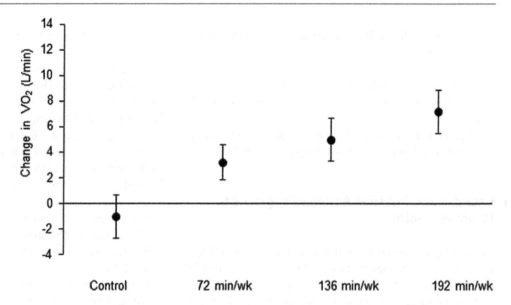

Fig. 13.3 Change in fitness level at 6 months across different levels of exercise training. VO_2 oxygen uptake

ies show, especially in very detrained individuals, a small, reproducible increase in CRF with resistance training. For example, in the STRRIDE aerobic training/resistance training (AT/RT) study, an increase ($\sim 4.6\%$) in VO_{2peak} was observed in the resistance training group alone [25]. However, the increase in CRF with resistance training is small compared to the increase from aerobic exercise alone ($\sim 11.7\%$). Somewhat different results have been observed in individuals with T2D from the Health Benefits of Aerobic and Resistance Training in individuals with T2D (HART-D) study [26, 27]. The increase in CRF (VO_{2peak}) was negligible with resistance training alone; however, the observed increase was 2-fold greater with the combination of aerobic and resistance training compared to aerobic training alone. Interestingly, exercise time during the graded exercise test (or maximal METs) was similar between the aerobic and combined groups inferring that, somehow, the resistance training promoted a different muscular adaptation to exercise when added to aerobic training. Whether this difference promotes greater or lesser health benefits is not known. In addition, the optimal aerobic intensity, as well as the optimal combination of sets and reps in the resistance training protocol, is not known.

Exercise and Physical Activity Programs to Improve Insulin Resistance and Type-2 Diabetes

Several well-designed and powered interventions aimed at improving the health of individuals at risk for T2D, or with overt disease, can be found in the literature.

While data on aerobic exercise intensity suggest that higher intensity is optimal to improve CRF, the effect of intensity on insulin resistance is more pronounced. Ross et al. [23] observed that high-intensity aerobic exercise improved

insulin resistance (2-h post-challenge blood glucose from an oral glucose tolerance test [OGTT]) while low-intensity exercise did not produce significant effects on insulin resistance in overweight/obese adults.

In individuals at risk for insulin resistance, aerobic and combined aerobic and resistance training are ideal compared to resistance training alone. The STRRIDE-AT/RT study showed that aerobic and combined training improved fasting blood glucose (FBG) levels compared to resistance training programs alone [28]. In individuals with T2D, combined aerobic and resistance exercise result in a greater decrease in glycated hemoglobin (A1C). Two major studies, the HART-D and Diabetes Aerobic and Resistance Exercise (DARE) studies, examined the effect of resistance training, alone and in combination with aerobic training on A1C, and observed the largest decrease in A1C in participants who completed the combined exercise training protocols [26, 29]. Greater specificity on the effectiveness of aerobic and resistance training can be seen if the two studies are contrasted. For example, about a 3-fold greater change in A1C was observed in the DARE study in the combined training group (approximately -1.0% compared with control) compared with the HART-D combined training group (approximately -0.35% compared to control), likely due to the way the training modalities were combined and the study protocol for changes in diabetes medications. The combined training group in the DARE study used the full prescription for the aerobic and resistance training groups while the HART-D study used a reduced aerobic stimulus (10 KKW instead of 12 KKW in the aerobic training alone group) and resistance training on 2 days with only one set of all exercises (instead of 3 days at two to three sets). In addition, the DARE study participants were not allowed to alter their diabetes medications during the study unless necessary, while the HART-D participants were allowed to do so. Combining these results provides additional support for the Guidelines in that combined exercise is better than either modality alone, and additional exercise above what is recommended may confer greater health benefits in individuals with T2D. Interestingly, in the HART-D study, participants were about three times more likely to have either a significant reduction in A1C ($> -0.5\%$) or reduce their diabetes medication use if they increased their CRF (maximal METs) and reduced their waist circumference compared to participants who decreased CRF and increased waist circumference [30].

Conclusions

The Federal Physical Activity Guidelines recommend that adults should participate in at least 150 min (2 h and 30 min) a week of moderate-intensity or 75 min (1 h and 15 min) a week of vigorous-intensity aerobic PA or an equivalent combination of moderate- and vigorous-intensity aerobic activity. In addition to aerobic activity, adults should also participate in muscle-strengthening activities (resistance training) that involve all major muscle groups on 2 or more days a week. It is very important to point out that while regular PA is important in preventing chronic diseases, it may be even more important in preventing adverse health events in those with existing chronic conditions. For example, within groups of individuals with diabetes, hypertension, dyslipidemia and/or obesity, regular PA greatly reduces the risk of CVD. While there remain many areas that need more research, the available literature strongly supports the current guidelines, and these guidelines should serve as foundation for clinical exercise prescription.

References

1. U.S. Department of Health and Human Services. 2008 physical activity guidelines for Americans. 2008. p. 1–3.
2. Haskell WL, et al. Physical activity and public health: updated recommendation for adults from the American college of sports medicine and the American Heart Association. Med Sci Sports Exerc. 2007;39(8):1423–34.
3. Go AS, et al. Heart disease and stroke statistics—2014 update: a report from the American heart association. Circulation. 2014;129(3):e28–92.
4. Sesso HD, Paffenbarger RS, Lee I-M. Physical activity and coronary heart disease in men. Circulation. 2000;102(9):975–80.
5. LaMonte MJ, Blair SN. Physical activity, cardiorespiratory fitness, and adiposity: contributions to disease risk. Curr Opin Clin Nutr Metab Care. 2006;9(5):540–6.
6. LaMonte MJ, Blair SN, Church TS. Physical activity and diabetes prevention. J Appl PHysiol (1985). 2005; 99:1205–13.
7. Erikssen G. Physical fitness and changes in mortality. Sports Med. 2001;31(8):571–6.
8. Blair SN, et al. Physical fitness and all-cause mortality: a prospective study of healthy men and women. JAMA. 1989;262(17):2395–401.
9. Li J, Siegrist J. Physical activity and risk of cardiovascular disease—a meta-analysis of prospective cohort studies. Int J Environ Res Public Health. 2012;9(2):391–407.
10. Swift DL, et al. Physical activity, cardiorespiratory fitness, and exercise training in primary and secondary coronary prevention. Circ J. 2013;77(2):281–92.
11. Lee CD, Blair SN, Jackson AS. Cardiorespiratory fitness, body composition, and all-cause and cardiovascular disease mortality in men. Am J Clin Nutr. 1999;69(3):373–80.
12. Blair Sn K, Kohl JB, H. W, et al. Influences of cardiorespiratory fitness and other precursors on cardiovascular disease and all-cause mortality in men and women. J Am Med Assoc. 1996;276(3):205–10.
13. Lee D-c, et al. Long-term effects of changes in cardiorespiratory fitness and body mass index on all-cause and cardiovascular disease mortality in men: the aerobics center longitudinal study. Circulation. 2011;124(23):2483–90.
14. American Diabetes Association. Economic costs of diabetes in the U.S. in 2012. Diabetes Care. 2013;36:1033–46.
15. Wei M, et al. The association between cardiorespiratory fitness and impaired fasting glucose and type 2 diabetes mellitus in men. Ann Intern Med. 1999;130(2):89–96.
16. Sui X, et al. A prospective study of cardiorespiratory fitness and risk of type 2 diabetes in women. Diabetes Care. 2008;31(3):550–5.
17. Carnethon MR, et al. Association of 20-year changes in cardiorespiratory fitness with incident type 2 diabetes. Diabetes Care. 2009;32(7):1284–8.
18. Wei M, Kampert JB, Barlow CE. Relationship between low cardiorespiratory fitness and mortality in normal-weight, overweight, and obese men. J Am Med Assoc. 1999;282(16):1547–53.
19. Church TS, et al. Exercise capacity and body composition as predictors of mortality among men with diabetes. Diabetes Care. 2004;27(1):83–8.
20. Church TS, et al. Cardiorespiratory fitness and body mass index as predictors of cardiovascular disease mortality among men with diabetes. Arch Intern Med. 2005;165(18):2114–20.
21. Church TS, et al. Effects of different doses of physical activity on cardiorespiratory fitness among sedentary, overweight or obese postmenopausal women with elevated blood pressure: a randomized controlled trial. JAMA. 2007;297(19):2081–91.
22. Duscha BD, et al. Effects of exercise training amount and intensity on peak oxygen consumption in middle-age men and women at risk for cardiovascular disease. Chest. 2005;128(4):2788–93.
23. Ross R, et al. Effects of exercise amount and intensity on abdominal obesity and glucose tolerance in obese adults: a randomized trial. Ann Intern Med. 2015;162(5):325–34.
24. American College of Sports Medicine. ACSM's Guidelines for Exercise Testing and Prescription. 9th ed. Philadelphia, PA: Lippincott Williams & Williams; 2014.
25. Bateman LA, et al. Comparison of aerobic versus resistance exercise training effects on metabolic syndrome (from the studies of a targeted risk reduction intervention through defined exercise—STRRIDE-AT/RT). Am J Cardiol. 2011;108(6):838–44.
26. Church TS, et al. Effects of aerobic and resistance training on hemoglobin A1c levels in patients with type 2 diabetes: a randomized controlled trial. JAMA. 2010;304(20):2253–62.
27. Johannsen NM, et al. Categorical analysis of the impact of aerobic and resistance exercise training, alone and in combination, on cardiorespiratory fitness levels in patients with type 2 diabetes: results from the HART-D study. Diabetes Care. 2013;36(10):3305–12.
28. Slentz CA, et al. Inactivity, exercise, and visceral fat. STRRIDE: a randomized, controlled study of exercise intensity and amount. J Appl Physiol (1985). 2005;99(4):1613–8.
29. Sigal RJ, et al. Effects of aerobic training, resistance training, or both on glycemic control in type 2 diabetes: a randomized trial. Ann Intern Med. 2007;147(6):357–69.
30. Senechal M, et al. Changes in body fat distribution and fitness are associated with changes in hemoglobin A1c after 9 months of exercise training: results from the HART-D study. Diabetes Care. 2013;36(9):2843–9.

Behavior Modification and Cognitive Therapy

John P. Foreyt and Craig A. Johnston

Abbreviations

AHEAD	Action for Health in Diabetes
DPP	Diabetes Prevention Program
HCPs	Health-care professionals
T2D	Type-2 diabetes
TOPS	Take off Pounds Sensibly

Introduction

What is behavior modification? We have all heard the term. What about cognitive therapy, behavior therapy, behavioral treatment, cognitive behavior therapy, and lifestyle modification? Are these terms all referring to the same principles, strategies, techniques, and procedures or is there something unique about each one?

As health-care professionals (HCPs), the terms can be thought of as reasonably synonymous. No matter what term is used, the approach to patients will be similar. At an academic and technical level, the terms differ slightly. Behavior modification generally refers to principles and strategies initially developed through research on rodents, pigeons, and other animals and applied to humans based on a number of related learning theories. Remembering back to introductory psychology courses in college, the work of B.F. Skinner, Ivan Pavlov, and others played a prominent role [1, 2]. Remember *Walden Two* [3]? When the principles and strategies are applied to humans during an intervention to modify lifestyle, they become known as behavior therapy or, with the addition of some of the newer cognitive strategies, cognitive behavioral therapy. Lifestyle modification generally refers to these approaches aimed at improving health through diet and physical activity.

Historically, behavior modification was based on both classical and operant conditioning. Becoming obese, for example, was viewed as the result of unhealthy behaviors that simply needed modifying using the principles of these learning theory conditioning models [4]. It was thought to be easy. Apply the principles developed through animal models, and then overeating and underexercising would be modified. There are many interesting papers published in the 1960s and 1970s attempting to modify these unhealthful patterns of behavior through learning theory models of changing schedules of reinforcement, modifying environmental triggers, or applying aversive stimuli [5–7]. Unfortunately, the published studies were usually case reports of a small number of individuals or trials of short duration with little or no follow-up [8]. Although the early studies provide a wonderful window into the development of our current behavior modification and cognitive therapies, we have learned that the development of unhealthy lifestyles is not just the result of bad habits but that our genetics, biochemistry, metabolism, hormones, culture, and emotion all play important roles in making changes difficult, both short- and long-term.

Behavior modification today involves the use of a number of empirically tested strategies aimed at helping individuals develop the skills needed to achieve and maintain a healthy lifestyle through improved diet and physical activity [9, 10]. The strategies are differentiated from other analytic approaches by focusing primarily on current behaviors. Behavior modification is not psychotherapy. It does not dwell on the patients' past relationships with their mothers or analyze their dreams. It is a here and now approach. It focuses on goal-setting and emphasizes small behavioral changes which are thought to be more easily maintained. Both tested cognitive and behavioral strategies are typically used by practitioners. Our preferred term is cognitive behavior therapy [11].

J. P. Foreyt (✉)
Behavioral Medicine Research Center, Baylor College of Medicine, 6655 Travis Street, Suite 320, Houston, TX 77030, USA
e-mail: jforeyt@bcm.edu

C. A. Johnston
Department of Medicine, Department of Pediatrics-Nutrition, USDA/ARS Children's Nutrition Research Center, Baylor College of Medicine, Houston, TX, USA

© Springer International Publishing Switzerland 2016
J. I. Mechanick, R. F. Kushner (eds.), *Lifestyle Medicine*, DOI 10.1007/978-3-319-24687-1_14

Table 14.1 Cognitive behavior therapy strategies

Strategy	Details
Goal-setting	Helps patients make specific, realistic plans for behavior change
Self-monitoring	Raises a patient's awareness of what needs to be changed by systematic observation, recording, and feedback of the behaviors needing modification
Stimulus control	Helps patients recognize triggers or cues in the environment that lead to undesired behaviors and then modify these environmental stimuli
Cognitive restructuring	Assists patients in identifying and changing unhealthy beliefs about themselves
Stress management	Teaches patients to use cognitive behavioral strategies to lessen and relieve negative affective states
Social support	Provides patients motivation for lifestyle change, role models, enhancement of self-acceptance, and confidence feelings
Behavioral contracting	Supports short-term motivation of a new behavior by first verbalizing the agreed healthful behavior and then signing a contract
Relapse prevention	Teaches patients that lapses are normal and manageable by developing behavior strategies to cope with and prevent them

Current Cognitive Behavior Therapy

Current cognitive behavior therapy involves a number of strategies, which are tailored to each patient's specific needs. These strategies include goal-setting, self-monitoring, stimulus control, cognitive restructuring, stress management, social support, behavioral contracting, and relapse prevention. Please refer to Table 14.1 for additional information regarding these strategies.

Goal-Setting

Cognitive behavior therapy typically begins by asking patients how the interventionist can help. Goal-setting then involves helping patients make specific, realistic plans for behavior change. The average patient with obesity oftentimes has unrealistic goals. One study reported that patients with obesity expect to lose more than 30% of their body weight [12]. Even explaining that such losses are unrealistic, patients frequently are not persuaded, which may lead to their early dropout. We acknowledge the patient's desire and explain that a 10% initial goal would be a good start; then the patient is reevaluated after that initial goal is reached. Behaviorally, the primary goal in behavioral interventions is a weight loss of 1–2 pounds (0.5–1.0 kg) per week. The prescribed diet may vary depending on the patient's initial weight, but typically will be about 1200 kcal/d for women and 1500 kcal/d for men. The prescribed physical activity goal also varies but is typically about 30 min of walking, 5 days a week [13]. With reasonable adherence, patients will lose about 8% of body weight over the first 24 weeks [14].

Goals need to be specific, time limited, and quantifiable. "I'll do better next week" is not a specific, quantifiable goal. But, "I will walk for 30 min before dinner on Tuesday, Thursday, and Saturday" is. Weekly goals are better than monthly goals. Somewhat challenging goals are better than easy ones. Achieving goals helps improve self-esteem, well-being, and a sense of accomplishment [15].

Self-Monitoring

If a practitioner encourages patients to adopt only one behavioral strategy, it should be self-monitoring. Self-monitoring is the most important of all cognitive behavioral approaches because it raises a patient's awareness of what needs to be changed. Self-monitoring involves the systematic observation, recording, and feedback of the behaviors needing modification. No matter what the behavior to be changed is, self-monitoring of that behavior is critical. For patients with obesity, the primary behaviors are obvious: food, physical activity, and weight. Those are the minimum. Sometimes, patients might be asked to record their hours of sleep, the times of the day they eat and exercise, their moods, including levels of stress before eating, or other behaviors influencing their intake and exercise. Self-monitoring, usually in a food and physical activity diary, can serve as a tool for the interventionist to discuss patients' successes and challenges since their last session [16]. Patients typically hate keeping food and physical activity diaries. They lie or forget to report what they ate, therefore underreport their intake, and likewise overreport their physical activity [17–19]. The lack of accuracy does not matter. Remember the primary goal of self-monitoring is to increase awareness of behaviors needing change, not trying to catch a patient in an inconsistency. Self-monitoring diaries do not work well as dependent variables (accuracy in reporting); they work well as independent variables (treatment strategies to raise awareness) [20]. One recent study reported that individuals with obesity who wrote the most words in their food diaries at the beginning of their intervention later were found to have lost the most weight 1 year later compared to those who initially wrote fewer words [21].

Self-monitoring can be tailored to individual patients. If weight gain results from the business person's travel, the food diary might only be needed during those times. If weekends or night eating are the primary problem, the diary might be used only then. This is called selective tracking. It is best that the feedback on the diary, whether it be calories, fat grams, or some point system, be completed by the patient, not the interventionist, again to help raise awareness.

There are currently many physical activity monitors that provide feedback in a variety of ways. However, tracking physical activity in a mechanized way is not required. Using 5 cal burned a minute of brisk walking is a reasonable, easy to figure standard, that is, count 30 min of walking as burning 150 cal [22]. Patients with obesity will burn more calories but the 5 cal burned per minute is an estimate for patients to use. Weighing should be on a regular schedule. Daily self-weighing has been shown to be especially useful for many but can be tailored to the individual. Again, if the practitioner incorporates only one behavioral strategy into the lifestyle intervention, research studies suggest it be self-monitoring [23, 24].

Stimulus Control

Patients often get themselves into trouble with their diet or exercise because of environmental triggers, cues, or stimuli. The identification of those triggers can be helpful in the behavioral change process. The subsequent modification of those triggers or cues is called stimulus control, that is, controlling the triggers that lead to one's downfall [25]. The behavior change strategy typically involves helping patients change their environment to make it easier for them to do what they want to do, that is, eat better and be more active. The hard part for the interventionist is to help the patient identify the major triggers. Food and physical diaries help. So does asking the patients about specific problems or challenges they faced since the last session. The stimulus control strategies are then usually pretty obvious and should come from the patient, not the interventionist. If the patient regularly stops at a fast-food restaurant driving to or from work, changing the route may help. If patients have trouble controlling what they eat for dinner because they are focused on watching television or checking their emails rather than on their food, the stimulus control strategy is apparent. The strategies are pretty straightforward, but again try to coax them out of the patient.

Cognitive Restructuring

Here's where the cognitive aspects of intervention come in. Early behavior modification relied almost entirely on self-monitoring and stimulus control. We subsequently learned that patients' beliefs, attitudes, and feelings about themselves also can play a major role in either success or failure in lifestyle modification programs. Cognitive restructuring strategies were added to classic behavior modification interventions and are aimed at helping patients identify and change unhealthy beliefs about themselves [11, 26, 27]. Typically, patients are asked to self-monitor any thoughts that may be interfering with their abilities to make healthy lifestyle changes. Self-affirmations can be used to help change unhealthy beliefs, thoughts, and feelings. We all have read about athletes psyching themselves up before a competition. It is the same thing here. Patients can be asked to repeat to themselves positive affirmations several times a day. It is best if the patients come up with their own affirmations ("one day at a time," "just do it," etc.) rather than the interventionist doing it for them. Although we use affirmations with some patients, cognitive restructuring strategies have less research support than other behavioral approaches, such as self-monitoring and stimulus control, suggesting the need for additional research in these cognitive strategies.

There are good self-help books or programs on the internet with helpful affirmations if the patient has trouble coming up with some personally relevant ones. The Lifestyle, Exercise, Attitudes, Relationships, and Nutrition (LEARN) Manual is an example of a self-help book for weight management that is based in behavior therapy [28]. This book outlines a widely used 17 lesson program, grounded in science, for weight loss and healthier eating through nutrition education, physical activity, and behavior modification.

Stress Management

Stress, tension, anxiety, depression, loneliness, anger, boredom, and other emotions can wreak havoc on one's best intentions and ruin a lifestyle intervention [29]. Stress can be an especially damaging emotion. It is oftentimes used as a coping mechanism for overeating. There are a number of cognitive behavioral strategies that can be used to help manage stress and other negative affective states when they interfere with progress in an intervention. Physical activity is a major intervention for those under high stress. It increases feelings of well-being and helps put matters in perspective. Meditation can help. Helping patients learn to meditate each day has been shown to keep negative feelings in check. Progressive muscle relaxation can help patients learn to achieve a relaxation response quickly when under stress. These cognitive behavioral strategies can also reduce other negative mood states. However, when feelings of depression or other negative feelings become too strong, referral to appropriate professionals should be done.

Social Support

Support from others can play an important role in the ultimate achievement of personal lifestyle goals. There is evidence that support from groups like Weight Watchers and Take off Pounds Sensibly (TOPS) can provide motivation for lifestyle change for some people [30, 31]. Attending support groups may help patients realize that if others can make positive change, so can they. Support systems can provide good role models, assist in overcoming challenges, and contribute to one's feelings of self-acceptance. Families, neighbors, good friends, colleagues at the job, and interventionists can all serve as potential sources of support for lifestyle change. Sometimes, however, these potential support persons, such as one's spouse or other family member, relative, or close friend, may, for reasons of their own, try to sabotage or undermine the change process. Choosing the right support person or group may make the difference between long-term lifestyle success and ultimate failure.

Behavioral Contracting

Behavioral contracting involves patients verbalizing one or more healthful behaviors they agree to do between sessions and putting pen to paper. The healthful behaviors chosen should be short-term, realistic, simple, a little challenging, but achievable. Increasing the days or the amount of time per day walking, or adding a vegetable to dinner, or skipping dessert each night for a week seem realistic, simple, but also achievable. Having the patient write down the agreed-upon behavior and then sign the "contract" along with the interventionist's signature tends to formalize the agreement. Contracting is most helpful in maintaining motivation short-term and a new behavior with a new contract at each session is recommended [32].

Relapse Prevention

We all stray from our good intentions from time to time. Relapse prevention involves helping patients understand that to err is human. Lapses are normal, expected, and can be managed. Interventionists can help patients anticipate the situations when lapses may occur, including holidays, vacations, even visiting Las Vegas and its buffets, and help them develop behavioral strategies to cope with the situation. The goal is not specifically to prevent all lapses, but to prevent them from becoming relapses [33].

Incorporating Cognitive Behavioral Therapy in the Office

The structure of cognitive behavioral counseling has evolved since the 1960s and 1970s. According to the recent obesity guidelines, the recommended intervention involves 60–90 min weekly sessions, either individual or group, for the first 6 months followed by biweekly, then monthly sessions [34]. A good size for a group is around eight participants. The interventionist, typically a registered dietitian, psychologist, nurse, or other HCP, should have received training in cognitive behavioral counseling strategies [35].

There are advantages and disadvantages to seeing patients in groups or individually. The primary advantage of group sessions is that larger numbers can receive intervention at the same time and members of the group can serve as role models and a source of support to each other. The primary disadvantage is that there is less time to tailor interventions to each person as the size of the group increases. Individual sessions obviously provide more time for tailoring, but patients lack support from others and fewer patients can be seen by the interventionist. Overall, we prefer group sessions. In a perfect world, lifestyle interventions are best delivered by a multidisciplinary team of HCPs, including physicians, registered dietitians, exercise physiologists, and behavioral specialists. In today's busy world, newer delivery systems, including the Internet, apps, and other technological approaches, are increasingly being tested and used to present the intervention.

Results of Cognitive Behavioral Interventions

Cognitive behavioral interventions are generally tested as a "package" of strategies, not as individual components. For example, there are only a few research studies that examined the efficacy of only stimulus control, cognitive restructuring, stress management, or relapse prevention as the sole intervention for lifestyle modification. The strategies are not used individually to improve diet or physical activity; they are used in combination to maximize behavioral changes. Published reviews of the research have documented the beneficial effects of their use in lifestyle modification. Randomized controlled trials, the gold standard in research, have shown that the combination, usually delivered in weekly group sessions for 24 weeks, result in an average weight loss of about 8.0 % (8 kg) [14]. A weight loss of 8 % will typically result in beneficial changes in blood pressure, blood glucose, blood lipids, insulin sensitivity, endothelial function, quality of life, well-being, and other risk factors [36]. Unfortunately, long-term maintenance of these initial results has been less successful. A recent review summarizing the results of about 30 randomized controlled behavioral studies usually of 6 months duration, with follow-ups of 2 years or more, showed that few patients with obesity managed to maintain all of their initial losses [35]. Most regain some of their losses over time. The data are much more encouraging when patients are seen for longer periods of time, usually biweekly or monthly following initial weekly interventions. The results suggest that with extended intervention, some patients maintain modest but clinically significant losses of 5 % or more for at least 2 years [35].

Perspective is important. Untreated, the average adult with obesity gains about 0.6 kg/year [37]. Although not everyone succeeds in maintaining all their weight losses, many do well and the behavioral skills they learn may serve them well in future attempts at lifestyle modification [38].

Examples of Long-term Cognitive Behavioral Interventions

Diabetes Prevention Program

The Diabetes Prevention Program (DPP) is an example of an intervention for preventing or delaying the onset of type-2 diabetes (T2D) in at-risk individuals who are overweight/obese [39]. A total of 3234 at-risk individuals were randomized to a lifestyle modification intervention, metformin, or placebo with a study goal of 7% weight loss and 150 min/week of physical activity. The lifestyle modification intervention included an initial 16 session curriculum of diet, physical activity, and behavior modification strategies including the ones summarized earlier in this chapter. Case managers initially saw participants individually during the first 24 weeks. Later, the individual sessions were held less frequently, usually on a monthly basis. Group sessions were also held occasionally to reinforce behavior change.

At the 1-year assessment, the mean weight loss for the lifestyle modification group was 6.7 kg, compared with 2.7 and 0.4 kg in the metformin and placebo groups, respectively. At the 4-year assessment, the lifestyle modification group maintained a mean loss of 3.5 kg, compared with 1.3 and 0.2 kg in the metformin and placebo groups, respectively. Remarkably, the lifestyle intervention group showed a 58% reduction in the incidence of T2D compared to the placebo group, whereas the incidence in the metformin intervention group was reduced by 31%. The lifestyle modification intervention was significantly more effective in reducing the incidence of T2D than both the placebo and metformin groups. The DPP demonstrates the efficacy of a lifestyle modification intervention for significantly improving long-term health [38].

Look AHEAD

The Look AHEAD (Action for Health in Diabetes) trial is a multicenter, randomized controlled trial designed to evaluate whether modest changes in weight through lifestyle modification would reduce cardiovascular morbidity and mortality in individuals who are overweight/obese and have T2D [40]. A total of 5145 individuals who were overweight/obese and had T2D were randomized to either a lifestyle modification intervention or a usual care group, with a study goal of 7% weight loss and 175 min of physical activity per week. During the first 6 months, the lifestyle modification condition consisted of 24 initial sessions of diet, physical activity, and behavior modification strategies similar to the ones used in DPP. Look AHEAD combined both individual and group sessions. Sessions became less frequent over time. Those who had difficulty meeting treatment goals were offered ad-

ditional interventions from a study "toolbox". The usual care group received three sessions a year on diabetes support and education but did not receive the cognitive behavioral intervention strategies.

At the 1-year assessment, the mean weight loss for the lifestyle intervention group was 8.6%, exceeding the study's goal, compared with 0.7% in the usual care group. The lifestyle intervention group showed beneficial changes in cardiovascular risk factors and reduced medication needs compared to the usual care group [41]. At the 9.6-year assessment, the mean weight loss for the lifestyle intervention was 6% compared to 3.5% in the usual care group [42]. At every annual assessment, the weight losses for the lifestyle intervention group were significantly greater than the usual care group. Although the study did not meet its primary goal of significantly reduced cardiovascular morbidity and mortality, it has demonstrated the efficacy of cognitive behavior modification for long-term weight loss and maintenance. The study is currently ongoing as an observational trial and is assessing additional benefits of the initial intervention.

Conclusion

Cognitive behavioral intervention is key to the development and maintenance of long-term health and well-being. Strategies utilized in this type of intervention include setting reasonable goals and expectations, raising awareness of the behaviors needing to be changed, confronting, and effectively dealing with environmental challenges, managing stress and negative affect, increasing social support, and preventing relapse. The challenge for HCPs is to incorporate the cognitive behavioral strategies utilized successfully in the DPP and the Look AHEAD intervention and adapt them to their own practices [43]. New delivery systems such as intervention over the Internet, apps, smart phones, and other mobile devices may help extend contact with patients and improve outcomes.

Acknowledgments The authors would like to thank the Children's Nutrition Research Center for their continued support. This manuscript was supported by a grant from the US Department of Agriculture (ARS 2533759353).

References

1. Ferster CB, Skinner BF. Schedules of reinforcement. Englewood Cliffs: Prentice-Hall; 1957.
2. Kazdin AE. History of behavior modification. Experimental foundation of contemporary research. Baltimore: University Park Press; 1978.
3. Skinner BF. Walden two. New York: Macmillan; 1976.

4. Ferster CB, Nurnberger JI, Levitt E. The control of eating. J Mathetics. 1962;1:87–109.

5. Foreyt JP. Behavioral treatments of obesity. New York: Pergamon Press; 1977.

6. Stuart RB. Behavioral control of overeating. Behav Res Ther. 1967;5:357–65.

7. Walen S, Hauserman NM, Lavin PJ. Clinical guide to behavior therapy. Baltimore: Williams & Wilkins; 1977.

8. Ullmann LP, Krasner L. Case studies in behavior modification. New York: Holt, Rinehart and Winston; 1965.

9. Berkel LA, Poston WS, Reeves RS, Foreyt JP. Behavioral interventions for obesity. J Am Diet Assoc. 2005;105(5 Suppl 1):S35–43.

10. Foreyt JP, Poston WS. What is the role of cognitive-behavior therapy in patient management? Obes Res. 1998;6:18S–22S.

11. Foreyt JP, Rathjen DP. Cognitive behavior therapy: research and application. New York: Plenum Press; 1978.

12. Foster GD, Wadden TA, Vogt RA, Brewer G. What is a reasonable weight loss? Patients' expectations and evaluations of obesity treatment outcomes. J Consult Clin Psychol. 1997;65(1):79–85.

13. Foreyt JP, Pendleton VR. Management of obesity. Primary Care Rep. 2000;6:19–30.

14. Jones LR, Wilson CI, Wadden TA. Lifestyle modification in the treatment of obesity: an educational challenge and opportunity. Clin Pharmacol Ther. 2007;81(5):776–9.

15. Bandura A, Simon K. The role of proximal intentions in self-regulation of refractory behavior. Cogn Ther Res. 1977;1(3):177–93.

16. Wadden TA, Letizia KA. Predictors of attrition and weight loss in patients treated by moderate and severe caloric restriction. In: Wadden TA, Van Itallie TB, editors. Treatment of the seriously obese patient. New York: Guilford Press; 1992. pp. 383–410.

17. de Vries JH, Zock PL, Mensink RP, Katan MB. Underestimation of energy intake by 3-d records compared with energy intake to maintain body weight in 269 nonobese adults. Am J Clin Nutr. 1994;60(6):855–60.

18. Lichtman SW, Pisarska K, Berman ER, et al. Discrepancy between self-reported and actual caloric intake and exercise in obese subjects. N Engl J Med. 1992;327(27):1893–8.

19. Tooze JA, Subar AF, Thompson FE, Troiano R, Schatzkin A, Kipnis V. Psychosocial predictors of energy underreporting in a large doubly labeled water study. Am J Clin Nutr. 2004;79(5):795–804.

20. Foreyt JP, Goodrick GK. Factors common to successful therapy for the obese patient. Med Sci Sports Exerc. 1991;23(3):292–7.

21. Tsai AG, Fabricatore AN, Wadden TA, et al. Readiness redefined: a behavioral task during screening predicted 1-year weight loss in the Look AHEAD study. Obesity (Silver Spring). 2014;22(4):1016–23.

22. U.S. Department of Health and Human Services and U.S. Department of Agriculture. Dietary Guidelines for Americans, 2005. 6th Edition, Washington, DC: U.S. Government Printing Office; January 2005.

23. Baker RC, Kirschenbaum DS. Self-monitoring may be necessary for successful weight control. Behav Ther. 1993;24:377–94.

24. Wing RR, Tate DF, Gorin AA, Raynor HA, Fava JL. A self-regulation program for maintenance of weight loss. N Engl J Med. 2006;355(15):1563–71.

25. McReynolds WT, Paulsen BK. Stimulus control as the behavioral basis of weight loss procedures. In: Williams BJ, Martin S, Foreyt JP, editors. Obesity: behavioral approaches to dietary management. New York: Brunner/Mazel; 1976. pp. 43–64.

26. Dobson KS. Handbook of cognitive-behavioral therapies. New York: Guilford Press; 2001.

27. Fabricatore AN. Behavior therapy and cognitive-behavioral therapy of obesity: is there a difference? J Am Diet Assoc. 2007;107(1):92–9.

28. Brownell KD. The LEARN Program for weight management. Dallas: American Health Publishing Co; 2000.

29. Ozier AD, Kendrick OW, Leeper JD, Knol LL, Perko M, Burnham J. Overweight and obesity are associated with emotion- and stress-related eating as measured by the eating and appraisal due to emotions and stress questionnaire. J Am Diet Assoc. 2008;108(1):49–56.

30. Wing RR, Jeffery RW. Benefits of recruiting participants with friends and increasing social support for weight loss and maintenance. J Consult Clin Psychol. 1999;67(1):132–8.

31. Johnston CA, Rost S, Miller-Kovach K, Moreno JP, Foreyt JP. A randomized controlled trial of a community-based behavioral counseling program. Am J Med. 2013;126(12):1143.e19–24.

32. Foreyt JP. Need for lifestyle intervention: how to begin. Am J Cardiol. 2005;96(4A):11E–14E.

33. Marlatt GA, Gordon JR. Relapse prevention. New York: Guilford Press; 1985.

34. Jensen MD, Ryan DH, Apovian CM, et al. 2013 ACC/AHA/TOS Guidelines for the management of overweight and obesity in adults: a report of the American college of cardiology/American heart association task force on practice guidelines and the obesity society. J Am Coll Cardiol. 2014;63(25 Pt B):2985–3023.

35. Anton SD, Foreyt JP, Perri MS. Preventing weight regain after weight loss. In: Bray GA, Bouchard C, editors. Handbook of obesity volume 2: clinical applications. 4th ed. New York: CRC Press; 2014. pp. 145–66.

36. Aronne LJ, Brown WV, Isoldi KK. Cardiovascular disease in obesity: a review of related risk factors and risk-reduction strategies. J Clin Lipidol. 2007;1(6):575–82.

37. Shah M, Hannan PJ, Jeffery RW. Secular trend in body mass index in the adult population of three communities from the upper midwestern part of the USA: the Minnesota heart health program. Int J Obes. 1991;15(8):499–503.

38. Kramer FM, Jeffery RW, Forster JL, Snell MK. Long-term follow-up of behavioral treatment for obesity: patterns of weight regain among men and women. Int J Obes. 1989;13(2):123–36.

39. Knowler WC, Barrett-Connor E, Fowler SE, et al. Reduction in the incidence of type 2 diabetes with lifestyle intervention or metformin. N Engl J Med. 2002;346(6):393–403.

40. Look AHEAD Research Group, Wadden TA, West DS, et al. The look AHEAD study: a description of the lifestyle intervention and the evidence supporting it. Obesity (Silver Spring). 2006;14(5):737–52.

41. Look AHEAD Research Group, Pi-Sunyer X, Blackburn G, et al. Reduction in weight and cardiovascular disease risk factors in individuals with type 2 diabetes: one-year results of the Look AHEAD trial. Diabetes Care. 2007;30(6):1374–83.

42. Look AHEAD Research Group, Wing RR, Bolin P, et al. Cardiovascular effects of intensive lifestyle intervention in type 2 diabetes. N Engl J Med. 2013;369(2):145–54.

43. Perri MG. Effects of behavioral treatment on long-term weight loss: lessons learned from the Look AHEAD trial. Obesity (Silver Spring). 2014;22(1):3–4.

Treating Tobacco Use in Clinical Practice

Allison J. Carroll, Anna K. Veluz-Wilkins and Brian Hitsman

"Cigarette smoking is the chief, single, avoidable cause of death in our society and the most important public health issue of our time."

C. Everett Koop, M. D. in 1982, former US Surgeon General

Abbreviations

AA	African-American
AAFP	American Academy of Family Physicians
ACA	Affordable Care Act
CI	Confidence interval
COPD	Chronic obstructive pulmonary disease
EHR	Electronic Health Record
ENDS	Electronic nicotine delivery systems
FAQ	Frequently Asked Questions
FDA	Food and Drug Administration
GED	General Educational Development
H	Hispanic
LGBTQ	Lesbian, gay, bisexual, transgender, and questioning
MAO	Monoamine oxidase
NRT	Nicotine replacement therapy
OB/GYN	Obstetrician/gynecological
OTC	Over-the-counter
PHS	Public Health Service
RCT	Randomized clinical trial
Rx	Prescription product
SES	Socioeconomic status
SIDS	Sudden infant death syndrome
SR	Sustained release
USPSTF	US Preventive Services Task Force

B. Hitsman (✉) · A. J. Carroll · A. K. Veluz-Wilkins
Department of Preventive Medicine, Northwestern University
Feinberg School of Medicine, 680 N. Lake Shore Dr., Suite 1400,
Chicago, IL 60611, USA
e-mail: b-hitsman@northwestern.edu

Introduction

Tobacco use has been well identified as the single most preventable cause of disease, disability, and death in the USA, accounting for one in every five deaths in the USA each year. Unfortunately, more than 30 years after C. Everett Koop's public condemnation of smoking, his statement continues to hold true today. First-, second-, and even third-hand smoking harm nearly every organ in the body, reduce quality of life and life expectancy, are causally linked to cancer at 18 different human organ sites and at least 13 chronic diseases across the cardiovascular, pulmonary, reproductive, and developmental systems as well as various orthopedic, ophthalmologic, and dental illnesses [1, 2]. Each year, more people in the USA die from smoking than from alcohol, cocaine, heroin, suicide, homicide, acquired immunodeficiency syndrome, motor-vehicle accidents, and fires combined [2]. Patients who smoke will die an average of 14 years earlier than their nonsmoking counterparts.

While awareness of the negative consequences of smoking has grown exponentially, and many former smokers have been able to quit, tobacco use rates have not significantly decreased in nearly a decade, with cigarette smoking hovering just under 18 % in the US population. Major disparities in tobacco use persist in particular populations, including psychiatric populations (44 % smoke across all psychiatric diagnoses, up to 90 % among populations in substance abuse treatment); certain racial/ethnic minorities (e.g., 26 % of those who self-identify as American Indian/Alaskan Native and 27 % of those who self-identify as multiple race); lesbian, gay, bisexual, transgender, and questioning (LGBTQ) populations (27 %); those who are economically disadvantaged (29 %); and populations with limited education (41 % of those with a General Educational Development, GED) [3].

© Springer International Publishing Switzerland 2016
J. I. Mechanick, R. F. Kushner (eds.), *Lifestyle Medicine*, DOI 10.1007/978-3-319-24687-1_15

Most smokers want to or know they should quit, but less than 5% of those attempting to quit use the most effective tools to do so (i.e., pharmacotherapy and/or counseling), and only around 3% of individuals who quit "cold-turkey" achieve long-term abstinence (i.e., 6 months or longer). Health-care providers are in a uniquely powerful position to educate their smoking patients about the best cessation approaches that are likely to increase quitting success. Advising a patient to quit smoking or simply asking about smoking status enhances a smoker's motivation to quit and increases quit rates [4], and brief (i.e., 3-min.) interventions significantly increase abstinence rates [5].

The health impact of continued tobacco use has a trajectory similar to that of other chronic diseases, and for this reason it should be treated as such by health-care providers. Specifically, tobacco use is a persistent behavior that typically involves multiple periods of relapse and remission, requiring regular screening and repeated intervention. Therefore, recommending long-term, intensive, and/or combination treatment beyond the typical 8-week course of nicotine replacement therapy (NRT) should be considered, especially for patients who are at highest risk for smoking relapse following a quit attempt. This includes providing assistance with evidence-based pharmacotherapy, incorporating behavioral counseling, and regularly following up with patients by asking about tobacco use and abstinence at every visit.

Here, we review tobacco use management in a clinical practice setting, with specific discussion on brief evidence-based pharmacological and counseling treatments for tobacco users who are willing to quit, unwilling to quit, and recently quit. The recommendations provided below come in large part from the Public Health Service (PHS) Guidelines for Treating Tobacco Use and Dependence (2008 update) [5]. These guidelines are based on more than 8700 peer-reviewed articles published between 1975 and 2007.

We further outline the adaptations of tobacco treatment approaches for special populations, including populations with comorbid medical and psychiatric illnesses, those that are socioeconomically disadvantaged, and light or intermittent smokers. Finally, we will address current issues that are affecting clinical treatment of tobacco use: e-cigarettes, alternative tobacco products, and the Affordable Care Act (ACA) parameters for tobacco treatment.

Pharmacological Treatment of Tobacco Dependence

Smoking cessation pharmacotherapies come in two forms: NRTs and non-nicotine medications. See Table 15.1 for the seven first-line pharmacotherapies currently available in the USA for treating nicotine dependence, additional combination pharmacotherapy options, and corresponding efficacy data.

Nicotine Replacement Therapies NRTs reduce physical withdrawal from nicotine by delivering either acute (gum, lozenge, inhaler, nasal spray) or continuous (patch) nicotine to the body. This route of nicotine delivery reduces some of the physical withdrawal symptoms associated with nicotine abstinence and blocks some of the immediate, reinforcing effects of tobacco smoke. By minimizing nicotine withdrawal, patients can then focus on learning the behavioral skills needed to quit, in the context of provider and other social support, and avoid relapse back to smoking. All five NRTs significantly increase a patient's likelihood of successful quitting, with a patient's likelihood of quitting ranging somewhere between 1.5 (nicotine gum for 6–14 weeks) and 2.3 times (high-dose nicotine patch and nasal spray) compared to placebo [5].

Non-nicotine Medications Two non-nicotine medications are Food and Drug Administration (FDA)-approved as first-line pharmacotherapies for treating nicotine dependence. Bupropion sustained release (SR; brand name: Zyban) works by enhancing central nervous system noradrenergic and dopaminergic release. Bupropion SR can also be prescribed as an antidepressant (brand name: Wellbutrin SR) and therefore should be considered for smokers who struggle with depression or depressed moods when trying to quit. The recommended duration of treatment with bupropion is 7–12 weeks but can be used for up to 6 months, with the longer duration likely contributing to maintenance of abstinence among patients who have successfully quit.

Varenicline tartrate (brand name: Chantix or Champix) is a partial agonist at the alpha-4 beta-2 subunit of the nicotinic acetylcholine receptor, the receptor that contributes to the reinforcing effects of nicotine. As a partial agonist, varenicline binds to and produces partial stimulation of alpha-4 beta-2 nicotine receptor, thereby reducing nicotine withdrawal symptoms, including depressed mood and cognitive impairment. Additionally, because it binds with high affinity, it works as a partial antagonist by blocking the nicotine from tobacco smoke, therefore reducing the subjective pleasurable effects of cigarette smoking. In prior randomized-controlled trials of varenicline, biochemically confirmed quit rates are more than three times those in the placebo group when used in conjunction with brief counseling, making it the most effective FDA-approved smoking cessation medication currently available. Varenicline is typically prescribed for a 12-week course but has been FDA-approved for use up to 24 weeks.

Both bupropion and varenicline currently carry black box warnings due to post-marketing reports of increased suicidality and other psychiatric symptoms. However, recent safety trials of varenicline, conducted after the black box warnings, have indicated that varenicline is both safe, even among individuals with a history of depression [6] or other serious mental illness [7]. Similarly, despite initial evidence from a meta-analysis that varenicline may increase the likelihood of cardiac events (including chest pain, heart attack, stroke,

Table 15.1 Food and Drug Administration (FDA)-approved medications for smoking cessation. (Adapted and reprinted with permission from: Rx for Change: Clinician-Assisted Tobacco Cessation. The Regents of the University of California)

	Nicotine replacement therapy (NRT) formulations					Bupropion SR	Varenicline
	Transdermal patch	Gum	Lozenge	Nasal spray	Oral inhaler		
Product	*NicoDerm CQ[a]*, generic OTC (NicoDerm CQ, generic) Rx (generic) 7, 14, and 21 mg (24-h release)	*Nicorette[a]*, generic OTC 2 mg, 4 mg original, cinnamon, fruit, mint, and orange	*Nicorette Lozenge[a]*, *Nicorette Mini Lozenge[a]*, generic OTC 2 mg, 4 mg cherry and mint	*Nicotrol NS[b]* Rx metered spray 0.5 mg nicotine in 50 mcL aqueous nicotine solution	*Nicotrol Inhaler[b]* Rx 10 mg cartridge delivers 4 mg inhaled nicotine vapor	*Zyban[a]*, generic Rx 150 mg sustained-release tablet	*Chantix[b]* Rx 0.5 mg, 1 mg tablet
Precautions	Recent (≤2 weeks) myocardial infarction Serious underlying arrhythmias Serious or worsening angina pectoris Pregnancy[c] (Rx formulations, category D) and breastfeeding Adolescents (<18 years)	Recent (≤2 weeks) myocardial infarction Serious underlying arrhythmias Serious or worsening angina pectoris Temporomandibular joint disease Pregnancy[c] and breastfeeding Adolescents (<18 years)	Recent (≤2 weeks) myocardial infarction Serious underlying arrhythmias Serious or worsening angina pectoris Pregnancy[c] and breastfeeding Adolescents (<18 years)	Recent (≤2 weeks) myocardial infarction Serious underlying arrhythmias Serious or worsening angina pectoris Underlying chronic nasal disorders (rhinitis, nasal polyps, sinusitis) Severe reactive airway disease Pregnancy[c] (category D) and breastfeeding Adolescents (<18 years)	Recent (≤2 weeks) myocardial infarction Serious underlying arrhythmias Serious or worsening angina pectoris Bronchospastic disease Pregnancy[c] (category D) and breastfeeding Adolescents (<18 years)	Concomitant therapy with medications or medical conditions known to lower the seizure threshold Severe hepatic cirrhosis Pregnancy[c] (category C) and breastfeeding Adolescents (<18 years) *Warning* Black-boxed warning for neuropsychiatric symptoms[d] *Contraindications* Seizure disorder Concomitant bupropion (e.g., Wellbutrin) therapy Current or prior diagnosis of bulimia or anorexia nervosa Simultaneous abrupt discontinuation of alcohol or sedatives/benzodiazepines MAO inhibitor therapy in previous 14 days	Severe renal impairment (dosage adjustment is necessary) Pregnancy[c] (category C) and breastfeeding Adolescents (<18 years) *Warnings* Black-boxed warning for neuropsychiatric symptoms[d] *Please see extended discussion in chapter regarding neuropsychiatric concerns and management* Cardiovascular adverse events in patients with existing cardiovascular disease Seizure-related adverse events in patients with seizure Hx or risk May lower alcohol tolerance

Table 15.1 (continued)

	Nicotine replacement therapy (NRT) formulations					Bupropion SR	Varenicline
	Transdermal patch	Gum	Lozenge	Nasal spray	Oral inhaler		
Dosing	≤10 cigarettes/day: 14 mg/day × 6 weeks 7 mg/day × 2 weeks >10 cigarettes/day: 21 mg/day × 4 weeks (generic) or 6 weeks (NicoDerm CQ) 14 mg/day × 2 weeks 7 mg/day × 2 weeks May wear patch for 16 h if patient experiences sleep disturbances (remove at bedtime) Duration: 8–10 weeks; can be longer under guidance of physician	1st cigarette >30 min after waking: 2 mg 1st cigarette ≤30 min after waking: 4 mg Weeks 1–6: 1 piece q 1–2 h Weeks 7–9: 1 piece q 2–4 h Weeks 10–12: 1 piece q 4–8 h Maximum: 24 pieces/day Chew each piece slowly Park between cheek and gum when peppery or tingling sensation appears (~15–30 chews) Resume chewing when tingle fades Repeat chew/park steps until most of the nicotine is gone (i.e., tingle does not return; generally 30 min) Park in different areas of mouth No food or beverages 15 min before or during use Duration: up to 12 weeks	1st cigarette ≤30 min after waking: 4 mg 1st cigarette 30 min after waking: 2 mg Weeks 1–6: 1 lozenge q 1–2 h Weeks 7–9: 1 lozenge q 2–4 h Weeks 10–12: 1 lozenge q 4–8 h Maximum: 20 lozenges/day Allow to dissolve slowly (20–30 min for standard; 10 min for mini) Nicotine release may cause a warm, tingling sensation Do not chew or swallow Occasionally rotate to different areas of the mouth No food or beverages 15 min before or during use Duration: up to 12 weeks	1–2 doses/h (8–40 doses/day) One dose = 2 sprays (one in each nostril) Each spray delivers 0.5 mg of nicotine to the nasal mucosa Maximum: 5 doses/h or 40 doses/day For best results, initially use at least 8 doses/day Do not sniff, swallow, or inhale through the nose as the spray is being administered Duration: 3–6 months	6–16 cartridges/day Individualize dosing; initially use 1 cartridge q 1–2 h Best effects with continuous puffing for 20 min Initially use at least 6 cartridges/day Nicotine in cartridge is depleted after 20 min of active puffing Inhale into back of throat or puff in short breaths Do not inhale into the lungs (like a cigarette) but "puff" as if lighting a pipe Open cartridge retains potency for 24 h No food or beverages 15 min before or during use Duration: 3–6 months	150 mg po q AM x 3 days, then 150 mg po bid Maximum: 300 mg/day Begin therapy 1–2 weeks prior to quit date Allow at least 8 h between doses Avoid bedtime dosing to minimize insomnia Dose tapering is not necessary Can be used safely with NRT Duration: 7–12 weeks, with maintenance up to 6 months in selected patients	Days 1–3: 0.5 mg po q AM Days 4–7: 0.5 mg po bid Weeks 2–12: 1 mg po bid Begin therapy 1 week prior to quit date; alternatively, the patient can begin therapy and then quit smoking between days 8–35 of treatment Take dose after eating and with a full glass of water Dose tapering is not necessary Dosing adjustment is necessary for patients with severe renal impairment Duration: standard is 12 weeks; an additional 12-week course may be used in selected patients
Adverse effects	Local skin reactions (erythema, pruritus, and burning) Headache Sleep disturbances (insomnia, abnormal/vivid dreams); associated with nocturnal nicotine absorption	Mouth/jaw soreness Hiccups Dyspepsia Hypersalivation Effects associated with incorrect chewing technique: Lightheadedness Nausea/vomiting Throat and mouth irritation	Nausea Hiccups Cough Heartburn Headache Flatulence Insomnia	Nasal and/or throat irritation (hot, peppery, or burning sensation) Rhinitis Tearing Sneezing Cough Headache	Mouth and/or throat irritation Cough Headache Rhinitis Dyspepsia Hiccups	Insomnia Dry mouth Nervousness/difficulty concentrating Rash Constipation Seizures (risk is 0.1%) Neuropsychiatric symptoms (rare; see precautions)	Nausea Sleep disturbances (insomnia, abnormal/vivid dreams) Constipation Flatulence Vomiting Neuropsychiatric symptoms (rare; see precautions)

Table 15.1 (continued)

	Nicotine replacement therapy (NRT) formulations					Bupropion SR	Varenicline
	Transdermal patch	Gum	Lozenge	Nasal spray	Oral inhaler		
Efficacy[e]	*Monotherapy—estimated odds ratio (95% CI)*						
	1.9 (1.7–2.2)	1.5 (1.2–1.7)	2.0 (1.4–2.8)[f]	2.3 (1.7–3.0)	2.1 (1.5–2.9)	2.0 (1.8–2.6)	3.1 (2.5–3.8)
	Combination therapy—estimated odds ratio (95 % CI)						
	All effective combinations contain the transdermal patch as one of the medications	Long-term (>14 weeks) nicotine gum + patch 3.6 (2.5–5.2)	Data not available	Long-term (>14 weeks) nicotine spray + patch 3.6 (2.5–5.2)	Nicotine inhale + patch 2.2 (1.3–3.6)	Bupropion SR + nicotine patch 2.5 (1.9–3.4)	Data not available
US$/day[g]	1.52–3.40 (1 patch)	1.90–5.48/day (9 pieces)	3.05–4.38/day (9 pieces)	4.32–6.48/day (8–12 doses)	7.74–20.64/day (6–16 cartridges)	2.54–6.22/day (2 tablets) OR 419.10–1026.30 (12-week course)	6.54/day (2 tablets) OR 1079.10 (12-week course)
Advantages	Provides consistent nicotine levels over 24 h Easy to use and conceal Once-daily dosing associated with fewer compliance problems	Might satisfy oral cravings Might delay weight gain Patients can titrate therapy to manage withdrawal symptoms Variety of flavors are available	Might satisfy oral cravings Might delay weight gain Nasal/throat irritation may be bothersome	Patients can titrate therapy to rapidly manage withdrawal symptoms Need for frequent dosing can compromise compliance Nasal/throat irritation may be bothersome	Patients can titrate therapy to manage withdrawal symptoms Mimics hand-to-mouth ritual of smoking (could also be perceived as a disadvantage) Need for frequent dosing can compromise compliance	Easy to use; oral formulation might be associated with fewer compliance problems Might delay weight gain Can be used with NRT Might be beneficial in patients with depression	Easy to use; oral formulation might be associated with fewer compliance problems Offers a new mechanism of action for patients who have failed other agents

Table 15.1 (continued)

Nicotine replacement therapy (NRT) formulations

	Transdermal patch	Gum	Lozenge	Nasal spray	Oral inhaler	Bupropion SR	Varenicline
Disadvantage	Patients cannot titrate the dose to acutely manage withdrawal symptoms Allergic reactions to adhesive might occur Patients with dermatologic conditions should not use the patch	Need for frequent dosing can compromise compliance Might be problematic for patients with significant dental work Patients must use proper chewing technique to minimize adverse effects Gum chewing may not be socially acceptable	Gastrointestinal side effects (nausea, hiccups, and heartburn) might be bothersome	Patients must wait 5 min before driving or operating heavy machinery Patients with chronic nasal disorders or severe reactive airway disease should not use the spray	Initial throat or mouth irritation can be bothersome Cartridges should not be stored in very warm conditions or used in very cold conditions Patients with underlying bronchospastic disease must use with caution	Seizure risk is increased Several contraindications and precautions preclude use in some patients (see precautions) Patients should be monitored for potential neuropsychiatric symptoms[d] (see precautions)	May induce nausea in up to one third of patients Patients should be monitored for potential neuropsychiatric symptoms[d] (see precautions)

For complete prescribing information, please refer to the manufacturers' package inserts

MAO monoamine oxidase, *NRT* nicotine replacement therapy, *OTC* over-the-counter (nonprescription product), *Rx* prescription product, *SR* sustained release, *q* every, *po* by the way of mouth, *bid* twice a day, *AM* before noon, *CI* confidence interval

[a] Marketed by GlaxoSmithKline

[b] Marketed by Pfizer

[c] The US Clinical Practice Guideline states that pregnant smokers should be encouraged to quit without medication based on insufficient evidence of effectiveness and theoretical concerns with safety. Pregnant smokers should be offered behavioral counseling interventions that exceed minimal advice to quit

[d] In July 2009, the FDA mandated that the prescribing information for all bupropion- and varenicline-containing products include a black-boxed warning highlighting the risk of serious neuropsychiatric symptoms, including changes in behavior, hostility, agitation, depressed mood, suicidal thoughts and behavior, and attempted suicide. Clinicians should advise patients to stop taking varenicline or bupropion SR and contact a health-care provider immediately if they experience agitation, depressed mood, and any changes in behavior that are not typical of nicotine withdrawal, or if they experience suicidal thoughts or behavior. If treatment is stopped due to neuropsychiatric symptoms, patients should be monitored until the symptoms resolve

[e] Efficacy: Odds ratio of abstinence relative to the placebo group; all medications were used in combination with behavioral cessation counseling; all numbers taken from meta-analysis published in the 2008 PHS Guidelines

[f] Odds ratio based on a single study included in the 2008 PHS Guidelines

[g] Wholesale acquisition cost from Red Book Online. Thomson Reuters, September 2013

shortness of breath, calf pain, numbness, or difficulty speaking) [8], a convincing reanalysis involving additional data indicated that there is no difference in cardiac event rates between varenicline and placebo groups [9]. These black box warnings have introduced considerable media frenzy and perhaps contributed to public misunderstanding. Therefore, it will be especially helpful to educate patients who may be prescribed either bupropion or varenicline about the evidence and likely misconceptions surrounding these medications.

Combination Pharmacotherapies Treatment with a combination of cessation medications can further reduce withdrawal symptoms and increase quit rates. The PHS Guidelines found that all cessation medication combinations increased the odds of quitting by 2.0–3.6 times compared to placebo [5]. For example, a nicotine patch can be used for continuous nicotine delivery in combination with nicotine gum to combat acute cravings (90 % increased odds of quitting using the combination compared to only using the nicotine patch).

Cessation Medications: Developing Patient "Buy-In"

When discussing treatment options with patients, health-care providers should explain that cessation medications target the physical addiction to nicotine and minimize nicotine withdrawal symptoms, a common reason for relapse. It is also important to review common physiological side effects of nicotine withdrawal, such as cravings, headaches, appetite and/or weight changes, and mood changes (e.g., irritability, anxiety, depressed mood), so that patients can anticipate and prepare for these potential symptoms and differentiate them from potential medication side effects. Withdrawal symptoms typically start 24–48 h after quitting, peak within the first week, and subside within 2–4 weeks [10]. This education piece is critical, particularly among certain higher-burden tobacco using populations who are more likely to hold strong misconceptions about NRT, thereby deterring their use [11]. Patients are significantly more likely to be abstinent at the end of a 12-week course of NRT if they demonstrate increased perceived control over withdrawal symptoms within the first 3 weeks of treatment [12]. By clearly emphasizing the time-limited nature of withdrawal, medical professionals can provide helpful self-talk that can be used by a patient to manage any initial cravings experienced and potentially prevent him/her from slipping back into smoking.

Cessation Medications: Compliance Concerns

Even when prescribed, there are many reasons why patients may not follow through with pharmacotherapy [13]. Having a frank discussion with your patients about compliance may help minimize these issues. First, patients may not fill the prescription due to lack of access or high cost (see below how the ACA may help to address this issue).

Second, patients may not use the medication in the most effective manner due to a misunderstanding or misconceptions about medication use, potential side effects, or the efficacy of the medications. Patients often misattribute common withdrawal symptoms, which, as noted above, typically pass in 2–4 weeks, to medication side effects. Likewise, patients who happen to slip and smoke a cigarette often discontinue useful pharmacotherapy due to concerns about side effects, thereby increasing the chances of the slip leading to a full relapse. To address this general issue, the FDA recently updated the instructions for nicotine patch use, indicating that it is safe to smoke while using the nicotine patch with the caveat that individuals may experience some negative side effects (e.g., nausea) if they do [14]. Therefore, health-care providers must educate the patient about the specific smoking cessation medication(s) recommended and/or prescribed, the potential efficacy, and how symptoms experienced may, in fact, be a withdrawal symptom from quitting that will likely pass in time rather than a persistent side effect of the prescribed medication.

"Aren't I Just Replacing One Addiction with Another?" Patients also express concern about becoming addicted to the pharmacotherapy they use in their quit attempt. In reality, the odds of a patient developing a physical addiction to NRTs are slim to none as the amount of nicotine delivered is quite small in comparison to a cigarette, and more critically, cessation medications have not been shown to have addictive properties. To address this issue, health-care providers can discuss the possibility for tapering off some of the medications; e.g., nicotine patches can be tapered from 21 mg (4 weeks) to 14 mg (2 weeks) to 7 mg (2 weeks) as the level of addiction decreases and patient confidence increases. Of note, while tapering is safe and recommended, research has not demonstrated an added overall benefit for tapering medication dose versus not tapering (e.g., 8 weeks 21 mg sustained dosing) to complete the course of cessation medication. However, it is possible that a patient may misattribute their successful abstinence solely to the medication and fear that stopping the medication will lead to increased cravings and withdrawal symptoms. This fear can be combated with education regarding the length of physical side effects and withdrawal symptoms as discussed above.

Evidence-Based Behavioral Counseling Interventions

Decades of intervention research have evaluated the most effective treatments for tobacco cessation. The PHS Guidelines identify behavioral counseling approaches for tobacco

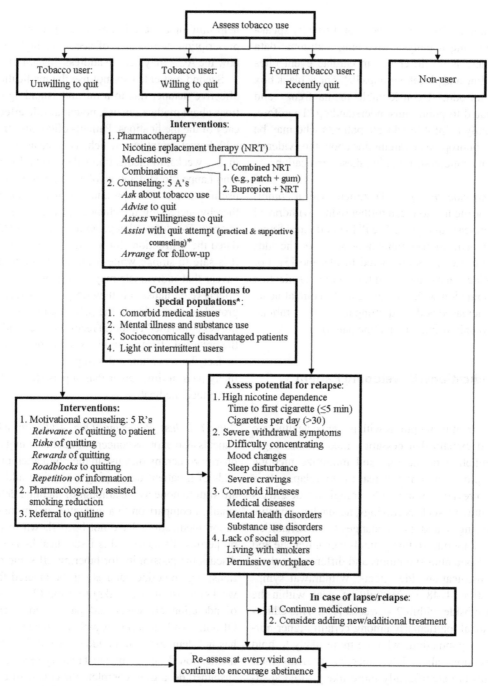

Fig. 15.1 Treatment algorithm for addressing tobacco use in clinical practice according to a patient's smoking status and motivational readiness to make a quit attempt. Ask, advise, and assess are necessary for all patients. For patients unwilling to make a quit attempt, motivational intervention (5 R's) or pre-quit smoking cessation medication can be effective. Patients willing to make a quit attempt should receive brief intervention (5 A's), including psychological (practical and supportive counseling) and pharmacological (cessation medication) support. For patients who have recently quit (past year), the potential for relapse to tobacco use should be assessed and relapse prevention intervention provided as needed. Patients who have not smoked within the past year should be reassessed at every visit and encouraged to stay smoke free. (Adapted from Hughes [16, p. 217])

users who (1) are willing to quit, (2) are currently unwilling to quit, and (3) have recently quit. Please see Fig. 15.1 for a summary algorithm of PHS Guideline-recommended cessation intervention approaches organized by patients' readiness to quit.

Tobacco Users Willing to Quit

The most effective treatments for patients who are willing to quit using tobacco are those that combine cessation medications to treat the physical addiction, as discussed above, with

Table 15.2 Practical and supportive cessation counseling strategies for smokers willing to quit

Strategy	Example
Practical counseling	
Education	Discuss potential withdrawal symptoms and expected length of withdrawal symptoms
Identify smoking triggers	*Behaviors:* drinking coffee/alcohol, spending time with other smokers *Thoughts:* *"Smoking will help me relax."* or *"A cigarette would make this meal taste better."* *Feelings:* depressed mood, stress, excitement, boredom
Develop coping skills	*Behavior:* avoiding trigger situations (e.g., alcohol), change routines (e.g., morning coffee), and increase smoking incompatible behaviors (e.g., wash dishes, brush/floss teeth) *Cognitive:* increase positive self-talk (e.g., *"This craving will pass. It's only 5 min."*), counter permission-giving thoughts (e.g., *"I've had a really hard day, I deserve a cigarette."*), and utilize distraction tactics (e.g., listen to music, do a crossword)
Supportive counseling	
Encourage quit attempt	Encourage the patient to identify his or her own reasons for quitting
Empathize	Acknowledge how difficult it can be to quit smoking and that many smokers fail several times before they are able to quit for good
Encourage discussion of the process	Ask about the patient's concerns about quitting (e.g., identity as a smoker), past difficulties, and failures

behavioral counseling to treat the psychological addiction that often maintains dependence. It is essential to educate patients about the importance of using *both* pharmacotherapy and behavioral counseling, as this combination significantly increases abstinence compared to either treatment approach alone [5, 15].

Cessation Counseling: The Five A's The PHS Guidelines outline the 5 A's for addressing nicotine dependence: Ask, Advise, Assess, Assist, and Arrange for follow-up (see Table 15.2 for practical and supportive counseling strategies and examples) [5]. In conjunction with pharmacotherapy, behavioral counseling is critical to address the psychological dependence on smoking that typically remains long after the physical addiction on nicotine has been broken. Individuals trying to quit smoking have to learn new behavioral patterns and coping strategies to adopt a smoke-free life. If left unaddressed, the psychological dependence and behavioral routines around smoking are most often the triggers that can lead to relapse.

At each and every visit, it is critical to *ask* patients about their tobacco use. If they report that they use any tobacco products, *advise* them to quit and then *assess* their willingness to quit. If patients are willing to consider making a quit attempt in the next two weeks, health-care providers should then *assist* their patients to make a quit attempt. The *assist* step includes both pharmacotherapy (as described above) and counseling techniques, which are described below in further detail.

In addition to pharmacotherapy, health-care providers should *assist* smoking patients by encouraging them to (1) set a quit date, (2) tell others about their quit attempt (as social support is predictive of successful quitting), (3) anticipate barriers to quitting and briefly discuss how they can overcome these barriers, and (4) remove all products related to smoking (e.g., ashtrays). It is also important for health-

care providers to be aware of the factors that may facilitate or impair an individual's success in quitting smoking, including high nicotine dependence, withdrawal symptoms, comorbid illnesses, and lack of social support. For instance, a simple measure to assess a patient's level of nicotine dependence is the Heavy Smoking Index [17] comprising two questions: (1) "How soon after waking do you smoke your first cigarette?" and (2) "How many cigarettes do you smoke per day?" Patients who report smoking within 5 min of waking and smoking > 30 cigarettes per day are categorized with the most severe dependence. For patients with more barriers to quitting smoking, more intensive and/or longer-term treatment is indicated to increase the likelihood of their achieving and maintaining abstinence.

Higher doses of counseling (overall time as well as number of contacts) tend to yield higher quit rates. It is for this reason that health-care providers should always *arrange* for follow-up after assisting a patient with a quit attempt. If time constraints or lack of expertise are of concern, there are many supplemental resources for smoking patients. Referrals to the national toll-free quitline (1-800-QUIT-NOW or 1-855-DEJELO-YA for Spanish speakers) connect patients to their local state quitline that, depending on current state funding, provides free behavior and supportive counseling and, in some cases, smoking cessation pharmacotherapy.

With the advent of technology and social media, many online resources and interactive modules are available to assist individuals when smoking, some of which are being paired with quitline services. These resources include online social support groups and chatrooms, and mobile phone applications to monitor smoking behaviors, which may serve as measures of accountability and support for patients between medical visits. Please see the resources section at the end of this chapter for a list of tobacco cessation information, tools, and interactive modules.

Tobacco Users Currently Unwilling to Quit

For smokers who are not willing to set a quit date within the upcoming month, different motivational interventions are appropriate. The PHS Guidelines outline a motivation approach called the 5 R's: Relevance, Risks, Rewards, Roadblocks, and Repetition [5]. When a health-care provider spends time with the patient providing education regarding reasons to quit that are *relevant* to the patient's personal situation, recognizing the *risks* and *rewards* of quitting smoking, and expressing understanding of the *roadblocks* faced by quitting, patients are more likely to contemplate smoking cessation and discuss it with health-care providers in the future *(repetition)* to receive help in quitting.

Evidence indicates that, for individuals who are currently unwilling or unable to quit smoking, reduction is an effective step toward abstinence [18], particularly when aided by pharmacotherapy (nicotine patch or varenicline) [14, 19]. Reduced tobacco consumption has been shown to predict successful abstinence. When individuals take charge of their behavior change, the sense of control over their own health that is gained during an initial stage of reduction can help them to achieve successful abstinence in the long run. However, this strategy comes with the caveat that reducing tobacco consumption in and of itself is not an effective strategy for reducing risk of tobacco-attributable disease occurrence or exacerbation. Therefore, while it is important to encourage and applaud any steps a patient is willing and able to make toward abstinence, it is also necessary to continue to educate patients about the importance of complete abstinence as the end goal.

Tobacco Users Who Have Recently Quit

As with other chronic diseases, it is important to continue to monitor and assess patients for relapse potential. Many smokers who relapse do so because they fail to anticipate and plan for difficult situations that could trigger a slip. It is not uncommon for patients to think that they can simply "be strong," "use will power," and just "make" themselves quit. In addition to recognizing patients with a high potential for relapse, high-risk situations to anticipate and discuss directly with patients include positive events (e.g., celebrations), negative mood states (e.g., depression, stress), and situations with alcohol (especially in social situations). By having frank discussions about these issues, patients can be better equipped to handle high-risk situations as they arise and thereby decrease their own risk for relapse.

Like patients who are still smoking, it is important to arrange for follow-up soon after their quit date, at the completion of treatment, and during subsequent contacts (either by phone or in the office), praise patients for continued success, and counsel patients regarding the potential for slips and re-

lapse as outlined above. Those who have recently quit should also be connected to resources in the community for additional support or their state quitline to help them maintain abstinence and stay quit.

Adapting Treatment to Special Populations

The pharmacotherapies and behavioral strategies outlined above have been demonstrated to be effective in the general population of smokers. However, there are myriad smokers whose sociodemographic, medical, and psychiatric histories negatively influence their chances of success. Populations that require special attention regarding tobacco treatment are those who (a) smoke at >10% higher rates than the general population, (b) experience greater tobacco-attributable health disparities, (c) have less access to treatment, or (d) have not been specifically studied [20]. It is useful to understand the treatments that are most effective or may be contraindicated for these special populations. The PHS recommendations for special populations [5] are summarized in Table 15.3 and outlined in further detail below.

Medical Populations

Patients with medical conditions related to or exacerbated by smoking often experience "teachable moments," or moments when patients feel vulnerable and are more likely to engage in behavior change, particularly if quitting smoking is known to reduce or completely ameliorate the problem. Behavior counseling and education regarding smoking cessation has been shown to be effective in hospitalized patients, though abstinence rates improve only when *at least 1 month* of follow-up is included [21]. There are unique considerations and barriers that require specific interventions and care for certain medical populations.

Chronic Disease Populations It is well-known that tobacco use causes and exacerbates chronic diseases, including cardiovascular disease, pulmonary diseases, cancer, and many others. Smoking cessation is more effective than medications for prevention of a secondary coronary event or cancer disease progression and recurrence, yet fewer than 50% of individuals quit smoking after experiencing a heart attack or being diagnosed with lung cancer. Barriers may arise from health-care providers, who do not want to place additional "pressure" or stress on their patients to quit smoking while they are dealing with their chronic disease, or they have concerns about giving smoking patients additional medications on top of an already complicated regimen.

While more research to develop effective, manageable interventions for these populations is warranted, smoking

Table 15.3 Evidence-based tobacco cessation pharmacotherapy and behavior counseling interventions and adaptations shown to be effective in special populations. (Adapted from the PHS Guidelines [5])

Population	Pharmacotherapy	Behavior counseling
Hospitalized patients	Patch is most common	Counseling and education (with at least 1 month of follow-up)
Cardiovascular diseases	Patch, gum, inhaler, bupropion	Psychosocial interventions, exercise
Pulmonary diseases (e.g., COPD)	NRT (patch and inhaler), bupropion	Behavior cessation counseling, behavioral relapse prevention
Cancers	Any of the 3 general classes of cessation medications (NRT, bupropion, varenicline) should be considered	Motivational interviewing, behavior cessation counseling, ideally initiated in the preoperative period prior to major oncological surgery and continued in the postoperative period
Pregnant women	Mounting evidence that NRT shown to be safe/effective, but more research is needed	Behavior cessation counseling, education
Disabilities	No RCTs conducted	No RCTs conducted
Depression	Bupropion, nortriptyline	Behavior cessation counseling
Severe mental illness (schizophrenia, bipolar disorder)	Varenicline, bupropion	Behavior cessation counseling with motivational enhancement therapy; specific counseling adaptations have not been tested
Substance use disorders (including alcohol)	Any of the cessation medications should be considered; varenicline requires monitoring for potential neuropsychiatric side effects	Behavior cessation counseling
LGBTQ	Bupropion or nicotine patch (when combined with behavior cessation counseling)	Non-tailored intensive behavior counseling combined with pharmacotherapy (when combined with pharmacotherapy)
Low SES/limited formal education	Patch specifically shown effective	Behavior cessation counseling, motivational interviewing, telephone counseling
Racial/ethnic minorities[a]	Bupropion (AA), nicotine patch (AA, H)	In person and phone; motivational interviewing, behavior counseling, tailored self-help/education, biofeedback (AA only), clinician advice
Light or intermittent smokers	No RCTs conducted	Behavior cessation counseling

COPD chronic obstructive pulmonary disease; *LGBTQ* lesbian, gay, bisexual, transgender, and questioning; *RCT* randomized clinical trial; *AA* African-American; *H* Hispanic; *NRT* nicotine replacement therapies; *SES* socioeconomic status

[a] No RCTs (medication) have been conducted specifically for American Indians/Alaska Natives, and no RCTs (medication or behavioral counseling) have been conducted specifically for Asian/Pacific Islanders

cessation interventions that are effective in the general population (e.g., those discussed above) have also been shown to be effective and safe in medical populations and should be employed. Intensive behavioral counseling alone has been found to significantly increase quit rates among all groups. In addition, NRTs and other first-line smoking cessation medications combined with behavioral counseling have been shown to be safe and effective for the majority of these populations.

It is important to monitor these patients closely for heightened psychological distress associated with both the burden of a chronic disease and smoking cessation. Health-care providers should emphasize that this distress is manageable and, in the case of nicotine withdrawal symptoms or medication side effects, time limited. Certain medications, such as varenicline and bupropion, appear to be effective in part through improving depressed mood and cognitive functioning and may be particularly effective for helping chronic disease patients to manage the stress associated with quitting tobacco.

Pregnant Women Although many women are strongly motivated to quit smoking when they are pregnant, nearly 12% of women report smoking in their third trimester of pregnancy,

and postpartum relapse rates are nearly 100%. Smoking during pregnancy is associated with higher rates of spontaneous abortion, premature birth, sudden infant death syndrome (SIDS), and developmental (cognitive, emotional, behavioral) issues.

All pregnant women should be asked regularly about their tobacco use. Strong social norms that discourage smoking among pregnant women can deter some women from disclosing their smoking behavior. Tobacco use can be assessed in clinical practice by asking the patient if she has ever smoked, if she was smoking when she first discovered that she was pregnant, if she has smoked in the past week (i.e., current smoking), and for a current smoker, how many cigarettes she smokes per day or week. There is an important role obstetrician/gynecological (OB/GYN), pediatrics, and primary-care providers to provide supportive counseling for women who are able to quit during pregnancy to help them prepare for postpartum stressors that may trigger relapse, and continue to encourage quit attempts in the context of their child(ren)'s health.

As pregnant and lactating women have traditionally been excluded from intervention and pharmacotherapy trials, the use and potential consequences of smoking cessation treatments in this population are not well understood. It is strongly believed that certain pharmacotherapies, particularly NRTs, would be less harmful than would be continued smoking, but there is currently insufficient evidence to suggest that NRT significantly increases cessation rates or improves birth outcomes [22]. Much more research is needed in this area; therefore, as of 2008 the PHS Guidelines strongly recommend increased psychosocial support for women throughout a pregnancy and postpartum [5]. As with the general population, community cessation resources or the state quitline are important referrals that should be provided.

Patients with Disabilities An emerging trend of increased smoking prevalence among populations with disabilities (i.e., any self-reported limitation in vision, hearing, cognition, movement, or activities of daily living) has been drawing attention of researchers, as the smoking rates approach/exceed 23% compared to 17% of individuals without a disability [3]. As this is a relatively new observation, randomized-controlled trials evaluating behavioral or pharmacological interventions for smoking cessation among these populations have not yet been conducted. However, given that these populations are more likely to seek regular medical care, it behooves health-care providers to be at the first line of intervention using the interventions outlined above by, at a minimum, asking about tobacco use, offering assistance with pharmacotherapy, connecting patients with additional resources, and following up at subsequent health-care visits.

Mental Health Populations

Smoking rates among people with a current or past mental health disorder are more than double the rates in the general population (>40% vs. 17%), particularly among those with schizophrenia and/or substance use (66–90%). Individuals with psychiatric conditions account for nearly half of the annual tobacco-attributable deaths in the USA, and psychiatric patients who smoke die on average 25 years earlier than the general population. Many health-care providers feel that they do not have the time or skills to address their patients' nicotine addiction. Given that smoking cessation can induce a variety of acute psychological effects, including agitation, irritability, and negative mood, it is important for medical providers to assess psychiatric patients' mental status (e.g., severity, stability) when discussing smoking cessation. Numerous studies have demonstrated that treating tobacco dependence does not interfere with treatment of other substance use, including alcohol and illicit substances, and may even improve mental health in the case of other conditions, such as depression.

As with medical conditions, health-care providers are sometimes hesitant to add smoking cessation pharmacotherapy to the often tenuous balance of psychiatric medications.

However, a recent study found that patients with severe mental illness (i.e., schizophrenia and bipolar disorder) assigned to behavioral counseling plus varenicline had higher abstinence rates than those in the placebo group; they also reported fewer psychiatric symptoms and serious adverse events. Moreover, these patients benefited even more from long-term (52 weeks) treatment [7]. These findings indicate that, contrary to common beliefs, psychiatric patients can be safely and effectively treated for nicotine dependence using a combination of behavioral counseling and pharmacotherapy, when their psychiatric symptoms are relatively stable. Of note, cigarette smoking can affect the metabolism of many psychotropic drugs (e.g., clozapine, fluvoxamine, olanzapine, haloperidol), usually by increasing clearance of these drugs from the body via the induction of hepatic cytochrome P450 enzymes (primarily CYP1A2). Therefore, smokers taking psychotropic medication that interacts with smoking may require higher dosages than nonsmokers. Conversely, once patients have quit smoking, they may require reduction in the dosage of an interacting medication.

Light and Intermittent Smokers

Between the increasing cost of cigarettes and the general recognition of the need to quit, a larger proportion of smokers have reduced their consumption and are smoking fewer cigarettes per day. There are many definitions in research and clinical practice of "light" or "intermittent" smokers, including individuals who smoke fewer than 10 cigarettes per day, fewer than 40 cigarettes per week, or individuals who only smoke in certain situations (e.g., "social smokers"). Regardless, individuals classified as light or intermittent smokers are not necessarily any less dependent on cigarettes and may require just as much help in quitting; in fact, research demonstrates that light smokers place greater value on each cigarette and de-emphasize the health consequences associated with light smoking. Contrary to popular belief, light and intermittent smoking confer risk for the same diseases as heavier smoking, including cardiovascular diseases, pulmonary dysfunction, lung and other cancers, and smoking-attributable complications of current chronic medical conditions, compared to individuals who have never smoked [23].

As such, it is still critical to identify these smokers, typically using a behavior-based question such as, *"Have you used a tobacco product in the past 30 days?"* rather than a labeling question such as, *"Are you a smoker?"* because many individuals who might be classified as light and intermittent smokers are unlikely to self-identify as such. Once recognized, it is important to strongly urge them to quit and to provide counseling treatment interventions using the same techniques as outlined above, with a particular emphasis on dispelling the beliefs about the relative safety of light or intermittent smoking. Behavioral counseling is the first-line treatment for light and intermittent smokers, but research is currently being conducted to evaluate the safety and efficacy of pharmacotherapy in light smokers.

Current Issues in Tobacco Treatment

The Potential of e-Cigarettes As a Treatment Strategy

Since their initial introduction to the USA in 2007, use of electronic nicotine delivery systems (ENDS), better known as electronic or e-cigarettes, has been rising dramatically while the research, clinical, and public health communities are struggling to evaluate their safety and efficacy. The term "e-cigarette" is slightly misleading, as these devices have more in common with pipes or inhalers (i.e., devices loaded with a drug). While there is no single definition of an e-cigarette, the devices recognized in this class typically comprise three components: the delivery device itself, a cartridge, and the contents or solutions to fill the cartridge. The solutions most often contain nicotine, though non-nicotinic solutions are also available, and many come in appealing flavors. Refillable e-cigarette cartridges are sold with, on average, around 20 mg of nicotine (compared to approximately 10 mg of nicotine in a traditional cigarette); however, when consumers refill their own cartridges the concentration of nicotine can be much higher and therefore maintain a stronger addiction.

Are ENDS Effective Aids to Smoking Cessation? Very little is known regarding the safety of e-cigarettes and consequences of long-term use. Initial evidence has demonstrated that e-cigarettes expose users to fewer carcinogens than do traditional cigarettes. This is not to say that e-cigarettes are without risk: Recent studies have demonstrated that the majority of e-cigarettes produce at least minimally detectable levels of carcinogens, and laboratory studies demonstrate that e-cigarettes induce physiological pulmonary reactions similar to the effects observed in cigarette smokers [24]. Long-term follow-up studies have yet to be conducted to assess the safety of extended e-cigarette use.

The clinical utility of e-cigarettes remains to be determined, and, as a result, the FDA has proposed to extend its tobacco authority to include e-cigarettes as drug delivery devices rather than as therapeutic agents (as of date this chapter was sent to press). Regardless, more and more smokers are turning to e-cigarettes to aid in cessation. At this time, the few randomized-controlled trials of e-cigarettes for cessation found that participants using e-cigarettes had equivalent abstinence rates to participants using the nicotine patch [25]. On the other hand, an observational study of individuals who utilized state tobacco quitlines found that individuals who used an e-cigarette were less likely to be abstinent at 6 months than those who did not use an e-cigarette [26].

Public Health Concerns There are several major clinical and public health concerns regarding the use of e-cigarettes [24]. First, there is concern that these devices will encourage dual use, that e-cigarettes will serve as a "bridge" between cigarettes when individuals are unable to smoke (e.g., during working hours), rather than replacing cigarettes with e-cigarette use. Health-care providers should educate patients about the risk for dual-use and warn against the possibility of increased nicotine dependence with dual use. Second, these technological and flavorful devices are appealing to adolescents and young adults, and because of the current lack of regulatory structure these devices are readily available and do not have minimum age limits for purchase. Third, it reintroduces smoking as an acceptable behavior, thus "renormalizing" cigarette use in society, directly contrary to the past 50 years of public health efforts. Therefore, until more research and guidelines are available on the clinical utility of e-cigarettes, health-care providers should continue to use only evidence-based and FDA-approved treatments for their smoking patients and, given how much is still unknown regarding the safety and quality control of e-cigarettes, caution patients regarding their use.

Alternative Tobacco Products

As rates of cigarette smoking are decreasing, rates of use of other tobacco products is on the rise. These products are similar to e-cigarettes in that many people view these products as safer than traditional cigarettes. Users may not classify themselves as smokers or tobacco users and thus may be more difficult to identify. Moreover, looser regulation can cause additional concern, particularly in regards to youth access. Fortunately, many of the same cessation treatment strategies may be employed for patients who use these products, particularly education regarding the negative health effects of continued use and supportive counseling strategies.

Smokeless Tobacco The rates of use of smokeless tobacco products, including snuff, chew, and snus have increased significantly in recent years. Many smokers use smokeless tobacco products as a way to reduce their cigarette consumption, as these products are taxed at far lower rates than cigarettes, and they may use these products as a bridge between cigarettes in situations in which they cannot smoke (e.g., during work hours). Similar to e-cigarettes, these products are often viewed as potential "harm reduction" therapeutics. While switching to smokeless tobacco decreases risk of developing some diseases (e.g., lung cancer), it also increases risk for others (e.g., oral cancer). Many of the same behavioral counseling strategies, as well as pharmacotherapy (especially varenicline) may be used to increase quit rates among smokeless tobacco users [27].

Water Pipes (Hookah) The use of water pipe tobacco smoking, commonly in the form of Hookah, is especially popular among youth, women, and minorities. It is commonly believed that, because it is water vapor, water pipes are safe and nonaddictive. In fact, one session of water pipe use is equivalent to smoking up to 50 cigarettes [28]. Though much of the research in this field is preliminary, most studies conducted thus far examining the negative health effects of water pipe smoking have found that water pipe use is associated with increased rates of lung cancer, respiratory diseases, and OB/GYN concerns (e.g., low birth weight) [29]. Currently, there are no published interventions for water pipe cessation treatment. Therefore, it is important to assess for water pipe use, provide education about the negative health effects of use, and encourage users to quit.

The ACA and Tobacco Cessation Treatment

Tobacco Cessation Benefits A major component of the ACA is recognition of the importance of chronic disease prevention to reduce health-care costs by providing preventive services at no or low cost to patients; tobacco cessation is especially emphasized for the primary prevention of chronic disease. In line with this mission, the ACA includes increased coverage for tobacco dependence treatments (medications and counseling) under Preventive Services and Essential Health Benefits, which include all preventive services recommended with an "A" or "B" rating by the US Preventive Services Task Force (USPSTF) like those identified in the PHS Tobacco Guidelines. Moreover, everyone is required to have health insurance, and patients currently without private insurance are eligible for coverage through health insurance marketplace exchanges. The Department of Health and Human Services issued a Frequently Asked Questions (FAQ) guidance document (May 2014) to translate the USPSTF recommendation into insurance coverage policy. For both private and marketplace insurance providers to be in compliance with the ACA requirement, plans must cover tobacco screening, counseling (phone, group, and individual), and all seven FDA-approved medications without cost sharing, i.e., no co-pays, coinsurance, or deductibles. The FAQ provided only an example for length and frequency of counseling services that should be covered: at least two cessation attempts per year, with one attempt viewed as "four cessation counseling sessions of at least 10 min each, without prior authorization." However, based on a report released on March 31, 2015, by the American Lung Association, only

17.2% of marketplace plans indicated full coverage of all seven cessation medications.

Of note, new grants are available for implementation of community services to make available preventive services like smoking cessation and other preventive services including physical activity, healthy diet, and emotional wellness. Please see the resources section at the end of this chapter for a list of websites that will provide more information regarding ACA tobacco cessation coverage information.

Required Reporting of Tobacco Treatment Use To assess implementation and progress of the ACA, providers will be required to report the percentage of individuals who are (1) assessed for smoking status within the past 24 months and (2) received a smoking cessation intervention if determined to be a current tobacco user. To assist in tobacco use and treatment reporting, the following recommendations are offered: (1) record smoking status in a form (rather than in free text) in the Electronic Health Record (EHR), (2) include smoking status as a vital sign; (3) use alerts to remind staff to record smoking status and offer cessation interventions,(4) enroll all health-care providers in documenting smoking status, (5) develop a protocol for offering tobacco cessation interventions (e.g., referral to a state quitline), and (6) increase physician comfort with cessation pharmacotherapies and/or provide resources within the EHR.

ACA Impact on Special Populations: Medicaid Coverage Under the ACA, tobacco cessation treatment is mandated to be covered for all Medicaid and Medicare patients. As of January 1, 2014, all state Medicaid programs are required to support all FDA-approved tobacco cessation pharmacotherapies without requiring co-pays or other financial barriers. Given that Medicaid and uninsured patients are of lower socioeconomic status, tend to have less education, and comprise greater proportions of minority populations, these new requirements ensure that a greater proportion of the population with higher rates of tobacco use, as discussed above, will now be covered. Medicare patients will now be offered an annual wellness visit designed to increase the amount of time health-care providers can spend addressing preventive measures such as tobacco cessation rather than simply treating acute presenting problems.

ACA Impact on Pregnant Women Another patient population that has newly expanded coverage under the ACA is pregnant women. Prior to the ACA, fewer than half of Medicaid programs included tobacco treatment (either medication or counseling) for pregnant women. Since the signing of the ACA in 2010, the ACA has covered tobacco cessation treatment for all pregnant women at no cost to the patient—100% of the programs cover medication, and nearly 85% of them cover behavior counseling services.

Overall, it appears as though the ACA will bring about positive changes for tobacco use treatment on many fronts. The ACA includes increased coverage of both pharmacotherapy and counseling services for important populations who smoke at higher rates and require more assistance in quitting smoking. Unfortunately, the exact parameters of coverage are still unclear; time will tell if the new coverage of cessation treatment will in fact increase utilization of tobacco dependence treatment and overall cessation rates.

Conclusion

Rates of tobacco use have stagnated over the past decade, and there are substantial disparities in tobacco use among the US population. It is important for health-care providers at all levels of care to be mindful of subgroups who smoke at high rates, experience greater difficulty quitting, and who have low access to effective treatment, as well as be familiar with appropriate techniques, strategies, and pharmacotherapies for cessation of cigarettes and other tobacco products. This includes behavioral counseling techniques for individuals who are willing to quit, not ready to quit, or recently quit, as well as specific adaptations for populations with comorbid medical and psychiatric illnesses that are often seen in primary-care settings. Finally, understanding how the field of tobacco cessation is changing with the advent of e-cigarettes, the rise of other tobacco products, and the ACA is critical for continuing to decrease smoking rates in the USA as an important strategy to prevent and decrease chronic disease morbidity and mortality.

Resources

Smoking Cessation Resources

1. National quitline:
   a. 1-800-QUIT-NOW (1–800-784–8669)
   b. 1-855-DÉJELO-YA (1-855-335-3569)
2. www.smokefree.gov
3. SmokefreeTXT: http://smokefree.gov/smokefreetxt
4. QuitSTART
5. NCI QuitPal

ACA Resources

1. www.healthcare.gov
2. *US Department of Health and Human Services FAQ document (See Q5 in FAQ Part XIX for Tobacco coverage):* http://www.dol.gov/ebsa/faqs/faq-aca19.html
3. American Academy of Family Physicians (AAFP): http://www.aafp.org/home.html
   For a succinct description of current provisions and coverage, including insurance coding references, the AAFP has compiled a summary of cessation benefits provided,

organized by plan (http://www.aafp.org/patient-care/public-health/tobacco-nicotine/ask-act/coding-reference.html, last accessed March 2015). At the time of press, the AAFP site contained more cessation coverage information than could be accessed on www.healthcare.gov
4. State Health Insurance Marketplace Plans: New Opportunities to Help Smokers Quit, American Lung Association report (March 31, 2015): http://www.lung.org/assets/documents/publications/other-reports/state-health-insurance-opportunities.pdf

Disclosures The authors have no conflicts of interest to disclose.

Dr. Hitsman receives medication and placebo free of charge from Pfizer for use in ongoing National Institutes of Health supported clinical trials; Dr. Hitsman has also served on a scientific advisory board for Pfizer.

References

1. USDHHS. How tobacco smoke causes disease: the biology and behavioral basis for smoking-attributable disease: a report of the Surgeon General. Rockville, MD, Washington, DC: United States Department of Health and Human Services, Public Health Service; 2010.
2. USDHHS. The Health Consequences of Smoking—50 Years of Progress: a Report of the Surgeon General, 2014. Atlanta, GA: United States Department of Health and Human Services, Centers for Disease Control and Prevention, National Center for Chronic Disease Prevention and Health Promotion, Office on Smoking and Health; 2014.
3. Jamal A, Agaku IT, O'Connor E, King BA, Kenemer JB, Neff L. Current cigarette smoking among adults—United States, 2005–2013. Morb Mortal Wkly Rep. 2014;63(47):1108–12.
4. Stead LF, Bergson G, Lancaster T. Physician advice for smoking cessation. Cochrane Database Syst Rev. 2008;16(2):CD000165.
5. Fiore M, Jaén C, Baker T, et al. Treating tobacco use and dependence: 2008 update. Rockville: United States Department of Health and Human Services; 2008.
6. MacPherson L, Tull MT, Matusiewicz AK, et al. Randomized controlled trial of behavioral activation smoking cessation treatment for smokers with elevated depressive symptoms. J Consult Clin Psychol. 2010;78(1):55–61.
7. Evins AE, Cather C, Pratt SA, et al. Maintenance treatment with varenicline for smoking cessation in patients with schizophrenia and bipolar disorder: a randomized clinical trial. JAMA. 2014;311(2):145–54.
8. Singh S, Loke YK, Spangler JG, Furberg CD. Risk of serious adverse cardiovascular events associated with varenicline: a systematic review and meta-analysis. CMAJ. 2011;183(12):1359–66.
9. Prochaska JJ, Hilton JF. Risk of cardiovascular serious adverse events associated with varenicline use for tobacco cessation: systematic review and meta-analysis. BMJ. 2012;4(344):e2856.
10. Hughes JR. Effects of abstinence from tobacco: valid symptoms and time course. Nicotine Tob Res. 2007;9(3):315–27.
11. Carpenter MJ, Ford ME, Cartmell K, Alberg AJ. Misperceptions of nicotine replacement therapy within racially and ethnically diverse smokers. J Natl Med Assoc. 2011;103(9–10):885–894.
12. Schnoll RA, Martinez E, Tatum KL, et al. Increased self-efficacy to quit and perceived control over withdrawal symptoms predict smoking cessation following nicotine dependence treatment. Addict Behav. 2011;36(1–2):144–7.

13. Vogt F, Hall S, Marteau TM. Understanding why smokers do not want to use nicotine dependence medications to stop smoking: qualitative and quantitative studies. Nicotine Tob Res. 2008;10(8):1405–13.

14. Fucito LM, Bars MP, Forray A, et al. Addressing the evidence for FDA nicotine replacement therapy label changes: a policy statement of the Association for the Treatment of Tobacco use and Dependence and the Society for Research on Nicotine and Tobacco. Nicotine Tob Res. 2014;16(7):909–14.

15. Stead LF, Lancaster T. Behavioural interventions as adjuncts to pharmacotherapy for smoking cessation. Cochrane Database Syst Rev. 2012;12(12):CD009670.

16. Hughes JR. An updated algorithm for choosing among smoking cessation treatments. J Subst Abuse Treat. 2013;45(2):215–21.

17. Heatherton TF, Kozlowski LT, Frecker RC, Rickert W, Robinson J. Measuring the heaviness of smoking: using self-reported time to the first cigarette of the day and number of cigarettes smoked per day. Br J Addict. 1989;84(7):791–9.

18. Lindson-Hawley N, Aveyard P, Hughes JR. Reduction versus abrupt cessation in smokers who want to quit. Cochrane Database Syst Rev. 2012;14(11):CD008033.

19. Ebbert JO, Hughes JR, West RJ, et al. Effect of varenicline on smoking cessation through smoking reduction: a randomized clinical trial. JAMA. 2015;313(7):687–94.

20. Borrelli B. Smoking cessation: next steps for special populations research and innovative treatments. J Consult Clin Psychol. 2010;78(1):1–12.

21. Rigotti NA, Clair C, Munafo MR, Stead LF. Interventions for smoking cessation in hospitalised patients. Cochrane Database Syst Rev. 2012;16(5):CD001837.

22. Coleman T, Chamberlain C, Davey MA, Cooper SE, Leonardi-Bee J. Pharmacological interventions for promoting smoking cessation during pregnancy. Cochrane Database Syst Rev. 2012;12(9):CD010078.

23. Schane RE, Ling PM, Glantz SA. Health effects of light and intermittent smoking: a review. Circulation. 2010;121(13):1518–22.

24. Cobb NK, Abrams DB. E-cigarette or drug-delivery device? Regulating novel nicotine products. N Engl J Med. 2011;365(3):193–5.

25. Bullen C, Howe C, Laugesen M, et al. Electronic cigarettes for smoking cessation: a randomised controlled trial. Lancet. 2013;382(9905):1629–37.

26. Vickerman KA, Carpenter KM, Altman T, Nash CM, Zbikowski SM. Use of electronic cigarettes among state tobacco cessation quitline callers. Nicotine Tob Res. 2013;15(10):1787–91.

27. Ebbert J, Montori VM, Erwin PJ, Stead LF. Interventions for smokeless tobacco use cessation. Cochrane Database Syst Rev. 2011;16(2):CD004306.

28. Cobb C, Ward KD, Maziak W, Shihadeh AL, Eissenberg T. Waterpipe tobacco smoking: an emerging health crisis in the United States. Am J Health Behav. 2010;34(3):275–85.

29. Akl EA, Gaddam S, Gunukula SK, Honeine R, Jaoude PA, Irani J. The effects of waterpipe tobacco smoking on health outcomes: a systematic review. Int J Epidemiol. 2010;39(3):834–57.

Alcohol Use and Management

Evan Goulding

Abbreviations

AUD	Alcohol use disorder
AUDIT	Alcohol Use Disorders Identification Test
CAGE	Cut down, Annoyed, Guilty, Eye opener
HCP	Health-care professional
IM	Intramuscular
NIAAA	National Institute on Alcohol Abuse and Alcoholism
NIDA	National Institute on Drug Abuse
NMDA	N-methyl-D-aspartate
NNT	Number needed to treat

Alcohol Use and Problems

In the USA, about 80 % of the population drinks at some time during their life and about 50 % of the population drinks alcohol regularly in any given year [1]. Individuals report a variety of reasons for drinking alcohol including celebrating special occasions, increased enjoyment of social situations, liking the positive feelings induced by use, and experiencing decreased negative feelings [2]. Consumption of alcohol may have beneficial or harmful effects depending on the amount consumed and individual characteristics. Relative to abstaining, moderate alcohol use (1–2 drinks daily) may slightly decrease morbidity and mortality primarily as a result of decreased cardiovascular problems [3, 4]. However, even light alcohol use (≤1 drink daily) increases the risk of developing cancer [5], and heavier use (≥2–4 drinks daily) significantly increases morbidity and mortality [1, 3, 4]. Overall alcohol use results in substantial public health problems: Alcohol consumption is the third leading cause of death from modifiable factors and produces significant morbidity and economic costs every year [6, 7].

Continuum of Harm

Problems related to alcohol consumption occur across a spectrum that is strongly associated with alcohol use levels [8]. As levels of intake increase, the probability of an individual developing problems such as an alcohol use disorder (AUD; Table 16.1), cirrhosis, seizures, certain types of cancer, hypertension, stroke, and injuries significantly increases [9, 10]. In addition, heavier use is associated with significant harm to others as a result of motor vehicle accidents, homicides, domestic violence, child abuse, and childhood neurodevelopment disorders [11–14]. It is important to note that the majority of these alcohol-related harms occur in drinkers who do not meet criteria for an AUD [11, 15, 16].

This important fact combined with the prevalence of alcohol use highlights the importance of screening for and addressing the risks of alcohol use in all individuals seeking medical treatment. In addition, AUD is not an acute illness. Progression from initial alcohol use to the development of AUD typically takes years, and even after diagnostic criteria for AUD are met, symptom severity often increases over time [17, 18]. Thus, the health-care professional (HCP) has an opportunity to intervene at early stages of alcohol use to: (1) reduce harm in the absence of AUD, (2) prevent development of AUD, and (3) decrease progression to more severe AUD. Because of these opportunities, the concept of addressing the entire continuum of unhealthy alcohol use (Table 16.2) is replacing the disease-oriented model that focuses on identifying and treating individuals who meet criteria for AUD [4, 7, 8, 19].

E. Goulding (✉)
Department of Psychiatry and Behavioral Sciences, Feinberg School of Medicine, Northwestern University, Chicago, IL, USA
e-mail: e-goulding@fsm.northwestern.edu

© Springer International Publishing Switzerland 2016
J. I. Mechanick, R. F. Kushner (eds.), *Lifestyle Medicine,* DOI 10.1007/978-3-319-24687-1_16

Table 16.1 Alcohol use disorder (DSM V)

Maladaptive pattern or use leading to clinically significant impairment or distress	
Two or more of the following within a 12-month period	
Recurrent use resulting in a failure to fulfill major role obligations at work, school, or home	DSM IV Alcohol Abuse
Recurrent use resulting in social or interpersonal problems	
Recurrent use in physically hazardous situations	
Craving, strong desire, or urge to use	
Often taken in larger amounts or over longer period than intended	DSM IV Alcohol Dependence
Continued use despite knowledge of recurrent physical or psychological problems caused by use	
Persistent desire or unsuccessful efforts to cut down or control use	
Great deal of time spent in activities to obtain use or recover from effects	
Important social, occupational, or recreational activities given up or reduced due to use	
Tolerance	
Withdrawal	
Severity: mild 2–3 symptoms, moderate 4–5 symptoms, severe ≥6 symptoms	

DSM IV & V Diagnostic and Statistical Manual of Mental Disorders, 4th Edition

Table 16.2 Unhealthy alcohol use [8, 19]

Category of use		Definition
At-risk or hazardous drinking		Men <65 years old: >4 drinks/day or >14 drinks/week
		Men >65 years old: >3 drinks/day or >7 drinks/week
		Women any age: >3 drinks/day or >7 drinks/week
Harmful or problem drinking		Presence of harm related to alcohol use in the absence of meeting criteria for alcohol use disorder
Alcohol use disorder	Mild	Meeting criteria for alcohol use disorder (see Table 16.1)
	Moderate	
	Severe	

Screening and Intervention

As a result of this disease model shift, increasing efforts are underway to provide screening and intervention earlier in the process of alcohol use. Since primary-care physicians are frequently the only medical professionals that individuals with unhealthy drinking encounter, the primary-care setting has been the main focus for the development of interventions to identify and treat unhealthy alcohol use that has not progressed to AUD [16, 20, 21]. These interventions are typically delivered by a primary-care physician during a standard consultation to drinkers who are seeking general medical care but not treatment for their alcohol use. The style of counseling is based on motivational interviewing: The primary-care physician in this case utilizes therapeutic empathy, feedback of risk, deals with ambivalence, assesses motivation to change, emphasizes patient responsibility and self-efficacy, and provides a menu of specific strategies to reduce alcohol use. However, brief interventions tend to be distinct from standard motivational interviewing as the primary-care physician utilizes clear directive advice to reduce alcohol consumption. Brief interventions also draw on cognitive behavioral therapy and general education strategies by utilizing contracting, goal setting, and written materials such as self-help manuals [22].

The time demands on primary-care physicians have driven an effort to make interventions efficient and time limited. As a result, these interventions are brief. A single short intervention (5–15 min) can be effective; however, multiple contact interventions with 2–4 short sessions (5–15 min) seem to be more effective [16, 21]. The emphasis is on increased patient insight and awareness of risk that leads to patient establishment and self-management of a reduced alcohol intake goal. A harm reduction goal of reduced intake is typically encouraged as opposed to a goal of abstinence that is more commonly recommended for individuals with AUD [19–21, 23]. For individuals in the primary-care setting who also meet criteria for AUD, brief intervention can still be delivered; however, a goal of abstinence is recommended and a referral to further treatment is provided [19–21, 23].

Brief interventions for unhealthy drinking in the absence of AUD are among the most cost-effective preventive services delivered in the primary-care setting with economic savings similar to screening for colorectal cancer and hypertension [24]. Compared with controls, drinkers receiving a brief intervention are twice as likely to moderate their drinking at 6–12 months [25] and significantly reduce alcohol intake by about four drinks per week at follow-up periods of 12 months or more [16, 21, 26]. In addition, the provision of brief interventions significantly decreases the proportion of individuals whose intake exceeds recommended levels [21]. While reductions in alcohol intake are the most commonly measured outcome in brief intervention studies, other outcomes have been examined, including reduced morbidity and mortality resulting from motor-vehicle crashes, falls, suicide attempts, domestic violence, assaults, and child abuse [11, 27]. Overall, brief interventions are among the best supported treatment for alcohol use problems [28].

Recommended Limits

Although there is no single threshold between safe and unsafe alcohol intake, internationally recognized guidelines have been established that address both maximum daily use (i.e., heavy or binge drinking) and average weekly consumption limits [15, 29]. The National Institute on Alcohol Abuse and Alcoholism (NIAAA) suggests that to avoid the risk of harm: men < 65 years old drink no more than 4 drinks/day and no more than 14 drinks/week; women of any age and men ≥65 years old drink no more than 3 drinks/day and no more than 7 drinks/week [23]. A standard drink is defined as 14 g of absolute ethanol (12 ounces of beer, 5 ounces of wine, and 1.5 ounces of distilled spirits). Drinking above the NIAAA levels is likely to result in harm and is frequently defined as hazardous or at-risk use [19, 21, 30]. The American Heart Association also suggests limiting intake to an average of 1–2 drinks/day for men and 1 drink/day for women, which is consistent with the NIAAA weekly limits. Moderate alcohol use (1–2 drinks daily) may slightly decrease morbidity and mortality primarily as a result of decreased cardiovascular problems [3, 4]. However, even light alcohol use (≤1 drink daily) increases the risk of developing cancer [5], and heavier use (≥2–4 drinks daily) significantly increases morbidity and mortality [1, 3, 4]. Given these and other risks, the American Heart Association cautions that, if they do not already drink alcohol, people should *not* start drinking for the purported cardiovascular benefits of alcohol.

A category of harmful or problematic use, defined as use that has already resulted in adverse mental or physical effects but that does not meet criteria for AUD, has also been described [19, 21, 30]. Using these definitions, the full spectrum of alcohol misuse includes at-risk or hazardous use, harmful or problematic use, and use in the presence of AUD (Table 16.2). In the USA, about 20% of the population exceeds the NIAAA-recommended alcohol intake guidelines without meeting criteria for an AUD and can be described as exhibiting at-risk or harmful drinking (Fig. 16.1) [19, 23]. A smaller proportion of the population (~8%) meets criteria for an alcohol use disorder and also typically exceeds the NIAAA-recommended limits [19, 23, 31, 32]. Although a substantial proportion of the population is engaged in unhealthy alcohol use, most of these individuals do not recognize that they have a problem nor do they seek treatment

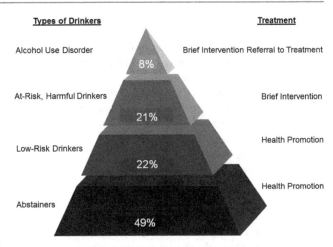

Fig. 16.1 Abstainers report no alcohol consumption in the past month or drink < 12 drinks a year. Low-risk drinkers report consuming alcohol below the daily and weekly NIAAA limits. Problem drinkers report consuming alcohol above the daily and/or weekly NIAAA limits but do not meet *Diagnostic and Statistical Manual of Mental Disorders*, 4th Edition, Text Revision (DSM-IV-TR) criteria for an alcohol use disorder. Almost all individuals in the 8% of the population who meet criteria for an alcohol use disorder in the last 12 months drink above the daily and/or weekly NIAAA limits. *NIAAA* National Institute on Alcohol Abuse and Alcoholism. [23, 41]

highlighting the need for effective screening and intervention [33].

Brief Intervention

Brief interventions for drinking are time-limited, patient-centered counseling strategies that focus on assisting people to reduce their drinking. Numerous studies support the efficacy and cost-savings resulting from these interventions [11, 16, 21, 24–27, 34]. Adults receiving brief (10–15 min) multi-contact behavioral interventions decrease their consumption by 13–34% more than controls (2.4–4.8 fewer drinks than controls) [21, 35]. In addition, among adults receiving these interventions, 12% fewer adults report heavy drinking episodes and 11% more adults report drinking less than the suggested limits [21, 35].

The exact nature of brief interventions varies somewhat across studies, but a set of general features characterizing brief interventions includes: (1) being directed at drinkers who do not have AUD, (2) being delivered by a primary-care HCP, (3) having a goal of reduced drinking as opposed to total abstinence, (4) addressing level of motivation to change drinking patterns, and (5) being patient self-directed [34]. An empathic professional behavior combined with an expression of nonjudgmental concern, a discussion of drinking likes/dislikes, and of life goals may increase patient engagement [36]. Clear, direct advice to reduce or stop drinking is provided along with a clarification of drinking norms and patient specific adverse effects. The use of (1) mutual

Table 16.3 5 As of brief intervention

Ask: Screen for use
- Do you sometimes drink beer, wine, or alcohol?
- In the past year, how many times have you had five or more drinks in a day?

Advise: Provide strong direct personal advice to change
- Empathic, non-confrontational feedback on drinking pattern and consequences
- Relate consequences to current health, family, social, and legal issues
- State concern and recommend change

Assess: Determine willingness to change
- Discuss drinking likes and dislikes
- Discuss life goals
- Discuss how willing and what willing to change
- Agree on a mutually acceptable goal

Assist: Help patient make a change if ready
- Mutually set specific goals (how many days, how many drinks)
- Encourage a written risk reduction agreement ("Rx")
- Provide techniques (diary cards, pace, space, switch, include food)
- Identify high-risk situations
- Identify supporters (family and friends)
- Self-help manual

Arrange: Reinforce change effort with follow-up
- Follow-up appointment
- Supportive telephone consult
- Referral to specialty treatment

Table 16.4 CAGE questions [40]

Cut down	"Have you ever felt you ought to cut down on your drinking?"
Annoyed	"Have people annoyed you by criticizing your drinking?"
Guilty	"Have you ever felt bad or guilty about your drinking?"
Eye opener	"Have you ever had a drink first thing in the morning to steady your nerves or get rid of a hangover?"

goal setting, (2) encouragement of a personal plan to reduce drinking, (3) a self-help booklet, (4) drinking dairy cards, and (5) follow-up phone calls or visits are also common features of brief interventions [20, 21, 30, 34, 37]. Screening and brief intervention guidelines suggest a standard approach for assessing and managing problem drinking and alcohol use disorders [23, 38]. This approach can be described by the "5 As of intervention" (Table 16.3) which reflects the different brief intervention strategies described in the literature [16, 19, 20, 23, 30, 34, 36, 38].

Ask

A prescreening question about any alcohol use provides a simple way to initiate a conversation ("Do you sometimes drink beer, wine, or other alcoholic beverages?"). Incorporating questions about alcohol consumption with questions about other health habits (diet, exercise, and/or smoking) may decrease defensiveness about drinking. In the event of alcohol use, a single-question screen to detect five plus drinks a day for men or four plus drinks a day for women

can be used (5+/4+: "In the past year, how many times have you had 5/4 or more drinks a day?"). Alcohol use at this level one or more times a year indicates a positive screen that provides good sensitivity and specificity for detecting unhealthy drinking [19, 39]. In the case of a positive screen, additional questions concerning weekly alcohol intake should be asked to determine the average frequency and quantity of alcohol consumption ("On average, how many days a week do you have an alcoholic drink?", "On a typical drinking day, how many drinks do you have?"). During screening, presenting a chart describing what constitutes a standard drink may be helpful. Additional questions from the widely used Cut down, Annoyed, Guilty, Eye opener (CAGE) screening test, which is focused on symptoms of AUD can also be used by the screening HCP [40] (Table 16.4). In clinics with a more formal screening protocol, patients are often requested to complete a written self-report such as the Alcohol Use Disorders Identification Test (AUDIT) [41] prior to seeing their primary-care HCP. This 10-question survey covers domains of at-risk and harmful use, as well as AUD symptoms (Table 16.5). It has been used in a number of brief intervention research studies [19, 30, 42]. In the presence

Table 16.5 Alcohol Use Disorders Identification Test (AUDIT)

Questions	0	1	2	3	4	Score
1. How often do you have a drink containing alcohol?	Never	Monthly or less	2–4 times a month	2–3 times a week	4 or more times a week	
2. How many drinks containing alcohol do you have on a typical day when you are drinking?	1 or 2	3 or 4	5 or 6	7 to 9	10 or more	
3. How often do you have six or more drinks on one occasion?	Never	Less than monthly	Monthly	Weekly	Daily or almost daily	
4. How often during the last year have you found that you were not able to stop drinking once you had started?	Never	Less than monthly	Monthly	Weekly	Daily or almost daily	
5. How often during the last year have you failed to do what was normally expected of you because of drinking?	Never	Less than monthly	Monthly	Weekly	Daily or almost daily	
6. How often during the last year have you needed a first drink in the morning to get yourself going after a heavy drinking session?	Never	Less than monthly	Monthly	Weekly	Daily or almost daily	
7. How often during the last year have you had a feeling of guilt or remorse after drinking?	Never	Less than monthly	Monthly	Weekly	Daily or almost daily	
8. How often during the last year have you been unable to remember what happened the night before because of your drinking?	Never	Less than monthly	Monthly	Weekly	Daily or almost daily	
9. Have you or someone else been injured because of your drinking?	No		Yes, but not in the last year		Yes, during the last year	
10. Has a relative, friend, doctor, or other health-care worker been concerned about your drinking or suggested you cut down?	No		Yes, but not in the last year		Yes, during the last year	
					Total	

0–7 Alcohol Education; 8–15 Advice, BI; 16–19 Advice, Brief Counseling, Monitoring; 20–40 Referral

of unhealthy drinking, further assessment to determine if an AUD is present would then complete a full evaluation of the alcohol use spectrum for a given individual.

Advise

In the presence of unhealthy alcohol use, the next step is to provide, in an empathic and nonconfrontational manner, feedback about the patient's drinking and its consequences along with clear recommendations ("You're drinking more than is medically safe, I strongly recommend that you cut down." "I believe you have a serious alcohol problem and strongly recommend that you quit drinking."). Providing feedback about the patient's drinking pattern in comparison to population norms may be helpful ("fewer than 20% of people drink as much as you") and charts to visualize this comparison are available [23, 38]. To the greatest extent possible, the consequences of the patient's drinking should be individualized to their use: tied to information discussed in their medical interview and related to their current physical, mental, family, social, and legal concerns. Feedback and suggestions for change should be conveyed empathically in the context of a HCP conveying health recommendations ("As your clinician, I am concerned about how much you drink and how it is affecting your health."). However to respect and maintain patient autonomy, the aim is to provide a medical recommendation rather than a directive ("As your clinician, I feel I should tell you" rather than "You should"). A clear message of a willingness to help should be conveyed along with the feedback and recommendations ("I am willing to help.").

Assess

The provision of feedback and recommendations is then followed by an assessment of readiness to change ("Given what we've talked about, are you willing to consider making changes in your drinking?"). Building bridges from individual alcohol use to personal consequences may improve patient engagement ("If you keep drinking at your current levels, do you think your goal of improving your grades will be easier, harder, or no effect?") [36]. If the patient is willing to make a change, a mutually agreed upon patient-specific goal should be negotiated. This might include reducing drinking to within the recommended limits, going from daily use to use only several times a week, or abstaining for a period of time. For patients who meet criteria for AUD, abstinence is advised and should be the primary treatment goal. If a patient is not willing to make a change, concern regarding the patient's drinking health-related consequences and the clinician's willingness to help should be restated.

Assist

Once a mutually agreed upon goal has been negotiated between the patient and the HCP, a discussion aimed at developing an individualized treatment plan for assisting the patient in achieving the goal should be pursued. The treatment plan should include specific steps that the patient will take to reduce or quit drinking and provision of tools that the patient may choose to use. The clinician can offer the patient educational handouts on standard drink sizes and limits, alcohol-associated harms, and strategies for cutting down or abstaining (pacing use, spacing use by including nonalcoholic beverages and food, plans to handle urges, engaging in other activities, and/or using alcohol money for other items), as well as calendars for tracking drinking (a drinking dairy). A discussion aimed at identifying situations where the patient is likely to have difficulty maintaining their drinking goal can be held along with strategies for avoiding or managing such situations. The patient can be asked to identify a family member or friend who can help them to achieve their goal. Patients with AUD should be referred to specialty treatment for AUD and encouraged to attend mutual self-help groups. A brief written change plan signed by both the patient and the HCP can be useful along with the recognition that the HCP will check in on treatment plan progress at the next visit.

If a patient is not willing to make a change, a discussion concerning the perceived benefits of continued drinking versus those associated with reducing or stopping drinking may be used to encourage reflection by the patient about their drinking patterns. Any potential barriers to change should be elicited and discussed. These discussions should be carried out with the recognition by the clinician that ambivalence and reluctance to change drinking patterns is common and that many patients are unaware of the risks of their alcohol use. The provision of information, advice, and discussion of drinking patterns may lead the patient to contemplate change at a later time.

Arrange

A follow-up appointment should be given to the patient to provide reinforcement including further support, feedback, and assistance in setting, achieving, and maintaining realistic goals. In the context of multi-contact brief interventions, a follow-up call might be made after 2 weeks by the physician or clinic staff to check on progress and a follow-up appointment might be made in 1 month. With the use of newer technology, clinical staff may have the opportunity to email or text message patients to check on progress between face-to-face clinic visits. At the follow-up appointment, it should be determined if the patient was able to meet and sustain the drinking goal. If so, the clinician should reinforce and support continued adherence, renegotiate drinking goals if indicated, and encourage follow-up with at least annual re-screening. With patients who were unable to meet their treatment goals, it should be acknowledged that change is difficult, any positive changes should be supported, and barriers to reaching the goal should be addressed. The HCP should reemphasize a willingness to help, reevaluate the diagnosis, treatment plan, and goals, and schedule close follow-up. Engaging significant others in the treatment process should be considered.

Referral to Treatment

Brief intervention appears most effective for at-risk drinkers, may be less effective for drinkers who are already experiencing harm, and may be ineffective for drinkers who meet criteria for AUD [35]. For nontreatment seeking at-risk drinkers, brief interventions exhibit a small to medium effect size (0.263) over 6–12 months of follow-up and provide a risk reduction of about 10% with a number needed to treat for benefit of 10 [21, 34]. In contrast, the effect size over 6–12 months for brief interventions delivered to treatment seeking drinkers is minimal (0.004) [34]. In addition, the presence of comorbid anxiety and depressive disorders may reduce the effectiveness of brief intervention [35]. Thus, while screening and brief interventions are an important component of managing unhealthy alcohol use, referral to treatment is also a mainstay of care and can be addressed in a similar manner as less severe unhealthy alcohol use by clearly communicating conclusions and recommendations in a nonjudgmental manner [19]. All patients with an AUD should be offered referral to treatment as even those who are not ready to begin treatment may benefit from referral to a specialist for confirmation of diagnoses and recommendations [8].

Specialty treatment of AUD with the goal of achieving and maintaining abstinence is effective particularly in the case of longitudinal treatments [43]. More extended brief treatment in the primary-care setting combined with referral to specialty care for those who screen positive for AUD has been shown to result in decreased frequency of alcohol use and drinking to intoxication [33, 44]. However, it is also clear that many individuals referred to specialty care often do not attend [45]. As a result, attention is shifting to developing treatments for AUD in primary care that capitalize on the ability of primary care to deliver the longitudinal, comprehensive, and coordinated care that has been effective in the treatment of other chronic diseases such as diabetes and hypertension [33, 35, 43–45]. The screening and brief intervention paradigm is also being extended to illicit substances (including the use of prescription medications in ways other than prescribed), suggesting that the approach to unhealthy alcohol use described here may be effectively adapted to address illicit substance use in primary-care settings [33, 44].

Pharmacotherapy

The core of treatment for the entire spectrum of unhealthy alcohol use rests with psychosocial interventions such as brief intervention, motivational interviewing, cognitive behavioral therapy, and 12-step facilitation [1]. However, systematic reviews and meta-analyses indicate that when used in conjunction with psychosocial interventions, medications are effective in enhancing relapse prevention in AUD [46]. To prevent one person from returning to any drinking, the number needed to treat (NNT) were 12 for acamprosate and 20 for oral naltrexone (50 mg/d) [46]. For return to heavy drinking, acamprosate was not associated with improvement, whereas oral naltrexone (50 mg/d) was associated with a NNT of 12 [46]. Acamprosate (N-methyl-D-aspartate (NMDA) modulator) and oral naltrexone (opioid antagonist) have the best evidence supporting their benefits in terms of increasing time to any drinking or heavy drinking and decreasing the percent of drinking days or heavy drinking days [46]. Acamprosate is somewhat less convenient to use (3 times daily) than oral naltrexone (once daily) and is contraindicated with severe renal disease. Naltrexone is contraindicated with acute hepatitis, liver failure, and concurrent or anticipated need for opioids. Overall, trials comparing these two medications have not established a difference in outcomes between them [46]. Factors such as dosing frequency, adverse effects, and availability of other treatments may therefore guide treatment choice. An extended release naltrexone (intramuscular (IM) injection) has been shown to increase time to first drink and decrease the number of drinking days and may be useful where adherence with oral naltrexone is an issue [47]. While disulfiram (acetaldehyde dehydrogenase inhibitor) is widely used, well-controlled trials do not show overall reductions in alcohol intake. However, disulfiram may be effective in certain populations, particularly when used under supervision [46, 47].

The vast majority of data examining pharmacologic treatment for unhealthy alcohol use has been carried out with individuals who meet criteria for AUD and who are engaged in specialty treatment with abstinence as the primary goal [46, 47]. While the ultimate treatment goal for those with AUD is usually stable abstinence promoted by relapse prevention in longitudinal specialty care, a clinically significant reduction in alcohol intake promoted by pharmacologic treatment and management in primary care may be a valid intermediate goal [47, 48]. Limited data suggest that naltrexone may be effectively used in the treatment of AUD in primary-care settings [45, 49]. In addition, naltrexone has also been used to successfully decrease heavy drinking in at-risk and harmful drinkers who do not meet criteria for AUD [50]. Thus, it is possible that naltrexone may be useful when combined with brief intervention in primary-care settings to assist at-risk and harmful drinkers in reducing their drinking levels.

Resources

- National Institute on Alcohol Abuse and Alcoholism (NIAAA). Helping Patients Who Drink Too Much: A Clinician's Guide. Updated 2005 Edition. NIH Publication No. 07–3769. Washington, DC: NIAAA, 2007. http://pubs.niaaa.nih.gov/publications/Practitioner/Clinicians-Guide2005/guide.pdf.
- National Institute on Drug Abuse (NIDA). Resource Guide: Screening for Drug Use in General Medical Settings. Published: April 2009: NIDA, Revised: March 2012. www.drugabuse.gov/publications/resource-guide.
- National Institute on Drug Abuse (NIDA). Screening for Drug Use in General Medical Settings Quick Reference Guide. Published: April 2009: NIDA. http://www.drugabuse.gov/sites/default/files/files/screening_qr.pdf.

References

1. Schuckit MA. Alcohol-use disorders. Lancet. 2009;373:492–501.
2. Cooper M. Motivations for alcohol use among adolescents: development and validation of a four-factor model. Psychol Assess. 1994;6:117–28.
3. Bergmann MM, et al. The association of pattern of lifetime alcohol use and cause of death in the European Prospective Investigation into Cancer and Nutrition (EPIC) study. Int J Epidemiol. 2013;42:1772–90.
4. Jayasekara H, English DR, Room R, MacInnis RJ. Alcohol consumption over time and risk of death: a systematic review and meta-analysis. Am J Epidemiol. 2014;179:1049–59.
5. Bagnardi V, et al. Light alcohol drinking and cancer: a meta-analysis. Ann Oncol. 2013;24:301–8.
6. Mokdad AH, Marks JS, Stroup DF, Gerberding JL. Actual causes of death in the United States, 2000. JAMA. 2004;291:1238–45.
7. Harwood, HJ, Fountain, D, Fountain, G. Economic cost of alcohol and drug abuse in the United States. a report. Addiction. 1992;94:631–5. (1999).
8. Saitz, R. Clinical practice. Unhealthy alcohol use. N Engl J Med. 2005;352:596–607.
9. Rehm J, et al. The relationship of average volume of alcohol consumption and patterns of drinking to burden of disease: an overview. Addiction. 2003;98:1209–28.
10. Dawson DA, Li TK, Grant BF. A prospective study of risk drinking: at risk for what? Drug Alcohol Depend. 2008;95:62–72.
11. Dinh-Zarr T, Goss C, Heitman E, Roberts I, DiGuiseppi C. Interventions for preventing injuries in problem drinkers. Cochrane Database Syst Rev (Online). 2004;3:CD001857.
12. Floyd RL, et al. Preventing alcohol-exposed pregnancies: a randomized controlled trial. Am J Prev Med. 2007;32:1–10.
13. Gmel G, Rehm J. Harmful alcohol use. Alcohol Res Health. 2003;27:52–62.
14. O'Connor MJ, Whaley SE. Brief intervention for alcohol use by pregnant women. Am J Public Health. 2007;97:252–8.
15. Bradley KA, Donovan DM, Larson EB. How much is too much? Advising patients about safe levels of alcohol consumption. Arch Intern Med. 1993;153:2734–40.
16. Kaner EF, et al. The effectiveness of brief alcohol interventions in primary care settings: a systematic review. Drug Alcohol Rev. 2009;28:301–23.
17. Schuckit MA, Anthenelli RM, Bucholz KK, Hesselbrock VM, Tipp J. The time course of development of alcohol-related problems in men and women. J Stud Alcohol. 1995;56:218–25.
18. Wagner FA, Anthony JC. From first drug use to drug dependence; developmental periods of risk for dependence upon marijuana, cocaine, and alcohol. Neuropsychopharmacology. 2002;26:479–88.
19. Willenbring ML, Massey SH, Gardner MB. Helping patients who drink too much: an evidence-based guide for primary care clinicians. Am Fam Physician. 2009;80:44–50.
20. Fleming M, Manwell LB. Brief intervention in primary care settings. A primary treatment method for at-risk, problem, and dependent drinkers. Alcohol Res Health. 1999;23:128–37.
21. Whitlock EP, Polen MR, Green CA, Orleans T, Klein J. Behavioral counseling interventions in primary care to reduce risky/harmful alcohol use by adults: a summary of the evidence for the U.S. Preventive Services Task Force. Ann Intern Med. 2004;140:557–68.
22. Fleming MF, et al. Brief physician advice for heavy drinking college students: a randomized controlled trial in college health clinics. J Stud Alcohol Drugs. 2010;71:23–31.
23. U.S. Department of Health and Human Services, N.I.o.H., National Institue on Alcohol Abuse and Alcoholism. Helping patients who drink too much: a clinician's guide. 2007. NIH publication no. 07-3769 http://pubs.niaaa.nih.gov/publications/Practitioner/CliniciansGuide2005/guide.pdf.
24. Solberg LI, Maciosek MV, Edwards NM. Primary care intervention to reduce alcohol misuse ranking its health impact and cost effectiveness. Am J Prev Med. 2008;34:143–52.
25. Wilk AI, Jensen NM, Havighurst TC. Meta-analysis of randomized control trials addressing brief interventions in heavy alcohol drinkers. J Gen Intern Med. 1997;12:274–83.
26. Bertholet N, Daeppen JB, Wietlisbach V, Fleming M, Burnand B. Reduction of alcohol consumption by brief alcohol intervention in primary care: systematic review and meta-analysis. Arch Intern Med. 2005;165:986–95.
27. Cuijpers P, Riper H, Lemmers L. The effects on mortality of brief interventions for problem drinking: a meta-analysis. Addiction. 2004;99:839–45.
28. Miller WR, Wilbourne PL. Mesa Grande: a methodological analysis of clinical trials of treatments for alcohol use disorders. Addiction. 2002;97:265–77.
29. Batty GD, Lewars H, Emslie C, Gale CR, Hunt K. Internationally recognized guidelines for 'sensible' alcohol consumption: is exceeding them actually detrimental to health and social circumstances? Evidence from a population-based cohort study. J Public Health (Oxf). 2009;31:360–5.
30. Fiellin DA, Reid MC, O'Connor PG. Outpatient management of patients with alcohol problems. Ann Intern Med. 2000;133:815–27.
31. Office of Applied Studies. National Survey on Drug Use and Health. SAMHSA. 2002. http://www.drugabusestatistics.samhsa.gov/nhsda/2k2nsduh/html/toc.htm.
32. Grant BF, et al. The 12-month prevalence and trends in DSM-IV alcohol abuse and dependence: United States, 1991–1992 and 2001–2002. Drug Alcohol Depend. 2004;74:223–34.
33. Madras BK, et al. Screening, brief interventions, referral to treatment (SBIRT) for illicit drug and alcohol use at multiple healthcare sites: comparison at intake and 6 months later. Drug Alcohol Depend. 2009;99:280–95.
34. Moyer A, Finney JW, Swearingen CE, Vergun P. Brief interventions for alcohol problems: a meta-analytic review of controlled investigations in treatment-seeking and non-treatment-seeking populations. Addiction. 2002;97:279–92.

35. Jonas DE, et al. Behavioral counseling after screening for alcohol misuse in primary care: a systematic review and meta-analysis for the U.S. Preventive Services Task Force. Ann Intern Med. 2012;157:645–54.
36. Grossberg P, et al. Inside the physician's black bag: critical ingredients of brief alcohol interventions. Subst Abus. 2010;31:240–50.
37. Fleming MF, et al. Brief physician advice for problem drinkers: long-term efficacy and benefit-cost analysis. Alcohol Clin Exp Res. 2002;26:36–43.
38. Babor TFH-B, J.C. Brief intervention for hazardous and harmful drinking: a manual for use in primary care. 2001. World Health Organisation, Document No. WHO/MSD/MSB/01.6b http://whqlibdoc.who.int/hq/2001/WHO_MSD_MSB_01.6b.pdf.
39. Dawson DA, Pulay AJ, Grant BF. A comparison of two single-item screeners for hazardous drinking and alcohol use disorder. Alcohol Clin Exp Res. 2010;34:364–74.
40. Ewing, JA. Detecting alcoholism. The CAGE questionnaire. JAMA. 1984;252:1905–7.
41. Babor TF, Higgins-Biddle JC, Saunders JB, Monteiro MG. AUDIT: the Alcohol Use Disorders Identification Test, guidelines for use in primary care. In: WHO, editor. 2001.
42. Saunders JB, Aasland OG, Babor TF, de la Fuente JR, Grant M. Development of the Alcohol Use Disorders Identification Test (AUDIT): WHO collaborative project on early detection of persons with harmful alcohol consumption–II. Addiction. 1993;88:791–804.
43. Saitz R, et al. Chronic care management for dependence on alcohol and other drugs: the AHEAD randomized trial. JAMA. 2013;310:1156–67.
44. Gryczynski J, et al. The relationship between services delivered and substance use outcomes in New Mexico's screening, brief intervention, referral and treatment (SBIRT) initiative. Drug Alcohol Depend. 2011;118:152–7.
45. Oslin DW, et al. A randomized clinical trial of alcohol care management delivered in Department of Veterans Affairs primary care clinics versus specialty addiction treatment. J Gen Intern Med. 2014;29:162–8.
46. Jonas DE, et al. Pharmacotherapy for adults with alcohol use disorders in outpatient settings: a systematic review and meta-analysis. JAMA. 2014;311:1889–900.
47. Franck J, Jayaram-Lindstrom N. Pharmacotherapy for alcohol dependence: status of current treatments. Curr Opin Neurobiol. 2013;23:692–9.
48. Gastfriend DR, Garbutt JC, Pettinati HM, Forman RF. Reduction in heavy drinking as a treatment outcome in alcohol dependence. J Subst Abuse Treat. 2007;33:71–80.
49. O'Malley SS, et al. Initial and maintenance naltrexone treatment for alcohol dependence using primary care vs specialty care: a nested sequence of 3 randomized trials. Arch Intern Med. 2003;163:1695–704.
50. O'Malley SS, O'Connor PG. Medications for unhealthy alcohol use: across the spectrum. Alcohol Res Health. 2011;33:300–12.

Sleep Management

Kelly Glazer Baron and Leland Bardsley

Abbreviations

AHI	Apnea–hypopnea index
CBT-I	Cognitive behavioral therapy for insomnia
CPAP	Continuous positive airway pressure
ECG	Electrocardiogram
EEG	Electroencephalogram
EMG	Electromyogram
EOG	Electrooculogram
ICSD3	International Classification of Sleep Disorders, third edition
OSA	Obstructive sleep apnea
PAP	Positive airway pressure
PSG	Polysomnogram
REM	Rapid eye movement
SCN	Suprachiasmatic nucleus
STOP	Snoring, Tired, Obesity, blood Pressure

Introduction

People spend a third of their lives sleeping and it is only in the past few decades that science has revealed the importance of sleep. It is estimated that 70 million Americans suffer from sleep disorders [1]. Sleep is an important topic in lifestyle medicine and is influenced by both biological and behavioral factors. For example, the time of day in which an individual sleeps best is biologically determined [2]. However, behavioral and social factors, such as social/family obligations and work schedules, can determine an individual's sleep opportunity. Furthermore, poor sleep can lead to poorer diet and lower exercise participation [3, 4]. A mismatch be-

tween biology, social drivers, and occupational factors can lead to sleep loss and thus contribute to the development of unhealthy behaviors. Sleep disorders, such as insomnia and obstructive sleep apnea (OSA), are common causes of sleep loss in the population. The first part of this chapter will review several causes of sleep loss and increased risk for physical and psychiatric diseases. The second part of the chapter will discuss common sleep disorders: insufficient sleep, insomnia, and OSA. Finally, the third part of the chapter will review general recommendations for good sleep habits and treatment approaches for common sleep disorders.

Basics of Sleep

Sleep is most simply defined as "a reversible state of perceptual disengagement from and unresponsiveness to the environment" [5]. The factors that control sleep are determined by both time spent awake and the internal biological rhythm. Two main processes have been proposed to contribute to the individual's sleep–wake propensity across the 24-h period (Fig. 17.1; [2]). The homeostatic sleep drive, or "Process S," is the drive or hunger for sleep that accumulates over the 24-h period. Longer wakefulness leads to a greater drive for sleep. The other process, the circadian rhythm, or "Process C," is determined by the internal biological rhythm generated by the suprachiasmatic nucleus (SCN) in the anterior hypothalamus. The SCN, or "master clock," generates an alerting signal throughout the day that promotes alertness despite the increasing sleep drive. There is a slight dip in the circadian alerting signal in the afternoon, then an increase in alertness to oppose the high sleep drive late in the day. In the evening, the alerting signal dissipates. Misalignment of these two sleep systems can lead to sleep problems. For example, sleep deprivation leads to an excess buildup of sleep drive. Then, waking at the normal time due to schedule constraints can cause the individual to have residual sleepiness. Also, a midday nap can lead to insufficient sleep drive in the evening, leading to insomnia.

K. G. Baron (✉)
Department of Neurology, Feinberg School of Medicine,
Northwestern University, Abbott Hall, Rm 523,
710 N. Lake Shore Dr., Chicago, IL 60611, USA
e-mail: k-baron@northwestern.edu

L. Bardsley
Illinois Institute of Technology, Chicago, IL, USA

© Springer International Publishing Switzerland 2016
J. I. Mechanick, R. F. Kushner (eds.), *Lifestyle Medicine,* DOI 10.1007/978-3-319-24687-1_17

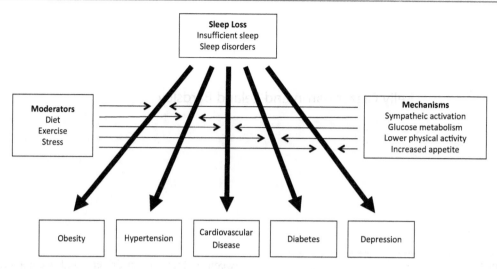

Fig. 17.1 Proposed relationships between sleep loss and health. Bidirectional pathways have been established between sleep and chronic physical and mental disorders. The relationships between sleep and development of chronic illness have been demonstrated. Mechanisms include multiple biological and behavioral factors such as sympathetic nervous system activation and changes in dietary behavior. The relationship between disturbed sleep and chronic illness is also well established, in that having chronic illness is a risk factor for the development of poor sleep

Table 17.1 Sleep hygiene recommendations

Schedule and time spent in bed	Do not go to bed unless sleepy
	Get out of bed if awake for 20 min
	Use the bed for sleep and intimacy only
	Get up at the same time each morning
	Avoid naps
	Allow yourself sufficient time for sleep; for most adults, 7–8 h per night
Presleep activities	Do not go to bed hungry, but also do not eat a large meal 2 h prior to bed
	Wind down in the evening, such as a warm bath or a few minutes of reading before bed
Bedroom environment	The bedroom should be cool, dark, and quiet. Use room-darkening shades or an eye mask to control light. For sound, a white noise machine or table fan may be helpful.
	Go "off the grid." Turn off cell phone, tablet, and other electronic media
Engage in healthy behaviors and avoid substances and behaviors that interfere with sleep	Avoid caffeine in the afternoon
	Avoid alcohol prior to bedtime
	Avoid cigarettes and nicotine before bedtime
	Avoid or limit use of sleeping pills
	Schedule "worry time"
	Turn alarm clock face away from the bed to resist the temptation to check the time
	Exercise regularly
	Manage stress and engage in relaxation

Sleep Evaluation

Clinicians should inquire about sleep among all patients, but a sleep history is particularly important to screen for OSA in high-risk populations (i.e., obese patients, hypertension, and diabetes) and insomnia in those with medical and psychiatric disorders. Sleep evaluation begins with a thorough sleep history (Table 17.1). Clinicians should begin by assessing the current sleep problem, including the perceived factors involved in the onset of the sleep problem (e.g., stressful event leading to insomnia) as well as the duration and course of the problem. Other contributing factors may include nighttime worry or cognitive hyperarousal or maladaptive beliefs about sleep. These include beliefs such as needing 8 h of sleep to function or significant worry about the consequences of their loss on their health. The assessment should also assess the consequences including effects on daytime function including job performance and social/family functioning. A sleep evaluation should also include a basic screening for symptoms of OSA or restless legs syndrome even among patients such as those with insomnia, as these disorders may either be comorbid with insomnia. In terms of sleep schedule, patients' weekday and weekend schedule should be assessed. Clinicians should also assess the bedtime environment as well as relevant health and sleep habits (e.g., timing and amount of alcohol, caffeine, and exercise). Finally, a thorough understanding of medical and psychiatric disorders as well as current medications is helpful in diagnosis and treatment planning for patients with sleep problems.

Among self-report measures, one of the most common instruments is a sleep diary. Sleep diaries are easy to administer and inexpensive. They also can evaluate the individual's sleep pattern over weeks or months. Many different standardized sleep diaries exist including those published by the Academy of Sleep Medicine and the National Sleep Foundation. Most sleep diaries include a bedtime, fall asleep time, awakenings in the night, estimated sleep duration, risetime, and naps. Patients can also include other behaviors that may affect sleep, including alcohol, caffeine intake, and exercise. Sleep diaries are limited by their reliance on patient self-report and can be burdensome to complete. Other brief self-report measures that may be useful include the STOP (**S**noring, **T**ired, **O**besity, blood**P**ressure) questionnaire [6] for assessment of risk for OSA, the Epworth Sleepiness Scale [7] to assess for self-reported sleepiness, and the Insomnia Severity Index [8] to assess for the criteria for insomnia.

Only a selection of patients will require a polysomnogram (PSG) or "sleep study." PSG typically includes electroencephalogram (EEG), electrooculogram (EOG), electromyogram (EMG), and electrocardiogram (ECG), as well as respiratory effort and oxygen saturation. Sleep states are divided into non-rapid eye movement stages (N1, N2, and N3, also referred to as slow-wave sleep) and rapid eye movement (REM). Sleep duration and the amount of time spent in each sleep stage change significantly across the lifespan. For example, slow-wave sleep comprises approximately 30% of the sleep period in midlife and declines with age. In adults aged 70 and above, the amount of slow-wave sleep decreases to 5% among men and 15–20% among women [9]. The percentage of non-REM to REM sleep remains fairly stable, in that the decline in slow-wave sleep is replaced by lighter stages of sleep (N1, N2) and wake. Sleep disorders such as OSA also affect sleep architecture. Apneas lead to frequent awakenings and a decrease in slow-wave sleep.

Clinically, PSG is most frequently used to diagnose sleep-disordered breathing, such as OSA, and titrate or adjust the appropriate pressure for positive airway pressure (PAP) treatment. PSG is also used to evaluate other abnormal nocturnal behaviors, including sleepwalking, periodic limb movements, and nocturnal seizures. It is not indicated for the assessment of insomnia. The benefits of the PSG (in laboratory or home) include increased monitoring of the participant during the study, such as video monitoring. The drawbacks of this approach are cost, burden to the patient, and limited number of nights assessed. Although the majority of PSG are conducted in the laboratory at this time, a growing number of clinics are offering ambulatory (home) studies. Currently,

many insurance programs as well as Medicare reimburse for ambulatory PSG. Particularly in the case of those at high risk for sleep apnea without other comorbidities, the cost savings of home PSG paired with increased comfort for the patient make this an attractive option [10]. For home PSG, patients typically come to the clinic to pick up equipment and receive instructions from clinic staff. The equipment includes respiratory effort belts, pulse oximeter, and nasal cannula. Some but not all ambulatory PSG units also include EEG. Patients then can return the equipment in person or by mail for download and evaluation. The greatest limitation to home PSG is that patient's sleep state is not known, since none of the units have a full EEG. Therefore, it can be difficult to determine whether events, such as limb movements, are occurring when awake or during sleep. Because of this limitation, ambulatory PSG is only indicated for diagnosis of OSA.

Another approach to monitoring sleep in the home environment is wrist actigraphy. In these types of devices, a monitor that measures movement is worn on the wrist. A movement-based algorithm determines sleep pattern and this information is often paired with a diary or marker to indicate sleep period. This technique is most useful in studying sleep patterns in insomnia and circadian rhythm disorders, or in populations that have difficulty reporting their sleep pattern (e.g., children and elderly). Some devices (e.g., Actiwatch Spectrum, Philips Inc.) have validated published algorithms for estimating sleep/wake states. Recently, consumer wrist-worn devices (e.g., Jawbone®, UP®, Fitbit®, BodyMedia FIT®, SenseWear®) have gained popularity among the public, suggesting that people are interested in their sleep patterns. At this time, comparisons between consumer devices with PSG and research actigraphy indicate these devices are far less accurate at estimating sleep. However, their usefulness for sleep intervention is only beginning to be explored. It is likely these devices can help motivate people to improve their sleep patterns and also demonstrate sensitivity to within-person changes. At the present time, they are not indicated in the assessment of sleep disorders.

Sleep Loss, Sleep Disorders, and Disease Risk

Sleep loss has been linked to cognitive performance, mood, and risk for disease. Epidemiologic studies have demonstrated a U-shaped relationship between sleep duration and poor health. Typically, those with less than 6 h and those with more than 9 h of sleep have increased risk for disease. This relationship has been demonstrated for risk of cardiovascular disease , hypertension, diabetes, obesity, and all-cause mortality [11–16]. The links between sleep loss and disease are not fully understood. Some of the proposed pathways are provided in Fig. 17.2. Sleep loss can be due to social or occupational constraints, or as a result of a sleep disorder. Sleep loss

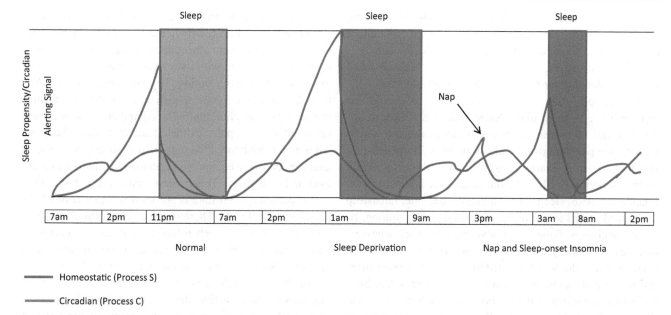

Fig. 17.2 Relationship between sleep drive, circadian rhythm, and sleep propensity. The above figure illustrates the two-process model of sleep. Process S represents the drive, or hunger, for sleep. Note that Process S decreases rapidly during periods of sleep. The body's circadian rhythm (Process C) is an "alerting" signal that promotes wakefulness. There is a natural dip for Process C in the afternoon between 1 and 3 p.m. in most people; however, Process C increases until around 11 p.m. in most people. The interaction of the peak in Process S and the decrease in Process C at night allows for restorative sleep at night. The *first panel* depicts normal sleep. In the *second panel,* sleep deprivation causes an increase in sleep drive at night. The *third panel* depicts a nap, where the sleep drive decreases and then is not high enough for sleep until later than the typical time

has also been associated with sympathetic nervous system hyperactivation [17]. This, in turn, affects glucose regulation and health behaviors, such as diet and physical activity. Diet and exercise can moderate the relationship between sleep and disease risk, as well as improve sleep disorders directly.

Common Sleep Disorders

Insufficient Sleep

The problem of insufficient sleep is one of the most common causes of daytime sleepiness [1]. The average sleep duration reported on weekdays is approximately 6.5 h in Americans, whereas they report needing 7.25 h to function at their best [18]. Approximately 50% of the Americans report they do not get sufficient sleep on weekdays. Most people are not aware that insufficient sleep is classified as a sleep disorder. According to the International Classification of Sleep Disorders, third edition (ICSD3; [19]), insufficient sleep syndrome is characterized by having daytime sleepiness (dozing off unintentionally) along with a chronic pattern of sleep time that is shorter than expected for their age and present for 3 months. The individual must sleep longer on weekends or vacations and symptoms may not be explained by another disorder.

Insomnia

Insomnia is one of the most prevalent sleep problems reported in primary care [20]. Chronic insomnia disorder affects 9–12% of the population and up to 30% of older adults [21, 22]. It is defined by the ICSD3 as difficulty initiating and/or maintaining sleep, or waking earlier than desired at least 3 times per week for at least 3 months [19]. This sleep disturbance must cause a negative consequence at least 3 days per week, such as fatigue, mood disturbance, daytime sleepiness, or concerns about sleep. It is differentiated from insufficient sleep because the individual must have adequate opportunity for sleep. Insomnia has been associated with poor quality of life, increased health-care unitization, and decreased work productivity [23, 24]. Recent evidence has linked insomnia, particularly insomnia combined with short sleep duration, to increased risk of hypertension, diabetes, and all-cause mortality [25–27].

Obstructive Sleep Apnea (OSA)

OSA is characterized by repeated pauses in breathing due to airway collapse [19]. This causes frequent nocturnal awakenings, intermittent hypoxia, and disruption of sleep architecture, such as frequent awakenings and decreased amounts of slow-wave sleep. Patients with OSA may have virtually no slow-wave (deep) sleep and hundreds of awakenings during the night. OSA is present in 2–4 % of middle-aged adults and up to 20 % of older adults [28, 29]. Older adults, men, African-Americans, Asians, and obese individuals are at increased risk for OSA. Among women, the rates of OSA double after menopause [30]. OSA is associated with daytime sleepiness, increased risk for cardiovascular events, stroke, poor glycemic control, and decreased quality of life [31–34].

Shift Work and Shift Work Disorder

At least 20 % of the population is involved in a job that requires shift work. The definition of shift work can include late night, overnight, and early morning shifts. Commute times also play a role. For example, a person who starts work at 6 a.m. may need to wake at 4 a.m. to get ready and drive into work. There are two interrelated factors involved in sleep problems experienced by shift workers. One factor is circadian disruption. Shift workers are often required to work during the biological night. Second, shift workers also report short sleep duration, typically 1–4 h less than day workers in similar jobs [35, 36]. Reasons for sleep curtailment include the fact that shift workers need to sleep during a nonoptimal time, a result of circadian misalignment of the sleep–wake cycle. Furthermore, shift workers often curtail their sleep because of social and family factors, such as childcare responsibilities.

Sleep Disorder Treatments: Considerations for Lifestyle Medicine

General Considerations for Good Sleep

The term "sleep hygiene" has come to mean a list of the common "do's and don'ts" of sleep habits. The term was first coined by Peter Hauri, one of the founders of the behavioral sleep medicine field [37]. Different variations of these rules have been published over the past 35 years. A review of the sleep hygiene rules by Stepanski and Wyatt [38] demonstrates the overlap between sleep hygiene rules and insomnia treatment recommendations (e.g., stimulus control), such as the advice to get out of bed if awake for more than 20 min.

Many of these recommendations focus on increasing homeostatic drive for sleep through restricting the time in bed and limiting napping. Other recommendations suggest wind-down time prior to bed and making the bedroom environment conducive to sleep. Social (e.g., Facebook and Twitter updates) and work demands (e.g., e-mail and text messages) should also be suspended to allow for uninterrupted sleep. Individuals should incorporate lifestyle changes that improve sleep (e.g., daytime light exposure) as well as those that ameliorate the negative impact of stress on sleep (e.g., relaxation). Finally, several recommendations focus on avoiding substances or behaviors that interfere with sleep, such as caffeine or cigarettes.

Exercise is an interesting topic in terms of sleep. Individuals who exercise tend to sleep better. However, it has been a common recommendation that evening exercise is detrimental to sleep even though several studies have demonstrated that evening exercise does not necessarily compromise sleep quality [39, 40].

Extending Sleep Duration

Interventions to extend sleep duration are clearly needed for a large percentage of the population. To date, there are two studies that have tested the effects of sleep extension interventions [41, 42]. These studies aimed to increase sleep duration by 1 h. This was accomplished by monitoring sleep and providing structure to the sleep schedule by setting a bedtime 30 min earlier and a wake time 30 min later than their typical times. For individuals who could not move their wake time because of work or school schedules, they were told to advance their bedtime 60 min rather than 30 min. One study assigned participants with prehypertension and short sleep duration (6.5 h on actigraphy) to a sleep extension protocol versus no change [41]. The results demonstrated a 35 min increase in sleep duration and a statistically significant 14 mmHg decrease in beat-to-beat systolic blood pressure in the sleep extension group compared to a 4 min increase in sleep and a statistically nonsignificant 7 mmHg decrease in the control group. Another study assigned adolescents with short sleep duration to a similar protocol of set bed/wake times but also added a more gradual change in sleep schedule, by gradually moving the bedtime earlier over the first week, to achieve a 55 min increase in their sleep opportunity [42]. This study demonstrated that this protocol was effective at improving sleep duration and reducing depressive symptoms among adolescents. Table 17.2 lists recommendations for increasing sleep duration based on these sleep extension protocols.

Insomnia Treatment

Cognitive behavioral therapy for insomnia (CBT-I) is a multi-component treatment that involves both cognitive and behavioral interventions aimed at changing the thoughts and

Table 17.2 Extending sleep duration

Prepare	Evaluate current average sleep/wake time by logging sleep patterns for 1 week
	Establish a goal for new sleep duration (e.g., increase sleep duration by 1 h); aim for 7–8 h per night
	Specify a consistent sleep and wake time that will last for the targeted duration of time; for those who cannot adjust wake time due to rigid conflicts (e.g., a work day start time), solely focus changes on advancing sleep time
Plan	Identify potential barriers to making changes to sleep/wake time
	For example
	If a favorite TV show conflicts with the new sleep schedule, consider recording the show and watching it the following day
	If the new wake time conflicts with a partner or roommate, negotiate a schedule that will permit both parties to complete morning routines simultaneously
	Note that current daily routines may need to be adjusted to allow for altered sleep/wake times; modify activities accordingly
	Discuss your plans with significant others, family members, and close friends; clearly communicate intention to increase sleep duration, alerting others of changes in availability for social commitments, phone calls, and other obligations
Implement	Gradually adjust sleep/wake time (e.g., over the course of 1 week, advance sleep time by 5 min per night and delay wake time by 5 min each morning)
	Fastidiously attend to sleep hygiene recommendations while attempting to extend sleep duration (see Table 17.1)
	Ensure that bedroom is conducive to sleep, wind down prior to bedtime, and avoid behaviors that will interfere with sleep
	Make use of natural sources of support (e.g., partner) who can assist with follow-through on the new commitment
Adapt	Be flexible and forgiving
	As with any behavior change, setbacks are a normal part of the process
	Employ positive thinking to combat negative cognitions about slips-ups
	Instead of catastrophizing and discounting the positives, focus on successes and long-term goals
	Expect some sleep periods to fall short of the established target.
	When these nights occur, recommit to the new sleep goal

behaviors that perpetuate insomnia. CBT-I has been demonstrated to be effective in multiple populations including adults, older adults, patients with hypnotic dependence, insomnia with comorbid conditions including depression, chronic pain, and heart disease. CBT-I is time limited and cost-effective [43]. The standard length of CBT-I treatments is six sessions but other brief CBT-I interventions designed to be implemented in primary care sessions by physicians or nurses have also been demonstrated to be effective [44, 45]. Many of these techniques can be used effectively in a primary care setting. However, patients with more severe insomnia, those who need further evaluation of their sleep for additional comorbid disorder and those patients who are interested in a more rigorous treatment (6 sessions vs. 1 or 2), should be referred to a specialist in behavioral sleep medicine. A list of certified behavioral sleep medicine specialists are listed on the website of the Society for Behavioral Sleep Medicine (www.behavioralsleep.org). The main components of CBT-I are described below.

Sleep Restriction

Sleep restriction [46] increases the drive to sleep by decreasing the time spent in bed. In this component of treatment, patients calculate their number of hours sleeping (total sleep time) and divide that number by the hours spent in bed. So, an individual who spends 8 h in bed but sleeps 6 h would have a sleep efficiency of 75%. Then, they set a sleep window for only the amount of time spent sleeping (minimum of 5 h). For someone who says they sleep only 5½ h between 9 p.m. and 7 a.m., they would then schedule a bedtime and

wake time allowing for 6 h. Those 6 h should be scheduled according to when the individual is most likely to be able to sleep (e.g., 12:00–6:00). Scheduling from 9 p.m. to 3 a.m. would be challenging for most people. The patient and clinician evaluate the sleep efficiency each week and adjust the time in bed 15 min at a time. The patient gains time in bed if sleep efficiency is 90, loses time in bed if sleep efficiency is 80%, and maintains the same time in bed if sleep efficiency is 80–90%.

Stimulus Control

In stimulus control [47], the goal is to spend only the time asleep in bed and avoid activities that are not sleep promoting in bed, including worrying, watching TV, eating, or reading. Individuals with insomnia are recommended to only use the bed for sleep and sex, and get out of bed if awake in the middle of the night for more than 15–20 min. Recommended activities when out of bed include non-stimulating but not unpleasant activities including light reading, watching TV, and listening to music.

Cognitive Interventions

The targets for cognitive interventions [48, 49], or restructuring, include catastrophizing next-day consequences of sleep loss and significant worry about sleep loss. Patients may also be instructed in techniques for reducing worry.

Exercise, Meditation, and Yoga

These activities have also been demonstrated to improve sleep quality. There is the most evidence for aerobic exercise

Table 17.3 Improving adherence to positive airway pressure (PAP)

Assessing expectancies	Evaluate patient's expectations about using continuous positive airway pressure (CPAP) device
	Are the patient's expectations realistic?
	Discuss with patient that CPAP treatment is not easy but the benefits are substantial (e.g., increased energy, reduced health risk, improvements in mood, etc.)
	Ask patient to share concerns or fears about starting the treatment
	Do the patient's concerns about treatment relate to areas that require special attention (e.g., worries that the device will impede intimacy with partner)?
Setting a solid foundation	Address adherence problems and other complications related to CPAP use early in the course of treatment. Early intervention will:
	Promote a good relationship between provider and patient
	Short-circuit the development of negative beliefs about CPAP treatment
	Prevent the formation of bad habits
Identifying strengths	Ask the patient to share specific examples of past successes with behavior change
	Allow the patient to home in on what will likely work as he/she attempts to make use of CPAP treatment
Education	Explore CPAP options with the patient
	Discuss differences in device type (e.g., air pressure application) and face masks variations (e.g., full, nasal, etc.)
	Explain the importance of adequate seal for effectiveness and comfort
	Prepare patient for a process that includes selection of a device, fitting, testing, adjustment, and changing devices when a selection is not working. The process may require numerous iterations
	Consider specific clinical concerns or patient preferences that may suggest a particular device would be the best match for the patient
Consider technological interventions	Assess the patient's comfort with the device
	Does the patient report that the mask is fitting poorly, causing a lot of leak at night, or causing skin breakdown?
	Does the CPAP adherence and efficacy download demonstrate a large leak for a significant portion of the night?
	Assess adequacy of the CPAP prescription
	Assess on the CPAP download if the OSA is adequately treated (apnea–hypopnea index <10)
	If still unable to wear the device, consider reevaluation with a sleep medicine specialist for desensitization or retitration to a bilevel machine

among individuals with insomnia or poor sleep quality. A few studies have also demonstrated that resistance training, tai chi, and yoga can improve sleep quality [50–52].

OSA Treatment

PAP is considered the gold standard for OSA treatment and is effective at eliminating apneas [53]. It is recommended that patients use PAP treatment all night, every night, and during naps. Medicare requires use of 4 h per night on 70% of the nights and patients must demonstrate adherence through a download from their machine within the first 90 days or it will not be covered. Data demonstrate that 4 h of use can improve blood pressure. Later publications demonstrate more is better when it comes to outcomes such as daytime sleepiness and quality of life [54]. However, approximately 50% of patients are nonadherent [54]. Patients with higher adherence have better neurocognitive and subjective outcomes [55]. Therefore, adherence is critical to the success of this treatment. It is now standard for PAP machines to include adherence data-recording capabilities. The specific data included on each download report vary based on machine and manufacturer but downloads include usage (average, per night, and on nights used) and efficacy (apnea

severity, presence of snoring, and mask leak). These data are helpful to clinicians in monitoring and encouraging patients' adherence. Table 17.3 provides suggestions for increasing PAP adherence based on recommendations from a task force of the American Academy of Sleep Medicine [56]. Evidence from numerous trials have demonstrated aspects of effective interventions for PAP adherence including education, assessing motivation and barriers, setting goals and a follow-up plan, and assessing the need for technological intervention, such as mask changes [57, 58].

There are other treatments for OSA beyond PAP. In particular, lifestyle interventions have been shown to lead to significant improvement in the severity of OSA as well as daytime symptoms. Due to the role of obesity in the etiology of OSA, weight loss can improve OSA for a large percentage of patients. Weight loss through behavioral interventions, pharmacotherapy, and bariatric surgery has been shown to reduce indices of apnea severity, including the number of apneic events (apnea–hypopnea index (AHI)) and oxyhemoglobin desaturations (desaturation index) per hour [59, 60]. However, it is important to note that despite weight loss, patients on average continue to have mild-to-moderate OSA, which typically requires additional treatment. For overweight or obese patients with mild OSA, weight loss may be the only treatment needed [61].

Several studies have also demonstrated that exercise can improve the symptoms of OSA [62]. In one randomized controlled trial, patients with moderate-to-severe sleep apnea were randomized to 12 weeks of exercise training (a combination of aerobic and resistance) or low-intensity stretching (control). Post intervention, participants in the exercise group had significantly greater reductions in AHI and oxygen desaturation indices, two measures of sleep apnea severity. Interestingly, improvements in apnea severity occurred despite participants not losing weight in this study, suggesting that exercise improves OSA through other mechanisms. This study did not identify a specific mechanism, but improvements in muscle strength or the stability of sleep may play a role.

There are also additional treatments that may benefit particular subgroups of patients. Patients with mild OSA also may benefit from the use of a dental appliance, which creates space in the airway through advancing the mandible [63], or positional therapy [64]—either purchased (e.g., side sleeping pillows and tennis ball t-shirts) or homemade devices (e.g., tennis balls in a backpack)—to help the patient avoid sleeping on their back. This may be particularly beneficial for patients in whom all or the majority of apneic episodes occur in the supine position as documented in the PSG report. In addition, surgical interventions to increase space in the airway are effective at improving OSA in some patients [65].

Shift Work Treatment

Lifestyle recommendations are often necessary in the treatment of shift work disorder as well as for the general health of shift workers. According to the American Academy of Sleep Medicine, there is the most evidence to support interventions in which shift workers plan their sleep schedule in a way that they can maximize sleep duration [66]. For overnight workers, for example, sleep is typically best before noon. Therefore, workers are recommended to sleep as early as possible after they get home. It is also recommended that night workers minimize the change in their sleep schedule from work and nonwork days, in order to reduce the number of hours shifted each week but also allow the individual to engage in daytime activities on their day off. For example, an overnight worker may sleep from 8 a.m. to 12 or 1 p.m. following work shifts. Then, on days off, it is recommended that the worker sleep from 2 or 3 a.m. to 10 a.m., in order to minimize the shift between work and nonwork days. This "compromise schedule" has been demonstrated to improve performance and mood in the laboratory [67]. Other evidence-based treatments are timed light exposure (specific timing dependent on the worker's hours), melatonin, use of hypnotics at night, and stimulant medications to promote alertness [68].

Conclusion

Sleep is an important health behavior due to the role of sleep in physical and emotional health. In addition, poor sleep may also influence other health behaviors, through decreasing participation in exercise and increasing appetite and poor-eating behaviors. Lifestyle interventions are critical to the treatment of sleep disturbances, including short sleep duration, insomnia, shift work, and OSA. Many of the interventions recommended to improve sleep include reducing stress, improving regularity of sleep/wake schedules, and improving health behaviors, such as limiting caffeine, nicotine, and alcohol, all of which have additional effects on overall health and well-being. Furthermore, other lifestyle interventions, such as weight loss and exercise, have been shown to improve sleep.

From the public health perspective, more research is needed on the high levels of chronic insufficient sleep in the population as well as interventions to improve sleep health at the population level. Although additional pressure to "have-it-all" and to sacrifice rest for perceived financial and career success is evident, a backlash resisting these sociocultural shifts has materialized. New measures of success have entered the public discourse, with an emphasis on vitality and emotional well-being.

As sleep is important for both emotional and physical well-being, it is a clear area of concern for the lifestyle medicine health-care professional. Assessment of and patient-centered discussions about sleep are essential elements of comprehensive lifestyle medicine. Although calls for more sleep are mounting, the prevailing attitude within today's fast-paced, hyper-connected society is that people must relentlessly push themselves to the point of exhaustion in an effort to race to the top. The best research on sleep and health tells us that losing out on sleep—either willfully or as a consequence of a sleep disorder—has substantial costs. Lifestyle medicine grants an opportunity to encourage patients to prioritize sleep as part of a transformation to a healthier state.

References

1. Colten HR, Altevogt BM, editors. Sleep disorders and sleep deprivation: an unmet public health problem. Washington, DC: National Academies Press; 2006.
2. Borbely AA. A two process model of sleep regulation. Hum Neurobiol. 1982;1(3):195–204. (Epub 1982/01/01).
3. Nedeltcheva AV, Kilkus JM, Imperial J, Kasza K, Schoeller DA, Penev PD. Sleep curtailment is accompanied by increased intake of calories from snacks. Am J Clin Nutr. 2009;89(1):126–33. (Epub 2008/12/06).
4. Baron KG, Reid KJ, Zee PC. Exercise to improve sleep in insomnia: exploration of the bidirectional effects. J Clin Sleep Med. 2013;9(8):819–24. (Epub 2013/08/16).
5. Carskadon MA, Dement WC. Normal human sleep: an overivew. In: Kryger MH, Roth T, Dement WC, editors. Principles and practice of sleep medicine. 5th ed. St. Louis: Elsevier Saunders.; 2011. pp. 16–26.

6. Chung F, Subramanyam R, Liao P, Sasaki E, Shapiro C, Sun Y. High STOP-Bang score indicates a high probability of obstructive sleep apnoea. Br J Anaesth. 2012;108(5):768–75. (Epub 2012/03/10).

7. Johns MW. Daytime sleepiness, snoring, and obstructive sleep apnea. The Epworth sleepiness scale. Chest. 1993;103(1):30–6. (Epub 1993/01/01).

8. Morin CM, Belleville G, Belanger L, Ivers H. The Insomnia Severity Index: psychometric indicators to detect insomnia cases and evaluate treatment response. Sleep. 2011;34(5):601–8. (Epub 2011/05/03).

9. Redline S, Kirchner HL, Quan SF, Gottlieb DJ, Kapur V, Newman A. The effects of age, sex, ethnicity, and sleep-disordered breathing on sleep architecture. Arch Intern Med. 2004;164(4):406–18. (Epub 2004/02/26).

10. Bruyneel M, Ninane V. Unattended home-based polysomnography for sleep disordered breathing: current concepts and perspectives. Sleep Med Rev. 2014;18(4):341–7. (Epub 2014/01/07).

11. Ayas NT, White DP, Manson JE, Stampfer MJ, Speizer FE, Malhotra A, et al. A prospective study of sleep duration and coronary heart disease in women. Arch Intern Med. 2003;163(2):205–9. (Epub 2003/01/28).

12. Chaput JP, Despres JP, Bouchard C, Tremblay A. Short sleep duration is associated with reduced leptin levels and increased adiposity: results from the Quebec family study. Obesity (Silver Spring). 2007;15(1):253–61. (Epub 2007/01/18).

13. Gottlieb DJ, Redline S, Nieto FJ, Baldwin CM, Newman AB, Resnick HE, et al. Association of usual sleep duration with hypertension: the sleep heart health study. Sleep. 2006;29(8):1009–14. (Epub 2006/09/02).

14. Patel SR, Malhotra A, White DP, Gottlieb DJ, Hu FB. Association between reduced sleep and weight gain in women. Am J Epidemiol. 2006;164(10):947–54. (Epub 2006/08/18).

15. Cappuccio FP, Cooper D, D'Elia L, Strazzullo P, Miller MA. Sleep duration predicts cardiovascular outcomes: a systematic review and meta-analysis of prospective studies. Eur Heart J. 2011;32(12):1484–92. (Epub 2011/02/09).

16. McNeil J, Doucet E, Chaput JP. Inadequate sleep as a contributor to obesity and type 2 diabetes. Can. J Diabetes. 2013;37(2):103–8. (Epub 2013/09/28).

17. Bonnet MH, Arand DL. Hyperarousal and insomnia: state of the science. Sleep Med Rev. 2010;14(1):9–15. (Epub 2009/07/31).

18. Foundation NS. 2013 Sleep in America poll. Arlington, VA: February 20, 2013. Report No.

19. American Academy of Sleep Medicine. International classification of sleep disorders. 3rd ed. Darien: American Academy of Sleep Medicine; 2014.

20. Alattar M, Harrington JJ, Mitchell CM, Sloane P. Sleep problems in primary care: a North Carolina Family Practice Research Network (NC-FP-RN) study. J Am Board Fam Med. 2007;20(4):365–74.

21. Foley DJ, Monjan AA, Brown SL, Simonsick EM, Wallace RB, Blazer DG. Sleep complaints among elderly persons: an epidemiologic study of three communities. Sleep. 1995;18(6):425–32. (Epub 1995/07/01).

22. Ohayon MM. Epidemiology of insomnia: what we know and what we still need to learn. Sleep Med Rev. 2002;6(2):97–111.

23. Fullerton DS. The economic impact of insomnia in managed care: a clearer picture emerges. Am J Manag Care. 2006;12(8 Suppl):S246–52.

24. Novak M, Mucsi I, Shapiro CM, Rethelyi J, Kopp MS. Increased utilization of health services by insomniacs—an epidemiological perspective. J Psychosom Res. 2004;56(5):527–36.

25. Vgontzas AN, Liao D, Bixler EO. Insomnia and hypertension. Sleep. 2009;32(12):1547. (Epub 2010/01/01).

26. Fernandez-Mendoza J, Vgontzas AN, Liao D, Shaffer ML, Vela-Bueno A, Basta M, et al. Insomnia with objective short sleep duration and incident hypertension: the Penn State Cohort. Hypertension. 2012;60(4):929–35. (Epub 2012/08/16).

27. Kripke DF, Garfinkel L, Wingard DL, Klauber MR, Marler MR. Mortality associated with sleep duration and insomnia. Arch Gen Psychiat. 2002;59(2):131–6.

28. Young T, Shahar E, Nieto FJ, Redline S, Newman AB, Gottlieb DJ, et al. Predictors of sleep-disordered breathing in community-dwelling adults: the Sleep Heart Health Study. Arch Intern Med. 2002;162(8):893–900.

29. Netzer NC, Hoegel JJ, Loube D, Netzer CM, Hay B, Alvarez-Sala R, et al. Prevalence of symptoms and risk of sleep apnea in primary care. Chest. 2003;124(4):1406–14.

30. Young T, Finn L, Austin D, Peterson A. Menopausal status and sleep-disordered breathing in the Wisconsin Sleep Cohort Study. Am J Respir Crit Care Med. 2003;167(9):1181–5.

31. Chervin RD. Sleepiness, fatigue, tiredness, and lack of energy in obstructive sleep apnea. Chest. 2000;118(2):372–9.

32. Marin JM, Carrizo SJ, Vicente E, Agusti AG. Long-term cardiovascular outcomes in men with obstructive sleep apnoea-hypopnoea with or without treatment with continuous positive airway pressure: an observational study. Lancet. 2005;365(9464):1046–53.

33. Chasens ER. Obstructive sleep apnea, daytime sleepiness, and type 2 diabetes. Diabetes Educ. 2007;33(3):475–82. (Epub 2007/06/16).

34. Baldwin CM, Griffith KA, Nieto FJ, O'Connor GT, Walsleben JA, Redline S. The association of sleep-disordered breathing and sleep symptoms with quality of life in the Sleep Heart Health Study. Sleep. 2001;24(1):96–105.

35. Akerstedt T. Work hours, sleepiness and the underlying mechanisms. J Sleep Res. 1995;4(S2):15–22. (Epub 1995/12/01).

36. Knauth P, Landau K, Droge C, Schwitteck M, Widynski M, Rutenfranz J. Duration of sleep depending on the type of shift work. Int Arch Occup Environ Health. 1980;46(2):167–77. (Epub 1980/01/01).

37. Hauri P. Current concepts: the sleep disorders. Kalamazoo: The Upjohn Company; 1977.

38. Stepanski EJ, Wyatt JK. Use of sleep hygiene in the treatment of insomnia. Sleep Med Rev. 2003;7(3):215–25. (Epub 2003/08/21).

39. Buman MP, Phillips BA, Youngstedt SD, Kline CE, Hirshkowitz M. Does nighttime exercise really disturb sleep? Results from the 2013 National Sleep Foundation Sleep in America Poll. Sleep Med. 2014;15(7):755–61. (Epub 2014/06/17).

40. Youngstedt SD, Kripke DF, Elliott JA. Is sleep disturbed by vigorous late-night exercise? Med Sci Sports Exerc. 1999;31(6):864–9. (Epub 1999/06/23).

41. Haack M, Serrador J, Cohen D, Simpson N, Meier-Ewert H, Mullington JM. Increasing sleep duration to lower beat-to-beat blood pressure: a pilot study. J Sleep Res. 2013;22(3):295–304. (Epub 2012/11/23).

42. Dewald-Kaufmann JF, Oort FJ, Meijer AM. The effects of sleep extension on sleep and cognitive performance in adolescents with chronic sleep reduction: an experimental study. Sleep Med. 2013;14(6):510–7. (Epub 2013/03/26).

43. McCrae CS, Bramoweth AD, Williams J, Roth A, Mosti C. Impact of brief cognitive behavioral treatment for insomnia on health care utilization and costs. J Clin Sleep Med. 2014;10(2):127–35. (Epub 2014/02/18).

44. Buysse DJ, Germain A, Moul DE, Franzen PL, Brar LK, Fletcher ME, et al. Efficacy of brief behavioral treatment for chronic insomnia in older adults. Arch Intern Med. 2011;171(10):887–95. (Epub 2011/01/26).

45. Edinger JD, Sampson WS. A primary care "friendly" cognitive behavioral insomnia therapy. Sleep. 2003;26(2):177–82. (Epub 2003/04/10).

46. Spielman AJ, Saskin P, Thorpy MJ. Treatment of chronic insomnia by restriction of time in bed. Sleep. 1987;10(1):45–56. (Epub 1987/02/01).

47. Bootzin RR, Stimulus control treatment for insomnia. American Psychological Association Proceedings; 395–6; 1972.

48. Morin CM. Insomnia: psychological assessment and management. New York: Guilford Press; 1993.

49. Harvey AG. A cognitive model of insomnia. Behav Res Ther. 2002;40(8):869–93. (Epub 2002/08/21).

50. Li F, Fisher KJ, Harmer P, Irbe D, Tearse RG, Weimer C. Tai chi and self-rated quality of sleep and daytime sleepiness in older adults: a randomized controlled trial. J Am Geriatr Soc. 2004;52(6):892–900. (Epub 2004/05/27).

51. Singh NA, Clements KM, Fiatarone MA. A randomized controlled trial of the effect of exercise on sleep. Sleep. 1997;20(2):95–101. (Epub 1997/02/01).

52. Mustian KM, Sprod LK, Janelsins M, Peppone LJ, Palesh OG, Chandwani K, et al. Multicenter, randomized controlled trial of yoga for sleep quality among cancer survivors. J Clin Oncol. 2013;31(26):3233–41. (Epub 2013/08/14).

53. Morgenthaler TI, Kapen S, Lee-Chiong T, Alessi C, Boehlecke B, Brown T, et al. Practice parameters for the medical therapy of obstructive sleep apnea. Sleep. 2006;29(8):1031–5.

54. Weaver TE, Grunstein RR. Adherence to continuous positive airway pressure therapy: the challenge to effective treatment. Proc Am Thorac Soc. 2008;5(2):173–8.

55. Weaver TE, Maislin G, Dinges DF, Bloxham T, George CF, Greenberg H, et al. Relationship between hours of CPAP use and achieving normal levels of sleepiness and daily functioning. Sleep. 2007;30(6):711–9.

56. Epstein LJ, Kristo D, Strollo PJ Jr, Friedman N, Malhotra A, Patil SP, et al. Clinical guideline for the evaluation, management and long-term care of obstructive sleep apnea in adults. J Clin Sleep Med. 2009;5(3):263–76. (Epub 2009/12/08).

57. Aloia MS, Arnedt JT, Strand M, Millman RP, Borrelli B. Motivational enhancement to improve adherence to positive airway pressure in patients with obstructive sleep apnea: a randomized controlled trial. Sleep. 2013;36(11):1655–62. (Epub 2013/11/02).

58. Wickwire EM, Lettieri CJ, Cairns AA, Collop NA. Maximizing positive airway pressure adherence in adults: a common-sense approach. Chest. 2013;144(2):680–93. (Epub 2013/08/07).

59. Greenburg DL, Lettieri CJ, Eliasson AH. Effects of surgical weight loss on measures of obstructive sleep apnea: a meta-analysis. Am J Med. 2009;122(6):535–42. (Epub 2009/06/03).

60. Mitchell LJ, Davidson ZE, Bonham M, O'Driskcoll DM, Hamilton GS, Truby H. Weight loss from lifestyle interventions and severity of sleep apnea: a systematic review and meta-analysis. Sleep Med. 2014;15:1173–83.

61. Tuomilehto HP, Seppa JM, Partinen MM, Peltonen M, Gylling H, Tuomilehto JO, et al. Lifestyle intervention with weight reduction: first-line treatment in mild obstructive sleep apnea. Am J Respir Crit Care Med. 2009;179(4):320–7. (Epub 2008/11/18).

62. Iftikhar IH, Kline CE, Youngstedt SD. Effects of exercise training on sleep apnea: a meta-analysis. Lung. 2014;192(1):175–84. (Epub 2013/10/01).

63. Sutherland K, Vanderveken OM, Tsuda H, Marklund M, Gagnadoux F, Kushida CA, et al. Oral appliance treatment for obstructive sleep apnea: an update. J Clin Sleep Med. 2014;10(2):215–27. (Epub 2014/02/18).

64. Oksenberg AS. Positional therapy for sleep apnea: a promising behavioral therapeutic option still waiting for qualified studies. Sleep Med Rev. 2014;18(1):3–5. (Epub 2013/10/09).

65. Kotecha BT, Hall AC. Role of surgery in adult obstructive sleep apnoea. Sleep Med Rev. 2014;18:405–13. (Epub 2014/04/08).

66. Morgenthaler TI, Lee-Chiong T, Alessi C, Friedman L, Aurora RN, Boehlecke B, et al. Practice parameters for the clinical evaluation and treatment of circadian rhythm sleep disorders. An American Academy of Sleep Medicine report. Sleep. 2007;30(11):1445–59. (Epub 2007/11/29).

67. Smith MR, Fogg LF, Eastman CI. Practical interventions to promote circadian adaptation to permanent night shift work: study 4. J Biol Rhythms. 2009;24(2):161–72. (Epub 2009/04/07).

68. Thorpy MJ. Managing the patient with shift-work disorder. J Fam Pract. 2010;59(1 Suppl):S24–S31. (Epub 2010/01/28).

Integrative Medicine

Melinda Ring and Leslie Mendoza Temple

Abbreviations

ANC	Academic naturopathic clinic
BMI	Body mass index
CAM	Complementary and alternative medicine
CI	Confidence interval
DNS	Diabetic neuropathy symptom
FFMQ	Five Facet Mindfulness Questionnaire
HPUS	Homeopathic Pharmacopeia of the United States
HT	Healing touch
IFM	Institute for Functional Medicine
LAc	Licensed acupuncturists
MBSR	Mindfulness-based stress reduction
MSQ	Medical Symptom Questionnaire
NCCAM	National Center for Complementary and Alternative Medicine
NCRCI	National Center for Research on Complementary and Integrative Health
NDs	Naturopathic doctors
PHS	Public Health Service
RCT	Randomized controlled trial
SDSC	Summary Diabetes Self-Care Activities Questionnaire
SF-12	Short Form 12
TCM	Traditional Chinese medicine
T2D	Type-2 diabetes
TM	Transcendental meditation
TT	Therapeutic touch

L. M. Temple (✉)
NorthShore University HealthSystem Integrative Medicine Program, University of Chicago Pritzker School of Medicine, 2400 Chestnut Ave, Glenview, IL 60026, USA
e-mail: lmendoza@northshore.org

M. Ring
Osher Center for Integrative Medicine at Northwestern University, Northwestern Feinberg School of Medicine, Chicago, IL, USA

Terminology in Integrative Medicine

Over the past 50 years, the field of integrative medicine has evolved in response to scientific, economic, and social factors from a grassroots movement of patients seeking out alternatives to the Western biomedical paradigm to a place where integrative medicine, in many settings, may be regarded as a part of mainstream medicine. Various terms that have been used to describe this phenomenon and new paradigm of care are described below.

Holistic Medicine

The growth of the whole foods and supplement industries in the 1950s, along with increased awareness of foreign treatment approaches (e.g., acupuncture) through media exposure, has contributed to the emergence of the holistic health movement in the 1970s [1–3]. Holistic practice emphasizes an attention to the whole person, including the physical, spiritual, psychological, and ecological dimensions of healing.

Complementary and Alternative Medicine (CAM)

Increasing patient use of unconventional health care practices, presumably in place of conventional health care, led to the adoption of the term "alternative medicine" in the USA and Europe in the late 1980s [4, 5]. Landmark surveys in the early 1990s, most notably "Trends in Alternative Medicine Use" by Harvard researcher David Eisenberg, MD, found that consumers were accessing a range of therapeutic and preventive options, both alternative and conventional, to essentially "complement" one another [6]. Subsequently the terms "complementary medicine" and "complementary and alternative medicine (CAM)" became designations for health care used as adjuncts to conventional health care. Congress applied the phrase to the National Institutes of Health's National Center for Complementary and Alternative Medicine (NCCAM), when the Office of Alternative Medicine was upgraded to the status of a coordinating research center in 1999. Studies found that many viewed CAM to be more aligned with "their own values, beliefs and philosophical orientation towards health and life than traditional medicine." [7]

Integrative Medicine or Integrative Health Care

The growth of research on CAM practices, as well as an evolving understanding that the change needed in health care was not only the inclusion of a broader range of disciplines but also a transformation in the paradigm of health and healing, led to a transition to the term "integrative medicine" or more recently "integrative health care." Integrative medicine has been described as:

> healing-oriented medicine that takes account of the whole person (body, mind and spirit), including all aspects of lifestyle. It emphasizes the therapeutic relationship and makes use of all appropriate therapies, both conventional and alternative. [8]

In this context, lifestyle medicine becomes a core aspect of integrative medicine. Indeed, any good integrative plan should fundamentally address the four pillars of health: nutrition, physical activity, stress management, and sleep. The use of dietary supplements or complementary medicine disciplines becomes a secondary line of defense.

The 2012 publication *Integrative Medicine in America: How Integrative Medicine Is Being Practiced in Clinical Centers Across the United States* documented strong affiliations of integrative medicine programs to hospitals, health care systems, and medical and nursing schools [9]. US hospitals report increasing percentages, up to 42% of respondents in a national survey in 2010, offering some form of CAM therapies as part of their inpatient or outpatient services [10]. Academic medicine is similarly embracing the importance of integrative medicine: As of 2014, there are 14 established integrative medicine fellowship programs, the American Board of Physician Specialties offered the first American Board of Integrative Medicine in November 2014, and the Consortium of Academic Health Centers for Integrative Medicine has grown from 8 to 65 (member institutions) over the past decade [11–13]. Congress similarly has acknowledged the field with a proposed name change for the NCCAM to the National Center for Research on Complementary and Integrative Health (NCRCI) [14].

With prevalence of use of integrative medicine among patients approaching 40% and even higher in some disease states, all health care practitioners should be aware of the current state of evidence of integrative approaches relevant to their area of interest [15, 16]. In particular, health care providers with an inherent interest in lifestyle and preven-

tive medicine should recognize the significant overlap and congruent philosophies between the fields.

The NCCAM Framework with a Focus on Diabetes

While integrative medicine contains, at its essence, a philosophy of how health care should be delivered, the inclusion of evidence-based CAM disciplines is intrinsic to an integrative care plan. The NCCAM developed a framework for categorizing these therapies:

- Biologically based therapies
- Mind–body medicine
- Energy medicine
- Manual therapies
- Whole healing systems

While in no way comprehensive of all existing evidence, the discussion of this framework using a patient with diabetes is intended to provide a basic understanding of how an integrative care plan might be constructed for a particular patient.

Biologically Based Therapies

A literature review based on 18 studies from nine countries suggested that the prevalence of CAM use among diabetics worldwide ranges from 17 to 72.8% [17]. The most widely used therapies among patients with diabetes were nutritional/dietary and herbal supplements, nutritional advice, spiritual healing, and relaxation techniques. A focus on the US population drawn from the 1997 National Health Interview Survey found that while 57% of patients with diabetes used a CAM therapy in the past year, excluding prayer, only 20% did so specifically to treat their diabetes [18]. The prevalence of CAM use reinforces that health care professionals need to be aware and incorporate this type of information into the processes of patient assessment and intervention.

- Chances are that patients are taking supplements or considering them while also taking multiple medications for diabetes and other conditions. Hence, there exists the potential for drug interactions leading to adverse events [19, 20]. Many patients do not inform their health providers that they are taking additional supplements, or they are not asked. This prospective lack of crucial information may impact clinical decision-making. Hence, it is imperative to perform a thorough interview and cross-check for herb-drug and herb-dietary supplement interactions. The evidence base is building for the use of certain natural products and may be considered safe additions to patient treatment plans. However, many products are still in need of a comprehensive review for safety and efficacy. It is important to note that overall, the evidence base for supplements and herbs needs further development with respect to scientific rigor and consistency of studied natural products. In the authors' experience, diabetes is best managed with a combination of pharmaceuticals, nutrition, lifestyle management, and the potential addition of herbs and supplements, depending on the individual and the clinician's experience. By the time the disease has reached clinical criterion for diabetes, herbs and supplements are typically not sufficient and to replace medications for glycemic control. However, natural products may be helpful in supporting conventional diabetes treatment, particularly in combination with a strong regimen of healthy diet, stress management and regular exercise, with the goal to potentially limit pharmaceutical dose escalation or addition of new pharmaceuticals.

- The decision to recommend supplements should be based on whether evidence exists regarding their safety

and efficacy. Questions about supplements may be initiated by the patient who learned of specific natural products from reliable or unreliable information sources. The claims can range from Food and Drug Administration (FDA)-allowed functional claims (i.e., "supports vascular health") to frank and inappropriate overstatements (i.e., "reverses diabetes"). It is helpful to review the marketing literature online with the patient, or to read through the written materials that the patient brings in to critically review the merit of the supplement. Then, the clinician can turn to one of several excellent, non-industry-sponsored natural products databases to review those same products for clinical decision-making. A summary of commonly used natural products for diabetes and insulin resistance is given in Table 18.1. Guidance on brands for purchasing decisions and recommendations may be found on the non-industry-sponsored Web site www.consumerlab.com.

Of the natural products listed in Table 18.1, alpha-lipoic acid has some evidence base for improving blood sugar lev-

Table 18.1 Diabetes medications and natural products. Many natural products are tried for diabetes, but very few have reliable evidence of efficacy. Inclusion in this list does *not* imply that these products are effective for diabetes. (Adapted with permission from *Natural Medicines in the Clinical Management of Diabetes.* [91])

Mechanism of action	Pharmaceutical agent	Natural product
Hypoglycemic	Chlorpropamide *(Diabinese)* Glimepiride *(Amaryl)* Glipizide *(Glucotrol)* Glyburide *(DiaBeta, Glynase, Micronase)* Nateglinide *(Starlix)* Repaglinide *(Prandin)* Tolazamide *(Tolinase)* Tolbutamide *(Orinase)*	Banaba *(Lagerstroemia speciosa)* Bitter melon *(Momordica charantia)* Fenugreek *(Trigonella foenum-graecum)* Gymnema *(Gymnema sylvestre)*
Insulin sensitizers	Metformin *(Glucophage)* Pioglitazone *(Actos)* Rosiglitazone *(Avandia)*	Agaricus mushroom *(Agaricus blazei)* American ginseng *(Panax quinquefolius)* Banaba *(Lagerstroemia speciosa)* Cassia cinnamon *(Cinnamomum aromaticum)* Chromium Magnesium Panax ginseng Prickly pear cactus *(Opuntia ficus-indica)* Soy *(Glycine max)* Vanadium
Carbohydrate absorption inhibitors	Acarbose *(Precose)* Miglitol *(Glyset)*	Bean pod *(Phaseolus vulgaris)* Blond psyllium *(Plantago ovata)* Fenugreek *(Trigonella foenum-graecum)* Glucomannan *(Amorphophallus konjac)* Guar gum *(Cyamopsis tetragonoloba)* Oat bran *(Avena sativa)* Prickly pear cactus *(Opuntia ficus-indica)* Soy *(Glycine max)* White mulberry *(Morus alba)*
Miscellaneous	Exenatide *(Byetta)*, Pramlintide *(Symlin)*, Liraglutide *(Victoza)*, Albiglutide *(Tanzeum)*, Dulaglutide *(Trulicity)* Saxagliptin *(Onglyza)*, Sitagliptin *(Januvia)*, Linagliptin *(Tradjenta)*, Alogliptin *(Nesina)* Canagliflozin *(invokana)*, Dapagliflozin *(farxiga)*, Empagliflozin *(jardiance)*	*Alpha lipoic acid* Chia *(Salvia hispanica)* Coenzyme Q10 Selenium Stevia *(Stevia rebaudiana)*

els in patients with type-2 diabetes (T2D) [21–26]. Alpha-lipoic acid is an endogenous coenzyme with antioxidant and insulin-sensitizing activity. As a supplement to augment conventional treatment for diabetes, alpha-lipoic acid may help reduce diabetic neuropathy symptoms of burning, tingling, and numbness; however, it may take a month or more of compliant usage for noticeable improvement. The dose range for diabetic neuropathy is between 600 and 1200 mg per day [21–26]. Again, It is important to note that supplements are not frank substitutes for conventional therapies in diabetes, but they may have potential to provide benefit as a supportive therapy in patients who are particularly interested in natural products.

Mind–Body Medicine

Mind–body medicine, based on the interdependence of our mental, emotional, and physical states, is reviewed in detail in Chap. 16. The inclusion of a mind–body approach for stress management is a core aspect of many integrative treatment plans. Diabetes is no exception since cortically mediated stress responses modulate glycemic control through immune-neuroendocrine activation, hyperinsulinemia, hyperlipidemia, inflammation, and with chronic exposure, compromised immunity, insulin resistance, and obesity. Research showing benefits of mind–body interventions in patients with diabetes is limited; however, risks are minimal. Movement-based mind–body approaches, such as yoga and Tai Chi, supplement the needed physical activity allotment for patients with diabetes, with the relative risk similar to that of other physical activities. The current evidence for five mind–body therapies in patients with T2D is reviewed below.

Biofeedback

Biofeedback is a self-regulation technique in which patients learn to have voluntary control over aspects of their physiology. Sensors that monitor physiological functions such as blood pressure, muscle tension, heart rate variability, and brain waves report back to the patient how active engagement in a relaxation approach is creating changes in their system, thereby reinforcing the benefits of the activity. Biofeedback in combination with standard care was found in a small randomized controlled trial (RCT) to improve glycemic control compared to standard care plus education [33]. Biofeedback-assisted relaxation training, measuring surface electromyography, and thermal feedback, provided via 10 weekly 45-min sessions, also showed significant improvement in glycemic control with a reduction in A1C levels from 7.4 to 6.8%; this improvement persisted at 3-month follow-up.

Biofeedback has also been studied for diabetic neuropathy, as this complication can produce clinically significant

toe temperature elevations. In patients with T2D, volitional warming has been associated with increased circulation, improved intermittent claudication pain, more rapid healing of diabetic ulcers, and improved functional status [34–36].

Yoga

Yoga is an ancient system of relaxation, exercise, and healing with origins in Indian philosophy. The word "yoga" comes from the Sanskrit root *yuj* or "to yoke," implying a uniting of the physical, spiritual, and mental bodies. The practice of yoga may include techniques of movement (*asanas* or poses), breathing *(pranayama),* meditation *(dhyan)*, chanting, and lifestyle change.

Two systematic reviews concluded that yoga is likely to provide benefits with lowered fasting blood glucose and A1C, improved lipid profiles, and reduced body weight and waist-to-hip ratio [37, 38]. A third more rigorous systematic review identified five trials that met the inclusion criteria [39]. The reviewers criticized the studies for having a medium to high risk of bias, small sample sizes, and different intervention characteristics. The studies' results showed improvement in short- to intermediate- term outcomes, such as fasting blood glucose and lipids. However, not all changes were statistically significant. Results of a qualitative study suggest that yoga may have ancillary benefits in terms of improved physical function, enhanced mental/emotional state, enriched sleep quality, and improved lifestyle choices, and, furthermore, that yoga may be useful as a health promotion strategy [40]. At this point, it is reasonable to recommend yoga as an option for patients as part of their physical activity routine.

Meditation

Meditation is a technique of mental concentration that involves the conscious direction of one's attention toward breathwork, a sustained or repeated sound or word, or some other object of focus, as a means to increase awareness of the present, reduce stress, promote relaxation, and attain personal growth. A variety of meditation techniques are commonly used and have extensive literature demonstrating benefits for stress reduction both in clinical and basic research studies. Meditation has been shown to affect the hypothalamic–pituitary–adrenal axis, as evidenced by reduced cortisol output with experimental stressors [41]. There are now several apps available for smartphones or Internet sites that can guide a patient through self-directed meditation.

A 16-week RCT examined the effects of transcendental meditation (TM) versus health education on components of metabolic syndrome and coronary heart disease [42]. At the end of the trial, patients in the TM group had significantly lower blood pressure, improved fasting blood glucose and insulin levels, and improved heart rate variability.

Mindfulness-Based Stress Reduction

The practice of mindfulness-based stress reduction (MBSR) seeks to establish and reinforce a nonreactive, nonjudgmental approach to thoughts and emotions and to cultivate acceptance through moment-to-moment awareness or "mindfulness." A small, prospective, observational study of 14 patients who completed the 8-week standardized MBSR course found a reduction in A1C of 0.5% and reduced mean arterial pressure of 6 mmHg, as well as decreases in depression, anxiety, and general psychological distress [43]. An extended randomized trial (mindfulness intervention vs. usual care) study will examine impact over 5 years; already at the 1-year follow-up mark, the MBSR group showed lower levels of depression and improved health status compared with the control group [44]. A 2014 systematic review and meta-analysis of mindfulness-based RCTs pertinent to lifestyle medicine concluded that partial evidence exists across a wide range of populations and outcomes, particularly in diet/weight management and symptom burden [45].

Tai Chi

Tai Chi is a mind–body practice from China with roots in martial arts and ancient healing traditions. Tai Chi consists of coordinated gentle movements with mental focus, breathing, and relaxation. A 2011 systematic review of Tai Chi and diabetes identified eight RCTs and three nonrandomized clinical trials [46]. While some studies showed trends toward benefits in both glycemic control and quality of life measures, few were statistically significant.

Energy Medicine

Energy medicine can be divided into two major categories. The first category relates to bioelectromagnetic energy therapies: the use of concrete energy interventions such as light therapy for seasonal affective disorder or magnet therapy for bone fracture healing. The second category refers to energy biofields: the concept that living things have energy fields that interact with their environment and influence health and disease states. While the scientific understanding of biofield therapies is in its infancy, the concept can be found in cultures across the world: therapeutic touch (TT) and healing touch (HT) in Western medicine, Reiki (ray-key) in Japan, and Qigong (chi-kung) in China. These practices are based on the belief that problems in the patient's energy field that cause illness and pain can be identified and rebalanced by a healer placing his/her hands either gently on the patient or above the patient in the biofield. A study done in 2007 by the National Health Interview Survey indicates that 1.2 million adults and 161,000 children received one or more sessions of energy healing therapy, such as Reiki, in the previous year

[47]. The use of biofield therapies remains controversial and the evidence is questionable. Nevertheless, light touch or no touch approaches carry little risk to the patient.

Western Touch Therapies

TT and HT are Western-born nursing-based interventions that have been used for more than 25 years to support and comfort patients [48]. In the 1970s, Delores Krieger, PhD, RN, developed TT. An American hospital survey conducted in 2005 noted that about 30% of 1400 responding hospitals offered TT [49]. Janet Mentgen, RN, founded HT in 1989 as a continuing education program for nurses, massage therapists, other health care professionals, and laypersons [50]. More than 90,000 nurses and other health professionals use HT in hospitals and in private practice, with at least 100 US hospitals offering the service in the past 15 years. The American Holistic Nurses Association's position statement on CAM endorses noninvasive energy work as valid nursing interventions to render holistic care [51].

Due to the nursing link, these approaches have been evaluated in more research than other energy medicine approaches. Early studies indicated efficacy in muscle relaxation, pain and stress, and anxiety reduction in a variety of settings, patients, and disease states, as well as physiological effects on blood pressure and temperature [52, 53]. Meta-analyses examining TT and HT as nursing interventions concluded that touch therapies have a positive, intermediate effect on physiological and psychological variables, but many of the studies had significant methodological issues that could significantly bias the reported results [54–56].

Reiki

Buddhist monks may have practiced this Eastern form of healing 2500 years ago. Reiki healing was formalized in Japan in 1920 and brought to the US in 1937. According to the American Hospital Association, in 2007, 15% or more than 800 American hospitals offered Reiki as part of hospital services [57]. A student can learn to provide level 1 Reiki during a weekend class, making the practice attractive to nurses and other health care practitioners as well as the lay public; advanced skills require additional training. There is no standardization or certification for Reiki practitioners and protocols, since hand positions can vary among teachers and lead to difficulty in conducting research.

Overall, high-quality research on Reiki is scant. A review summarizing investigations using Reiki for effects on stress, relaxation, depression, pain, and wound healing concluded that results in all areas were inconsistent [58]. One study explored the efficacy of Reiki to control peripheral diabetic neuropathy. Global pain scores and walking distance improved from baseline in both the Reiki and mimic-Reiki groups, with no significant differences at the final visit [59].

Manual Therapy

Chiropractic is a health care profession that focuses on the relationship between the body's structure, mainly the spine, and its ability to function. Although practitioners may use a variety of treatment approaches, they primarily perform adjustments (manipulations) to the spine or other parts of the body.

Osteopathic medicine is a distinct form of medical practice in that it provides all the aspects of conventional medicine (i.e., pharmaceuticals, surgery, and diagnostic testing) while additionally offering hands-on diagnosis and treatment through osteopathic manipulative medicine. Since both chiropractic and osteopathic manipulation utilize manual therapies, it is important to recognize the distinction in the professions. The goal of manual therapies is to correct alignment, alleviate pain, improve function, and support the body's natural ability to heal itself.

Patients with and without diabetes may have concomitant musculoskeletal and neurological dysfunction. The use of manual manipulation may help manage these conditions when performed appropriately. The "UK Evidence Report" on manual therapies is a systematic review of 46 RCTs and 16 evidence-based clinical guidelines by Bronfort et al. [27]. The report concluded that spinal and joint manipulation and mobilization were effective in adults for acute, subacute, and chronic low back pain, migraine and cervicogenic headache, cervicogenic dizziness, several extremity joint conditions, and acute and subacute neck pain. An updated review of the 2010 UK Report by Clar et al. [28] additionally supported manual manipulation for shoulder pain and dysfunction, plantar fasciitis, and myofascial release for cancer care. Mild-to-moderate adverse events of transient nature (e.g., worsening symptoms, increased pain, soreness, headache, dizziness, tiredness, nausea, and vomiting) may occur with manipulation and mobilization procedures. The risk of major adverse events is very low and includes vertebrobasilar artery stroke, lumbar disc herniation, and cauda equina syndrome [27, 29, 30].

Massage therapy encompasses many different techniques where therapists apply pressure and rub or otherwise manipulate the muscles, connective tissue, tendons, and ligaments of the body to promote relaxation, reduce pain and stiffness, and enhance well-being. The evidence base for massage therapy in improving chronic low back pain appears promising [31, 32]. For diabetes, however, there are not enough quality studies to support use, specifically for this condition. Positive effects of anxiety reduction, deep relaxation, increased body awareness, and pain reduction with low risk to the patient may merit prescription of massage therapy for patients with diabetes dealing with chronic anxiety, stress, or pain.

Whole Healing Systems

Naturopathic Medicine

Naturopathic medicine is a holistic approach based on the following six principles of healing:

1. The body has the inherent ability to maintain and restore health.
2. The physician aims to identify and treat the cause rather than the symptoms.
3. Methods designed to suppress the symptoms and not the cause are considered harmful and should be avoided or minimized.
4. The physician treats the whole person—taking into account the physical, spiritual, mental, and social aspects of the individual.
5. The physician plays a role in educating and encouraging the patient to take responsibility for his/her health.
6. The physician assesses risk factors and hereditary susceptibility to disease to make appropriate interventions to avoid further harm or risk to the patient.

Naturopathic doctors (NDs) are trained as primary care physicians in 4-year, accredited doctoral-level naturopathic medical schools; there are eight accredited naturopathic colleges in North America [60]. The 4-year graduate level program includes about 4500 h of academic and clinical training in topics such as clinical nutrition, homeopathic medicine, botanical medicine, psychology, and counseling. Following graduation, an ND takes rigorous professional board exams; currently 17 states, the District of Columbia, Puerto Rico, and the Virgin Islands have licensing or regulation laws for NDs [61].

Several recent studies have examined the impact of a naturopathic approach as an adjunct to conventional care on clinical outcomes.

- A retrospective analysis of medical records from an academic naturopathic clinic (ANC) investigated treatment recommendations and levels of evidence. Naturopathic physicians prescribe comprehensive therapeutic lifestyle change recommendations supported by a high level of evidence consistent with existing scientific guidelines from national organizations such as the ADA, JNC, and NCEP. Among patients receiving naturopathic care, 100% received dietary counseling, 69% were taught stress reduction techniques, and 94% were prescribed exercise. All patients additionally received prescriptions for botanical and nutritional supplementation, often in combination with conventional medication [62].
- Forty patients with poorly controlled T2D (A1C 7.5–9.5%) were invited from a large integrated health care

system to receive up to eight naturopathic visits. In addition to clinical markers, standardized questionnaires were administered by telephone to collect outcome data on self-care, self-efficacy, diabetes problem areas, perceived stress, motivation, and mood. These results were compared to a cohort of 329 eligible, nonparticipating patients using electronic medical records data. Participants made an average of 3.9 ANC visits. At 6 months, significant improvements were found in most patient-reported measures, including glucose testing, diet, physical activity, mood, self-efficacy, and motivation to change lifestyle, with improvements in all (except physical activity and diet) persisting at 12 months. Compared to usual care, there was a significant decrease in mean A1C at 6 months (-0.90% ($P=0.02$)) in the ANC cohort at 6 months, a -0.51% mean difference compared to usual care ($P=0.07$), which did not persist at 12 months [63].

- A multisite RCT of enhanced usual care (usual care plus biometric measurement) compared with enhanced usual care plus naturopathic care. Postal workers aged 25–65 years with an increased risk of cardiovascular disease were invited to participate. Participants in both groups received care from their family physicians. Those in the naturopathic group also received individualized care (health promotion counseling, nutritional medicine, or dietary supplementation) at seven preset times in work-site clinics by licensed naturopathic doctors. Of the 246 participants randomly assigned to a study group, 207 completed the study. Compared with the control group, at 1 year, those in the naturopathic group had a reduced adjusted 10-year cardiovascular risk based on the Framingham Risk Score (control: 10.81%; naturopathic group: 7.74%; risk reduction -3.07% [95% confidence interval (CI) -4.35% to -1.78%], $p<0.001$) and a lower adjusted frequency of metabolic syndrome (control group: 48.48%; naturopathic care: 31.58%; risk reduction -16.90% [95% CI -29.55% to -4.25%], $p=0.002$.) [64]. A follow-up evaluation of the economic impact showed that these risk reductions had average net study-year savings of $1138 in societal costs and $1187 in employer costs [65].

These preliminary findings suggest that the addition of naturopathic care to usual care may be an option for supporting patients through lifestyle behavior changes. The personalized, holistic approach may appeal to some patients. Licensing and insurance coverage remain issues that may be barriers to access.

Functional Medicine

In 1990, Dr. Jeffrey Bland formulated the concept of functional medicine, subsequently forming the Institute for Functional Medicine (IFM) to educate and support the implementation of functional medicine across disciplines [66]. According to the IFM Web site, (www.functionalmedicine.org, accessed on June 1, 2014) functional medicine is:

> a systems-biology approach to the prevention and management of chronic disease utilizing appropriate tools including nutrition, lifestyle, exercise, environment, structural, cognitive, emotional, and pharmaceutical therapies to meet the individual needs of the patient. …by shifting the traditional disease-centered focus of medical practice to a more patient-centered approach, functional medicine addresses the whole person, not just an isolated set of symptoms. Functional medicine practitioners spend time … looking at the interactions among genetic, environmental, and lifestyle factors that can influence long-term health and complex, chronic disease.

Training through the IFM, and more recently some competing organizations, is available internationally to licensed health care professionals. The Accreditation Council for Continuing Medical Education accredits the IFM to provide continuing medical education for physicians. According to the IFM, more than 100,000 practitioners from 91 countries have been introduced to the principles and practices of functional medicine [66]. Faculty members from one fifth of all US medical schools have attended the foundational training course, *Applying Functional Medicine in Clinical Practice.*

Clinicians are trained to first, based on the patient's story, identify possible predisposing factors, triggering events, and mediators, as well as assess five categories of modifiable personal lifestyle factors: sleep and relaxation, exercise and movement, nutrition, stress, and relationships [67]. The next step involves evaluation of seven functional/biological systems to understand possible functional imbalances that underlie the disease: assimilation, defense and repair, energy, biotransformation and elimination, transport, communication, and structural integrity. Assessments of these areas are often accomplished through the use of specialized testing. Then, customized interventions are created using tools from both conventional and integrative medicine, as well as lifestyle adjustments.

Despite the escalating popularity of functional medicine among both health care professionals seeking a new way to care for patients and patients seeking a more personalized and holistic approach, there exist little data on the benefits of a functional medicine systematic approach. A pilot study of a functional medicine program, including a longitudinal comprehensive mindfulness-based therapeutic lifestyle change program in 26 patients with diabetes over 6 months, shows significant improvements in weight, waist circumference, body mass index (BMI), and patient-reported outcome measures (Five Facet Mindfulness Questionnaire (FFMQ) and Medical Symptom Questionnaire (MSQ); EuroQol's EQ5D and Short Form 12 (SF-12); and the Summary Diabetes Self-Care Activities Questionnaire (SDSC)). The publication does not provide additional information regarding how this functional medicine intervention differs from usual recommended counseling on lifestyle factors [68].

While frequently offered in private practices, a national survey of integrative medicine physicians in academic health centers reported that 34% use some degree of functional medicine in their practices as well [69]. The functional medicine movement is a growing player in the options available to patients. Additional research is needed to validate individual, programmatic, and economic components of this care option.

Homeopathy

Homeopathy is a system of medicine developed by the German doctor Samuel Hahnemann in the early 1800s based on the law of similars, often described as "like cures like" [70]. For example, a substance known to cause vomiting, such as ipecac, may be thought to prevent emesis when used in extremely small doses. Additional core principles include those of using the minimum dose possible and the use of "potentization" whereby a substance is sequentially diluted and vigorously shaken between each dilution. Homeopathic products may be made from plants, minerals, and organic compounds. The 1938 Federal Food, Drug, and Cosmetic Act recognized all homeopathic preparations described in the *Homeopathic Pharmacopeia of the United States* (HPUS) as drugs. In addition to legalizing the manufacture and sale of homeopathic remedies in the USA, this Act permitted them to be regulated in the same manner as nonprescription, over-the-counter drugs. The US FDA currently regulates the manufacturing of homeopathic remedies but does not evaluate their safety or effectiveness [71]. Licensure and scope of practice is determined by each state in the USA. Homeopathic preparations are generally considered safe, although reports of contamination with heavy metals or medication have been reported [72].

Worldwide, the use of homeopathy for diabetes issues is quite common. In a study of children with type 1 diabetes in Germany, 42% received CAM treatment, most commonly homeopathy (14.5%) [73]. Among patients with diabetes attending a public primary care clinic in Malaysia, homeopathy was one of two most often cited natural therapies [74]. In contrast, a survey of a subset of academic health centers in the USA lists homeopathy among the least common prescribed integrative therapies [75].

Despite the high international prevalence of use, there are few studies on the impact of homeopathy on clinical outcomes in diabetes. Animal studies of the homeopathic preparations of *Syzygium jambolanum* and *Cephalandra indica* in rats with experimentally induced T2D reported beneficial effects on fasting blood glucose, serum insulin and insulin signaling molecules in the skeletal muscle (gastrocnemius), and lipid profiles after treatment [76, 77]. Two recent prospective observational studies examined the benefit of individualized prescriptions of homeopathic medications for patients with diabetic neuropathy. In one pilot study, comparing 32

patients receiving homeopathic remedies to 29 controls, the treatment group reported significant improvements in the diabetic neuropathy symptom (DNS) score, as well as decreased cost of needed conventional drugs [78]. In a subsequent multicenter study ($n = 247$), a significant improvement in symptom scores was noted at 12 months, but not identified in objective measures such as conduction studies [79].

Traditional Chinese Medicine

The overarching principle in the practice of traditional Chinese medicine (TCM) is the achievement of a natural balance between Yin and Yang, the two opposing forces of the body represented in the ancient Chinese Taoism philosophy, dating more than 2500 years. When Yin and Yang become unbalanced, disease and dysfunction may occur. TCM encompasses many different practices in Asian medicine, including acupuncture (insertion of fine needles into specific body points), moxibustion (burning a herb above the skin to apply heat to acupuncture points), herbal medicine, tui na (Chinese therapeutic massage), dietary therapy, and Tai Chi and Qigong (movements, postures, coordinated breathing, and mental focus). Traditional systems of medicine also exist in other eastern and southern Asian countries, including Japan (where the traditional herbal medicine is called Kampo) and Korea. Acupuncture is the most methodically studied aspect of TCM.

A systematic review of RCTs for manual acupuncture to treat diabetic peripheral neuropathy showed benefits from the use of acupuncture and select B vitamins. The analysis included 25 trials with 1649 participants but had generally poor methodological quality and a high risk of bias. The meta-analysis showed that manual acupuncture had a greater effect on global symptom improvement compared with B1 and B12 vitamins, a combination of acupuncture and B vitamins, or no treatment. Adverse events were not reported in any trials [80].

In another systematic review regarding acupuncture and diabetic gastroparesis, 14 RCTs suggested that acupuncture treatment had a higher response rate than controls in significantly improving dyspeptic symptoms like nausea, vomiting, loss of appetite, and stomach fullness. There was no difference in solid gastric emptying between acupuncture and control groups. However, most studies had a high risk of bias and small sample size (median = 62). The majority of the RCTs reported a positive effect of acupuncture in improving dyspeptic symptoms [81].

The TCM approach to diabetes is multipronged and individualized to the patient's constitution and diagnosed imbalance of Yin and Yang, identified through the patient's history, tongue appearance, and radial pulse palpation. Weekly or semiweekly treatments are recommended to start, with a course of 10 or more treatments performed before assessing the overall effect on the patient and deciding to continue therapy. Side effects are rare and can include vasovagal syncope, infection, pain at needling sites, bruising, and organ puncture (extremely rare). Licensed acupuncturists (LAc) achieve the highest level of training in the field. Other health care providers, usually physicians and chiropractors, may pursue shorter courses of training in acupuncture to enhance their clinical practice and patient outcomes.

Ayurvedic Medicine

Ayurveda, which means "science of life," is derived from the Sanskrit words *ayur* meaning life and *veda* meaning knowledge. In Ayurveda, all objects and living bodies are composed of five basic structural elements, or *panchamahabhutas,* namely earth, water, fire, air, and vacuum (ether). Ayurveda espouses the theory of *tridoshas,* namely *vata* (ether and air), *pitta* (fire), and *kapha* (earth and water) that are physiological entities in living beings. Good health is achieved when the five structural elements and the three *doshas* are in a state of equilibrium. Any imbalance due to internal or external factors may cause disease. Ayurvedic treatment seeks to balance these elements with medicines (plant, animal, metal, or mineral derived), diet, exercise, yoga, breathing exercises, and lifestyle.

Ayurvedic practitioners also treat diabetes with a multipronged approach, including herbal medicine. For example, *shilajit,* turmeric, *neem, coccinea indica, amalaki, triphala,* bitter gourd, rose apple, leaves of *bilva,* cinnamon, *gymnema,* fenugreek, bay leaf, and aloe vera are some Ayurvedic diabetes medicines [82, 83].

A systematic review looked at several Ayurvedic herbal formulas and a whole-systems approach. Significant glucose-lowering effects were seen with the use of some herbal mixtures, but the studies had methodological deficiencies and small sample sizes [84].

There are reports of heavy metal contamination (such as lead) in herbal preparations resulting in intoxication [85]. There are also reports of some herbal products contaminated with oral hypoglycemic agents that could lead to adverse effects, such as hypoglycemic episodes [86].

Economics of CAM Use in the USA

Integrative medicine therapies are mostly spent out of pocket. In the National Health Interview Study in 2007 [16], more than 30 million adults reported out-of-pocket expenditures on CAM services, and of these individuals, 7.2 million were heavy CAM spenders with a mean annual expenditure of $1385. The top 25% of CAM spenders accounted for $10 billion of the $13.9 billion spent nationally on CAM in 2007[16]. Of the $13.9 billion spent in 2007, 60% was spent on manipulative and body-based therapies, 24% on mind–body therapies, 10% on alternative medical systems,

and 6.4% on biologically based therapies and energy healing therapy [87].

Adults in the highest quartile were more likely to reside in the Northeast or the West and less likely to reside in the Midwest, and were more likely to be older, female, non-Hispanic white, unmarried, and more educated. When compared to the $2.6 trillion spent on conventional health care [88], total expenditures on CAM ($13.9 billion) are small yet impressive.

Health Policy and Integrative Medicine

Public Health Service (PHS) Act Sect. 2706(a) in the Affordable Care Act states that a "group health plan and a health insurance issuer offering group or individual health insurance coverage shall not discriminate with respect to participation under the plan or coverage against any healthcare provider who is acting within the scope of that provider's license or certification under applicable state law." The law does not require "that a group health plan or health insurance issuer contract with any healthcare provider willing to abide by the terms and conditions for participation established by the plan or issuer," and nothing in the provision prevents "a group health plan, a health insurance issuer, or the Secretary from establishing varying reimbursement rates based on quality or performance measures." This provision does not require plans to accept all types of providers into a network nor does it govern provider reimbursement rates [89, 90]. The intent of this provision is to give consumers greater choices among the types of health care providers they visit, particularly holistic health care providers such as acupuncturists, chiropractors, massage therapists, and naturopathic physicians with the potential for insurance coverage, should these therapies gain inclusion in the individual's health plan.

Conclusion

With the great variety of diabetes therapies to choose from, whether conventional or complementary, the clinician has the daunting task of weighing the optimal treatment plan for his/her patient to achieve the best possible outcome. Various resources are available to physicians and other health care professionals to assist with this decision-making and are provided in Table 18.2. Glycemic control, symptom relief, reduction of morbidity and mortality, and enhancement of quality of life with a greater sense of well-being describe true success in managing the whole person with diabetes. In addition to weighing the evidence base for complementary and conventional therapies, factors such as time, finances, insurance coverage, cultural values, disease severity, and wellness objectives must come together to inform clinicians on designing the most sensible and effective treatment packages

Table 18.2 Resources for clinicians

Professional development for physicians[a]
Arizona Center for Integrative Medicine: 1000 h, 2-year distance learning program at the University of Arizona—www.integrativemedicine.arizona.edu
American Board of Integrative and Holistic Medicine—www.abihm.org
Clinical homeopathy: Center for Education and Development of Homeopathy—www.cedhusa.org
Institute for Functional Medicine—www.functionalmedicine.org
Medical acupuncture: Helms Medical Institute—www.hmieducation.com
Natural products databases
Consumer Lab: www.consumerlab.com
Memorial Sloan-Kettering (oncology): www.mskcc.org
Natural Medicines Comprehensive Database: www.naturaldatabase.com
Natural Standard: www.naturalmedicines.therapeuticresearch.com
Policy, research
National Center for Complementary and Integrative Health (NCCIH): https://nccih.nih.gov/
Academic Consortium for Integrative Medicine and Health: www.imconsortium.org
Academic Consortium for Complementary and Alternative Healthcare—www.accahc.org
International Society for Complementary Medicine Research—www.iscmr.org
Integrative and complementary medicine practitioner databases
Ayurveda: National Ayurvedic Medical Association—www.ayurvedanama.org
Chiropractic: American Chiropractic Association—www.acatoday.org
Healing Touch; Directory of Healing Touch practitioners—www.htpractitioner.com
Massage: American Massage Therapy Association—www.amtamassage.org
Naturopathy: American Association of Naturopathic Physicians—www.naturopathic.org
Traditional Chinese Medicine (TCM): National Certification Commission for Acupuncture and Oriental Medicine—www.nccaom.org
Board certification for integrative medicine
American Board of Physician Specialties: www.abpsus.org

[a] Some offerings are available for nurse practitioners and allied health professionals

for their patients. In a nutshell, the role of integrative medicine is consistent with the definition of lifestyle medicine as the nonpharmacological and nonsurgical management of chronic disease. The critical point, however, is whether the particular integrative medicine modality being considered is deemed safe and effective for the target indication.

References

1. Now RJ. Let me tell you about my appendectomy in Peking. NY Times. 26 July 1971;1(6).
2. Berliner HS, Salmon JW. The holistic alternative to scientific medicine: history and analysis. Int J Health Serv. 1980;10:133–47.
3. Lowenberg JS. Caring and responsibility: the crossroads between holistic practice and traditional medicine. Philadelphia: University of Pennsylvania Press; 1989.
4. Furnham A, Smith C. Choosing alternative medicine: a comparison of the beliefs of patients visiting a general practitioner and a homoeopath. Soc Sci Med. 1988;26(7):685–9.
5. Murray J, Shepherd S. Alternative or additional medicine? A new dilemma for the doctor. J R Coll Gen Pract. 1988;38(316):511–4.
6. Eisenberg DM, Kessler RC, Foster C, Norlock FE, Calkins DR, Delbanco TL. Unconventional medicine in the United States: prevalence, costs, and patterns of use. N Engl J Med. 1993;328:246–52.
7. Astin JA. Why patients use alternative medicine: results of a national study. JAMA. 1998;279(19):1548–53.
8. Rakel D, Weil A. Philosophy of integrative medicine. In: Rakel D, editor. Integrative medicine. 3rd ed. Philadelphia: Elsevier Inc.; 2012. p. 2–11.
9. Integrative Medicine in America. How integrative medicine is being practiced in clinical centers across the United States [Internet]. [cited 2014 May 27]. http://www.bravewell.org/current_projects/mapping_field/.
10. Ananth S. 2010 Complementary and Alternative Medicine Survey of Hospitals: Summary of Results [Internet]. Health Forum American Hospital Association and the Samueli Institute. 2011 Sept. http://www.siib.org/our-research/integrative-medicine/im-publications.
11. Ring M, Brodsky M, Low Dog T, Sierpina V, Bailey M, Locke A, Kogan M, Rindfleisch JA, Saper R. Developing and implementing core competencies for integrative medicine fellowships. Acad Med. 2014;89(3):421–8.
12. Integrative Medicine [Internet]. Tampa (FL): The American Board of Physician Specialties; c2014 [cited 2014 May 31]. http://www.abpsus.org/integrative-medicine.
13. IMConcortium.org [Internet]. Consortium of Academic Health Centers for Integrative Medicine; [updated 2013 Nov 5; cited 2014 May 29]. http://www.imconsortium.org.
14. Doctor's Page [Internet]. Bethesda (MD): National Center for Complementary and Alternative Medicine; [cited 2014 May 31]. http://nccam.nih.gov/about/offices/od/comments.
15. Eisenberg DM, Davis RB, Ettner SL, Appel S, Wilkey S, Van Rompay M, et al. Trends in alternative medicine use in the United States, 1990–1997: results of a follow-up national survey. JAMA. 1998;280(18):1569–75.
16. Barnes PM, Bloom B, Nahin R. The use of complementary and alternative medicine in the United States: findings from the 2007 National Health Interview Survey (NHIS) conducted by the National Center for Complementary and Alternative Medicine (NCCAM) and the National Center for Health Statistics. CDC Natl Health Statistics Rep #12 [Internet]. 2008 Dec [cited 2014 May 31]. http://nccam.nih.gov/news/camstats/2007/camsurvey_fs1.htm.

17. Chang HY, Wallis M, Tiralongo E. Use of complementary and alternative medicine among people living with diabetes: literature review. J Adv Nurs. 2007;58:307–19.

18. Yeh GY, Eisenberg DM, Davis RB, Phillips RS. Use of complementary and alternative medicine among persons with diabetes mellitus: results of a national survey. Am J Public Health. 2002;92(10):1648–52.

19. Kennedy DA, Seely D. Clinically based evidence of drug–herb interactions: a systematic review. Expert Opin Drug Saf. 2010;9:79–124.

20. Gardiner P, Graham RE, Legedza AT, Eisenberg DM, Phillips RS. Factors associated with dietary supplement use among prescription medication users. Arch Intern Med. 2006;166:1968–74.

21. Ziegler D, Hanefeld M, Ruhnau KJ, Hasche H, Lobisch M, Schütte K, et al. Treatment of symptomatic diabetic polyneuropathy with the antioxidant alpha-lipoic acid: a 7-month, multicenter, randomized, controlled trial (ALADIN III Study). Diabetes Care. 1999;22:1296–301.

22. Reljanovic M, Reichel G, Rett K, Lobisch M, Schuette K, Möller W, et al. Treatment of diabetic polyneuropathy with the antioxidant thioctic acid (alpha-lipoic acid): a 2-year, multicenter, randomized, double-blind, placebo-controlled trial (ALADIN II). Alpha Lipoic Acid in Diabetic Neuropathy [abstract]. Free Radic Res. 1999;31:171–7.

23. Ziegler D, Hanefeld M, Ruhnau KJ, Meissner HP, Lobisch M, Schütte K, et al. Treatment of symptomatic diabetic peripheral neuropathy with the antioxidant alpha-lipoic acid: a 3-week, multicentre randomized controlled trial (ALADIN Study). Diabetologia. 1995;38:1425–33.

24. Ruhnau KJ, Meissner HP, Finn JR, Reljanovic M, Lobisch M, Schütte K, et al. Effects of 3-week oral treatment with the antioxidant thioctic acid (alpha-lipoic acid) in symptomatic diabetic polyneuropathy. Diabet Med. 1999;16:1040–3.

25. Ametov AS, Barinov A, Dyck PJ, Hermann R, Kozlova N, Litchy WJ, et al. The sensory symptoms of diabetic polyneuropathy are improved with alpha-lipoic acid. Diabetes Care. 2003;26:770–6.

26. Ziegler D, Nowak H, Kempler P, Vargha P, Low PA. Treatment of symptomatic diabetic polyneuropathy with the antioxidant alpha-lipoic acid: a meta-analysis. Diabet Med. 2004;21:114–21.

27. Bronfort G, Haas M, Evans R, Leininger B, Triano J. Effectiveness of manual therapies: the UK evidence report. Chiropr Osteopat. 2010;18:3.

28. Clar C, Tsertsvadze A, Court R, Hundt GL, Clarke A, Sutcliffe P. Clinical effectiveness of manual therapy for the management of musculoskeletal and non-musculoskeletal conditions: systematic review and update of UK evidence report. Chiropr Man Therap. 2014;22:12. Epub 2014 March 28.

29. Rubinstein SM. Adverse events following chiropractic care for subjects with neck or low-back pain: do the benefits outweigh the risks? J Manipulative Physiol Ther. 2008;31:461–4.

30. Ernst E. Adverse effects of spinal manipulation: a systematic review. J R Soc Med. 2007;100:330–8.

31. Furlan AD, Imamura M, Dryden T, Irvin E. Massage for low-back pain. Cochrane Database Syst Rev. 2008;(4).

32. Kumar S, Beaton K, Hughes T. The effectiveness of massage therapy for the treatment of nonspecific low back pain: a systematic review of systematic reviews. Int J Gen Med. 2013;6:733–41.

33. McGinnis RA, McGrady A, Cox SA, Grower-Dowling KA. Biofeedback-assisted relaxation in type 2 diabetes. Diabetes Care. 2005;28:2145–9.

34. Shulimson AD, Lawrence PL, Iacono CU. Diabetic ulcers: the effect of thermal biofeedback-mediated relaxation training on healing. Biofeedback Self Regul. 1986;11(4):311–9.

35. Rice BI, Schindler JV. Effect of thermal biofeedback–assisted relaxation training on blood circulation in the lower extremities of a population with diabetes. Diabetes Care. 1992;15:853–9.

36. Fiero PL, Galper DI, Cox DJ, Phillips LH, Fryburg DA. Thermal biofeedback and lower extremity blood flow in adults with diabetes: is neuropathy a limiting factor? Appl Psychophysiol Biofeedback. 2003;28:193–203.

37. Alexander GK, Taylor AG, Innes KE, Kulbok P, Selfe TK. Contextualizing the effects of yoga therapy on diabetes management. Fam Community Health. 2008;31:228–39.

38. Innes KE, Vincent HK. The influence of yoga-based programs on risk profiles in adults with type 2 diabetes mellitus: a systematic review. Evid Based Complement Alternat Med. 2007;4:469–86.

39. Aljasir B, Bryson M, Al-Shehri B. Yoga practice for the management of type II diabetes mellitus in adults: a systematic review. Evid Based Complement Alternat Med. 2010;7:399–408.

40. Alexander GK. "More than I expected": perceived benefits of yoga practice among older adults at risk for cardiovascular disease. Complement Ther Med. 2013;21(1):14–28.

41. Pace TWW, Negi LT, Adams DD, Cole SP, Sivilli TI, Brown TD, Issa MJ, Raison CL. Effect of compassion meditation on neuroendocrine, innate immune and behavioral responses to psychosocial stress. Psychoneuroendocrinology. 2009;34(1):87–98.

42. Paul-Labrador M, Polk D, Dwyer JH, Velasquez I, Nidich S, Rainforth M, et al. Effects of a randomized controlled trial of transcendental meditation on components of the metabolic syndrome in subjects with coronary heart disease. Arch Intern Med. 2006;166(11):1218–24.

43. Rosenzweig S, Reibel DK, Greeson JM, Edman JS, Jasser SA, McMerty KD, et al. Mindfulness-based stress reduction is associated with improved glycemic control in type 2 diabetes mellitus: a pilot study. Altern Ther Health Med. 2007;13:36–8.

44. Hartmann M, Kopf S, Kircher C, Faude-Lang V, Djuric Z, Augstein F, et al. Sustained effects of a mindfulness-based stress-reduction intervention in type 2 diabetic patients: design and first results of a randomized controlled trial (the Heidelberger Diabetes and Stress-study). Diabetes Care. 2012;35:945–7.

45. Victorson D, Kentor M, Maletich C, Lawton RC, Kaufman VH, Borrero M, Languido L, Lewett K, Pancoe H, Berkowitz C. A systematic review and meta-analysis of mindfulness-based randomized controlled trials relevant to lifestyle medicine. Am J Lifestyle Med. Published online July 10, 2014 before print.

46. Lee MS, Choi TY, Lim HJ, Ernst E. Tai Chi for management of type 2 diabetes mellitus: a systematic review. Chin J Integr Med. 2011;17(10):789–93.

47. Barnes PM, Bloom B, Nahin R. Complementary and alternative medicine use among adults and children: United States, 2007. CDC National Health Statistics Report #12. 2008.

48. Engebretson J, Wardell D. Energy based modalities. Nurs Clin North Am. 2007;42:243–59.

49. Latest Survey Shows More Hospital Offering Complementary and Alternative Medicine Services [Internet]. American Hospital Association; c2006-14 [cited 2014 May 26]. www.aha.org/presscenter/pressrel/2008/080915-pr-cam.shtml.

50. HealingBeyondBorders.org [Internet]. Healing Touch International; c1997 [cited 2014 May 26]. www.healingbeyondborders.org.

51. Position Statements [Internet]. American Nurses Association; c2014 [cited 2014 May 26]. www.ahna.org/Resources/Publications/Position-Statements.

52. Quinn JF. Building a body of knowledge: research on therapeutic touch 1974–1986. J Holist Nurs. 1988;6(1):37–45.

53. Gagne D, Toye R. The effects of therapeutic touch and relaxation therapy in reducing anxiety. Arch Psychiatr Nurs. 1994;8:184–9.

54. Winstead-Fry P, Kijek J. An integrative review and meta-analysis of therapeutic touch research. Alternative. 1999;5(6):58–67.

55. Peters RM. The effectiveness of therapeutic touch: a meta-analytic review. Nurs Sci Q. 1999;12(1):52–61.

56. Anderson JG, Taylor AG. Effects of healing touch in clinical practice: a systematic review of randomized clinical trials. J Holist Nurs. 2011;29:221–8.

57. Firth K, Smith K. 2007 survey of healing environments in American hospitals: nature and prevalence. Samueli Institute, 2011. www.samueliinstitute.org/file%20library/our%20research/ohe/ohe-hospital-survey-final-report-2007.pdf. Accessed 6 Aug 2014.

58. Vitale A. An integrative review of Reiki touch therapy research. Holist Nurs Pract. 2007;21(4):167–79.

59. Gillespie E, Gillespie B, Stevens M. Painful diabetic neuropathy: impact of an alternative approach. Diabetes Care. 2007;30:999–1001.

60. AANMC.org [Internet]. Washington (DC): Association of Accredited Naturopathic Medical Colleges; c2014 [cited 2014 May 27]. http://aanmc.org.

61. Licensed States & Licensing Authorities [Internet]. American Association of Naturopathic Physicians; c2014 [cited 2014 May 27]. http://www.naturopathic.org/content.asp?contentid=57.

62. Bradley R, Oberg EB. Naturopathic medicine and type 2 diabetes: a retrospective analysis from an academic clinic. Altern Med Rev. 2006;11(1):30–9.

63. Bradley R, Sherman KJ, Catz S, Calabrese C, Oberg EB, Jordan L, et al. Adjunctive naturopathic care for type 2 diabetes: patient-reported and clinical outcomes after one year. BMC Complement Altern Med. 2012;12:44.

64. Seely D, Szczurko O, Cooley K, Fritz H, Aberdour S, Herrington C, et al. Naturopathic medicine for the prevention of cardiovascular disease: a randomized clinical trial. CMAJ. 2013;185(9):E409–16.

65. Herman PM, Szczurko O, Cooley K, Seely DA. Naturopathic approach to the prevention of cardiovascular disease: cost-effectiveness analysis of a pragmatic multi-worksite randomized clinical trial. J Occup Environ Med. 2014;56(2):171–6.

66. FunctionalMedicine.org [Internet]. Institute for Functional Medicine; c2014 [cited 2014 May 27]. www.functionalmedicine.org/.

67. Functional Medicine Matrix [Internet]. Institute for Functional Medicine; c2013 [cited 2014 May 27]. www.functionalmedicine.org/files/library/ifm-matrix-teaching.pdf.

68. Franic D, Snapp C, DeBusk R. Newly developed functional medicine program in diabetes: impact on clinical and patient reported outcomes—functional medicine and quality of life. BMC Complementary Altern Med. 2012;12(Suppl 1):S1.

69. Gillian E, Callender T, Gaster B. Integrative medicine at academic health centers: a survey of clinicians' educational backgrounds and practices. Fam Med. 2013;45(5):330–4.

70. Reilly D. The puzzle of homeopathy. J Altern Complement Med. 2001;7(Suppl 1):S103–9.

71. CPG Sec. 400.400 Conditions Under Which Homeopathic Drugs May be Marketed [Internet]. Silver Spring (MD): U.S. Food and Drug Administration; [updated 2010 Jan 12; cited 2014 May 26]. www.fda.gov/iceci/compliancemanuals/compliancepolicyguidancemanual/ucm074360.htm.

72. Cuesta Laso LR, Alfonso Galan MT. Possible dangers for patients using homeopathy: may a homeopathic medicinal product contain active substances that are not homeopathic dilutions? Med Law. 2007;26(2):375–86.

73. Dannemann K, Hecker W, Haberlan H, Herbst A, Galler A, Schafer T, et al. Use of complementary and alternative medicine in children with type 1 diabetes mellitus—prevalence, patterns of use, and costs. Pediatr Diabetes. 2008;9(3 Pt 1):228–35.

74. Remli R, Chan SC. Use of complementary medicine amongst diabetic patients in a public primary care clinic in Ipoh. Med J Malaysia. 2003;58(5):688–93.

75. Ehrlich G, Callender T, Gaster B. Integrative medicine at academic health centers: a survey of clinicians' educational backgrounds and practices. Fam Med. 2013;45(5):330–4.

76. Sampath S, Narasimhan A, Chinta R, Nair KR, Khurana A, Nayak D, et al. Effect of homeopathic preparations of *Syzygium jambolanum* and *Cephalandra indica* on gastrocnemius muscle of high fat and high fructose-induced type-2 diabetic rats. Homeopathy. 2013;102(3):160–71.

77. Maiti S, Ali KM, Jana K, Chatterjee K, De D, Ghosh D, Ameliorating effect of mother tincture of Syzygium jambolanum on carbohydrate and lipid metabolic disorders in streptozotocin-induced diabetic rat: Homeopathic remedy. J Nat Sci Biol Med. 2013;4(1):68–73.

78. Pomposelli R, Piasere V, Andreoni C, Costini G, Tonini E, Spalluzzi A, et al. Observational study of homeopathic and conventional therapies in patients with diabetic polyneuropathy. Homeopathy. 2009;98(1):17–25.

79. Nayak C, Oberai P, Varanasi R, Baig H, Ch R, Reddy GR, et al. A prospective multi-centric open clinical trial of homeopathy in diabetic distal symmetric polyneuropathy. Homeopathy. 2013;102(2):130–8.

80. Chen W, Yang GY, Liu B, Manheimer E, Liu JP. Manual acupuncture for treatment of diabetic peripheral neuropathy: a systematic review of randomized controlled trials. PLoS ONE. 2013;12:8(9). eCollection 2013.

81. Yang M, Li X, Liu S, Li Z, Xue M, Gao D, et al. Meta-analysis of acupuncture for relieving non-organic dyspeptic symptoms suggestive of diabetic gastroparesis. BMC Complement Altern Med. 2013;13:311.

82. McWhorter LS. Biological complementary therapies: a focus on botanical products in diabetes. Diabetes Spectr. 2001;14:199–208.

83. Saxena A, Vikram NK. Role of selected Indian plants in management of type 2 diabetes: a review. J Altern Complement Med. 2004;10:369–78.

84. Sridharan K, Mohan R, Ramaratnam S, Panneerselvam D. Ayurvedic treatments for diabetes mellitus. Cochrane Database Syst Rev. 2011;(12).

85. Keen RW, Deacon AC, Delves HT, Moreton JA, Frost PG. Indian herbal remedies for diabetes as a cause of lead poisoning. Postgrad Med J. 1994;70:113–4.

86. Kulambil Padinjakara RN, Ashawesh K, Butt S, Nair R, Patel V. Herbal remedy for diabetes: two case reports. Exp Clin Endocrinol Diabetes. 2009;117:3–5.

87. Davis MA, Weeks WB. The concentration of out-of-pocket expenditures on complementary and alternative medicine in the United States. Altern Ther Health Med. 2012;18(5):36–42.

88. Nahin RL, Barnes PM, Stussman BJ, Bloom B. Costs of complementary and alternative medicine (CAM) and frequency of visits to CAM practitioners: United States, 2007. Natl Health Stat Report. 2009;(18):1–14.

89. HealthCare [Internet]. Washington (DC): US Department of Health and Human Services; [cited 2014 June 1]. www.hhs.gov/healthcare.

90. FAQs about the Affordable Care Implementation Part XV. [Internet]. Washington (DC): U.S. Department of Labor; 2013 Apr 29 [cited 2014 June 1]. www.dol.gov/ebsa/faqs/faq-aca15.html.

91. Jellin JM, Gregory PJ, et al. Natural medicines comprehensive database. www.naturaldatabase.com. Accessed 10 June 2014.

Transcultural Applications to Lifestyle Medicine

Osama Hamdy and Jeffrey I. Mechanick

Abbreviations

A1C	Glycated hemoglobin
BMI	Body mass index
CVD	Cardiovascular disease
DASH	Dietary Approaches to Stop Hypertension
EDC	Endocrine disrupting compounds
GI	Glycemic index
HCP	Health-care professionals
MUFA	Monounsaturated fatty acids
n-3 PUFA	Omega-3 polyunsaturated fatty acids
PA	Physical activity
T2D	type-2 diabetes
tDNA	Transcultural Diabetes Nutrition Algorithm
WC	Waist circumference
WHR	Waist-to-hip ratio

Introduction

The successful implementation of lifestyle medicine as a public health initiative depends on an effective population-based disease screening and risk stratification program, availability of a broad range of interventions, an educational system that increases the number of well-trained health-care professionals (HCP), and an infrastructure capable of funding, performing, and completing high-quality research. However, a critical element of this plan is to have a lifestyle medicine program nimble enough to manage people from different cultures, in whom chronic disease is expressed differently and interventions can have a wide range of targeted effects. The recognition of these cultural influences is generally excluded from mainstream medical practice, education, and research and poses a threat to the success of this burgeoning field of lifestyle medicine. Nonetheless, the basic principles of transcultural adaptation of health care can be provided to optimize lifestyle medicine.

What Is Transculturalization?

The term "culture" generally refers to the clustering of nonphysical attributes that distinguish categories, or populations, of people (Table 19.1). This is differentiated from race, which is a clustering of physical or genetic characteristics common to a group of people but can include ethnicity, which is based on ancestry and genealogy. In any medical discussion of culture, the concept of *cultural relativism* is recognized, that is, having no superiority or inferiority of one culture over another. As a corollary, *ethnocentrism* (the judgment of another culture based on one's own culture) is avoided. Furthermore, the widespread and fixed conceptualization of another's culture is described as a *stereotype* (cognitive), with or without an element of *prejudice* (affective/emotional) and/or *discrimination* (behavioral/action). Hence, even though cultural sensitivity is critical for effective lifestyle medicine, it also poses challenges for HCP comportment: the HCP must engage, listen, think, understand, and then act, without bias, appropriately and sensitively.

Important cultural factors that bear on medical decision-making include gender roles, language barriers, and attitudes toward food, physical activity, and exposures to environmental toxins. Socio-economic factors are a prime driver of cultural differences. This is particularly evident when considering the care of low-income patients. Poverty is associated with fatalism, loss of control and autonomy, greater need for governmental assistance, drug and alcohol abuse, dysfunctional family life and difficulties with socialization, low self-esteem, community disengagement, and a lower overall level of health [1]. In fact, there is a vicious cycle wherein poor

J. I. Mechanick (✉)
Division of Endocrinology, Diabetes and Bone Disease, Icahn School of Medicine at Mount Sinai, 1192 Park Avenue, New York, NY 10128, USA
e-mail: jeffreymechanick@gmail.com

O. Hamdy
Joslin Diabetes Center, Harvard Medical School, Boston, MA, USA
e-mail: osama.hamdy@joslin.harvard.edu

© Springer International Publishing Switzerland 2016
J. I. Mechanick, R. F. Kushner (eds.), *Lifestyle Medicine,* DOI 10.1007/978-3-319-24687-1_19

Table 19.1 Cultural attributes and relevance

Attribute	Relevance to lifestyle interventions
Genetic/epigenetic system interactions and laboratory values	Different responses to nutrients, stress, and/or other environmental cues
Anthropometrics (e.g., BMI, WC and WHR)	Body composition changes that are associated with chronic disease risk and responses to therapy (e.g., sarcopenic obesity)
Religion, ancestry, linguistics, political ideology, gender roles, and personal space orientation	Contributes to behaviors and attitudes
Food sourcing, availability, policy, politics, and culinary styles	Individually or in aggregate affect healthy or unhealthy eating patterns
Socio-economics	Strong driver for need and adoption of lifestyle interventions
Climate, geography, crime, and environmental safety	Affect type and levels of physical activity and stress
Use of dietary supplements, nutraceuticals, and other forms of alternative care	Introduce risks and benefits into a comprehensive lifestyle intervention
Exposure to pollutants, endocrine disruptors, tobacco, and excess alcohol	Mitigate benefits and/or cause occult or overt harm
Local health-care practices and public advocacy programs	Affect early detection of chronic disease, accessibility to care, and implementation of interventions
Medical school curricula and continuing education	Determines number of qualified HCP in lifestyle medicine
Infrastructure for scientific medical research	Improved evidence base to develop improved and novel lifestyle interventions

BMI body mass index, *HCP* health-care professional, *WC* waist circumference, *WHR* waist-to-hip ratio

health also contributes to poverty [1]. This ultimately manifests as increased risk for disease and their complications, longer recovery times and health-care expenses, greater post-illness morbidity, and decreased accessibility to health care. The complex interactions of each of the attributes in Table 19.1 create unique cultures and subcultures both inside and outside of the USA necessitating a formalized approach to tailor culture-specific lifestyle interventions—a process newly referred to as "transculturalization."

The nascent term *transculturalization* denotes the process of adapting concepts and recommendations for a specific culture. This process is differentiated from *acculturation*, which describes changes that occur when two or more cultures interact. As a result of acculturation, there may be a loss of one culture, or *deculturation*, and formation of a new culture, or *neoculturation*. Another related term for the creation of a new culture from the merging of two or more cultures is *transculturation* (to be differentiated from *transculturalization*).

With respect to lifestyle medicine, the importance of transculturalization is to enable adaptation of recommendations based on evidence from one culture or study population to be implemented for an individual patient of a different culture. A methodology for transculturalization has been detailed in a recent "transcultural Diabetes Nutrition Algorithm (tDNA)" program initiated in 2010, templated in 2012 [2], reported for six regions in 2012–2014 (Canada, India, Malaysia, Mexico, Southeast Asia, and Venezuela) [3–8], and content-validated in 2014 [9]. In this tDNA protocol, scientific evidence is vetted, integrating local cultures when possible, and then adapted by local thought leaders in diabetes and nutrition. The salient transcultural features for lifestyle intervention for these six regions are provided in Table 19.2 and reviewed in 2015 by Hegazi et al. [10].

Biological Drivers for Cultural Differences in Chronic Disease

In the mitochondrial haplotype model championed by Wallace [11], a rapid mitochondrial DNA mutational rate adapts to a rapidly changing environment. Specifically, as humans migrated north from the southern African continent, some populations split off and ventured further northeast through what is now Siberia, crossing the land-bridge over the Bering Strait into North America. These colder climes affected mitochondrial gene expression and cellular energetics affecting glycemic status, adiposity, lipid metabolism, and even risk for cardiovascular disease (CVD) [11]. Thus, mitochondrial haplotypes may prove to be markers of cardio-metabolic risk that segregate among specific cultures.

Exposure to pollutants and endocrine disrupting compounds (EDC) has also been associated with the development of various chronic diseases, especially those that are metabolic in nature [12–14]. These agents exert effects via certain molecular targets, such as PPAR, RXR, and steroid receptors [15]. Some EDC, such as bisphenol A [16], as well as artificial sweeteners [17, 18], are associated with overweight/obesity possibly through mechanisms that involve intestinal taste receptors, microbiota, entero-insular, and neuronal pathways.

Allostasis is an adaptive response to stress that incorporates different *(allo-)*pathways and signals to achieve a new stable physiological state. In other words, *allostasis* reflects "stability through change" and is contrasted with *homeostasis*, which reflects "resistance to change." In a rapidly changing environment, that may be unique for a particular culture, survival depends on the ability to adapt. In the allostasis model of stress, this process of adaptation is complex and necessarily involves the brain, with the endocrine system

Table 19.2 Select transcultural lifestyle medicine adaptations in eight regions of the world

Attribute[a]	Parameter	USA	Canada	India	Malaysia	Mexico	Southeast Asia	Venezuela
Reference		[2]	[6]	[4]	[5]	[8]	[3]	[7]
A	BMI cutoffs[b]	25	25	23	23	25	23	25
		30	30	25	23	30	25	27.5
A	WC cutoffs[c]	101.6 M	101.6 M	90 M	90 M	90 M	90 M	94 M
		88.9 F	88.9 F	80 F	80 F	80 F	80 F	90 F
E	PA	75–150 min/week	150 min/week	60 min/day	5 day/week	60 min/day	150 min/week	30 min/d 5–7 day/week
F	Fat[d]	<30	<35	20–25	25–35	<30	25–30	25–30
		<7	<7	<7	<7	<7	<7–10	<7
		200	–	<200	<200	<200	<200–300	<200
F	Carbohydrate[e]	45–65 low GI	60 low GI	60–70	45–65 low GI	45–65 low GI	45–65	45–55
F	Protein[f]	15–20	15–20	12–18	15–20	15–20	15–20	15–20
G	A1C% cutoffs[g]	5.7	6.0	5.7	–	–	–	–
		6.5–7.0	6.5	6.5	6.5	7.0	–	7.0

BMI body mass index, *GI* glycemic index, *PA* physical activity, *WC* waist circumference, *A1C* glycated hemoglobin

[a] A—anthropometric, E—environment, F—food, G—genetic-epigenetic-laboratory

[b] Overweight (top) and obese (bottom) lower limit values (kg/m^2)

[c] Low-high risk; M male; F—female (in cm)

[d] Amounts of total fat (%; top), saturated fat (%; middle), and cholesterol (mg/d; bottom); for Canada—eating patterns are emphasized and no specifications for dietary cholesterol

[e] % carbohydrate of total daily intake

[f] % protein of total daily intake

[g] Prediabetes (top) and diabetes (bottom) lower-limit values; not diagnostic by itself for any region

figuring prominently. The physiological cost of adaptation is expressed as *allostatic load,* and when there is an excessive amount or duration of stress response which may not be repayable, there is *allostatic overload* and expression of disease. Examples of specific allostatic models include ß-cell function and diabetes (via MicroRNA regulation [19], mitochondrial toxins, inflammation, aging [20], alcohol use [21], critical illness [22], changes in neuro-circuitry with mental illness and addiction [23], network complexity with nutrient excess [24], and obesity in pregnancy [25]).

Eating Patterns

One of the key components of a healthy lifestyle is healthy nutrition. Unfortunately, there are many perspectives of what exactly constitutes healthy nutrition. For instance, is it the consumption of:

- proper amounts of macronutrients (e.g., carbohydrate, fat, and protein) according to population-based guidelines,
- a scientifically proven diet for a specific population with a specific endpoint according to interventional studies, or…
- "good" foods and not "bad" foods based on opinion or anecdotal evidence?

Alternatively, is it a more holistic approach to the whole foods consumed, especially with respect to the biochemical and molecular composition of the entire diet? This last viewpoint describes the concept of *eating patterns,* which are a representation of the totality of nutrients consumed over a particular time period rather than just at a single meal [26]. Other attributes of eating patterns include:

- aggregate of different diets with combinatorial and averaging effects among individual components,
- context of chronic disease risk reduction,
- multiple scales, ranging from individual foods, to nutrients, to individual molecules,
- influence on a physiological steady state that may require years to achieve, rather than instantaneous effects [26].

There is a relationship between increased CVD risk as typified by the Western diet that is high in saturated fats from processed and red meat, butter, and dairy, as well as refined grains, eggs, and French fries compared with decreased CVD risk with a prudent diet that is composed of fruits, vegetables, whole grains, legumes, and vinegar salad [27]. In a study by Appel et al. [28], a plant-based eating pattern, high in fruits and vegetables, along with reduced saturated fat (similar to the Dietary Approaches to Stop Hypertension (DASH) diet) was associated with improved control of hypertension [28]. Janssen et al. [29] found that sweets consumption was associated with increased obesity risk among 34 different countries. Another important example is the Mediterranean eating pattern that is high in monounsaturated

Table 19.3 Culture and region specific eating pattern problems for targeted intervention and reference healthy eating pattern

Culture/Region	Unhealthy eating pattern component	Reference
Western	High protein, saturated fat, processed meats, refined grains, sugar, sugar and artificially sweetened beverages, alcohol, fast foods, excess calories, with energy dense foods, social pressure	[2, 6, 27]
Asian	Glutinous (polished) rice, lower protein, high sodium, alcohol, frequent snacking and festivals (India), social pressure	[3–5]
Latin American	High alcohol and sweetened soda, low in fresh fruits and vegetables, high starch, high fast foods, excess calories, social pressure	[7, 8]
Reference: healthy	High MUFA, n-3 PUFA, fiber, pulses, plant-based, low-fat dairy, high antioxidant, whole grains, seafood and lean meats, farm-to-table sourcing, organic	[2, 6, 26, 27]

MUFA monounsaturated fatty acids, *n-3 PUFA* omega-3 polyunsaturated fatty acids

fatty acids and associated with reduction in CVD risk [30, 31]. A summary of unhealthy eating pattern components for targeted intervention among different cultures is provided in Table 19.3.

Transcultural effects of eating patterns incorporate several important principles. Food sourcing, food policy, and food politics issues result from socio-economic and political infrastructures within a particular region where one or several cultures reside. Although these attributes are not biologically grounded, they inevitably trump all other variables in determining final eating patterns for the majority of a society. Therefore, efforts to improve health and lifestyle for cultures of vulnerable, impoverished regions will undoubtedly require the arduous task of political and social reform. Imposing regulatory changes such as reducing or eliminating *trans* fats or sugar sweetened beverages are not likely to succeed on their own—a much greater commitment and critical mass of legislative acts, on a systems level, may be necessary, though this is certainly not going to be an easy chore [32].

On the other hand, food preferences (e.g., taste, flavor, mouthfeel, chemesthesis, texture, aroma, visual impact, and auditory impact) and preparation (including safe practices and the culinary arts) are based on ancestral, social, and familial cues, and in many cases, cannot be gleaned simply from studying written material but must be experienced and contemplated for a pragmatic understanding [33]. Lastly, food-body interactions at the molecular level play a role in the expression of eating pattern effects on chronic disease metrics and outcomes. More specifically, the portfolio of molecules in whole foods that comprise a person's eating pattern interact in a complex fashion with that person's own epigenome and metabolome to produce clinical events [34]. In sum, the manifold interactions of these descriptors can theoretically produce unique culturally specific eating pattern effects on chronic disease, but this novel model will require validation in order to optimize personalized interventions.

Physical Activity

Physical activity, and the implicit antonym "sedentary lifestyle," affects chronic disease risk independent of other lifestyle interventions. The incentive and practice of particular physical activities is also subject to a host of cultural factors, such as climate, terrain, safety, socialization, availability, logistics, and economics. Moreover, ethnicity- and culture-related body composition types, such as leanness, sarcopenia, obesity, and fat distribution modulate the physiological effects and comfort associated with publicly performing physical activity.

Perhaps the best example is India where sarcopenic obesity, or over-and-under malnutrition, is evident among many people at higher risk for CVD [4]. In this condition, owing to a relatively lower median daily protein consumption (about 8% of the total diet, compared with 15–20% in other cultures), there is relatively less muscle mass. Note that the lower protein consumption is in large part due to economic factors and a high prevalence rate of poverty. With economic change among a sector of the Indian population ("transitional economy"), there is increased consumption of a Western-type unhealthy eating pattern and consequent increase in fat mass. Therefore, even with normal or near-normal BMI (18.5–22.9 kg/m^2 for Asian Indians), the decreased muscle and increased fat mass can produce a state of insulin resistance and increased CVD risk.

In another example, those living in the Persian Gulf states have decreased vitamin D nutriture [35]. This rather counterintuitive finding is due to the avoidance of outdoor activities or donning of protective clothing as a result of the very hot and sunny environment or religious (Islamic) custom. In addition, the high and still increasing prevalence rates of type-2 diabetes (T2D) and obesity may be due in part to downstream effects of vitamin D undernutrition, further illustrating not only complex interactions of various lifestyle drivers (nutrition, physical activity, and behavior) but also culturally sensitive aspects.

In a third example, people living in Venezuela, a region also prone to increased obesity, T2D, and CVD risk, exhibit unhealthy lifestyles. This is now a society in political turmoil on the verge of economic collapse with increasing poverty. But among the multitude of emerging unhealthy habits is a realization that decreased levels and amounts of outdoor physical activity stem from fears relating to safety and major crimes; chief among these are express kidnappings and staged, planned kidnappings [7]. Here, one can appreciate the impact of allostatic stress responses on human

Table 19.4 Transcultural physical activity factors and reference healthy profile

Culture/region	Physical activity factors	Reference
Western	Sedentary lifestyle and spectator participation in sports. Obesity and stigmatization in gyms and outdoor facilities. Increased screen time for children (video, computer, games). Insufficient urban planning (running/walking trails, etc.)	[2, 6]
Asian	Transitional economy and urbanization, alcohol Increased mechanization, increased screen time. Increasing sedentary lifestyle, poverty Sarcopenia (India). Bias that "obesity" = "health" = "wealthy". Extreme heat and sunlight (southern climes). Protective clothing (religious, sun exposure)	[3–5]
Latin American	Sedentary lifestyle, poverty, alcohol, crime. Increased television viewing. Urban planning (not conducive to walking)	[7, 8]
Reference: healthy	At least 150 min/week moderate activity. Include progressive resistance training	[2, 6]

behavior and the appearance of unhealthy lifestyle practices and chronic disease. Various transcultural physical activity factors are provided in Table 19.4.

Case Studies

Latino Culture

Patient Presentation A 16-year-old Mexican American boy is seen at the request of his parents for weight gain; the mother is currently being treated for her T2D. The patient is quiet during the interview and does not volunteer much information, even though he speaks English very well. The parents verbalize great problems with increased screen time (television viewing, computer games, and surfing the Internet) with very little outdoor playtime. The patient does not eat well at family mealtimes but is seen by his parents eating chips and other high calorie snack foods at home and is suspected of eating out at Mexican and American fast food restaurants with his friends. He is not doing well in school, and the teachers have reported various behavioral problems. The family recently moved to New York City from Mexico and lives in a community with other Mexican Americans. Past medical history is negative and the patient does not take any medication. The parents are unaware of any tobacco or drug use. There is a strong family history of T2D, obesity, and heart disease. The exam is remarkable for increased adiposity and BMI without evidence of hypothyroidism or hypogonadism. He is neurologically and cognitively normal. There is mild acanthosis nigricans behind the neck.

Cultural Factors Insulin resistance and T2D are prevalent among Mexican Americans and are particularly serious issues among Mexican children [8]. The patient here is clearly at higher risk for insulin resistance and developing T2D, necessitating an effective preventive lifestyle medicine approach despite the "Hispanic Paradox," that is, Hispanics have the longest life expectancy among the three major main ethnic/race groups in the USA despite their higher prevalence of CVD risk factors and socio-economic disadvantages [36]. Although he has retained some Mexican cultural behaviors, it appears he is acculturating to an American way of life but

without access to healthy lifestyle behaviors. Further discussion with the patient alone (the parents were asked to leave the examination room) demonstrates a more verbal patient who admits to consuming a high-starch, high-refined-sugar (including sugared soda), and low-fiber (very little fresh fruit or vegetables) eating pattern. He also admits to going out to eat locally with friends for pizza and other American-style fast foods late at night but also some traditional tortilla, beans/rice-based cuisine. He admits that he would like to participate in group sports but is uncomfortable with his appearance and feels funny running at school. Overall, the impression is that he wants to be healthy.

Transculturalized Recommendations Again, without the parents in the room, educational materials are provided and discussed regarding good nutrition and different types of physical activity, including just walking or climbing stairs more often. The patient was afforded the majority of the time to speak, and at opportune times, small changes in eating were suggested. These included incorporating an apple, pear, or berries for a snack instead of chips, substituting diet or no sugar beverages instead of sugared sodas, and including some more vegetables. It was further explained that the American culture does not always consist of fast foods and watching TV, rather there is an increased interest in being healthy, and specific places to go to for healthy eating as well as ways to augment physical activity without formal exercise were provided. His parents were invited back into the room, and all the information was summarized with the patient playing a greater role in the discussion, reflecting an acceptance of responsibility. Labs were drawn to evaluate for other aspects of metabolic syndrome, and the possible use of metformin was discussed but deferred for this initial consultation. The patient continues to be seen in follow up with good response. The key points here are:

- Childhood obesity and prediabetes/T2D are major problems in the Mexican American community.
- Acculturation can be directed to a healthy American way of life and away from more stereotypical unhealthy American practices.
- Shifting eating patterns away from high starch and sugar content are a high priority.

- Increasing physical activity is a high priority.
- Lifestyle education and conversation in a culturally sensitive fashion is very important.

Asian Indian Culture

Patient Presentation A 30-year-old Asian Indian American presents with "brain fog." He is a very successful businessman, and until recently had a stable relationship with his girlfriend and happy life. He was complaining of some scalp hair loss and started on branded finasteride therapy without adverse effects. Approximately 3 months ago, he was changed to a generic finasteride formulation and within a few weeks developed symptoms of lightheadedness, progressive through the day, difficulty concentrating, decreased libido, some agitation and anxiety, moodiness, shakes, and just not feeling well. This was progressive, possibly related to meals, and after seeing numerous specialists with negative findings was referred by friends in the Asian Indian community. He consumes more of a typical American diet than a typical Asian Indian diet (rice-based with vegetables fully cooked). Nevertheless, he enjoys a New York bagel each morning, and overall, his eating pattern is high in starch and sugar. The past medical history was negative and the family history remarkable only for his mother who had T2D. Examination was unremarkable; specifically, there were no clinical signs of hypothyroidism, hypogonadism, orthostasis, acanthosis nigricans, adrenal disease, or significant mood alteration. He was lean with a normal BMI. Biochemically, the evaluation was positive only for a subtle A1C elevation to 5.7% and increased insulin response with oral glucose tolerance testing. The patient telephoned numerous times with symptom exacerbation (without any interventions) and wanted to return within the week to review all the findings. He explicitly said he would do anything that was recommended to feel better.

Cultural Factors There is an increased and increasing prevalence rate among Asian Indians for T2D with certain qualifiers: more postprandial > fasting hyperglycemia, association with lower BMI and sarcopenic obesity, and a context of high-carbohydrate–low-protein eating patterns (primarily due to increased glutinous (polished) rice [4]. In this case presentation, there was a suspicion of an idiopathic postprandial syndrome accounting for the symptoms, supported historically and with subtle biochemical findings of prediabetes. A careful review of his eating pattern revealed a generally healthy profile with a trend for symptoms occurring after incorporation of high glycemic index starches.

Transculturalized Recommendations Based on a presumptive diagnosis of prediabetes, structure and some hard rules were suggested to incorporate protein with each meal, minimize simple starches and sugars, eat raw or lightly steamed vegetables, and snack between meals. This afforded some relief. In a subsequent follow-up visit, he was accompanied by friends and family—more typical of the Asian Indian community practice when visiting doctors. The conversation dwelled on symptoms, behaviors, and mood. Family and friends all played an important role in supporting the doctor's counseling. Further inquiry confirmed and focused on the clear association of symptom development with the transition from branded to generic finasteride, and the possibility of post-finasteride syndrome [37] was raised. Finasteride, a synthetic 5α-reductase inhibitor (to decrease the conversion of testosterone to dihydrotestosterone, DHT), is associated with the persistence of the following symptoms, among others, even after medication discontinuation: brain fog and cognitive impairment, decreased libido and erectile dysfunction, and depressed mood [37]. The pathophysiology of post-finasteride syndrome is unclear. In this clinical case, the medication was stopped, and after another month, symptoms improved. However, even with dietary changes, anxiety over a deteriorating relationship with his girlfriend and fear of lifelong symptoms persisted. At this point, spiritualism and traditional Asian Indian healing practices were discussed through direct face-to-face, engaged communication and caring. He was referred for yoga and transcendental meditation training while also encouraged to participate in regular, daily exercise, including progressive resistance training to increase muscle mass. After another month, his symptoms were 90% abated, and he was very pleased that additional medications were not used. He continues to feel well, despite restarting a low dose of branded finasteride, along with his new healthy eating pattern, Eastern healing practices, and increased physical activity. The key points here are:

- Recognition that insulin resistance and cardio-metabolic risk factors are prevalent in Asian Indians but with certain differences compared with Caucasians.
- More extensive history-taking, detailed empathetic conversation, and consideration of spirituality, especially in a supportive setting with family and friends present, is an effective method of information gathering and for designing therapeutics.
- Consider various complementary medicine practices, such as meditation and yoga.
- Probe the dietary history for sources of high-glycemic index foods, such as glutinous rice and well-cooked starchy vegetables, and gradually replace with other carbohydrates, such as raw/steamed vegetables, pulses (lentils, beans, peas, and nuts), and/or whole grains.
- Increase high biological quality protein and resistance training to increase muscle mass and improve eating patterns.

Conclusions

Transculturalization should be viewed as yet another cognitive layer in lifestyle medicine practice, education, and research, recognizing that people are different, not only among different foreign regions on a global scale but also among different ethnicities and cultures within a domestic target population. Optimizing the transcultural approach to lifestyle medicine in chronic disease management would involve acquisition of local, relevant scientific evidence. At present, the scientific substantiation for implementing a transculturalization approach is primarily epidemiologic in nature and not yet validated with interventional studies. HCPs should take extra care to converse and think about these factors with each routine patient encounter prior to presenting recommendations. This creates an improved understanding of cultural factors and more efficiently incorporates beliefs and nuances into structured lifestyle medicine practice.

References

1. Mowafi M, Khawaja M. Poverty. J Epidemiol Community Health. 2005;59:260–4.
2. Mechanick JI, Marchetti AE, Apovian C, et al. Diabetes-specific nutrition algorithm: a transcultural program to optimize diabetes and prediabetes care. Curr Diab Rep. 2012;12:180–94.
3. Su HY, Tsang MW, Huang SY, et al. Transculturalization of a diabetes-specific nutrition algorithm: Asian application. Curr Diab Rep. 2012;12:213–9.
4. Joshi SR, Mohan V, Joshi SS, et al. Transcultural diabetes nutrition therapy algorithm: the Asian Indian application. Curr Diab Rep. 2012;12:204–12.
5. Hussein Z, Hamdy O, Chia YC, et al. Transcultural diabetes nutrition algorithm: a Malaysian application. Int J Endocrinol. 2013. doi.org/10.1155/2013/679396.
6. Gougeon R, Sievenpiper JL, Jenkins D, et al. The transcultural diabetes nutrition algorithm: a Canadian perspective. Int J Endocrinol. 2014. doi.org/10.1155/2014/151068.
7. Nieto-Martinez R, Hamdy O, Marante D, et al. Transcultural diabetes nutrition algorithm (tDNA): Venezuelan application. Nutrients. 2014;6:1333–63.
8. Bolio Galvis A, Hamdy O, Escalante Pulido M, et al. Transcultural diabetes nutrition algorithm: the Mexican application. J Diabetes Metab. 2014;5:1–10. http://dx.doi.org/10.4172/2155-6156.1000423.
9. Hamdy O, Marchetti A, Hegazi RA, et al. The transcultural diabetes nutrition algorithm toolkit: survey and content validation in the United States, Mexico, and Taiwan. Diab Technol Therapeut 2014;16. doi:10.1089/dia.2013.0276.
10. Hegazi RA, DeVitt AA, Mechanick JI. The transcultural diabetes nutrition algorithm: from concept to implementation. In: Watson RR, Dokken BB, editors Glucose intake and utilization in prediabetes and diabetes. Boston: Elsevier, pp. 269–280.
11. Wallace DC. A mitochondrial paradigm of metabolic and degenerative diseases, aging, and cancer: a dawn for evolutionary medicine. Annu Rev Genet. 2005;39:359–410.
12. Sanchez-Guerra M, Perez-Herrera N, Quintanilla-Vega B. Organophosphorous pesticides research in Mexico: epidemiological and experimental approaches. Toxicol Mech Meth. 2011;21:681–91.
13. Schell LM, Burnitz KK, Lathrop PW. Pollution and human biology. Ann Hum Biol. 2010;37:347–66.
14. Villarreal-Calderon A, Acuna H, Villarreal-Calderon J, et al. Assessment of physical education time and after-school outdoor time in elementary and middle school students in south Mexico City: the dilemma between physical fitness and the adverse health effects of outdoor pollutant exposure. Arch Environ Health. 2002;57:450–60.
15. Casals-Casas C, Desvergne B. Endocrine disruptors: from endocrine to metabolic disruption. Annu Rev Physiol. 2011;73:135–62.
16. Xu X, Tan L, Himi T, et al. Changed preference for sweet taste in adulthood induced by perinatal exposure to bisphenol A—a probable link to overweight and obesity. Neurotoxicol Teratol. 2011;33:458–63.
17. Lange FT, Scheurer M, Brauch HJ. Artificial sweeteners—a recently recognized class of emerging environmental contaminants: a review. Anal Bioanal Chem. 2012;403:2503–18.
18. Payne AN, Chassard C, Lacroix C. Gut microbial adaptation to dietary consumption of fructose, artificial sweeteners and sugar alcohols: implications for host-microbe interactions contributing to obesity. Obes Rev. 2012;13:799–809.
19. Plaisance V, Waeber G, Regazzi R, et al. J Diabetes Res; 2014. http://dx.doi.org/10.1155/2014/618652.
20. Picard M, Juster RP, McEwen BS. Mitochondrial allostatic load puts the 'gluc' back in glucocorticoids. Nat Rev. 2014;10:303–10.
21. Welcome MO, Pereverzev VA. Glycemic allostasis during mental activities on fasting in non-alcohol users and alcohol users with different durations of abstinence. Ann Med Health Sci Res. 2014;4(Suppl 3):S199–S207.
22. Mechanick JI. Metabolic mechanisms of stress hyperglycemia. J Parenter Enteral Nutr. 2006;30:157–63.
23. Pettomuso M, De Risio L, Di Nicola M, et al. Allostasis as a conceptual framework linking bipolar disorder and addiction. Front Psychiat. 2014;5:1–10.
24. Baffy G, Loscalzo J. Complexity and network dynamics in physiological adaptation: an integrated view. Physiol Behav. 2014;131:49–56.
25. Power ML, Schulkin J. Maternal obesity, metabolic disease, and allostatic load. Physiol Behav. 2012;106:22–8.
26. Zhao S, Mechanick JI, Jacques PF. Eating patterns. In: Mechanick JI et al., editors. Molecular nutrition. Washington D.C.: Endocrine Press; 2015. pp. 52–62.
27. Hu FB, Rimm EB, Stampfer MJ, Ascherio A, Spiegelman D, Willett WC. Prospective study of major dietary patterns and risk of coronary heart disease in men. Am J Clin Nutr. 2000;72(4):912–21.
28. Appel LJ, Moore TJ, Obarzanek E, et al. A clinical trial of the effects of dietary patterns on blood pressure. DASH Collaborative Research Group. N Engl J Med. 1997;336(16):1117–24.
29. Janssen I, Katzmarzyk PT, Boyce WF, et al. Comparison of overweight and obesity prevalence in school-aged youth from 34 countries and their relationships with physical activity and dietary patterns. Obes Rev. 2005;6(2):123–32.
30. Mitrou PN, Kipnis V, Thiébaut ACM, et al. Mediterranean dietary pattern and prediction of all-cause mortality in a US population: results from the NIH-AARP diet and health study. Arch Intern Med. 2007;167(22):2461–8.
31. Salas-Salvadó J, Fernández-Ballart J, Ros E, et al. Effect of a Mediterranean diet supplemented with nuts on metabolic syndrome status: one-year results of the PREDIMED randomized trial. Arch Intern Med. 2008;168(22):2449–58.
32. Trivedi NJ, Fields J, Mechanick CH, et al. Lack of correlation between antiobesity policy and obesity growth rates: review and analysis. Endocr Pract. 2012;18:737–44.
33. Solomon R, Via MA, Piqueras R, et al. Dietetics, the culinary arts, and molecular gastronomy. In: Mechanick JI et al., editors. Molecular nutrition. Washington D.C.: Endocrine Press; 2015. pp. 29–51.

34. Zhao S, Mechanick JI. Targeting Foodome-metabolome interactions: a combined modeling approach. In: Mechanick JI et al., editors. Molecular nutrition. Washington D.C.: Endocrine Press; 2015. pp. 181–204.

35. Fields J, Trivedi NJ, Horton E, et al. Vitamin D in the Persian Gulf: integrative physiology and socioeconomic factors. Curr Osteoporos Rep. 2011;9:243–50.

36. Lopez-Jimenez F, Lavie CJ. Hispanics and cardiovascular health and the "Hispanic Paradox": what is known and what needs to be discovered? Prog Cardiovasc Dis. 2014;57:227–9.

37. Ganzer CA, Jacobs AR, Iqbal F. Persistent sexual, emotional, and cognitive impairment post-finasteride: a survey of men reporting symptoms. Am J Mens Health. 2014. doi:10.1177/1557988314538445.

Community Engagement and Networks: Leveraging Partnerships to Improve Lifestyle

20

Juliette Cutts, Mary-Virginia Maxwell, Robert F. Kushner and Jeffrey I. Mechanick

Abbreviations

ADHD	Attention deficit hyperactivity disorder
BHCs	Behavioral Health Consultants
FQHCs	Federally qualified health centers
CAM	Complementary and alternative medicine
CBPR	Community-based participatory research
CDC	Centers for Disease Control and Prevention
HCPs	Health care professionals
YMCA	Young Men's Christian Association

Introduction

Community partnerships are a key component of translating lifestyle medicine into a patient's daily life. However, it is not often clear how to approach the development of these community partnerships. This chapter will provide a framework to address the needs of a diverse population and rationale for how to include cultural factors. Recommendations will be based on lessons learned from working in two federally qualified health centers (FQHCs) where resources are quite limited and community partnerships are becoming an increasingly important aspect of removing barriers to patient care.

J. I. Mechanick (✉)
Division of Endocrinology, Diabetes and Bone Disease,
Icahn School of Medicine at Mount Sinai, 1192 Park Avenue,
New York, NY 10128, USA
e-mail: jeffreymechanick@gmail.com

J. Cutts
Yakima Valley Farm Workers Clinic, Salud Medical Center,
Woodburn, OR, USA

M.-V. Maxwell
Catholic Family and Child Service, Yakima, WA, USA

R. F. Kushner
Northwestern University Feinberg School of Medicine, Northwestern Comprehensive Center on Obesity, 750 North Lake Shore Drive, Rubloff 9-976, Chicago, IL 60611, USA
e-mail: rkushner@northwestern.edu

The ability to work with community agencies (appropriate community referral resources that support the implementation of healthy lifestyles) has been identified as one of the core competencies for lifestyle medicine [1]. Accessing community-based resources is also one of the key components of the Chronic Care Model [2]. The use of these resources is critical in moving health behavior changes beyond a short-term programmatic intervention and can also serve an important role in expanding the treatment team beyond the clinic walls.

Community partnerships can serve a dual purpose in that they reinforce lifestyle changes in the patient's daily life and direct the community toward a larger goal of improving a population's overall health. Ideally, community-based programs are situated near a person's neighborhood and local environment, incorporating group members who are integral to positive behavioral change [3]. The programs expand services that a clinic can offer while assuring services are convenient and relevant to the community at large. This can help identify and alleviate cultural factors that might otherwise serve as a barrier to patient engagement. Identifying the assets of a community, that is, focusing on the existing strengths that exist within a community, by using one of many asset mapping tools is one of the first steps in conducting a community-health needs assessment [4].

Community partnerships and coalitions derive from community organization and community engagement, which is part of the "built environment" and represents a key contextualization element of health promotion, chronic disease management, and lifestyle medicine implementation, research, and policy-making. Community organization describes the initial natural, usually spontaneous, and local process of forming a community. Community engagement is a policy initiative; it is the dynamic process of constructing relationships, or partnerships, as part of a global strategy to improve life within the community, oftentimes in response to hazards, undesirable events, or adverse derived metrics about the population. Rather than being tokenistic, community engagement has recently been formalized, backed by

Table 20.1 Community-based participatory research (CBPR) attributes. (Adapted from [10])

Attribute	Comment
Collaborative	Everyone participates in some fashion with a fair division of labor
Culture	Representation, personnel, and activities are culturally sensitive with respect to all aspects of the community;
Diversity	Representation from different components of the community across scales (e.g., local and integrated health care systems, academia, and "at-large" members)
Durability	The process is scalable: starting small and building infrastructure and credibility over time
Equitableness	Involving multiple tools (e.g., questionnaires) and groups (e.g., committees and boards)
Feedback	Process evaluation regarding CBPR adherence to assess, modify, and improve
Leadership	Part of a governance strategy including steering committee, subcommittees, representatives, organizers, and advocacy groups
Scientific	To be incorporated at design, content, and implementation levels
Tangible	Support and incentives for participation and action (e.g., academic partners, grants, and gift certificates)
Trust	Establish early in the process

various levels of government support, and requiring acceptance and *bona fide* involvement of health care professionals (HCPs) [5].

There are many models and theories that comprise the philosophical framework for community engagement. Enhancing participation in relationships through volunteerism is a critical component for these models to build community-based networks [6]. The Centers for Disease Control and Prevention (CDC) social ecological model of health promotion programs describes four levels: individual, relationship, community, and societal [7]. In this model, the role of the individual is considered within the context of society and culture and consists of multiple levels, or scales, of networking: intrapersonal, interpersonal, community, organizational, and, finally, social systems [8]. The SaludABLEOmaha initiative incorporates the triad of social cognitive, social network, and social movement theories; the last one includes community readiness [9]. In the community readiness model, there are nine stages:

- no awareness,
- denial or resistance,
- vague awareness,
- preplanning,
- preparation,
- initiation,
- stabilization,
- confirmation or expansion,
- high level of community ownership [7].

Community-based participatory research (CBPR) is an approach with growing acceptance to address health and well-being issues, especially in disadvantaged communities [10] (Table 20.1). Key aspects of CBPR include a participatory nature, partnerships based on equitable collaboration, co-learning and sharing of expertise within a network of partnerships, systems development and durability, fair empowerment for decision-making, and data-driven action or implementation [10].

Community-based relationships incorporate specific attributes. Examples include improvements in neighborhood design, accessibility of recreational spaces and facilities, walkability, and nutritional resources; these and other attributes comprise the social determinants of health or the built environment. Developing these relationships in the rural setting is a particular challenge and has been addressed by Kilpatrick [11]. Some specific health promoting assets and liabilities in the community are summarized in Table 20.2. Community engagement also incorporates cultural factors: nonphysical attributes shared by members of a group, including behaviors, socioeconomics, religion, attitudes, politics, etc. Virtual communities are Internet-based or incorporate other modalities of social networking and also qualify as a means for engagement.

A continuum of community involvement has been advanced by McCloskey et al. [12] and migrates from outreach, to consult—involve—and collaborate, and ends with shared leadership. Community engagement improves project design and logistics, translating results into change, ethics, public involvement, and collaboration with organizations and academia [12]. Although many benefits are aspirational and realized, there are some participants who experience negative effects of community engagement, such as fatigue, stress, and disappointment [13]; thus, the role of community engagement is complex and needs further research and clarification for optimization.

Prioritization Using Maslow's Hierarchy

One of the challenges for working in an FQHC, particularly in a rural area, is addressing the needs that potentially impair patient engagement in care models. One remedy incorporates Maslow's hierarchy of needs, wherein patients are less able to engage in high-level needs until baseline needs are met [14]. In order to improve the outcomes of interventions, it is beneficial to develop a network of partnerships with community agencies.

Working with local agencies increases community participation with the dividend of addressing cultural factors that impact patient–community engagement. The population of the USA is becoming more diverse [15], and in order to meet

Table 20.2 Community-based assets and liabilities for lifestyle medicine implementation

Factor	Asset	Liability
Neighborhood design	Promotes physical activity, walkability, and safety	Increased need to drive; proximity of fast food restaurants dangerous areas
Nutritional resources	Healthy eating restaurants Improves healthy eating patterns Grocery stores are accessible and affordable	Unhealthy foods may also be cheap and easy to access (e.g., small markets or gas stations) and impair healthy eating patterns
Physical centers		Transportation and timing logistics: strict routine may discourage long-term use
Recreational spaces	Easy access, fun, variation Increases physical activity	Hard to access; limited variation
Virtual centers	Internet and other social media access facilitates recruitment and retention	Older adults and other groups may not have access

the varied needs of the population, health care delivery must incorporate cultural factors [16]. A fully functioning network of providers would include community members providing a wide variety of services, such as indigenous healing, alternative forms of care, and mental health care.

Physical Needs

Physical needs can pose a significant obstacle to patient engagement. Examples include access to healthy and nutritious food, access to clean water, and restorative sleep. It is difficult, for example, to engage a patient in healthy eating when he/she do not have access to healthy foods due to his/her dependence on food pantries that frequently stock cheap, highly processed food. At a patient-centered medical home in Woodburn, OR, local food pantries are engaged and can identify where patients may obtain fresh fruits and vegetables. Patients with diabetes are also provided with a list of locations that will provide a "Better Box" that contains foods that are appropriate for their dietary needs. The Food Research and Action Center outlines a variety of factors that make food availability a priority for any lifestyle intervention [17]. It is important to integrate agencies that patients rely on for healthy foods, particularly when working with a population that is food insecure.

Security Needs

Security takes on various forms. Food security (high-, marginal-, low-, or very low food security) depends on the following attributes:

- food access: anxiety over adequacy, availability, shortages, etc.,
- food quality, variety, desirability, issues of spoilage, etc.,
- food affordability,
- skipped or missed meals, hunger, weight loss, and/or illness as a result of above shortcomings [18].

Once resources are available to address patients' physical needs, it will be important to coordinate services to address other security needs. For example, in Woodburn, OR, patients have difficulty engaging in behavior change due to high levels of domestic violence, as well as insecurity due to being undocumented immigrants. This can be addressed by developing a partnership with the local women's crisis center and providing space for an advocate to meet with women in the clinic where their partners are more likely to allow them to come for a visit. The advocate is able to help extricate women from their abusive relationships by promoting access to legal, housing, and financial resources.

In addition to basic safety, it is also important to consider partnerships with agencies that can provide emergency services. This includes emergency housing, psychiatric evaluation and treatment, and employment services, and it can help improve access for the truly needy by reducing overutilization.

Social Needs

Social support and positive state of mind improve patient adherence with lifestyle interventions [19]. Komiti et al. [20] found that being in an intimate relationship and being employed were protective factors while substance abuse and stress were depressive factors. These findings are also consistent with findings that patients with strong social support mechanisms have better adherence with treatment recommendations [21]. Conclusions from the CDC indicate that incorporating community partnerships into lifestyle interventions will increase adherence with clinical recommendations [22].

Establishing an extended referral network may be beneficial in order to account for all the services patients may be using. Depending on the cultural background and belief system of the community, a fully functioning network of providers may include indigenous healing, hypnosis, herbs, acupuncture, and mental health care. Together these additional treatment options are referred to as complementary and alternative medicine (CAM). Population shifts and an increasing number of immigrants from countries that adhere to different medical models and approaches have increased awareness of these practices.

When working with underserved populations, the treatment team may need to include family or community leaders. Medically underserved areas or populations, quantitatively described by the Index of Medical Underservice, are determined by the following factors:

- primary care physicians rate,
- infant mortality rate,
- poverty rate,
- prevalence rate of persons over 65 years of age [23].

Fadiman [24] described how by working through the familial or community hierarchy parents of patients can be receptive to change without "loss of face." This integrated approach acknowledges the community and family structure in order to provide care that is both effective and cohesive.

Partnering with traditional healers, within a sound evidence-based medical model, would provide more culturally relevant interventions and a higher level of cultural competence. In 2009, *The New York Times* reported that a sign of increased cross-cultural health care was the use of certified Hmong shamans, Navajo medicine men, and *curanderos* in medical centers across the USA [25].

Establishing a network of community and religious leaders as well as CAM providers will allow treatment teams to engage patients in their own care on a deeper level. They will be able to deliver more culturally competent care through strategic partnerships with multiple providers. Inclusion of these community members will also allow the care team to take an active role in identifying which practitioners are qualified and willing to work as part of the primary care team. At the same time, these community members will help coordinate interventions into daily life. The inclusion of patients' social networks in lifestyle interventions cannot only improve individual outcomes but community outcomes as well [26]. These networks include, but are not limited to, religious organizations, community groups, and local businesses.

Higher Level Needs

There is also a need for partnerships to address high-level needs: those pertaining to esteem and self-actualization. These needs must be addressed at individual as well as societal levels. Lifestyle medicine HCPs will benefit their patients and the efficacy of their program by supporting and advocating for programs and policies that also focus on these needs.

The Department of Health and Human Services report on Racial and Ethnic Health Disparities advocates for community-based interventions to address health care disparities, based on systematically experienced social and economic disadvantages by specific population sectors [27]. Efforts to increase community engagement, improve neighborhoods, and integrate cultural factors can be expected to reduce many of these disparities and improve overall health care.

High-level needs also occur at a political level. In order to incite beneficial change in society, one must be willing to speak out about food taxes, crop subsidies, food manufacturing, labeling regulations, and other (sometimes unpopular) politically and economically driven agendas [3]. There is only so much that can be done at a local level and HCPs will need to network with their communities to achieve effective and durable societal change.

Patients who are ready to address their highest level of need, that is, self-actualization, will benefit from referrals to programs that assist patients and their communities to fulfill their potential. This can be accomplished by working with local community colleges, universities, and religious organizations to provide a variety of options for self-exploration and skill building. These partnerships may also include organizations that can help patients to become leaders in the process of addressing lifestyle issues in their communities.

Implementation in Clinical Practice

Case Study

A successful example of community engagement and partnership is with a patient-centered medical home in Yakima, WA, which created a community childhood fitness program. In March 2012, Behavioral Health Consultants (BHCs) were funded through a grant to start integrated behavioral health services at a small pediatric clinic. The nine providers identified four main concerns that they believed would benefit from co-located and collaborated mental health services: behavior problems (temper tantrums, school refusal, and attention deficit hyperactivity disorder (ADHD)), anxiety, depression, and obesity.

Pediatricians were especially alarmed by the rates of children who were overweight and obese that they were treating daily, as well as the lack of services available to address the problem. Their observations were consistent with the observation that obesity is one of the most stigmatizing and least socially acceptable conditions in childhood [28]. HCPs at Yakima Pediatrics were seeing the negative psychosocial complications of childhood obesity including depressive symptoms, poor body image, low self-concept, behavior, and learning problems. They also observed poor health outcomes including type-2 diabetes, precocious puberty, hypertension, asthma, and exercise intolerance.

When Yakima County was ranked the eighth fattest city in the USA [29], it was time for action. Yakima Pediatrics hired BHCs who were given the task of removing barriers to adapting a healthy lifestyle. These barriers included how to increase children's exposure to healthy food (physical need), how to encourage the family to make healthy lifestyle changes (social needs), and how to engage them in moving their body's more (esteem needs). After 2 months in the clinic,

BHCs identified five barriers that were repeatedly mentioned when healthy lifestyle changes were suggested: cost, time, transportation, internalized shame ("no one looks like me, I can never do this"), and feelings of intimidation ("I don't know what to do" or "I don't how to use the equipment").

The BHC team approached a small, private gym with less than 300 members that was half a block from the pediatric clinic to establish a partnership to address these barriers. Thanks to a small grant, patients were offered a 45-min functional fitness class for youth twice a week. The classes included cardiovascular exercise and strength training and began in June 2012.

The model for this class is effective because the process is simple. A provider will ask the BHC to meet with a family and then make a referral to the gym, including brief information about any medical/behavioral concerns regarding exercise. The family will immediately walk or drive down the street to meet with the owner/trainer to complete the youth's assessment. When possible, the BHC will even accompany the family to the gym. Many family members will stay and watch their child in class. As a result, about 25% of the families referred to this program opt to obtain a gym membership for the entire family. This program is provided based on grant-funded scholarships.

In the first 2 years since the childhood fitness program began, it has served over 100 families with children between 6 and 13 years old. Each class typically has 18 participants who meet twice weekly to learn ways to enjoy moving their bodies and how to adopt healthy eating habits. They earn incentives along the way, such as gym t-shirts, water bottles, and healthy snacks. After 8 weeks, participants return to Yakima Pediatrics where they meet with the BHC to review their attendance and assess for attitude and self-esteem changes. Youth may continue in the program indefinitely on scholarship as long as they have an 80% attendance rate.

This program represents a fundamental way to address the social needs of youths. The gym is now viewed as a part of their neighborhood due to its proximity to the youth's homes. Many of the youth can walk to the gym from school or home and some parents have established friendships and now carpool together. The gym is also an extension of the clinic in that it is within a residential area, one block from the pediatric clinic. Moreover, HCPs and BHCs from the pediatric clinic can exercise at the gym where the youth will recognize and greet them.

Evidence and Other Examples

Scarinci et al. [30] reported the results of a cluster randomized controlled trial in six counties in rural Alabama involving African- American women ($N=565$) using the CBPR framework and found that a culturally relevant intervention improved and maintained healthy eating patterns. In a large diabetes prevention study by UnitedHealth Group (a health

Table 20.3 Barriers and enablers for recruitment and retention of adolescents for a community-based healthy lifestyle program. (Adapted from [34])

	Recruitment	Retention
Enabler	Proper advertising and promotion; positive messaging; free; government subsidized	Positive experience for child and parent; fun; practical; family involvement electronic media role models; good facilitators; realistic and measurable goals; transition into community
Barrier	Anxiety and embarrassment; denial; lack of HCP expertise; decreased pediatric services; economics and program costs	Location and transportation logistics; finding the time commitment; isolation and stigmatization; lack of centers or activities

HCP health care professional

system), the Young Men's Christian Association (YMCA) of the USA (a community-based program), and the CDC, the National Diabetes Prevention Program was scaled up within 2 years to 46 communities in 23 states, training 500 coaches, and enrolling 2369 participants (1723 completers), finding a cost-effective average weight loss of about 5% [31]. In England, Morton et al. [32] reported that although community-based pharmacists were uniquely and ideally positioned to deliver lifestyle advice to patients with cardiovascular disease, semi-structured interviewing demonstrated several challenges to more widespread implementation, such as proper training and appropriate remuneration. Along these lines, there remain perception issues regarding the role of health trainers in marginalized communities, primarily due to current professional culture expectations in health care [33].

Implementation of community-based healthy lifestyle programs for adolescents with overweight/obesity depends on enabling factors for recruitment and retention (Table 20.3) [34]. Many of these strategies can be extrapolated to other settings and clinical problems when developing and utilizing community-based programs. In the Agewell trial of older adults, a community-based brief low-cost goal-setting intervention was developed to address physical activity, cognitive activity, diet, and overall health, and was found to be feasible and acceptable [35]. Other innovations to enhance community engagements on a practical level include text messaging [36], culturally sensitive radio novella development [37], lifestyle questionnaires in local houses of worship [38], and booster intervention using face-to-face or telephone-based motivational interviewing [39].

Conclusion

Establishing community-based partnerships to address patient needs is a key component of increasing adherence and effective implementation of lifestyle medicine interventions.

An effective network of community referral sources can not only improve outcomes of an individual program but also expand those benefits to the entire community. Establishing sustainable and practical lifestyle medicine interventions that encourage, promote, and support families with healthy and attainable change is a prime target. Based on work at FQHCs, patients who need lifestyle medicine intervention the most have difficulty accessing these interventions due to barriers to basic needs.

Lifestyle medicine is much larger than an individual patient or even an individual program. The process of community engagement is organic and can scale up or down depending on relationships and productivity rather than a dependency on external organizations or power structures. Specifically, program participants become examples of success as others observe the benefits they have achieved. Successful programs become examples for other communities and can inform government policy. When lifestyle interventions are implemented at the community level as one part of a larger systemic effort, an entire community and, ultimately, society will benefit.

References

1. Lianov L, Johnson M. Physician competencies for prescribing lifestyle medicine. JAMA. 2010;304:202–3.
2. Bodenheimer T, Wager EH, Grumbach K. Improving primary care for patients with chronic illness. JAMA. 2002;288:1775–9.
3. Dysinger WS. Lifestyle medicine competencies for primary care physicians. Virtual Mentor. 2013;15:306–10.
4. Goldman KD, Schmalz KJ. "Accentuate the Positive!"; Using an asset-mapping tool as part of a community-health needs assessment. Health Promot Pract. 2005;6:125–8.
5. Kenyon L, Gordon F. Community engagement: from a professional to a public perspective. Community Pract. 2009;82:22–5.
6. Parisi JM, Kuo J, Rebok GW, et al. Increases in lifestyle activities as a result of Experience Corps® participation. J Urban Health. 2015;92:55–66.
7. Centers for Disease Control and Prevention. The social-ecological model. A framework for prevention Atlanta (GA): Centers for Disease Control and Prevention. http://www.cdc.gov/violenceprevention/overview/social-ecologicalmodel.html. Accessed 29 March 2015.
8. Weinstein LC, Plumb JD, Brawer R. Community engagement of men. Prim Care Office Pract. 2006;33:247–59.
9. Frerichs L, Brittin J, Robbins R, et al. SaludABLEOmaha: improving readiness to address obesity through healthy lifestyle in a Midwestern Latino Community, 2011–2013. CDC—Prev Chronic Dis. 2015;12:1–9.
10. Shalowitz MU, Isacco A, Barquin N, et al. Community-based participatory research: a review of the literature with strategies for community engagement. J Dev Behav Pediatr. 2009;30:350–61.
11. Kilpatrick S. Multi-level rural community engagement in health. Aust J Rural Health. 2009;17:39–44.
12. McCloskey DJ, McDonald MA, Cook J, et al. Community engagement: definitions and organizing concepts from the literature. In Clinical and Translational Science Awards Consortium Community Engagement Key Function Committee Task Force on the Principles of Community Engagement. Principles of Community
13. Engagement, Second Edition. NIH Publication No. 11–7782, Printed June 2011 pp. 3–41.
13. Attree P, French B, Milton B, et al. The experience of community engagement for individuals: a rapid review of evidence. Health Social Care Commun. 2011;19:250–60.
14. Maslow AH."Higher" and "lower" needs. J Psychol Interdiscip Appl 1948;25:433–436.
15. Humes KR, Jones NA, Ramirez RR. Overview of race and hispanic Origin, 2010. United States Census 2011; http://www.census.gov/prod/cen2010/briefs/c2010br-02.pdf. Accessed 29 March 2015.
16. Armstrong T, Swartzman L. Cross-cultural differences in illness models and expectations for the health care provider-client/patient interaction. In Kazarian SS, Evans DR, editors, Cultural health psychology 2001. San Diego: Academic, pp. 45–61.
17. Food Research and Action Center. Why low-income and food insecure people are vulnerable to overweight and obesity. Food Research and Action Center (FRAC); 2010. http://frac.org/initiatives/hunger-and-obesity/why-are-low-income-and-food-insecure-people-vulnerable-to-obesity/. Accessed 29 March 2015.
18. U.S. Department of Agriculture. Definitions of food security. http://www.ers.usda.gov/topics/food-nutrition-assistance/food-security-in-the-us/definitions-of-food-security.aspx. Accessed 29 March 2015.
19. Gonzalez JS, Pinedon FJ, Antoni MH, et al. Social support, positive states of mind, and HIV treatment adherence in men and women living with HIV/AIDS. Health Psychol. 2004;23:413–8.
20. Komiti A, Judd F, Grech P, et al. Depression in people living with HIV/AIDS attending primary care and outpatient clinics. Aust NZ J Psychiatry. 2003;37:70–7.
21. Tawalbeh LI, Tubaishat A, Batiha AM, et al. The relationship between social support and adherence to healthy lifestyle among patients with coronary artery disease in the north of Jordan. Clin Nurs Res. 2015;24:121–38.
22. Centers for Disease Control and Prevention (CDC). Healthy communities program. http://www.cdc.gov/nccdphp/dch/programs/healthycommunitiesprogram/. Accessed 29 March 2015.
23. U.S. Department of Health and Human Services. Medically underserved areas/populations. http://www.hrsa.gov/shortage/mua/. Accessed 29 March 2015.
24. Fadiman A. The spirit catches you and you fall down: a Hmong child, her American doctors, and the collision of two cultures. New York: Farrar, Straus and Giroux; 1997.
25. Brown PL. A doctor for disease, a shaman for the soul. The New York Times. 2009 Sept 20, p. A20.
26. Woolf SH, Dekker MM, Byrne FR, et al. Citizen-centered health promotion: building collaborations to facilitate healthy living. Am J Prev Med. 2011;40(1 Suppl 1):S38–47.
27. U.S. Department of Health and Human Services. HHS action plan to reduce racial and ethnic disparities: a nation free of disparities in health and health care. Washington, D.C.: U.S. Department of Health and Human Services; 2011. http://minorityhealth.hhs.gov/npa/files/Plans/HHS/HHS_Plan_complete.pdf. Accessed 29 March 2015.
28. Schwimmer JB, Burwinkle TM, Varni JW. Health-related quality of life of severely obese children and adolescents. JAMA. 2003;289:1813–9.
29. Banner V. 10 fattest cities in America. Quality Health 2008. http://www.qualityhealth.com/10-fattest-cities-in-america-8/featured-Article. Accessed 29 March 2015.
30. Scarinci IC, Moore A, Wynn-Wallace T. A community-based, culturally relevant intervention to promote healthy eating and physical activity among middle-aged African American women in rural Alabama: findings from a group randomized controlled trial. Prevent Med. 2014;69:13–20.
31. Vojta D, Koehler TB, Longjohn M, et al. A coordinated national model for diabetes prevention. Am J Prev Med. 2013;44:S301–6.

32. Morton K, Pattison H, Langley C, et al. A qualitative study of English community pharmacists' experiences of providing lifestyle advice to patients with cardiovascular disease. Res Social Adminst Pharm. 2015;11:e17–29.

33. Cook T, Wills J. Engaging with marginalized communities: the experiences of London health trainers. Persp Public Health. 2012;132:221–7.

34. Smith KL, Straker LM, McManus A, et al. Barriers and enablers for participation in healthy lifestyle programs by adolescents who are overweight: a qualitative study of the opinions of adolescents, their parents and community stakeholders. BMC Pediatr. 2014;14:53–66.

35. Claire L, Nelis SM, Jones IR, et al. The Agewell trial: a pilot randomised controlled trial of a behaviour change intervention to promote healthy ageing and reduce risk of dementia in later life. BMC Psychiatr. 2015;15:25–43.

36. Albright K, Krantz MJ, Jarquin PB, et al. Health promotion text messaging preferences and acceptability among the medically underserved. Health Promot Pract. 2015. doi:10.1177/1524839914566850.

37. Frazier M, Massingale S, Bowen M, et al. Engaging a community in developing an entertainment—education Spanish-language radio novella aimed at reducing chronic disease risk factors, Alabama, 2010–2011. CDC—Prev Chronic Dis. 2012;9:1–9.

38. Evans KR, Hudson SV. Engaging the community to improve nutrition and physical activity among houses of worship. CDC—Prev Chronic Dis. 2014;11:1–8.

39. Goyder E, Hind D, Breckon J, et al. A randomised controlled trial and cost-effectiveness evaluation of 'booster' interventions to sustain increases in physical activity in middle-aged adults in deprived urban neighbourhoods. Health Technol Assess. 2014;18:1–242.

Lifestyle Therapy as Medicine for the Treatment of Obesity

Jamy D. Ard and Gary D. Miller

Abbreviations

α-MSH	Alpha-Melanocyte-stimulating hormone
ARGP	Agouti-related peptide
AEE	Activity energy expenditure
BMI	Body Mass Index
CMR	Complete meal replacements
CVD	Cardiovascular disease
DHEA	Dehydroepiandrosterone
EOSS	Edmonton Obesity Staging System
GERD	Gastroesophageal reflux disease
GLP-1	Glucagon-like polypeptide-1
HIIT	High-intensity interval training
LCTs	Long-chain triglycerides
MCTs	Medium-chain triglycerides
MI	Motivational interviewing
MRs	Meal replacements
NCEP	National Cholesterol Education Program
NHANES	National Health and Nutrition Examination Survey
NPY	Neuropeptide Y
NTS	Nucleus Tractus Solitaries
PMR	Partial meal replacements
POMC	Proopiomelanocortin
RCT	Randomized controlled trial
REE	Resting energy expenditure
T2D	Type-2 diabetes
TEE	Total energy expenditure
TEF	Thermic effect of feeding
VAT	Visceral adipose tissue
VLCD	Very low-calorie diet

J. D. Ard (✉)
Department of Epidemiology and Prevention, Wake Forest University, Winston-Salem, NC, USA
e-mail: jard@wakehealth.edu

G. D. Miller
Department of Health and Exercise Science, Wake Forest University, Winston-Salem, NC, USA

© Springer International Publishing Switzerland 2016
J. I. Mechanick, R. F. Kushner (eds.), *Lifestyle Medicine,* DOI 10.1007/978-3-319-24687-1_21

Defining Obesity

Obesity is defined as a condition of excess accumulation and storage of body fat. We know that the presence of body fat serves critical functions related to hormonal balance, energy reserves, and thermoregulation. However, as with most biological systems, there is a continuum from normal to abnormal, and the challenge for obesity becomes identifying the point at which the accumulation of body fat reaches a point of being abnormal. Historically, increased body weight was deemed abnormal based on increased risk of death from all causes. This was previously defined by insurance tables that assessed death risk based on body weight at a given height [1]. Since the first Obesity Expert Panel report in 1998, body mass index (BMI) has been widely adopted as the standard for identifying excess body fat [1]. BMI accounts for weight based on height using the formula of body weight (kg)/height squared (m^2) [2]. BMI is highly correlated with total body fat based on studies of body composition using various techniques in the general population [2]. BMI is also positively associated with morbidity and mortality from excess body fat [3]. However, BMI has a number of limitations that should be acknowledged. Because older adults lose lean mass and accumulate fat mass with age, BMI can underestimate body fat in this population [4]. Conversely, very lean individuals with high amounts of muscle mass, such as highly trained athletes, will have less body fat than predicted by their BMI [1]. Additionally, as with any attempt to categorize a continuous phenomenon, the association with other disease risks in the lower ranges of abnormal BMI (i.e., overweight) are not as consistent on an individual level [5]. Finally, BMI does not provide any information about the distribution of the body fat, which can alter risk associations. With these caveats, this chapter will use the conventional definition of obesity for Caucasians based on a BMI of 30 kg/m^2 or greater, with class 2 obesity beginning at 35 kg/m^2 and class 3 beginning at a BMI of 40 kg/m^2. Overweight in Caucasians is defined as a BMI of 25–29.9 kg/m^2 [1].

Prevalence of Obesity

Nearly two-thirds of US adults are at least overweight [6]. The prevalence of obesity in the USA has increased from 22.3% in the 1988–1992 National Health and Nutrition Examination Survey (NHANES) III sample [1] to 34.9% of all adults in the NHANES 2011–2012 sample [6]. The increase in obesity has been even higher in some specific subgroups of Americans, with Hispanic Americans and African Americans having rates of 42.5 and 47.8%, respectively [6]. Globally, the increase in obesity is becoming more widespread. Estimates from 2008 place the number of individuals with obesity at approximately 500 million, representing 10–14% of the world's population [7]. North America, Latin American, North Africa, and the Middle East all have a prevalence of obesity that is greater than 30% [7]. The shift in body weight is affecting low- and middle-income countries as well, resulting in significant decreases in the proportions of people who are underweight and even greater increases in the proportions of those who are overweight and obese [8].

Obesity as a Disease

With the increased recognition of obesity in the USA and beyond, efforts to understand the pathology of excess accumulation of fat mass have grown. This increased emphasis on understanding obesity has led to greater recognition of the condition as a disease [9, 10]. Classifying obesity as a disease shifts the focus from simple personal factors that drive energy imbalance, like being inactive or simple overconsumption, to a more sophisticated examination of the interplay between the obesogenic environment, genetic predispositions, and the physiological adaptations that occur to counterbalance attempts to lose weight and maintain weight loss. As a disease, the pathology of excess adiposity has a variety of possible etiologies, ranging from medication-induced weight gain to monogenetic mutations, which all ultimately result in a period of sustained energy imbalance and accumulation of excess body weight, expanding the number (hyperplasia) and size (hypertrophy) of fat cells [9]. A positive energy imbalance can only occur via two pathways: increases in energy intake and/or alterations/decreases in energy expenditure. Modulators of food intake include peripherally secreted adipokines like leptin, gut peptides such as ghrelin, glucagon-like peptide-1 and cholecystokinin, monoamine neurochemicals like serotonin and dopamine, and neuropeptides like neuropeptide Y and agouti-related peptide. Table 21.1 shows many of these factors, how they interact with each other, and the related impact on energy intake. On the energy expenditure side of the equation, total energy expenditure (TEE) equals the sum of resting energy expenditure (REE), activity energy expenditure (AEE), and the thermic effect of feeding (TEF) [11]. AEE is the voluntary component of TEE, typically accounting for 30% of TEE but is highly variable based on the level of physical activity [12]. The remaining components of TEE are involuntary, which includes REE and TEF. REE accounts for approximately 60% of TEE and is largely determined by the volume of lean mass, including muscle and organ mass. Highly metabolically active organs like brain, heart, and kidneys make up a disproportionate amount of REE by weight, accounting for 60% of REE [13]. Overall, REE varies based on life stage and generally declines with age by approximately 1–2% per decade due to loss of quantity and composition of metabolically active fat-free mass [14]. TEF, energy consumed in the digestion and absorption of nutrients, contributes approximately 10% to TEE on a daily basis.

The Impact of the Environment

The voluntary contribution to the homeostasis equation, such as choices around AEE (e.g., exercise and physical activity) or eating pattern, can override biological mechanisms to a large extent. Further, the environment's influence on these voluntary components is an even larger force that may not be readily recognized at the individual level, but is likely critical to trends in body weight at the population level. There is evidence to suggest that the environment has fostered an increase in access to calories that has overwhelmed the biological mechanisms that promote dietary restraint. In the past century, improvements in technology for food production and manufacturing have decreased food scarcity. As of 2011, each American had a much larger quantity of food available for consumption compared to 1970 [15].

Over the past four decades, the average calorie intake for an American adult has increased from an estimated 2064 to 2538 calories/day, with grains accounting for 38.2% of this increase. Added fats and oils account for 224 calories of the increase, or 47.3% of the total [15]. There are few mechanisms to self-regulate calorie intake when faced with highly palatable foods that elicit a strong hedonic response [16]. This means that even in the context of a strong cognitive desire to limit caloric intake, there are significant overriding neurophysiologic systems that combine previous sensory and emotional experiences in the presence of strong food cues [17].

Further Defining Obesity

Although obesity is often described as a singular entity, there are genotypic and phenotypic patterns of expression of the disease that correspond to varying levels of risk and pathology. Aside from monogenic obesity syndromes, such

Table 21.1 Key appetite and energy regulation hormones, peptides, and neurotransmitters

Hormone/peptide/neurotransmitter	Increases with	Decreases with	Targets	Impact on energy intake/expenditure	Regulation/feedback
Leptin	Increased fat mass	Reduced caloric intake, starvation	POMC (↑) NPY (↓) AGRP (↓)	Decreases food intake	Sensitivity to leptin decreases with increasing weight gain
Insulin	Feeding, glucose, GLP-1	Glucagon, hypoglycemia	POMC (↑) NPY (↓) AGRP (↓)	Decrease food intake	Insulin resistance may be sentinel event in obesity, leading to higher insulin levels
Glucagon-like peptide-1	Food intake	Fasting	Glucagon (↓) insulin (↑)	Decreases food intake; delays gastric emptying	
PYY	Food intake; proportional to caloric intake	Fasting	Vagus/sympathetic nervous system NTS-activating POMC neurons	Decreases food intake; decreases between-meal hunger	
Alpha-melanocyte-stimulating hormone	POMC	Action blocked by AGRP	Melanocortin receptors	Decreased food intake	
Cholecystokinin	Nutrients being sensed in the small intestine	Fasting	Vagus/sympathetic nervous system NTS	Signal satiety	Opposes the action of ghrelin
Proopiomelanocortin	Weight gain	Weight loss	α-MSH (↑)	Decreases food intake	
Ghrelin	Fasting; upward surge before meal	Food intake, more responsive to carbohydrate intake than protein or fat	NPY (↑) AGRP (↑)	Initiation of meal	Regulates meal initiation and hunger; acts as a signal of starvation
Neuropeptide Y	Low leptin or insulin levels, hypoglycemia, negative energy balance	Leptin or insulin	Neurons of the hypothalamus	Increased food intake; decreased energy expenditure from brown adipose tissue	Potent stimulator of food intake
Agouti-related peptide	Low leptin or insulin levels, negative energy balance	Leptin or insulin	Melanocortin receptor antagonist	Increased food intake	
Dopamine		Leptin		Food seeking	Involved in reward associated with food intake
Serotonin	Increased carbohydrate and fat intake		NPY (↓) activates POMC neurons	Suppresses hunger and signals satiation; enhances energy metabolism	May be link between stress response and food-seeking behavior

POMC Proopiomelanocortin, *ARGP* Agouti-related peptide, *NPY* Neuropeptide Y, *GLP-1* Glucagon-like polypeptide-1, *α-MSH* Alpha-Melanocyte-stimulating hormone, *NTS* Nucleus Tractus Solitaries

as leptin deficiency, the most common forms of obesity are polygenetic and considered as complex traits [9, 18]. Understanding the spectrum of obesity presentations leads to better matching of treatment strategy with overall risk and comorbid resolution or control.

Beyond the assessment of BMI, the next consideration is the distribution of body fat. Accumulation of excess fat in different fat depots can have significant implications for disease in risk. The preponderance of fat in the truncal/abdominal space is classified as android (or male) distribution, while the preponderance of fat in the lower extremities is classified as gynoid (or female) distribution [19]. Abdominal fat can be located in the subcutaneous layer or centrally around the organs as visceral adipose tissue (VAT). VAT is considered to be highly active as a promoter of systemic inflammation and insulin resistance via the secretion of cytokines [20, 21]. This contributes to the increase in risk of cardiovascular disease (CVD), type-2 diabetes (T2D), and cancers of various sites [5]. While VAT has received much of the focus as a promoter of chronic disease risk, emerging evidence suggests that subcutaneous fat accumulation in the abdominal area is also associated with contributing to insulin resistance and inflammation [22]. Peripheral fat distribution (i.e., upper and lower extremities) is generally in the subcutaneous compartment, and in some studies, a predominance of fat in these areas has been associated with lower risks of hyperglycemia and hyperlipidemia when adjusting for BMI and age [23, 24]. Obesity can be further classified by considering the level of BMI (class I–III) or combining the distribution of excess fat and BMI with assessments of disease risk and functional status. Proposed staging systems such as the Edmonton Obesity Staging System (EOSS) and the American Association of Clinical Endocrinologist Staging algorithm go further to combine assessments of physical function and associated comorbid conditions with BMI to provide a broader classification scheme of obesity [25, 26]. These types of staging systems integrate the effects of obesity with weight class, highlighting the complexity of obesity as a multisystem disease. Ultimately, the goal of classifying the severity and risk associated with obesity is to determine the intensity of treatment strategies in a way that is more nuanced than simply considering overall size (i.e., BMI) and directly addresses associated risk.

Behavioral Health and Obesity

The behavioral health considerations within the staging of obesity are also critical to directing treatment strategies. These considerations range from comorbid mental health disease to disordered eating behaviors. The prevalence of mood disorders in patients with obesity seeking treatment is common, but the relationship can be bidirectional and complex in nature [27]. It is important to understand how mental health can affect the presentation of obesity and alter treatment effectiveness with lifestyle therapy. Disorders of emotional regulation like depression and anxiety can lead to emotional eating, where people choose to eat as a way to regulate their mood or cope with anxiety [28, 29]. When severe, altered mood states can also negatively affect thought patterns and decision making, limiting engagement in treatment and rational problem solving necessary for lifestyle change. Those taking a variety of mood stabilizers and atypical antipsychotics may experience medication-induced weight gain and develop insulin resistance, with varying rates of weight gain and risk for T2D [30]. Eating disorders such as binge eating may require specific psychotherapy with or without pharmacotherapy to improve outcomes for sustained weight reduction [31, 32]. Poorly managed behavioral health concerns can increase the severity of the initial obesity presentation and negatively affect the implementation of an otherwise appropriate treatment strategy. Therefore, it is incumbent on the provider to identify comorbid mental health disorders to effectively implement lifestyle therapy for obesity treatment.

The Risk Associated with Obesity and Implications for Lifestyle Therapy

In addition to associated mental health conditions, obesity has pleiotropic effects on disease risk and overall health. Some of the major conditions that are directly or partially attributable to obesity are shown in Table 21.2. Excess adiposity leads to both mechanical (e.g., joint destruction and hypoventilation) and physiologic derangements (e.g., T2D and dyslipidemia). These comorbid conditions ultimately

Table 21.2 Major diseases and conditions associated with or caused by obesity

Type-2 diabetes
Metabolic syndrome
Cancers of the uterus, breast, and colon
Nonalcoholic fatty liver disease
Cholelithiasis
Gastroesophageal reflux disease
Polycystic ovarian syndrome
Urinary incontinence
Obstructive sleep apnea
Obesity hypoventilation
Osteoarthritis
Gout
Pseudotumor cerebri
Dyslipidemia
Coronary heart disease
Congestive heart failure
Hypertension
Stroke
Depression

contribute to poor self-perception of overall health status and quality of life [33, 34]. Studies of various groups of individuals with obesity, either in community, research, or dedicated treatment settings, have demonstrated that obesity negatively affects a number of quality of life domains. To further underscore the relationship between obesity and quality of life, treatment of obesity by a variety of methods leads to significant improvements in quality of life [35, 36].

Understanding the effects of obesity on the individual patient can be informative for tailoring lifestyle therapy. As a result of defining the effects that obesity has on the patient and the associated disease processes attributable to obesity, therapy should be directed at ameliorating the underlying obesity as well as treating the comorbid conditions. Reducing body weight through calorie restriction will improve a range of risk factors such as blood pressure, lipids, and blood glucose. However, additional maneuvers beyond calorie restriction such as changes in diet composition, increases in physical activity, and behavioral strategies can augment these outcomes, at times independent of weight change. These outcomes can be targeted based on the associated comorbidities and intervention strategies designed accordingly. The focus of the remainder of this chapter is on delineating the expected outcomes and responses to specific intervention maneuvers so that practitioners can prescribe lifestyle interventions as medicine for the treatment of obesity in a tailored fashion.

Key Principles for Treatment of Obesity

Creating a Negative Energy Balance

Obesity develops from an energy imbalance resulting in the storage of excess energy as fat. The reduction in body fat can be established by addressing this energy imbalance through changes in energy intake and/or energy expenditure. Simplistically, energy balance is a thermodynamic process. However, it becomes complex once the dynamic physiological adaptations that occur with reducing body weight are considered [37]. These include alterations in REE, which is largely a factor of lean body mass, as well as changes in the energy expended during physical activity with weight loss. With this said, the same basic principle is supported, *weight loss occurs when the energy balance scale is tipped to negative*, irrespective of whether the effective intervention is based on individual application or some combination of eating patterns, physical activity, behavior, medication, or surgery.

Research continues to explore components of the energy balance equation, particularly as it relates to weight loss and weight loss maintenance. A guiding principle for continued weight loss is to reduce energy intake and/or increase energy expenditure by 3500 kcal to lose 1 pound [38]. Thus, a 500 kcal/day negative energy imbalance would theoretically create a 1 pound per week loss in body weight. However, without compensating for physiological adaptations during weight loss, this 3500 rule overestimates weight loss results. More complex mathematical models have been developed that account for these metabolic adjustments during negative energy balance [37]. Hall et al. [37] show over a 10 kg difference in weight loss using the static linear model of the 3500 rule versus their dynamic model that incorporates energy expenditure changes with weight loss. Thus, when utilizing the 3500 kcal value, it should not be surprising that patients typically fail to reach their expected weight loss or their weight loss goals, even for those strictly adhering to their diet program.

As part of weight loss, it is important to consider the partitioning of weight loss into body fat and lean tissue. Whereas fat mass contains 9404 kcals per kg, the equivalent mass in lean tissue is 1809 kcals, nearly a fivefold difference between tissues. A general rule of thumb is that during weight loss, ~80% comes from fat mass and ~20% from lean mass [39]. However, a number of factors influence this ratio including initial adiposity levels (body composition), participation in exercise, level of energy restriction, rate of weight loss, and protein level in the diet [40]. Because of the increased energy cost in maintaining lean body mass versus fat mass, the loss of lean body mass during negative energy balance further decreases REE.

Interestingly, Hall's prediction model comparing a 250–500 kcal daily negative energy balance created by diet restriction versus an energetically similar increase in physical activity shows a higher and more rapid weight loss with physical activity versus diet restriction [37]. However, this model does not account for the effect of physical activity on food intake. Furthermore, this model has not been confirmed in a strictly controlled randomized trial.

Compensation for the Negative Energy Balance

Alterations in the energy balance components do not happen independently of each other. Compensatory changes occur when another component is changed. There is a strong biological action to protect against a negative energy balance that occurs with energy restriction. Energy restriction reduces energy expenditure components, including REE and physical AEE in weight-dependent activities. In contrast, there is less compensatory change with overfeeding; together, our biology protects us more against weight loss than weight gain.

The weight loss plateau observed in most studies after ~6 months of weight loss is attributed to metabolic adaptations to energy expenditure, as energy expenditure decreases to equate intake. Thus, the negative energy balance is mitigated. Resting metabolic rate is the largest component of total daily energy expenditure, and even before significant weight occurs, RMR decreases substantially with energy restriction [41–43]. In a 12-week weight loss program consisting of a very low-calorie energy-restricted diet (565–650 kcals/day) and exercise training, weight loss averaged 67% of the predicted values; this has been attributed to a 11% decrease in RMR during the first month of the study, as well as reductions in the dietary-induced thermogenesis, the proportions of loss of fat mass and lean body mass, and decrease in AEE with the weight loss [39]. Using prediction equations modeled from weight loss studies, the early weight loss plateau that occurs is likely due to intermittent poor adherence to lifestyle changes [44].

When a Calorie is Not Necessarily a Calorie

The frequently referenced Atwater physiological fuel values of fats, carbohydrates, and protein considers the heat of combustion of the nutrient as well as its digestibility. These values of 9, 4, and 4 kcals/gram for fat, carbohydrates, and protein, respectively, are commonly used to estimate the metabolizable energy of food. However, the energy availability for these macronutrients is not constant, and other constituents in foods will alter the bioavailability and subsequent energy value for the macronutrients. For example, the Atwater physiological fuel values overestimate the available energy in a low-fat, high-fiber diet by ~10%, independent of whether the fiber is from cereal or fruit and vegetable sources [45]. A modified Atwater approach separates the carbohydrates into available and unavailable (dietary fiber) carbohydrates; each of these have their own energy values with the energy value for dietary fiber taken to be 2 kcal/g [46]. This is mostly the result of fermentation of undigested dietary carbohydrates in the large intestine to short-chain fatty acids, which supply a lower physiological fuel value.

Besides the presence of fiber in foods/diet, other foods and chemical components in foods that potentially have been shown to alter energy balance through changes in dietary energy availability and energy expenditure in different models include dehydroepiandrosterone (DHEA), nuts, microbiota, medium-chain triglycerides (MCTs), and green tea. In an experimental model utilizing aged rats, DHEA administered in the diet for 13 weeks decreased the digestibility of dietary protein [47]. A recent review [48] presented evidence from epidemiological studies of an inverse relationship between body weight (BMI) and nut consumption (peanuts and tree nuts) [49–52]. Clinical studies also showed that inclusion of nuts into a diet resulted in no weight change. These results are similar to those found with pecans [53] and almonds [54]. Although nuts are high in energy density, this lack of weight gain with chronic consumption indicates that: (1) the energy intake provided by the nuts is offset by a reduction in the energy intake from other foods; (2) an increase in energy expenditure occurs with nut consumption; and/or (3) there is a decrease in available energy from the nuts [48]. In an energy balance study, consumption of whole peanuts increased fecal fat excretion [55]. The amount of fat loss was about one-third of the fat contained in the peanuts.

The microbiota contained in the human gut are also being investigated regarding their effect on nutrient digestion and absorption. The short-chain fatty acids formed from the digestion of complex and indigestible carbohydrates by selected bacteria have been shown to activate G-protein-coupled receptors in gut epithelial cells [56]. The effect from this is a reduction in gut motility and a subsequent increase in nutrient absorption. This action is thought to be involved in the pathology of metabolic disorders, such as T2D. Presently, the specific microbes that lead to disorders or protect against these conditions are not known. Use of probiotics, prebiotics, antibiotics, bariatric weight loss surgery, energy restriction, and exercise modifies the gut microbial population, and these are currently being investigated for new strategies for obesity and metabolic disease treatment [57]. However, at this time, it is premature to recommend or include probiotics in the obesity treatment regimen in an attempt to alter the patients' microbiota.

MCTs, containing 8–12 carbon atoms, have different metabolic pathways than long-chain triglycerides (LCTs). MCT are more soluble and therefore have preferential absorption into the portal vein compared to LCT. They undergo rapid metabolism by beta-oxidation gaining mitochondrial entry without the carnitine shuttle. Research has shown that MCT increase energy expenditure and lipid oxidation, and some studies present data for increased satiety and reduction in food intake versus LCT [58–60]. Hence, MCT have the potential to create a negative energy balance with long-term weight loss. The current intake in the USA is about 1.3 g/day, mostly as coconut oil and palm kernel oil [61]. In a meta-analysis of 13 studies on the effects of MCT on weight loss, Mumme et al. [62] found modest reductions in body weight and body fat by replacing LCT with MCT. However, this group identified several factors that may have affected the quality of the results, including the level of dietary restriction, dosage of MCT (ranging from 2 up to 54 g/day), and study duration (1–4 months).

Several studies have shown that tea, specifically green tea and oolong tea, influences energy balance through increasing energy expenditure and fat oxidation [63, 64]. The polyphenols found in tea have been investigated as the mechanism responsible for the modest increase in energy output [65]. A recent systematic review demonstrated that the use of green tea extracts (primarily catechins and caffeine) exposed individuals to higher concentrations of the active ingredients as compared to drinking tea prepared from steeping a tea bag in hot water. This paves the way for the use of a supplement containing the purported active ingredients from tea.

Although the level of weight loss ranged from 0.3 to 3.5 kg over about 3 months [66], this magnitude of weight loss does not approach the 5–10% weight loss deemed to be clinically significant. Furthermore, an alternative mechanism for tea catechins promoting weight loss lies in a suppression of energy nutrient absorption [67].

Behavior Modification Approaches for Lifestyle Therapy in Obesity

Successful behavior modification interventions have several key components in common. These components and strategies are often employed in other disease treatment strategies as well. Some of the most commonly used strategies include frequent contact, self-monitoring, stimulus control, group support, and goal setting. The most recent guidelines on the treatment of obesity suggest that high-frequency contact schedules (at least 14 contacts in a 6-month period) are associated with the highest amounts of weight loss on average with behavioral interventions [5]. In many traditional weight loss interventions, one source of contact is the group counseling session. Research has demonstrated that attendance at behavioral counseling sessions is highly correlated with successful weight reduction [68, 69]. The group counseling session becomes a setting for social support that provides opportunities for group interaction with other participants. This approach naturally leads to participants modeling behavior for each other and helping each other solve problems.

In addition to providing a source of social support, group counseling can be used to teach skills and behavioral strategies such as goal setting, problem solving, and stimulus control. For goal setting, emphasis is placed on the individual's ability to regulate his/her own behavior by setting goals and monitoring progress towards the goals [70]. Goals should be short-term, specific, and matched to the participant's priorities and preferences. The practitioner can also assess the patient's confidence to achieve a particular goal (i.e., self-efficacy) and modify goals where self-efficacy is perceived to be low. Problem solving is a common skill that most people use regularly in a range of areas in daily life; in this context, it refers to helping the patient in identifying his/her own barriers and generating alternative responses/solutions. In this way, the provider is not playing the "expert" role and offering solutions to problems identified by the patient, but facilitating the process whereby the patient devises solutions for him/herself.

The behavior that is most often correlated with a high degree of successful behavior modification is self-monitoring [71]. Self-monitoring of dietary intake and physical activity behaviors leads to an increased awareness of actual behavior and allows the patient to identify patterns, triggers, and thought errors that lead to deviations from the prescribed plan. Additionally, in the setting of supervised behavioral counseling, review of the food or activity diary can be instructive for the participant and the practitioner, leading to identification of implementation errors or provide insight for additional adjustments to the plan necessary to optimize adherence and effectiveness.

Counseling Strategies for Obesity

Several strategies or approaches to behavioral counseling for obesity treatment have been popularized since the early 2000s, including motivational interviewing (MI) and the 5 A's approach. MI is a behavioral counseling strategy that was derived from substance abuse counseling paradigms and applied in obesity interventions [72]. MI provides a client-centered approach to counseling that allows the patient to identify his or her values and define action steps that are then consistent with those values [72]. Using an MI framework, the practitioner engages in reflective listening and facilitates the goal setting agenda by offering clarifying statements and probing with key questions.

The 5 A's approach is similar to the MI framework in that it has been adapted from the smoking cessation treatment paradigm and applied to general behavioral counseling schemes for lifestyle change [73]. However, the 5 A's approach is different from MI in that it is more structured, listing a series of actions for the provider to take in a counseling encounter with a patient that include assess, advise, agree, assist, and arrange (follow-up) [74]. With this framework, the practitioner is guided to assess weight status and associated risk, followed by a conversation to advise the patient of this risk and the implications of the risk. The patient and practitioner then agree upon goals and behavioral targets to change to reach the goals. The practitioner is then responsible for assisting the patient in developing a plan or accessing resources that help to achieve the behavior change. Finally, the practitioner arranges for follow-up to provide accountability, monitor progress, and adjust the plan as needed.

There have been very few studies that have compared the effectiveness of one behavioral counseling approach to another, making it difficult to say which technique lends to better outcomes. Ultimately, we recommend that the practitioner have some familiarity with these types of techniques and apply them as necessary in a given situation. In many instances, each one of these types of techniques can be used synergistically to accomplish effective behavioral counseling.

Strategies for Implementing Energy Restriction

Total energy intake is typically reduced by 500–1000 kcals per day to result in a 3500–7000 kcal weekly deficit, or a 1–2 pound per week weight loss. It has already been described that this static model results in less than predicted weight loss based on physiological adaptations that occur with weight loss. Reducing daily energy intake can be accomplished through several dietary changes. These include reducing portion sizes, choosing more nutrient-dense and less energy-dense foods, utilizing meal replacements (MRs), or altering macronutrient composition, glycemic index/load, meal frequency, or eating pattern.

Macronutrient Restriction

In conjunction with a restriction of total energy intake to produce a negative energy balance, alterations in macronutrient content is often considered a key factor in weight loss promotion. Since proteins, carbohydrates, and lipids have different effects on energy metabolism, appetite, and satiety, it is intuitive to consider that altering the proportion of macronutrients in diets with similar total calories will impact weight loss and body composition changes. Furthermore, altering diet composition may also change the energy density of the diet. A theoretical basis for the role diet composition plays in obesity treatment and prevention was presented by Flatt [75]. Because of the finite capacity for storing protein and carbohydrate in the body, and the nearly limitless capacity for fat storage, the body must have an ability to acutely regulate protein and carbohydrate balance. In contrast, the regulation of fat balance can occur chronically. The impact of macronutrient content of the diet on the body's energy balance depends to some extent on the energy state of the body, that is, in a negative, positive, or neutral energy balance. When in negative energy balance, there is no significant difference between reducing the fat or carbohydrate content of the diet as long as the total calorie reduction is similar. In contrast, if the energy intake is not fixed between diets, that is, ad libitum intake, differences in weight loss occur between high- versus low-fat diets [76–78]. This supports the theory that the macronutrient composition of the diet impacts feeding behaviors during weight loss. Furthermore, in energy balance conditions (stable weight), low-fat diets are associated with a reduced body weight, which may be based on the higher dietary-induced thermogenesis and lower energy intake with carbohydrates and proteins versus fat [79, 80]. Conventional wisdom dictated that a high-carbohydrate, low-fat diet produced more favorable weight loss and improvements in cardiovascular metabolic risk factors than a low-carbohydrate, high-fat diet. However, this approach was challenged when a well-publicized clinical trial showed that women following a low-carbohydrate, high-fat (Atkins pattern) diet lost more weight and had better improvements in cardiovascular metabolic risk factors than those following a diet higher in carbohydrates (Ornish pattern) [81]. In this randomized controlled trial (RCT), the calorie distribution intake from fat, carbohydrates, and protein at 12 months was 44, 35, and 21 % for Atkins compared to 30, 52, and 18 % for the Ornish diet.

More recently, high-protein diets have gained attention as a dietary strategy for weight loss and post-weight-loss regain. Generally, high-protein diets contain 25–35 % of energy as protein. In theory, a high-protein diet causes changes in both sides of the energy balance equation by increasing dietary-induced thermogenesis as well as reducing energy intake through altering satiety hormones [82–85]. Evidence from RCTs has supported the favorable outcome of a high-protein diet on weight management [86, 87]. Due et al. [86] showed that a diet composed of 25 % of energy from protein resulted in greater weight loss at 6 months than a diet containing 12 % of energy from protein. By 12 months, there was no difference in mean weight loss between diet groups; however, more individuals lost at least 10 kg in the higher protein diet. Ankarfeldt et al. [88] provided further evidence that a high-protein diet may be beneficial for weight loss in individuals who were overweight or obese. These data are consistent with findings from a meta-analysis of 24 studies that showed energy-restricted high-protein (mean of 1.25 g protein/kg body weight) versus standard-protein (mean of 0.72 g protein/kg body weight) diets produced greater decreases in body weight (-0.79 kg) and fat mass (-0.87 kg), as well as reduced decreases in fat-free mass (0.43 kg) [89]. However, these were generally short-term trials with the mean duration of ~ 12 weeks. Furthermore, there was greater satiety from the high-protein diets. Although this meta-analysis was confined to studies that included diets with the same amount of calories, there were still advantages with regards to weight loss and body composition changes, indicating that the effect was not based on lowering energy intake.

However, there is also support indicating that clinically meaningful weight loss can occur across a broad range of macronutrient composition [90]. In a study that examined four diets that varied in content of fat (20–40 %), protein (15–25 %), and carbohydrates (35–65 %), there was similar weight loss among the interventions over a 2-year period [91]. At the end of the trial, weight loss was modest at 4 kg on average across all groups. There were no differences in hunger and satiety ratings for all diets. Overall, trials comparing a wide variety of macronutrient distributions have found weight loss success in nearly all types of hypocaloric diets [92]. Thus, the weight loss success of a diet may, in part, be dependent on the ability of the individual to adhere to the hypocaloric diet.

Dietary Energy Density

The notion that energy density (kcals per gram of food) plays a role in energy intake, such that over time there would be a reduction in body weight, is based on evidence that humans eat a certain volume of food, independent of total energy content. If energy density increases, and the volume of food stays constant, a greater number of calories will be ingested [92–94]. Increasing fruit and vegetable consumption, which are high in water content and dietary fiber as well as reducing high-fat- and sugar-containing foods will decrease the energy density of the diet. If dietary compensation does not occur, there will be a decrease in total energy intake with subsequent weight loss. Over the short term, consuming a low-energy-dense food, such as soup or salad, before a meal reduces total energy intake for a single meal and for multiple meals when consumed over 1–2 days [95–98]. Rolls et al. further expanded this and found that consumption of two daily servings of a low-energy-dense soup compared to an isocaloric high-energy-dense snack lead to 50% greater weight loss up to 12 months [99]. Furthermore, counseling to lower energy density through increasing fruit and vegetable intake, along with fat intake, lead to greater weight loss than a group only instructed on reducing fat intake [100]. This was further supported in a 3-month weight loss study that showed that individuals randomized to an ad libitum low-energy-density diet prescription lost more weight than a calorie-restricted, low-fat group [101]. There is also evidence to suggest that a low-energy-dense diet will prevent regain of lost weight for up to 2 years of follow-up [102]. Taken together, increasing nutrient density through consuming low-energy-dense foods will promote greater weight loss and potentially less weight regain during weight maintenance. This evidence formed the basis for the 2010 Dietary Guidelines recommendation to consume an eating pattern low in energy density to manage body weight.

Glycemic Index

There has been substantial interest investigating the effect of the glycemic load of a diet, which is defined as the product of the glycemic index and grams of carbohydrates in a food, on weight loss. The rationale is that a high-carbohydrate intake, specifically refined carbohydrates, will have a larger insulin response, thereby stimulating hunger and inhibiting fat oxidation. Not only would this enhance energy storage, but it also increases the risk for T2D and the metabolic syndrome. Consumption of a lower carbohydrate and higher protein diet could provide favorable alterations in energy expenditure, blood lipids, and glucose homeostasis. In a recent meta-analysis comparing low- versus high-glycemic-index diet on weight loss, adults on the low-glycemic-index diet had 1.1 kg more weight loss than the high-glycemic index diet after 5 weeks to 6 months of intervention [103]. Conversely, Esfahani et al. [104] suggest there were significant inconsistencies in the clinical trials that compared low-glycemic-index and glycemic load diets on weight loss. In this

review, only 4 of the 19 controlled trials favored low-glycemic-index or glycemic load diets compared to controls. Although most studies showed a trend for increased weight loss with a low-glycemic-index or glycemic load diet, this effect did not reach statistical significance. Similarly, the glycemic index and glycemic load diets showed only nonsignificant effects on changes in body composition variables compared to control groups. These findings by Esfahani et al. [104] are consistent with the meta-analysis by Ajala et al. [105] who found that in comparison with control diets, a low-glycemic-index diet showed no difference in weight loss. In a large multisite trial in Europe, high-protein diets (>25% of total energy consumed) and low-glycemic-index diets showed the most resistance to weight regain following a mean 11 kg loss in body weight (~0.95 kg less weight regained over a 26-week period) [87]. Only the high-glycemic-index and low-protein diet combination showed significant weight regain. Low- and high-glycemic-index diets were targeted to differ by 15 glycemic index units. Additionally, during this weight maintenance phase of the study, the diets were not intentionally restricted but were ad libitum. Finally, McMillan-Price et al. [106] completed an RCT examining four different diets that varied in carbohydrates, protein, and glycemic index and load, and all with similar fat and dietary fiber intake. Although all four diets produced the same amount of weight loss across the 12-week study, the high-carbohydrate, low-glycemic-index diet, and the high-protein, high-glycemic-index diet had a higher proportion of participants achieving the clinically significant 5% weight loss goal. Thus, it is uncertain whether reducing the glycemic index and glycemic load of a diet leads to greater weight loss. Notwithstanding this conclusion, there may be other health advantages for consuming a low-glycemic-index or glycemic load diet, as well as other dietary manipulations, beyond weight loss.

Adopting Different Eating Patterns

Vegetarian

Studies show that individuals who adhere to a vegetarian dietary pattern have lower BMI and are leaner than nonvegetarians; this may be attributed to vegetarians consuming nearly 500 fewer kcals per day. This also provides a basis that this type of dietary pattern may be effective for weight loss in individuals who are overweight or obese [107–109]. Although there are risks for nutrient deficiencies with following a vegetarian eating pattern, such as protein, calcium, iron, and vitamin B12 [110], the diet is also rich in dietary fiber, whole grains, fruits, vegetables, and legumes. This high-nutrient-dense diet contains a high volume of fiber and water content, and this increases satiety and reduces hunger [111]. In an RCT that compared two calorie- and fat-restricted diets—one was from vegetarian sources and the other a standard omnivorous diet—both diets resulted in 8% weight loss at 18 months, indicating that a vegetarian dietary pattern could be sustained for a long period and that weight loss results are comparable to a standard diet over the long term [112]. A recent study that compared weight loss in overweight postmenopausal women showed that 14 weeks of behavioral counseling for a vegan diet resulted in greater weight loss at 1 and 2 years of follow-up than those on a National Cholesterol Education Program (NCEP) diet (−4.9 kg vs. −1.8 kg at year 1, respectively, and −3.1 kg vs. −0.8 kg at year 2, respectively) [113]. Turner-McGrievy et al. also performed a comparison study between four different types of plant-based diets (vegan [no animal products], vegetarian [no meat but allowed eggs and dairy], pesco-vegetarian [no meat but allowed eggs, dairy, and fish], and semi-vegetarian [allowed red meat ≤ 1 times/week and poultry ≤ 5 times/week]), and an omnivorous diet. Although this was conducted in overweight adults, calorie restriction and weight loss was not emphasized in the regular group meetings. At 6 months, all groups lost weight, but individuals following the vegan diet lost more than the pesco-vegetarian, semi-vegetarian, and omnivorous diets: −7.5% for vegan, −6.3% for vegetarian, −3.2% for pesco-vegetarian, −3.2% for semi-vegetarian, and −3.1% for omnivorous. This study is consistent with the notion that a nutrient-dense vegan diet can lead to greater weight loss than other less nutrient-dense plant-based and omnivorous diets [114]. In addition, it indicates that less stringent vegetarian eating patterns are at least comparable to omnivorous diets with regards to nutrient content and weight loss.

Mediterranean

Mediterranean diets are rich in olive oil, legumes, unrefined cereals, fruit, and vegetables, moderate in dairy, fish, and wine (when not proscribed for religious reasons) as well as being low in meat and meat products. This eating pattern has been extensively studied for cardiovascular health and results consistently show benefits with regard to cardiovascular metabolic risk factors, morbidity, and mortality. Although not frequently investigated solely as a weight loss diet, a recent meta-analysis of RCTs showed a − 1.86 kg better weight loss for Mediterranean diets than control diets. These data were derived from three trials lasting 6–12 months. In this eating pattern, the increase in whole grains, fruits, vegetables, and nuts likely contribute to the weight loss as these foods have a low energy and high-nutrient density [115, 116]. Several observational studies have also supported the weight loss effects of the Mediterranean diets [117–120]. There are also data to suggest that this eating pattern reduces risk for weight gain in adults [119, 121, 122]. Higher adherence to a Mediterranean eating pattern was associated with reduced weight gain and lower risk to develop obesity [123].

Paleo

A popular eating pattern that is only recently being researched in a systematic way is the Paleolithic (or "Paleo") diet. This diet comprises foods likely consumed during the Paleolithic period. Staple foods in the Paleolithic diet are lean meats, fish, shellfish, fruits, vegetables, roots, eggs, and nuts, with the avoidance of grains, dairy products, salt, and refined fats and sugar. Studies have found improvements in health indicators for individuals with T2D and CVD, including hemoglobin A1c (A1C), glucose tolerance, insulin sensitivity, inflammation, blood pressure, clotting factors, and blood lipid profiles [124–133]. Although several of these reports maintained body weight [133], there are a few studies that show reduction in body weight and waist circumference with this diet [129, 134]. Compared to a standard "diabetes diet," following a Paleolithic diet for 3 months resulted in 3 kg greater weight loss and a 4 cm reduction in waist circumference. Along with being lower in total energy, energy density, carbohydrates, glycemic load, calcium, and saturated fat, the Paleolithic diet was higher in unsaturated fat, cholesterol, selected vitamins, fruits, vegetables, meat, and eggs [134]. This reduction in total calories was accompanied by increased ratings of satiety at meal times, although participants reported difficulty in adhering to the diet [134].

Meal Replacements

Controlling portion sizes is a component of most dietary weight loss interventions. Research has shown that individuals increase their food, beverage, and total energy intake when they are provided larger portions at meals [135–137]. By limiting food exposure using proportioned foods, energy and food intake can be reduced. This is consistent with the 2010 Dietary Guidelines Advisory Committee reports [138]. Utilizing MRs is a strategy that has been utilized in a number of large-scale clinical weight loss trials [139–141]. MR are mostly liquid products and may be partial (PMR) or complete (CMR). For PMR, one to two meals a day are from the liquid meal, with one to two meals from conventional foods. In contrast, a program utilizing CMR has no conventional foods added to their diet. Both PMR and CMR add structure to the program and minimize decisions made by the individual on the amount and type of food to eat. By using a product with a balanced nutrient profile, nutrient intake is actually enhanced compared to an ad libitum weight-stable group [142].

The success for MR in weight loss programs has been highlighted in two recent reviews [143, 144]. Over a 12-month period, there was improved weight loss and compliance with liquid PMR versus lifestyle-change programs. In the Look AHEAD trial, the amount of weight loss at 1 year was related to the number of MR [139]. Another approach to portion control encompasses using preportioned foods, a more general paradigm for liquid MR. These preportioned foods are typically conventional foods that are packaged for single meals or snacks. This still provides the same general concept of portion control that a liquid MR has, but it incorporates a variety by using solid foods. Solid food products have been shown to enhance satiety as compared to liquid MR [145, 146]. A recent systematic review and meta-analysis of effectiveness trials showed that a commercial program that provided MR produced 6.83 kg greater weight loss at 12 months compared to a control group [147, 148]. This difference continued at the 24-month follow-up. Together, this may lead to enhanced continued use with preportioned solid foods. While the number of studies using these products are limited, weight loss was greater up to 1 year when preportioned solid foods comprised the diet plan compared to a self-selected diet that was targeted as being isocaloric to the preportioned foods [149, 150].

Based on its use of liquid products, a very low-calorie diet (VLCD) program is often a part of a CMR strategy. With this diet, up to 800 calories are provided per day, mostly using commercial formulas in the form of liquid shakes, soups, or bars. This type of diet requires medical supervision and is most frequently used to promote quick weight loss for a short time period. A loss of 1.5–3 kg per week is expected with this diet. Importantly, there can be rapid improvements in comorbidities of obesity, including T2D, hypertension, dyslipidemia, and reducing liver volume [151–153]. The most serious side effect is gallstones, although there are frequent reports of fatigue and gastrointestinal distress. To help preserve the loss of lean body mass on this diet, a minimum of 50 g of protein is included in the diet. In a recent review of commercial VLCD, the difference in mean percentage weight from the VLCD and comparison group ranged from −1.0 to −22.1% over a 3 to 9 month period.

Alternate Day Fasting

The reduction of energy intake through alternate day fasting is an eating pattern that is currently being investigated. This takes several different forms, but one method that was recently studied was alternating days of ad libitum intake followed by consuming 25–30% of energy needs in a fasting day [152, 153]. In these nonrandomized longitudinal trials, 4–6 weeks of alternate day fasting decreased weight by 5–6 kg, a rate of about 0.67 kg/week. Additionally, CVD

metabolic risk factors improved in both studies with reductions in systolic blood pressure, total and LDL cholesterol as well as triglyceride concentrations. This alternate form of dietary restriction was developed primarily to increase adherence. Instead of a daily reduction of 15–40% in an individual's energy needs, this provides a model where they are limiting their intake only every other day. Varady et al. [153] demonstrated that participants were able to adhere to this program on 85% of the days throughout the 8-week study. A recent study also showed that the timing of the meal(s) for the alternate day fasting has little impact on weight loss and CVD risk factors and may provide more flexibility for the individual [154]. Further research is necessary in this area to see if adherence remains high and if the weight loss is maintained over an extended period of time.

Strategies to Increase Physical Activity Energy Expenditure and Decrease Sedentary Behaviors

Intensity of Exercise and Interval Training

Epidemiological evidence from observational trials indicates declining levels of physical activity in the USA. Without adjusting energy intake, the decline in energy expenditure would lead to a positive energy balance. As a component of a lifestyle weight loss intervention, physical activity provides an additive effect to dietary restriction. By itself, a moderate increase in physical activity can achieve up to a 3 kg weight loss [155–162]. Part of the response is obviously related to level of exercise. Individuals engaging in 225–420 min of activity each week lost from 5 to 7.5 kg, whereas 2–3 kg was lost when minutes of activity per week was greater than 150 [163].

Frequently, physical activity is attributed to prevention of weight regain from previous dietary restriction. Some have reported that it just takes a small increase in physical activity to prevent weight gain [164]; however, much more activity is required to avoid weight regain after previous weight loss [165]. In a number of trials, the level of physical activity (reported as kcals expended in activity or minutes of activity per week) is related to weight loss at long-term (18–36 months) follow-up. Women that achieved at least a 10% weight loss after 24 months reported activity levels of 275 min per week (1515 kcals per week) [166]. In contrast, those achieving less than from 0 to 5% weight loss at 24 months reported an increase in physical activity of less than 500 kcals per week. Furthermore, a study that investigated components of behavioral weight loss interventions showed that engaging in high levels of physical activity was important for sustaining at least a 10% weight loss over 24 months [167]. The 2259 kcals/week expended through exercise by those that maintained > 10% weight loss at 24 months is similar to the amount of activity reported in the National Weight Control Registry [165]. The ACC/AHA/TOS obesity guidelines from 2014 also suggest that exercise reduces weight regain with VLCDs [5]. These same guidelines prescribe at least 150 min of aerobic physical activity per week for weight loss with 200–300 min per week for maintaining lost weight or reducing weight regain. These recommendations are derived from a review of ten RCTs (citations for these are provided in the ACC/AHA/TOS obesity guidelines) that investigated comprehensive interventions in this area. Unfortunately, most of these data are from secondary analyses from RCTs or from observational studies and do not fully answer the question of the role for physical activity in weight loss maintenance or the regain of lost weight.

To address the role of intensity of physical activity on weight loss, Jakicic et al. [166] randomized nearly 200 women (BMI 27–40 kg/m^2) into one of four groups: Vigorous Intensity/High Duration; Moderate Intensity/High Duration; Moderate Intensity/Moderate Duration; and Vigorous Intensity/Moderate Duration. The moderate and high duration groups had an estimated energy expenditure of 1000 and 2000 kcals/week, respectively. By 12 months, each of the moderate and high duration groups had lost 8–10% of their initial body weight, which was not statistically different. This nonsignificance between intervention groups remained at 24 months. Interestingly, the intensity of the exercise did not appear to affect weight loss; however, the low adherence to the exercise intensity prescription may have left this question unanswered. Similarly, others have shown that exercise intensity and duration have minimal impact on weight loss [168]. In this study, weight loss was similar in a 24-week program comparing combinations of low or high amount of activity and low- or high-intensity exercise. Participants were told to maintain similar calorie intake to baseline measures throughout the study. Although the exercising groups had greater reductions in waist circumference and weight loss than the non-exercising controls, there were no differences among the exercise groups. Thus, these studies showed that exercise intensity and duration had minimal impact on weight loss and weight maintenance.

One mode of exercise that is gaining popularity for weight loss as well as overall health is to engage in high-intensity interval training (HIIT). With this type of exercise program, individuals engage in a high-intensity bout of exercise for 30 s to several minutes, followed by 1–5 min of recovery. This is repeated at a minimum of four times, giving 2–5 min of exercise at maximum intensity and 15–25 min of low-intensity exercise for each session. The advantage is that it is time efficient and has increased patient compliance. There is improvement in cardiometabolic risk factors in both healthy and at-risk populations. Studies show that HIIT lowers body weight, regional fat deposits in the subcutaneous and abdominal depots, insulin resistance, and blood cholesterol as well as raises cardiovascular fitness compared to continuous moderate aerobic exercise [169–173]. Because a frequent barrier for exercise is time constraints, an HIIT program has been well received by individuals and it leads to less boredom [174, 175]. A major limitation with this type of program is the potential higher risk for injuries, especially for elderly and sedentary individuals. Nevertheless, one study found no differences in injuries between those performing HIIT and other forms of exercise [176].

Modality of Exercise

The modality of exercise that provides the greatest benefits in weight loss is continually being studied as research indicates that alternate formats like resistance training have benefits beyond aerobic training. The position from the American College of Sports Medicine touts the benefits of resistance training as part of a weight loss program [163]. A common theme in this area though is that the evidence for these recommendations has not been the primary aim in RCTs, but instead the data from observational studies and secondary analyses. In a recent randomized trial (STRRIDE AT/RT), aerobic training, resistance training, and their combination were compared for their effect on body weight and body fat loss [177]. There was no specific dietary restriction employed in the study. The aerobic training prescription consisted of treadmill, elliptical trainers, and cycle ergometers for a total time of about 130 min per week at 65–80% of peak VO$_2$. The resistance training consisted of 3 days/week for 3 sets/day with 8–12 repetitions/set for both upper and lower body training. The combination group performed both the aerobic and resistance training. Weight loss and fat mass (kg) change was similar between the aerobic training and combination group, and both were greater than the resistance training only group. The lean body mass change was similar for the two resistance training groups, which was greater than for the aerobic-only training group. Both aerobic and resistance training provided benefits to weight loss and body composition with aerobic training reducing body fat and resistance training increasing lean body mass and decreasing percent body fat. Their combination showed effects on both reduction in body fat and increase in lean body mass. Thus, both training modes provide beneficial effects on body composition. However, if exercise time is limited and the primary focus is loss of body weight and fat mass, then aerobic training is the optimal mode. This is supported by an earlier trial that kept weekly exercise constant between groups [178].

As patients turn to holistic medical options for health and well-being, yoga has become more mainstream. If effective, it has the potential to be an economical alternative that has few adverse effects and high levels of adherence and home practice. A number of studies have investigated yoga and weight management, yielding promising results with the reduction in body weight and body fat, and increase in lean body mass observed in several observational and RCT studies [179–190]. The majority of trials were in India, but a few have been in other areas, including the USA, Thailand, and Sweden. Because of the high variability in the study design and methodological concerns, it is difficult to draw conclusive findings, but there does seem to be some promise with this type of lifestyle change to benefit weight loss and body composition.

Reduction of Sedentary Behaviors

Sedentary behaviors are frequently defined as a waking behavior that expends less than 1.5 METS (metabolic equivalents; 1 MET equals energy expended during resting conditions). This usually includes sitting or reclining, such as in a car, or screen time, that is, using a computer or tablet, or viewing television [191]. Individuals that have high levels of sedentary behaviors, even when they are meeting physical activity guidelines, have poor health consequences [192, 193]. Thus, reducing sedentary behaviors in conjunction with increasing physical activity may be an approach for weight management. In testing post-bariatric surgery patients over a 2–16-year follow-up, there is an association between weight loss and high levels of sitting time [194, 195]. Furthermore, interrupting sedentary behaviors with 1–5 min-walking bouts throughout the day is associated with beneficial effects on metabolic risk and body composition [196]. The mechanism underlying the detrimental effects of these sedentary behaviors may reside in changes in muscle metabolism and/or energy expenditure. Animal studies indicate that lack of muscle contractions decreases skeletal muscle lipoprotein metabolism and glucose uptake [197,198]. Furthermore, clinical trials indicate that regular physical activity improves glucose metabolism [199]. Additionally, a 5-min walking break every hour throughout an 8-h workday would lead to an additional daily expenditure of 132 kcals. This equates to a yearly expenditure of 33,000 additional kcals, not a trivial amount. Taking short breaks throughout the day during sedentary behaviors has been shown to affect total daily energy expenditure and may lead to improved muscle metabolism.

Maintenance of Weight Loss

A plan for long-term weight loss is only as good as the strategies designed to maintain the weight loss once a goal is reached. The maintenance of weight loss is the ultimate challenge of lifestyle therapy for obesity. The reasons that maintenance of weight loss is so difficult for many are multifactorial. From a physiological perspective, intentional weight loss is not a naturally occurring phenomenon and is unique among the animal world to humans. Our homeostatic controls of body weight are most sensitive to signals produced by a body that is losing mass, leading to a cascade of physiological adaptations designed to minimize the further loss of mass and restore the body to the previous weight [200, 201]. These adaptations include a lowering of the resting metabolic rate with induction and maintenance of calorie restriction, decreased production of bioactive thyroid hormone, decreased heat generation, decreased circulating leptin, and improvements in muscle efficiency (i.e., burning fewer calories per unit of work) [201]. All of these maneuvers are designed to economize energy usage and lower the demand for energy needs in the setting of energy deficits. In addition to these energy-saving processes, hormonal signals begin to target the central nervous system to increase the sense that energy intake should increase. This is done via increases in hormones that increase hunger sensations and preferences for high-energy-dense foods [202]. Appetite-regulating hormones like ghrelin, cholecystokinin, insulin, peptide YY, gastric inhibitory polypeptide, and leptin all change in response to sustained weight loss, leading to effects that increase the perception of hunger and food-seeking behavior [202]. In the context of these biological changes, the individual is still subjected to an environment that supports a high-energy intake and provides ample energy-saving devices that promote sedentary behavior. The obesogenic environment must be resisted at a point when the internal drivers for overconsumption and energy conservation are at their strongest.

Studies of long-term weight loss reveal some of the effects that are associated with this complex systemic response to the induction of weight loss. Over time, individuals generally have a gradual decrease in overall adherence to the initial dietary prescription. This typically results in a gradual increase in their reported calorie intake, slowly increasing back to a pretreatment level of calorie intake. There is also a gradual return to the pretreatment macronutrient profile or eating pattern. One example of this phenomenon is clearly seen in a study of four popular dietary strategies for calorie restriction that included Atkins, Ornish, Weight Watchers, and Zone diets over 12 months. After the first month, self-rated adherence decreased each month during the study, while calorie intake and macronutrient profiles trended towards baseline no matter what treatment was assigned [203]. In addition to the dietary recidivism, physical activity levels also regress over time. This is especially problematic because more physical activity is required in the maintenance phase as a result of the efficiencies in AEE that occur with weight loss [5]. Studies by Weinsier et al. [204, 205] suggest that in overweight women who were weight reduced to a normal weight with a low-calorie diet and exercise program, a significant proportion of weight regain is attributed to low levels of AEE.

It is difficult to avoid the behavioral aspects of long-term weight control, even though these physiological and environmental forces are so dominant. As the changes in diet and physical activity tend to regress over time, so do the behaviors that are associated with successful induction of weight loss. For example, self-monitoring frequency tends to decrease in people who experience significant weight regain. Several studies have shown that a higher frequency of self-monitoring, including food intake and body weight, is associated with better maintenance of weight loss [71, 206, 207]. The decrease in the practice of these behaviors often corresponds to either a withdrawal or decrease in the frequency of treatment contacts, such as group or individual counseling [208]. As noted previously, higher frequency contact during the induction of weight loss is associated with larger amounts of weight loss; likewise, the longer the duration of this high-frequency contact, the longer the weight loss curve extends [209]. In the end, it is difficult to know which factors come first and the interplay of these systems. For instance, does the persistent hormonal counter-regulatory response decrease the mental resolve to engage in behaviors over time, or does the loss of focused concentrated effort on maintaining behavioral engagement make one more susceptible to the physiological and environmental cues to resume previous behaviors?

Even though the general tendency is for weight regain, there is evidence regarding lifestyle interventions that are associated with maintenance of lost weight. From observational data, we have reports of the behaviors that people consistently use to assist with maintenance of a lower body weight. The National Weight Control Registry includes a self-selected sample of adults who report having maintained at least 30 lb weight loss for more than 1 year [210–212]. Behaviors commonly reported by these individuals include consumption of a low-calorie dietary intake, maintenance of high levels of physical activity (i.e., greater than 200 min per week of at least moderate-intensity physical activity), self-monitoring (e.g., weighing regularly), and limited intake of fast food [213]. While such data are limited due to the nature of self-selection and self-report, there are some consistencies in the potential mechanisms that one would expect to be associated with countering the tendency for weight regain based on the known physiology. A lower calorie intake is necessary to be consistent with the lower body weight achieved and the improvements in energy efficiency. Higher levels of physical activity are also needed to counter the improvements in fitness and energy efficiency that are gained with weight loss. Dietary restraint, demonstrated by limiting fast food or high-energy-dense sweets, is likely required to limit the potential to indulge in highly rewarding food intake behaviors that have negative consequences for weight status.

From controlled trials of weight loss maintenance, we understand that with persistent intervention, a higher proportion of people can be successful at maintaining clinically meaningful amounts of weight loss. Few studies have been conducted with a true maintenance design, where the individual is weight reduced using a standardized or common approach followed by randomization to weight loss maintenance or control interventions. The largest such study to date was the Weight Loss Maintenance Trial, where 1032 individuals who lost at least 4.0 kg during a 6-month-weight loss intervention phase were randomly assigned to an interactive technology-based intervention, a personal contact intervention, or a self-directed intervention (control) and followed for 30 months [214]. A higher proportion of those assigned to the personal contact group (42.2%) compared to the control group (33.9%) maintained at least 5% weight loss at 30 months. The proportion of people who were at or below their post-intervention weight at 30 months was 76.7% in the personal contact group and 69.3% in the interactive technology group. In analyses of predictors of weight loss maintenance success, initial percent weight change and changes in dietary pattern were the only predictors associated with long-term weight changes. For every 1% weight loss achieved in the initial weight loss phase, there was an associated 0.66% weight loss over the course of the 36-month study [215]. Ultimately, the WLM trial demonstrates that short-term weight loss is important for weight loss maintenance, and long-term lifestyle therapy is beneficial and necessary for the treatment of obesity. With a long-term approach to obesity treatment that considers this as a chronic, relapsing disease, there is potential to provide effective therapy that leads to sustainable outcomes.

Developing and Implementing a Treatment Strategy for Obesity

Evaluation

The evaluation of the patient interested in pursuing lifestyle modification to lose weight should include some basic components to establish a clear baseline, provide proper staging of obesity, and identification of risk factors that may modify the treatment approach. The evaluation can include the following components:

- Vital signs including weight, height, BMI, waist circumference, blood pressure,
- Physical examination,
- Laboratory assessments including fasting blood glucose, lipids and insulin, A1C, thyroid-stimulating hormone, and

Weight history including weight trajectory, previous weight loss attempts, eating behaviors, mood assessment, psychiatric history, current activity patterns and limitations, and sleep pattern.

Goal Setting

Setting weight loss goals is a negotiated process that involves the clinician partnering with the patient to identify goals that are well informed and have a reasonable chance of being achieved based on the treatment options available. At a minimum, the clinician should help guide the patient on what may be an appropriate time frame to achieve a weight loss goal.

- Goals should be consistent with the type of strategy utilized (e.g., an MR strategy will generally lead to a faster rate of weight loss, while a food-based deficit diet may require a longer period of time to achieve similar volume of weight loss).
- Frequent feedback on progress towards goals is important.
- Goals should be modified based on the situation and circumstances of the patient; alternatively, treatment can be modified to improve the possibility of reaching goals.
- Include non-weight-specific goals (e.g., improvements in physical function or risk factors, quality of life indices).

Designing Dietary Targets

Based on the identified risk factors, weight loss and risk factor modification goals, and resources available, the dietary strategy can be selected for maximal efficiency in achieving the specified goals. As noted previously, any number of dietary strategies can be successful in producing weight loss as long as the patient can adhere to it and the dietary prescription creates a sufficient calorie deficit.

- Match dietary strategy to the identified risk factors to improve the chances that risk factor improvement will occur even with only modest weight reduction (e.g., low-carbohydrate diet for someone with T2D to improve blood glucose control).
- Understand the lifestyle factors that will affect the patient's ability to adhere to a given dietary strategy (e.g., unlikely to cook or do a lot of food preparation and/or identify convenience-focused strategies).
- Discuss long-term implications of the dietary strategy because the maintenance pattern will likely resemble the initial weight loss strategy.

Designing Fitness Targets

The physical activity plan contributes to the creation of the targeted energy deficit in a significant way and should be emphasized for optimal weight loss. As with dietary strategies, physical activity should be prescribed in a way that the patient can have a sense of confidence about achieving the target with reasonable effort.

- A gradual increase in physical activity to the target goal is preferable.
- Some focus should be given to limiting sedentary activities.
- Emphasis should be on increasing overall activity, but specific goals for moderate to vigorous physical activity are critical.
- Patients should not expect to dramatically increase the rate of weight loss by simply increasing exercise duration.

Follow-Up and Refinement

Providing a support system that gives the patient frequent contact and follow-up is important for success of the patient. It also gives the clinician a chance to intervene early when there are unexpected problems or difficulties implementing the prescribed plan.

- Early follow-up is important to identify problems, typically within a couple of weeks of initiating the plan.
- Short-term weight loss is predictive of longer term weight loss, therefore getting off to a good start is important.
- Be flexible in modifying the plan to address elements that are not working.
- Avoid instructing the patient to just try harder; define more specific plans that have measurable outcomes.

Maintenance Strategies

Once goals have been achieved, a specific maintenance plan should be considered paramount. Because a number of factors have changed and new behaviors can wane over time, the maintenance plan should help the patient understand the new requirements for weight control and the behaviors critical to maintaining a lower weight.

- A repeat of the initial assessment can provide the patient with a clear assessment of the changes achieved, including the REE.
- Refine the dietary prescription based on the new TEE.

- The physical activity prescription should be adjusted to include about a 20–25 % increase in AEE during maintenance.
- Goals should be set for some frequency of behaviors that are associated with long-term weight loss (e.g., weigh at least weekly, journal food intake 3–4 days per week).
- Long-term follow-up can help provide support for the patient, setting the expectation that help is available in cases of lapses.

Case Study

BR is a 59-year-old male with a history of osteoarthritis of his knees, obstructive sleep apnea, gastroesophageal reflux disease (GERD), and obesity. He presents to the office for routine care and raises the concern that his knee pain is worsening for the past several months. He describes more soreness after working in the yard or walking for more than 15 min at a time. He wants to know if there is anything else he can do to limit his knee pain to avoid having to take anti-inflammatory medications persistently.

On examination, his weight is 275 lb, up 10 lb from 6 months ago. His BMI is 39.5 kg/m^2. His blood pressure is 142/89 mmHg. The exam is otherwise unchanged from previous and generally unremarkable except for an android body habitus with predominant excess weight at the midsection and some crepitus in his knees bilaterally. Laboratory assessment shows normal fasting blood glucose, A1C of 5.8 %, and LDL cholesterol of 148 mg/dL.

In reviewing the laboratory results with BR and addressing his ongoing concerns about his knee pain, you point out that most of his medical issues can be addressed by focusing on losing some weight. You make the link between his sleep apnea, knee pain, and GERD, pointing out that when his weight was lower 10 years ago, he did not have any of these issues. He states that his new job that he began around that time has led to him having less time for exercise. He has also developed the habit of eating out two times per day to give him more time for work. He has not tried to lose weight before, but is interested in trying something, especially if he can address a number of health concerns at once.

You start by suggesting that he set some goals. He is interested in losing about 30 lb. He would also like to see if he could get off of his reflux medication. You advise him that losing 30 lb should have positive health benefits. He is agreeable to trying a 1600 kcal/day meal plan that will lower his carbohydrate intake to < 40 % of his overall calorie intake (< 160 g/day). One of your staff members gives him a crash course on tracking his food intake in one of the recommended electronic food journals and identifying high-carbohydrate foods that are part of his typical routine. He also believes that he can manage walking at a brisk pace for 15 min on 3 days/week right now. Anything more than that will lead to more knee pain. He says that his company recently provided him with a fitness tracking device that he can use to track his daily steps. For now, he will just track this to see his usual activity levels. You agree that he will follow up in 2 weeks to have a quick visit to assess his initial progress and make plan adjustments as needed.

He returns in 2 weeks for follow-up. At this point, he has recorded his food intake on a daily basis in a journal. He has also exceeded his exercise goal by an additional 1 day per week. His weight is down 5 lb. He is not sure if his dietary plan is working as well because he is really busy at work. He is just trying to watch portions, but this leads to him still consuming 50 % of his calories from carbohydrate based on his food journal. Further discussion reveals that time constraints are a key barrier for adequate planning. You suggest that he consider using a couple of MR to help avoid dining out during the work day and poor choices in those situations. You schedule a phone visit with the nurse in 2 more weeks to see how this new strategy is working and a 1 month follow-up clinic visit.

In 2 weeks, he reports that use of the MR is making a significant difference in his ability to meet carbohydrate goals and easily stay within his calorie prescription. At his 1 month follow-up visit (6 weeks into the plan), his weight is 260 lb. He notices that his knees are not sore if he walks up to 20–25 min; he is averaging approximately 7500 steps per day on his fitness tracker. He is also noticing that he has less reflux symptoms, especially later in the evening. He is interested in continuing with the plan.

Over the next 4 months, he continues to lose weight steadily until he reaches his goal of 245 lb. At this point he is exercising 4 days per week, walking for 30 min at a 3.5 mph pace. He has not needed any medication for reflux symptoms in the past 2 weeks. A repeat assessment of the previous labs shows improvements in LDL and A1C. You suggest that as a part of maintenance that he weighs himself weekly with a goal of maintaining 245–250 lb. If his weight goes above 250 lb, he should make an appointment to come into the office to update his plan so that he can get back within range quickly. He will continue to use his fitness tracker daily while journaling food intake at least a few days a week. You advise that adding strength training 2 days/week to his exercise program at this point would be beneficial. You recommend that he continue to limit his carbohydrate intake to 40 % of his calories. He can gradually increase his calories each week by approximately 100 kcal until his weight stabilizes. Finally, you set a follow-up appointment with the nurse in 3 months to check his weight and review his lifestyle program.

In summary, this case provides an example of some key aspects of how lifestyle medicine for obesity treatment can be applied in a practical way for common medical problems. First, it is important to note that the patient did not inquire directly about losing weight, but instead he was more focused on daily function and general health concerns. The provider takes the time to make a link for the patient between his weight and his primary health concerns, pointing out that improvement in body weight is an effective way to manage many of his concerns. This interaction is critical because many patients may not be aware of the direct impact of their weight on their health or may underestimate the amount of benefit that may be gained by losing even relatively small amounts of weight. Second, it is essential to engage the patient in collaborative goal setting to ensure that the patient is internally motivated to achieve the stated goals. If the provider sets the goals, the patient may have only a limited amount of external motivation to modify behaviors to please the provider. Third, the impact of self-monitoring and frequent follow-up cannot be underestimated. A key component of consistent achievement and progress towards goals is getting feedback to assess performance. Feedback can come from several sources, including any qualified member of the medical office team. This type of feedback is limited without monitoring tools and regular interactions to provide timely guidance. Finally, using this information to modify the original treatment strategy is important to maintain engagement and enhance efficacy, particularly early in the treatment process. In this case, addressing time constraints is a practical need and a barrier that if not addressed may lead to less than optimal outcomes or worse—disinterest and disengagement.

References

1. National Institutes of Health. Clinical guidelines on the identification. Evaluation and treatment of overweight and obesity in adults—the evidence report. Obes Res. 1998;6(Suppl 2):51S–209S.
2. Garrow JS, Webster J. Quetelet's index (W/H2) as a measure of fatness. Int J Obes. 1985;9(2):147–53.
3. Prospective Studies Collaboration, Whitlock G, Lewington S, et al. Body-mass index and cause-specific mortality in 900 000 adults: collaborative analyses of 57 prospective studies. The Lancet. 2009;373(9669):1083–96.
4. Villareal DT, Apovian CM, Kushner RF, Klein S, American Society for Nutrition, NAASO, The Obesity Society. Obesity in older adults: technical review and position statement of the American Society for Nutrition and NAASO, the Obesity Society. Obes Res. 2005;13(11):1849–63.
5. Jensen MD, Ryan DH, Apovian CM, et al. 2013 AHA/ACC/TOS guideline for the management of overweight and obesity in adults: a report of the American College of Cardiology/American Heart Association Task Force on Practice Guidelines and the Obesity Society. Circulation. 2014;129(25 Suppl 2):102–38.
6. Ogden CL, Carroll MD, Kit BK, Flegal KM. Prevalence of childhood and adult obesity in the United States, 2011–2012. JAMA. 2014;311(8):806–14.
7. Malik VS, Willett WC, Hu FB. Global obesity: trends, risk factors and policy implications. Nat Rev Endocrinol. 2013;9(1):13–27.
8. Popkin BM, Slining MM. New dynamics in global obesity facing low- and middle-income countries. Obes Rev. 2013;14(Suppl 2):11–20.
9. Bray GA. Obesity: the disease. J Med Chem. 2006;49(14):4001–7.
10. American Medical Association. Ama adopts new policies on second day of voting at annual meeting. http://www.ama-assn.org/ama/pub/news/news/2013/2013-06-18-new-ama-policies-annual-meeting.page2013.
11. Goran MI. Variation in total energy expenditure in humans. Obes Res. 1995;3(Suppl 1):59–66.
12. Weinsier RL, Hunter GR, Heini AF, Goran MI, Sell SM. The etiology of obesity: relative contribution of metabolic factors, diet, and physical activity. Am J Med. 1998;105(2):145–50.
13. Javed F, He Q, Davidson LE, et al. Brain and high metabolic rate organ mass: contributions to resting energy expenditure beyond fat-free mass. Am J Clin Nutr. 2010;91(4):907–12.
14. Bosy-Westphal A, Eichhorn C, Kutzner D, Illner K, Heller M, Muller MJ. The age-related decline in resting energy expenditure in humans is due to the loss of fat-free mass and to alterations in its metabolically active components. J Nutr. 2003;133(7):2356–62.
15. Economic Research Service. Food availability (per capita) data system summary findings. 2014.
16. Zheng H, Lenard NR, Shin AC, Berthoud HR. Appetite control and energy balance regulation in the modern world: reward-driven brain overrides repletion signals. Int J Obes (Lond). 2009;33(Suppl 2):S8–S13.
17. Appelhans BM, Whited MC, Schneider KL, Pagoto SL. Time to abandon the notion of personal choice in dietary counseling for obesity? J Am Diet Assoc. 2011;111(8):1130–6.
18. Bray GA. Obesity is a chronic, relapsing neurochemical disease. Int J Obes Relat Metab Disord. 2004;28(1):34–8.
19. Garg A. Regional adiposity and insulin resistance. J Clin Endocrinol Metab. 2004;89(9):4206–10.
20. Kershaw EE, Flier JS. Adipose tissue as an endocrine organ. J Clin Endocrinol Metab. 2004;89(6):2548–56.
21. Lee MJ, Wu Y, Fried SK. Adipose tissue heterogeneity: implication of depot differences in adipose tissue for obesity complications. Mol Aspects Med. 2013;34(1):1–11.
22. Patel P, Abate N. Role of subcutaneous adipose tissue in the pathogenesis of insulin resistance. J Obes. 2013;2013:489187.
23. Snijder MB, Visser M, Dekker JM, et al. Low subcutaneous thigh fat is a risk factor for unfavourable glucose and lipid levels, independently of high abdominal fat. The Health ABC Study. Diabetologia. 2005;48(2):301–8.
24. Snijder MB, Zimmet PZ, Visser M, Dekker JM, Seidell JC, Shaw JE. Independent and opposite associations of waist and hip circumferences with diabetes, hypertension and dyslipidemia: the AusDiab Study. Int J Obes Relat Metab Disord. 2004;28(3):402–9.
25. Garvey WT, Garber AJ, Mechanick JI, et al. American Association of Clinical Endocrinologists and American College of Endocrinology position statement on the 2014 advanced framework for a new diagnosis of obesity as a chronic disease. Endocr Pract. 2014;20(9):977–89.
26. Sharma AM, Kushner RF. A proposed clinical staging system for obesity. Int J Obes (Lond). 2009;33(3):289–95.
27. McElroy SL, Kotwal R, Malhotra S, Nelson EB, Keck PE, Nemeroff CB. Are mood disorders and obesity related? A review for the mental health professional. J Clin Psychiatry. 2004;65(5):634–51. quiz 730.
28. Leehr EJ, Krohmer K, Schag K, Dresler T, Zipfel S, Giel KE. Emotion regulation model in binge eating disorder and obesity—a systematic review. Neurosci Biobehav Rev. 2015;49:125–34.
29. Scott KM, McGee MA, Wells JE, Oakley Browne MA. Obesity and mental disorders in the adult general population. J Psychosom Res. 2008;64(1):97–105.
30. Das C, Mendez G, Jagasia S, Labbate LA. Second-generation antipsychotic use in schizophrenia and associated weight gain: a critical review and meta-analysis of behavioral and pharmacologic treatments. Ann Clin Psychiatry. 2012;24(3):225–39.

31. Reas DL, Grilo CM. Review and meta-analysis of pharmacotherapy for binge-eating disorder. Obesity (Silver Spring). 2008;16(9):2024–38.

32. Masheb RM, Grilo CM, Rolls BJ. A randomized controlled trial for obesity and binge eating disorder: low-energy-density dietary counseling and cognitive-behavioral therapy. Behav Res Ther. 2011;49(12):821–9.

33. Kolotkin RL, Meter K, Williams GR. Quality of life and obesity. Obes Rev. 2001;2(4):219–29.

34. Fontaine KR, Barofsky I. Obesity and health-related quality of life. Obes Rev. 2001;2(3):173–82.

35. Fontaine KR, Barofsky I, Andersen RE, et al. Impact of weight loss on health-related quality of life. Qual Life Res. 1999;8(3):275–7.

36. Williamson DA, Rejeski J, Lang W, et al. Impact of a weight management program on health-related quality of life in overweight adults with type 2 diabetes. Arch Intern Med. 2009;169(2):163–71.

37. Hall KD, Sacks G, Chandramohan D, et al. Quantification of the effect of energy imbalance on bodyweight. Lancet. 2011;378(9793):826–37.

38. Wishnofsky M. Caloric equivalents of gained or lost weight. Am J Clin Nutr. 1958;6(5):542–6.

39. Byrne NM, Wood RE, Schutz Y, Hills AP. Does metabolic compensation explain the majority of less-than-expected weight loss in obese adults during a short-term severe diet and exercise intervention? Int J Obes (Lond). 2012;36(11):1472–8.

40. Hall KD, Jordan PN. Modeling weight-loss maintenance to help prevent body weight regain. Am J Clin Nutr. 2008;88(6):1495–503.

41. Weinsier RL, Hunter GR, Zuckerman PA, et al. Energy expenditure and free-living physical activity in black and white women: comparison before and after weight loss. Am J Clin Nutr. 2000;71(5):1138–46.

42. Grande F, Anderson JT, Keys A. Changes of basal metabolic rate in man in semistarvation and refeeding. J Appl Physiol. 1958;12(2):230–8.

43. James WP, Shetty PS. Metabolic adaptation and energy requirements in developing countries. Hum Nutr Clin Nutr. 1982;36(5):331–6.

44. Thomas DM, Martin CK, Redman LM, et al. Effect of dietary adherence on the body weight plateau: a mathematical model incorporating intermittent compliance with energy intake prescription. Am J Clin Nutr. 2014;100(3):787–95.

45. Zou ML, Moughan PJ, Awati A, Livesey G. Accuracy of the Atwater factors and related food energy conversion factors with low-fat, high-fiber diets when energy intake is reduced spontaneously. Am J Clin Nutr. 2007;86(6):1649–56.

46. Brown J, Livesey G, Roe M, et al. Metabolizable energy of high non-starch polysaccharide-maintenance and weight-reducing diets in men: experimental appraisal of assessment systems. J Nutr. 1998;128(6):986–95.

47. de Heredia FP, Cerezo D, Zamora S, Garaulet M. Effect of dehydroepiandrosterone on protein and fat digestibility, body protein and muscular composition in high-fat-diet-fed old rats. Br J Nutr. 2007;97(3):464–70.

48. Mattes RD, Kris-Etherton PM, Foster GD. Impact of peanuts and tree nuts on body weight and healthy weight loss in adults. J Nutr. 2008;138(9):1741S–45S.

49. Fraser GE, Sabate J, Beeson WL, Strahan TMA. Possible protective effect of nut consumption on risk of coronary heart disease. The Adventist Health Study. Arch Intern Med. 1992;152(7):1416–24.

50. Hu FB, Stampfer MJ, Manson JE, et al. Frequent nut consumption and risk of coronary heart disease in women: prospective cohort study. BMJ. 1998;317(7169):1341–5.

51. Albert CM, Gaziano JM, Willett WC, Manson JE. Nut consumption and decreased risk of sudden cardiac death in the physicians' health study. Arch Intern Med. 2002;162(12):1382–7.

52. Ellsworth JL, Kushi LH, Folsom AR. Frequent nut intake and risk of death from coronary heart disease and all causes in postmenopausal women: the Iowa Women's Health Study. Nutr Metab Cardiovasc Dis. 2001;11(6):372–7.

53. Hudthagosol C, Haddad EH, McCarthy K, Wang P, Oda K, Sabate J. Pecans acutely increase plasma postprandial antioxidant capacity and catechins and decrease LDL oxidation in humans. J Nutr. 2011;141(1):56–62.

54. Ellis PR, Kendall CW, Ren Y, et al. Role of cell walls in the bioaccessibility of lipids in almond seeds. Am J Clin Nutr. 2004;80(3):604–13.

55. Traoret CJ, Lokko P, Cruz AC, et al. Peanut digestion and energy balance. Int J Obes (Lond). 2008;32(2):322–8.

56. Brown AJ, Goldsworthy SM, Barnes AA, et al. The Orphan G protein-coupled receptors Gpr41 and Gpr43 are activated by propionate and other short chain carboxylic acids. J Biol Chem. 2003;278(13):11312–9.

57. Erejuwa OO, Sulaiman SA, Ab Wahab MS. Modulation of gut microbiota in the management of metabolic disorders: the prospects and challenges. Int J Mol Sci. 2014;15(3):4158–88.

58. St-Onge MP, Ross R, Parsons WD, Jones PJ. Medium-chain triglycerides increase energy expenditure and decrease adiposity in overweight men. Obes Res. 2003;11(3):395–402.

59. Dulloo AG, Fathi M, Mensi N, Girardier L. Twenty-four-hour energy expenditure and urinary catecholamines of humans consuming low-to-moderate amounts of medium-chain triglycerides: a dose-response study in a human respiratory chamber. Eur J Clin Nutr. 1996;50(3):152–8.

60. Van Wymelbeke V, Himaya A, Louis-Sylvestre J, Fantino M. Influence of medium-chain and long-chain triacylglycerols on the control of food intake in men. Am J Clin Nutr. 1998;68(2):226–34.

61. Agricultural Research Service. Nutrient intakes from food: mean amounts consumed per individual. One day 2005–2006. U.S. Department of Agriculture; 2008.

62. Mumme K, Stonehouse W. Effects of medium-chain triglycerides on weight loss and body composition: a meta-analysis of randomized controlled trials. J Acad Nutr Diet. 2015;115(2):249–63.

63. Rumpler W, Seale J, Clevidence B, et al. Oolong tea increases metabolic rate and fat oxidation in men. J Nutr. 2001;131(11):2848–52.

64. Komatsu T, Nakamori M, Komatsu K, et al. Oolong tea increases energy metabolism in Japanese females. J Med Invest. 2003;50(3–4):170–5.

65. Dulloo AG, Seydoux J, Girardier L, Chantre P, Vandermander J. Green tea and thermogenesis: interactions between catechin-polyphenols, caffeine and sympathetic activity. Int J Obes Relat Metab Disord. 2000;24(2):252–8.

66. Jurgens TM, Whelan AM, Killian L, Doucette S, Kirk S, Foy E. Green tea for weight loss and weight maintenance in overweight or obese adults. Cochrane Database Syst Rev. 2012;12:CD008650.

67. Unno T, Osada C, Motoo Y, Suzuki Y, Kobayashi M, Nozawa A. Dietary tea catechins increase fecal energy in rats. J Nutr Sci Vitaminol (Tokyo). 2009;55(5):447–51.

68. Jeffery RW, Bjornson-Benson WM, Rosenthal BS, Lindquist RA, Kurth CL, Johnson SL. Correlates of weight loss and its maintenance over two years of follow-up among middle-aged men. Prev Med. 1984;13(2):155–68.

69. Wadden TA, Foster GD, Wang J, et al. Clinical correlates of short- and long-term weight loss. Am J Clin Nutr. 1992;56(1 Suppl):271S–274S.

70. Bodenheimer T, Lorig K, Holman H, Grumbach K. Patient self-management of chronic disease in primary care. JAMA. 2002;288:2469–75.

71. Burke LE, Wang J, Sevick MA. Self-monitoring in weight loss: a systematic review of the literature. J Am Diet Assoc. 2011;111(1):92–102.

72. DiLillo V, West DS. Motivational interviewing for weight loss. Psychiatr Clin North Am. 2011;34(4):861–9.

73. Glynn TJ, Manley MW. How to help your patients stop smoking: a manual for physicians. Bethesda: National Cancer Institute; 1989.

74. Whitlock EP, Orleans CT, Pender N, Allan J. Evaluating primary care behavioral counseling interventions: an evidence-based approach. Am J Prev Med. 2002;22(4):267–84.

75. Flatt JP. Importance of nutrient balance in body weight regulation. Diabetes Metab Rev. 1988;4(6):571–81.

76. Samaha FF, Iqbal N, Seshadri P, et al. A low-carbohydrate as compared with a low-fat diet in severe obesity. N Engl J Med. 2003;348(21):2074–81.

77. Stern L, Iqbal N, Seshadri P, et al. The effects of low-carbohydrate versus conventional weight loss diets in severely obese adults: one-year follow-up of a randomized trial. Ann Intern Med. 2004;140(10):778–85.

78. Foster GD, Wyatt HR, Hill JO, et al. A randomized trial of a low-carbohydrate diet for obesity. N Engl J Med. 2003;348(21):2082–90.

79. Astrup A, Ryan L, Grunwald GK, et al. The role of dietary fat in body fatness: evidence from a preliminary meta-analysis of ad libitum low-fat dietary intervention studies. Br J Nutr. 2000;83(Suppl 1):S25–S32.

80. Thomas CD, Peters JC, Reed GW, Abumrad NN, Sun M, Hill JO. Nutrient balance and energy expenditure during ad libitum feeding of high-fat and high-carbohydrate diets in humans. Am J Clin Nutr. 1992;55(5):934–42.

81. Gardner CD, Kiazand A, Alhassan S, et al. Comparison of the Atkins, Zone, Ornish, and Learn diets for change in weight and related risk factors among overweight premenopausal women: the A to Z Weight Loss Study: a randomized trial. JAMA. 2007;297(9):969–77.

82. Halton TL, Hu FB. The effects of high protein diets on thermogenesis, satiety and weight loss: a critical review. J Am Coll Nutr. 2004;23(5):373–85.

83. Paddon-Jones D, Westman E, Mattes RD, Wolfe RR, Astrup A, Westerterp-Plantenga M. Protein, weight management, and satiety. Am J Clin Nutr. 2008;87(5):1558S–61S.

84. Abete I, Astrup A, Martinez JA, Thorsdottir I, Zulet MA. Obesity and the metabolic syndrome: role of different dietary macronutrient distribution patterns and specific nutritional components on weight loss and maintenance. Nutr Rev. 2010;68(4):214–31.

85. Pesta DH, Samuel VT. A high-protein diet for reducing body fat: mechanisms and possible caveats. Nutr Metab (Lond). 2014;11(1):53.

86. Due A, Toubro S, Skov AR, Astrup A. Effect of normal-fat diets, either medium or high in protein, on body weight in overweight subjects: a randomised 1-year trial. Int J Obes Relat Metab Disord. 2004;28(10):1283–90.

87. Larsen TM, Dalskov SM, van Baak M, et al. Diets with high or low protein content and glycemic index for weight-loss maintenance. N Engl J Med. 2010;363(22):2102–13.

88. Ankarfeldt MZ, Angquist L, Stocks T, et al. Body characteristics, [corrected] dietary protein and body weight regulation. Reconciling conflicting results from intervention and observational studies? PLoS ONE. 2014;9(7):e101134.

89. Wycherley TP, Moran LJ, Clifton PM, Noakes M, Brinkworth GD. Effects of energy-restricted high-protein, low-fat compared with standard-protein, low-fat diets: a meta-analysis of randomized controlled trials. Am J Clin Nutr. 2012;96(6):1281–98.

90. Sacks FM, Bray GA, Carey VJ, et al. Comparison of weight-loss diets with different compositions of fat, protein, and carbohydrates. N Engl J Med. 2009;360(9):859–73.

91. Johnston BC, Kanters S, Bandayrel K, et al. Comparison of weight loss among named diet programs in overweight and obese adults: a meta-analysis. JAMA. 2014;312(9):923–33.

92. Stubbs RJ, Ritz P, Coward WA, Prentice AM. Covert manipulation of the ratio of dietary fat to carbohydrate and energy density: effect on food intake and energy balance in free-living men eating ad libitum. Am J Clin Nutr. 1995;62(2):330–7.

93. Stubbs RJ, Harbron CG, Murgatroyd PR, Prentice AM. Covert manipulation of dietary fat and energy density: effect on substrate flux and food intake in men eating ad libitum. Am J Clin Nutr. 1995;62(2):316–29.

94. Kral TV, Roe LS, Rolls BJ. Combined effects of energy density and portion size on energy intake in women. Am J Clin Nutr. 2004;79(6):962–8.

95. Rolls BJ, Bell EA, Thorwart ML. Water incorporated into a food but not served with a food decreases energy intake in lean women. Am J Clin Nutr. 1999;70(4):448–55.

96. Rolls BJ, Roe LS, Meengs JS. Salad and satiety: energy density and portion size of a first-course salad affect energy intake at lunch. J Am Diet Assoc. 2004;104(10):1570–6.

97. Bell EA, Castellanos VH, Pelkman CL, Thorwart ML, Rolls BJ. Energy density of foods affects energy intake in normal-weight women. Am J Clin Nutr. 1998;67(3):412–20.

98. Bell EA, Rolls BJ. Energy density of foods affects energy intake across multiple levels of fat content in lean and obese women. Am J Clin Nutr. 2001;73(6):1010–8.

99. Rolls BJ, Roe LS, Beach AM, Kris-Etherton PM. Provision of foods differing in energy density affects long-term weight loss. Obes Res. 2005;13(6):1052–60.

100. Ello-Martin JA, Roe LS, Ledikwe JH, Beach AM, Rolls BJ. Dietary energy density in the treatment of obesity: a year-long trial comparing 2 weight-loss diets. Am J Clin Nutr. 2007;85(6):1465–77.

101. Raynor HA, Looney SM, Steeves EA, Spence M, Gorin AA. The effects of an energy density prescription on diet quality and weight loss: a pilot randomized controlled trial. J Acad Nutr Diet. 2012;112(9):1397–402.

102. Lowe MR, Butryn ML, Thomas JG, Coletta M. Meal replacements, reduced energy density eating, and weight loss maintenance in primary care patients: a randomized controlled trial. Obesity (Silver Spring). 2014;22(1):94–100.

103. Thomas DE, Elliott EJ, Baur L. Low glycaemic index or low glycaemic load diets for overweight and obesity. Cochrane Database Syst Rev. 2007;(3):CD005105.

104. Esfahani A, Wong JM, Mirrahimi A, Villa CR, Kendall CW. The application of the glycemic index and glycemic load in weight loss: a review of the clinical evidence. IUBMB Life. 2011;63(1):7–13.

105. Ajala O, English P, Pinkney J. Systematic review and meta-analysis of different dietary approaches to the management of type 2 diabetes. Am J Clin Nutr. 2013;97(3):505–16.

106. McMillan-Price J, Petocz P, Atkinson F, et al. Comparison of 4 diets of varying glycemic load on weight loss and cardiovascular risk reduction in overweight and obese young adults: a randomized controlled trial. Arch Intern Med. 2006;166(14):1466–75.

107. Kennedy ET, Bowman SA, Spence JT, Freedman M, King J. Popular diets: correlation to health, nutrition, and obesity. J Am Diet Assoc. 2001;101(4):411–20.

108. Newby PK, Tucker KL, Wolk A. Risk of overweight and obesity among semivegetarian, lactovegetarian, and vegan women. Am J Clin Nutr. 2005;81(6):1267–74.

109. Spencer EA, Appleby PN, Davey GK, Key TJ. Diet and body mass index in 38000 EPIC-Oxford meat-eaters, fish-eaters, vegetarians and vegans. Int J Obes Relat Metab Disord. 2003;27(6):728–34.

110. Haddad EH, Tanzman JS. What do vegetarians in the United States eat? Am J Clin Nutr. 2003;78(3 Suppl):626S-632S.

111. Howarth NC, Saltzman E, Roberts SB. Dietary fiber and weight regulation. Nutr Rev. 2001;59(5):129–39.

112. Burke LE, Warziski M, Styn MA, Music E, Hudson AG, Sereika SM. A randomized clinical trial of a standard versus vegetarian diet for weight loss: the impact of treatment preference. Int J Obes (Lond). 2008;32(1):166–76.

113. Turner-McGrievy GM, Barnard ND, Scialli AR. A two-year randomized weight loss trial comparing a vegan diet to a more moderate low-fat diet. Obesity (Silver Spring). 2007;15(9):2276–81.

114. Turner-McGrievy GM, Davidson CR, Wingard EE, Wilcox S, Frongillo EA. Comparative effectiveness of plant-based diets for weight loss: a randomized controlled trial of five different diets. Nutrition. 2015;31(2):350–8.

115. Mozaffarian D, Hao T, Rimm EB, Willett WC, Hu FB. Changes in diet and lifestyle and long-term weight gain in women and men. N Engl J Med. 2011;364(25):2392–404.

116. Good CK, Holschuh N, Albertson AM, Eldridge AL. Whole grain consumption and body mass index in adult women: an analysis of nhanes 1999–2000 and the usda pyramid servings database. J Am Coll Nutr. 2008;27(1):80–7.

117. Goulet J, Lamarche B, Nadeau G, Lemieux S. Effect of a nutritional intervention promoting the Mediterranean food pattern on plasma lipids, lipoproteins and body weight in healthy French-Canadian women. Atherosclerosis. 2003;170(1):115–24.

118. Andreoli A, Lauro S, Daniele N D, Sorge R, Celi M, Volpe SL. Effect of a moderately hypoenergetic Mediterranean diet and exercise program on body cell mass and cardiovascular risk factors in obese women. Eur J Clin Nutr. 2008;62(7):892–7.

119. Beunza JJ, Toledo E, Hu FB, et al. Adherence to the Mediterranean diet, long-term weight change, and incident overweight or obesity: the Seguimiento Universidad de Navarra (SUN) cohort. Am J Clin Nutr. 2010;92(6):1484–93.

120. Martinez-Gonzalez MA, Garcia-Arellano A, Toledo E, et al. A 14-Item Mediterranean diet assessment tool and obesity indexes among high-risk subjects: the Predimed trial. PLoS One. 2012;7(8):e43134.

121. Romaguera D, Norat T, Vergnaud AC, et al. Mediterranean dietary patterns and prospective weight change in participants of the Epic-Panacea project. Am J Clin Nutr. 2010;92(4):912–21.

122. Mendez MA, Popkin BM, Jakszyn P, et al. Adherence to a Mediterranean diet is associated with reduced 3-year incidence of obesity. J Nutr. 2006;136(11):2934–8.

123. Garcia-Fernandez E, Rico-Cabanas L, Rosgaard N, Estruch R, Bach-Faig A. Mediterranean diet and cardiodiabesity: a review. Nutrients. 2014;6(9):3474–500.

124. Lindeberg S, Jonsson T, Granfeldt Y, et al. A Palaeolithic diet improves glucose tolerance more than a Mediterranean-like diet in individuals with ischaemic heart disease. Diabetologia. 2007;50(9):1795–807.

125. Howlett J, Ashwell M. Glycemic response and health: summary of a workshop. Am J Clin Nutr. 2008;87(1):212S–6S.

126. Livesey G, Taylor R, Hulshof T, Howlett J. Glycemic response and health–a systematic review and meta-analysis: relations between dietary glycemic properties and health outcomes. Am J Clin Nutr. 2008;87(1):258S–68S.

127. Riccardi G, Rivellese AA, Giacco R. Role of glycemic index and glycemic load in the healthy state, in prediabetes, and in diabetes. Am J Clin Nutr. 2008;87(1):269S–74S.

128. Thomas D, Elliott EJ. Low glycaemic index, or low glycaemic load, diets for diabetes mellitus. Cochrane Database Syst Rev. 2009;(1):CD006296.

129. Osterdahl M, Kocturk T, Koochek A, Wandell PE. Effects of a short-term intervention with a Paleolithic diet in healthy volunteers. Eur J Clin Nutr. 2008;62(5):682–5.

130. Frassetto LA, Schloetter M, Mietus-Synder M, Morris RC Jr, Sebastian A. Metabolic and physiologic improvements from consuming a Paleolithic, hunter-gatherer type diet. Eur J Clin Nutr. 2009;63(8):947–55.

131. Jonsson T, Ahren B, Pacini G, et al. A Paleolithic diet confers higher insulin sensitivity, lower c-reactive protein and lower blood pressure than a cereal-based diet in domestic pigs. Nutr Metab (Lond). 2006;3:39.

132. Jonsson T, Granfeldt Y, Lindeberg S, Hallberg AC. Subjective satiety and other experiences of a Paleolithic diet compared to a diabetes diet in patients with type 2 diabetes. Nutr J. 2013;12:105.

133. Boers I, Muskiet FA, Berkelaar E, et al. Favourable effects of consuming a Palaeolithic-type diet on characteristics of the metabolic syndrome: a randomized controlled pilot-study. Lipids Health Dis. 2014;13:160.

134. Jonsson T, Granfeldt Y, Ahren B, et al. Beneficial effects of a Paleolithic diet on cardiovascular risk factors in type 2 diabetes: a randomized cross-over pilot study. Cardiovasc Diabetol. 2009;8:35.

135. Rolls BJ, Morris EL, Roe LS. Portion size of food affects energy intake in normal-weight and overweight men and women. Am J Clin Nutr. 2002;76(6):1207–13.

136. Rolls BJ, Roe LS, Kral TV, Meengs JS, Wall DE. Increasing the portion size of a packaged snack increases energy intake in men and women. Appetite. 2004;42(1):63–9.

137. Rolls BJ, Roe LS, Meengs JS. Larger portion sizes lead to a sustained increase in energy intake over 2 days. J Am Diet Assoc. 2006;106(4):543–9.

138. Report of the Dietary Guidelines Advisory Committee on the Dietary Guidelines for Americans. 2010. In: U.S. Department of Agriculture UDoHaHS, editor. Washington, DC: U.S. Department of Agriculture. US Department of Health and Human Services; 2010.

139. Wadden TA, West DS, Neiberg RH, et al. One-year weight losses in the look ahead study: factors associated with success. Obesity (Silver Spring). 2009;17(4):713–22.

140. Ryan DH, Espeland MA, Foster GD, et al. Look ahead (action for health in diabetes): design and methods for a clinical trial of weight loss for the prevention of cardiovascular disease in type 2 diabetes. Control Clin Trials. 2003;24(5):610–28.

141. Messier SP, Legault C, Mihalko S, et al. The intensive diet and exercise for arthritis (idea) trial: design and rationale. BMC Musculoskelet Disord. 2009;10:93.

142. Miller GD. Improved nutrient intake in older obese adults undergoing a structured diet and exercise intentional weight loss program. J Nutr Health Aging. 2010;14(6):461–6.

143. Heymsfield SB, van Mierlo CA, van der Knaap HC, Heo M, Frier HI. Weight management using a meal replacement strategy: meta and pooling analysis from six studies. Int J Obes Relat Metab Disord. 2003;27(5):537–549.

144. Heymsfield SB. Meal replacements and energy balance. Physiol Behav. 2010;100(1):90–4.

145. Tieken SM, Leidy HJ, Stull AJ, Mattes RD, Schuster RA, Campbell WW. Effects of solid versus liquid meal-replacement products of similar energy content on hunger, satiety, and appetite-regulating hormones in older adults. Horm Metab Res. 2007;39(5):389–94.

146. Stull AJ, Apolzan JW, Thalacker-Mercer AE, Iglay HB, Campbell WW. Liquid and solid meal replacement products differentially affect postprandial appetite and food intake in older adults. J Am Diet Assoc. 2008;108(7):1226–30.

147. Hartmann-Boyce J, Johns DJ, Jebb SA, Summerbell C, Aveyard P, Behavioural Weight Management Review Group. Behavioural weight management programmes for adults assessed by trials conducted in everyday contexts: systematic review and meta-analysis. Obes Rev. 2014;15(11):920–32.

148. Rock CL, Flatt SW, Sherwood NE, Karanja N, Pakiz B, Thomson CA. Effect of a free prepared meal and incentivized weight loss program on weight loss and weight loss maintenance in obese and overweight women: a randomized controlled trial. JAMA. 2010;304(16):1803–10.

149. Foster GD, Wadden TA, Lagrotte CA, et al. A randomized comparison of a commercially available portion-controlled weight-loss intervention with a diabetes self-management education program. Nutr Diabetes. 2013;3:e63.

150. Cheskin LJ, Mitchell AM, Jhaveri AD, et al. Efficacy of meal replacements versus a standard food-based diet for weight loss

in type 2 diabetes: a controlled clinical trial. Diabetes Educ. 2008;34(1):118–27.

151. Leeds AR. Formula food-reducing diets: a new evidence-based addition to the weight management tool box. Nutr Bull. 2014;39(3):238–46.

152. Eshghinia S, Mohammadzadeh F. The effects of modified alternate-day fasting diet on weight loss and cad risk factors in overweight and obese women. J Diabetes Metab Disord. 2013;12(1):4.

153. Varady KA, Bhutani S, Church EC, Klempel MC. Short-term modified alternate-day fasting: a novel dietary strategy for weight loss and cardioprotection in obese adults. Am J Clin Nutr. 2009;90(5):1138–43.

154. Hoddy KK, Kroeger CM, Trepanowski JF, Barnosky A, Bhutani S, Varady KA. Meal timing during alternate day fasting: impact on body weight and cardiovascular disease risk in obese adults. Obesity (Silver Spring). 2014;22(12):2524–31.

155. Committee on Physical Activity Guidelines for Americans. 2008 Physical activity guidelines for Americans: be active, healthy, and happy! Washington, DC: U.S. Dept. of Health and Human Services; 2008.

156. Messier SP, Loeser RF, Miller GD, et al. Exercise and dietary weight loss in overweight and obese older adults with knee osteoarthritis: the arthritis, diet, and activity promotion trial. Arthritis Rheum. 2004;50(5):1501–10.

157. Messier SP, Mihalko SL, Legault C, et al. Effects of intensive diet and exercise on knee joint loads, inflammation, and clinical outcomes among overweight and obese adults with knee osteoarthritis: the idea randomized clinical trial. JAMA. 2013;310(12):1263–73.

158. Jakicic JM, Otto AD, Lang W, et al. The effect of physical activity on 18-month weight change in overweight adults. Obesity (Silver Spring). 2011;19(1):100–9.

159. Hagan RD, Upton SJ, Wong L, Whittam J. The effects of aerobic conditioning and/or caloric restriction in overweight men and women. Med Sci Sports Exerc. 1986;18(1):87–94.

160. Wing RR, Venditti E, Jakicic JM, Polley BA, Lang W. Lifestyle intervention in overweight individuals with a family history of diabetes. Diabetes Care. 1998;21(3):350–9.

161. Goodpaster BH, Delany JP, Otto AD, et al. Effects of diet and physical activity interventions on weight loss and cardiometabolic risk factors in severely obese adults: a randomized trial. JAMA. 2010;304(16):1795–802.

162. Curioni CC, Lourenco PM. Long-term weight loss after diet and exercise: a systematic review. Int J Obes Relat Metab Disord. 2005;29(10):1168–74.

163. Donnelly JE, Blair SN, Jakicic JM, Manore MM, Rankin JW, Smith BK. American College of Sports Medicine Position Stand. Appropriate physical activity intervention strategies for weight loss and prevention of weight regain for adults. Med Sci Sports Exerc. 2009;41(2):459–471.

164. Hill JO, Wyatt HR, Reed GW, Peters JC. Obesity and the environment: where do we go from here? Science. 2003;299(5608):853–5.

165. Klem ML, Wing RR, McGuire MT, Seagle HM, Hill JO. A descriptive study of individuals successful at long-term maintenance of substantial weight loss. Am J Clin Nutr. 1997;66(2):239–246.

166. Jakicic JM, Marcus BH, Lang W, Janney C. Effect of exercise on 24-month weight loss maintenance in overweight women. Arch Intern Med. 2008;168(14):1550–9; (discussion 1559–1560).

167. Unick JL, Jakicic JM, Marcus BH. Contribution of behavior intervention components to 24-month weight loss. Med Sci Sports Exerc. 2010;42(4):745–53.

168. Ross R, Hudson R, Stotz PJ, Lam M. Effects of exercise amount and intensity on abdominal obesity and glucose tolerance in obese adults: a randomized trial. Ann Intern Med. 2015;162(5):325–34.

169. Boutcher SH. High-intensity intermittent exercise and fat loss. J Obes. 2011;2011:868305.

170. Perry CG, Heigenhauser GJ, Bonen A, Spriet LL. High-intensity aerobic interval training increases fat and carbohydrate metabolic capacities in human skeletal muscle. Appl Physiol Nutr Metab. 2008;33(6):1112–23.

171. Tjonna AE, Lee SJ, Rognmo O, et al. Aerobic interval training versus continuous moderate exercise as a treatment for the metabolic syndrome: a pilot study. Circulation. 2008;118(4):346–54.

172. Helgerud J, Hoydal K, Wang E, et al. Aerobic high-intensity intervals improve Vo2max more than moderate training. Med Sci Sports Exerc. 2007;39(4):665–71.

173. Trapp EG, Chisholm DJ, Freund J, Boutcher SH. The effects of high-intensity intermittent exercise training on fat loss and fasting insulin levels of young women. Int J Obes (Lond). 2008;32(4):684–91.

174. Davidson LE, Hudson R, Kilpatrick K, et al. Effects of exercise modality on insulin resistance and functional limitation in older adults: a randomized controlled trial. Arch Intern Med. 2009;169(2):122–31.

175. Bartlett JD, Close GL, MacLaren DP, Gregson W, Drust B, Morton JP. High-intensity interval running is perceived to be more enjoyable than moderate-intensity continuous exercise: implications for exercise adherence. J Sports Sci. 2011;29(6):547–53.

176. Nielsen RO, Buist I, Sorensen H, Lind M, Rasmussen S. Training errors and running related injuries: a systematic review. Int J Sports Phys Ther. 2012;7(1):58–75.

177. Willis LH, Slentz CA, Bateman LA, et al. Effects of aerobic and/or resistance training on body mass and fat mass in overweight or obese adults. J Appl Physiol (1985). 2012;113(12):1831–7.

178. Davidson LE, Hudson R, Kilpatrick K, et al. Effects of exercise modality on insulin resistance and functional limitation in older adults: a randomized controlled trial. Arch Intern Med. 2009;169(2):122–131.

179. Rioux JG, Ritenbaugh C. Narrative review of yoga intervention clinical trials including weight-related outcomes. Altern Ther Health Med. 2013;19(3):32–46.

180. Thomley BS, Ray SH, Cha SS, Bauer BA. Effects of a brief, comprehensive, yoga-based program on quality of life and biometric measures in an employee population: a pilot study. Explore (NY). 2011;7(1):27–9.

181. Telles S, Naveen VK, Balkrishna A, Kumar S. Short term health impact of a yoga and diet change program on obesity. Med Sci Monit. 2010;16(1):CR35–C40.

182. Benavides S, Caballero J. Ashtanga yoga for children and adolescents for weight management and psychological well being: an uncontrolled open pilot study. Complement Ther Clin Pract. 2009;15(2):110–4.

183. Sivasankaran S, Pollard-Quintner S, Sachdeva R, Pugeda J, Hoq SM, Zarich SW. The effect of a six-week program of yoga and meditation on brachial artery reactivity: do psychosocial interventions affect vascular tone? Clin Cardiol. 2006;29(9):393–8.

184. Manchanda SC, Narang R, Reddy KS, et al. Retardation of coronary atherosclerosis with yoga lifestyle intervention. J Assoc Physicians India. 2000;48(7):687–94.

185. Murugesan R, Govindarajulu N, Bera TK. Effect of selected yogic practices on the management of hypertension. Indian J Physiol Pharmacol. 2000;44(2):207–10.

186. Mahajan AS, Reddy KS, Sachdeva U. Lipid profile of coronary risk subjects following yogic lifestyle intervention. Indian Heart J 1999;51(1):37–40.

187. Raju PS, Prasad KV, Venkata RY, Murthy KJ, Reddy MV. Influence of intensive yoga training on physiological changes in 6 adult women: a case report. J Altern Complement Med Fall. 1997;3(3):291–5.

188. Bera TK, Rajapurkar MV. Body composition, cardiovascular endurance and anaerobic power of yogic practitioner. Indian J Physiol Pharmacol. 1993;37(3):225–8.

189. Telles S, Nagarathna R, Nagendra HR, Desiraju T. Physiological changes in sports teachers following 3 months of training in Yoga. Indian J Med Sci. 1993;47(10):235–8.

190. Satyanarayana M, Rajeswari KR, Rani NJ, Krishna CS, Rao PV. Effect of Santhi Kriya on certain psychophysiological parameters: a preliminary study. Indian J Physiol Pharmacol. 1992;36(2):88–92.

191. Sedentary Behaviour Research Network. Letter to the editor: standardized use of the terms "sedentary" and "sedentary behaviours". Appl Physiol Nutr Metab. 2012;37(3):540–2.

192. Booth FW, Gordon SE, Carlson CJ, Hamilton MT. Waging war on modern chronic diseases: primary prevention through exercise biology. J Appl Physiol (1985). 2000;88(2):774–87.

193. Hamilton MT, Hamilton DG, Zderic TW. Role of low energy expenditure and sitting in obesity, metabolic syndrome. type 2 diabetes, and cardiovascular disease. Diabetes. 2007;56(11):2655–67.

194. Herman KM, Carver TE, Christou NV, Andersen RE. Keeping the weight off: physical activity, sitting time, and weight loss maintenance in bariatric surgery patients 2 to 16 years postsurgery. Obes Surg. 2014;24(7):1064–72.

195. Herman KM, Carver TE, Christou NV, Andersen RE. Physical activity and sitting time in bariatric surgery patients 1–16 years post-surgery. Clin Obes. 2014;4(5):267–76.

196. Healy GN, Dunstan DW, Salmon J, et al. Breaks in sedentary time: beneficial associations with metabolic risk. Diabetes Care. 2008;31(4):661–6.

197. Bey L, Hamilton MT. Suppression of skeletal muscle lipoprotein lipase activity during physical inactivity: a molecular reason to maintain daily low-intensity activity. J Physiol. 2003;551(Pt 2):673–82.

198. Hamilton MT, Hamilton DG, Zderic TW. Exercise physiology versus inactivity physiology: an essential concept for understanding lipoprotein lipase regulation. Exerc Sport Sci Rev. 2004;32(4):161–6.

199. Zanuso S, Jimenez A, Pugliese G, Corigliano G, Balducci S. Exercise for the management of type 2 diabetes: a review of the evidence. Acta Diabetol. 2010;47(1):15–22.

200. Major GC, Doucet E, Trayhurn P, Astrup A, Tremblay A. Clinical significance of adaptive thermogenesis. Int J Obes (Lond). 2007;31(2):204–12.

201. Rosenbaum M, Leibel RL. Adaptive thermogenesis in humans. Int J Obes (Lond). 2010;34(Suppl 1):S47–S55.

202. Sumithran P, Prendergast LA, Delbridge E, et al. Long-term persistence of hormonal adaptations to weight loss. N Engl J Med. 2011;365(17):1597–604.

203. Dansinger ML, Gleason JA, Griffith JL, Selker HP, Schaefer EJ. Comparison of the Atkins, Ornish, Weight Watchers, and Zone diets for weight loss and heart disease risk reduction: a randomized trial. JAMA. 2005;293(1):43–53.

204. Weinsier RL, Hunter GR, Zuckerman PA, et al. Energy expenditure and free-living physical activity in black and white women: comparison before and after weight loss. Am J Clin Nutr. 2000;71(5):1138–46.

205. Weinsier RL, Hunter GR, Desmond RA, Byrne NM, Zuckerman PA, Darnell BE. Free-living activity energy expenditure in women successful and unsuccessful at maintaining a normal body weight. Am J Clin Nutr. 2002;75(3):499–504.

206. Bartfield JK, Stevens VJ, Jerome GJ, et al. Behavioral transitions and weight change patterns within the PREMIER trial. Obesity (Silver Spring). 2011;19(8):1609–15.

207. Steinberg DM, Levine EL, Lane I, et al. Adherence to self-monitoring via interactive voice response technology in an eHealth intervention targeting weight gain prevention among black women: randomized controlled trial. J Med Internet Res. 2014;16(4):e114.

208. Fitzpatrick SL, Bandeen-Roche K, Stevens VJ, et al. Examining behavioral processes through which lifestyle interventions promote weight loss: results from PREMIER. Obesity (Silver Spring). 2014;22(4):1002–7.

209. Perri MG, Nezu AM, Patti ET, McCann KL. Effect of length of treatment on weight loss. J Consult Clin Psychol. 1989;57(3):450–2.

210. Catenacci VA, Odgen L, Phelan S, et al. Dietary habits and weight maintenance success in high versus low exercisers in the National Weight Control Registry. J Phys Act Health. 2014;11(8):1540–8.

211. Thomas JG, Bond DS, Phelan S, Hill JO, Wing RR. Weight-loss maintenance for 10 years in the national weight control registry. Am J Prev Med. 2014;46(1):17–23.

212. Daeninck E, Miller M. What can the national weight control registry teach us? Curr Diab Rep. 2006;6(5):401–4.

213. Klem ML, Wing RR, McGuire MT, Seagle HM, Hill JOA. Descriptive study of individuals successful at long-term maintenance of substantial weight loss. Am J Clin Nutr. 1997;66(2):239–46.

214. Svetkey LP, Stevens VJ, Brantley PJ, et al. Comparison of strategies for sustaining weight loss: the weight loss maintenance randomized controlled trial. JAMA. 2008;299(10):1139–48.

215. Svetkey LP, Ard JD, Stevens VJ, et al. Predictors of long-term weight loss in adults with modest initial weight loss, by sex and race. Obesity (Silver Spring). 2012;20(9):1820–8.

Lifestyle Therapy for Diabetes Mellitus

W. Timothy Garvey and Gillian Arathuzik

Abbreviations

ALA	α-linolenic acid
AACE	American Association of Clinical Endocrinologists
ADA	American Diabetes Association
AHA	American Heart Association
BMI	Body Mass Index
CVD	Cardiovascular disease
CDE	Certified Diabetes Educator
CPAP	Continuous positive airway pressure
DASH	Dietary approaches to stop hypertension
DHA	Docosahexaenoic acid
DSME&S	Diabetes self-management education and support
ECG	Electrocardiogram
EPA	Eicosapentaenoic acid
ER	Extended release
FDA	Food and Drug Administration
GI	Glycemic Index
HDL	High-density lipoprotein
IFG	Impaired fasting glucose
IGT	Impaired glucose tolerance
IOM	Institute of Medicine
LADA	Latent autoimmune diabetes of adults
LAGB	Laparoscopic adjustable gastric banding
LDL	Low-density lipoprotein
MNT	Medical nutrition therapy
OGTTs	Oral glucose tolerance tests
RD	Registered dietitian
SGLT2	Sodium/glucose cotransporter-2
STAMPEDE	Surgical Treatment And Medications Potentially Eradicate Diabetes Efficiently
T1D	Type-1 diabetes
T2D	Type-2 diabetes
TDD	Total daily dose
VLCDs	Very-low-calorie diets

Introduction

This chapter will discuss the practice of lifestyle therapy in both type-2 diabetes (T2D) and type 1 diabetes (T1D). Management of T2D has traditionally been centered on the control of glycemia through periodic blood glucose monitoring, lifestyle and nutritional modifications, and use of medications that augment insulin secretion or improve insulin sensitivity [1]. In T1D, the combined use of exogenous basal and rapid-acting insulin delivery is needed to mimic endogenous insulin secretion during fasting and in response to meals, which is no longer possible due to autoimmune destruction of insulin-producing pancreatic β cells. Lifestyle therapy is critically important for the management of both T2D and T1D and has undergone an evolution over the past decade. The conventional approach to lifestyle therapy includes several components including diabetes self-management education and support (DSME&S), medical nutrition therapy (MNT), and physical activity [2]. DSME&S has been shown to improve glycemic control, self-care behaviors, clinical outcomes, and quality of life, and there is increasing evidence that community health workers and peer coaching can play an effective role in this process [3–8]. National standards for DSME&S are periodically updated by a task force representing multiple key organizations [9]. Similarly, MNT and physical activity for diabetes are critical for effective control of glycemia, prevention of vascular complications, and reductions in cardiovascular risk factors.

W. T. Garvey (✉)
Department of Nutrition Sciences, University of Alabama at Birmingham, GRECC, Birmingham VA Medical Center, UAB Diabetes Research Center, Birmingham, AL 35294-3360, USA
e-mail: garveyt@uab.edu

G. Arathuzik
Addison Gilbert Hospital, Gloucester, MA, USA

Lahey Outpatient Center, Danvers, MA, USA

© Springer International Publishing Switzerland 2016
J. I. Mechanick, R. F. Kushner (eds.), *Lifestyle Medicine*, DOI 10.1007/978-3-319-24687-1_22

There are two developments that have impacted the overall approach to lifestyle therapy. First, lifestyle therapy has shifted away from a universal standard prescription to a more individualized, patient-focused model, with the patient at the center working in collaboration with a team of health-care professionals. Lifestyle therapy is tailored to the individual patient's needs, values, and preferences within a context demonstrated to improve outcomes, and the patient participates in therapeutic decisions together with the health-care team. This concept is called patient centeredness. Thus, MNT and physical activity should be individualized based on individual needs, access, health literacy, and willingness and ability for behavioral change.

The second development in lifestyle therapy for treatment of diabetes involves advances in treatment options for obesity that can be employed in patients who are overweight or obese [10]. Weight loss has long been known to enhance insulin sensitivity and improve glycemia in overweight and obese patients with T2D [11, 12]. While the conventional practice of MNT and lifestyle intervention in diabetes recognizes the benefits of weight loss, the approach has lacked a concerted approach in optimally using therapeutic options directed at weight loss as a primary treatment goal. This chapter will emphasize lifestyle therapy designed to achieve and sustain clinically meaningful weight loss as a primary objective. Despite the demonstrated benefits of weight loss, the underemphasis of weight loss therapy in the treatment and prevention of T2D may relate to difficulties in maintaining clinically meaningful reductions in body weight through diet and lifestyle changes alone [13] and to the previous paucity of effective and safe weight loss medications. However, in recent years, randomized clinical trials have demonstrated not only the efficacy of lifestyle therapy and the marked clinical benefits of weight loss but also those components and practices that are most effective in producing and sustaining weight loss. In addition, since 2012, four new weight loss medications have become available, which, together with refinements in bariatric surgical techniques and patient management, have dramatically augmented therapeutic options for obesity. These developments have enabled the development of more effective strategies and medical models for treatment of obesity as a disease including weight-related complications such as T2D [10, 14]. For example, the complications-centric approach of the American Association of Clinical Endocrinologists (AACE) emphasizes that the presence and severity of weight-related complications such as T2D, rather than body mass index (BMI) per se, should be the primary factor in selecting weight loss treatment modality and intensity [15]. Furthermore, in patients with either T2D or T1D, lifestyle therapy must be individualized to work synergistically with glucose-lowering medications as part of an integrated therapeutic plan designed to prevent vascular complications and hypoglycemia. Therefore, a new reconfigured approach to lifestyle therapy is proposed for overweight/obese patients with diabetes, which emphasizes weight loss as a primary therapeutic strategy for prevention and treatment. This approach to lifestyle therapy incorporates evidence-based practices involving diet, physical activity, behavioral interventions, and multidisciplinary care, with demonstrated effectiveness for weight loss.

Diabetes Mellitus

Prevalence rates of T2D have been increasing worldwide, resulting in a huge burden of patient suffering and social costs, which underscores the importance of finding effective strategies for both treatment and prevention [16, 17]. T2D is an end-stage manifestation of a cardiometabolic pathophysiological process that produces both metabolic and vascular diseases. As discussed in the chapter on cardiometabolic risk, insulin resistance begins early in life, progresses to the clinically identifiable high-risk states of metabolic syndrome and prediabetes, and culminates in overt T2D, cardiovascular disease (CVD), or both in single patients [18, 19]. Obesity can worsen insulin resistance and impel disease progression to T2D. While the relationship between obesity and pathogenesis of T2D is complex, weight loss represents highly effective therapy for glycemic control and improves cardiovascular risk factors in overweight/obese individuals with T2D.

Diabetes mellitus is a group of disorders characterized by abnormal glucose metabolism that affects over 10% of the US adult population [20]. In adults, diabetes is the leading cause of kidney failure, new cases of blindness, and nontraumatic lower-limb amputations in the USA. Medical costs for those with diabetes are two to four times higher than expenditures for those without diabetes [21]. The diagnosis of diabetes mellitus is based on measurements of blood glucose at levels of hyperglycemia that have been shown to place patients at risk for vascular complications. These thresholds have traditionally involved blood glucose determinations under fasting conditions, during oral glucose tolerance tests (OGTTs), or random measurements. However, recently a criterion for the diagnostic use of hemoglobin A1c (A1C) has been added, primarily to identify patients who have diabetes on the basis of elevated 2-h OGTT glucose levels, who may have gone undiagnosed due to the failure of health professionals to perform OGTTs on a more widespread basis [22]. Measurement of glycosylated hemoglobin is used as a chronic indicator of blood glucose that integrates or averages glucose values over approximately a 1–3-month duration. In the body, glucose becomes attached to hemoglobin, a major protein constituent of red blood cells, through a nonenzymatic reaction to a degree that is determined by ambient blood glucose levels over time.

Table 22.1 ADA diagnostic criteria for categories of glucose tolerance

	Fasting glucose	Two-hour glucose during OGTT	A1C (%)	Random glucose
Diabetes	≥126 mg/dL (7.0 mmol/L)	≥200 mg/dL (11.1 mmol/L)	≥6.5	≥200 mg/dL (11.1 mmol/L) with symptoms
Prediabetes	Impaired fasting glucose (IFG) 100–125 mg/dL (5.6–6.9 mmol/L)	Impaired glucose tolerance (IGT) 140–199 mg/dL (7.8–11.0 mmol/L)	5.7–6.4	
Normoglycemic	< 100 mg/dL (5.6 mmol/L)	< 140 mg/dL (7.8 mmol/L)	< 5.7	

A1C hemoglobin A1c, *ADA* American Diabetes Association, *OGTT* oral glucose tolerance test

The diagnostic criteria for diabetes are shown in Table 22.1. Symptoms of uncontrolled diabetes include excessive thirst, polyuria and nocturia, fatigue, blurred vision, and unintended weight loss. A classification scheme for the group of metabolic diseases known as diabetes mellitus has been established by the American Diabetes Association (ADA) [22]. This classification broadly discriminates between diseases caused by primary dysfunction of insulin-producing pancreatic β cells and diseases characterized by a combination of insulin resistance and an impairment in insulin secretion that renders the insulin secretory capacity unable to fully compensate for the prevailing degree of insulin resistance. T2D and T1D are the major types of diabetes encountered clinically. Other classifications of diabetes include gestational diabetes, severe insulin resistance and acanthosis nigricans, monogenic forms of diabetes (neonatal diabetes, maturity-onset diabetes of the young), diabetes associated with mitochondrial syndromes, diseases of the exocrine pancreas (cystic fibrosis, pancreatectomy, pancreatic diabetes), and drug- or chemical-induced diabetes.

T1D Formerly known as insulin-dependent diabetes mellitus or juvenile-onset diabetes, T1D is due to deficient insulin secretion resulting from autoimmune destruction of pancreatic β cells. Patients with T1D require exogenous insulin to avoid ketoacidosis and sustain life. While often presenting in children and adolescents, it can occur at any age. The rate of β cell destruction is variable, with some patients presenting with acute hyperglycemia and ketoacidosis, while others may preserve some insulin secretion for years before becoming dependent on exogenous insulin therapy. T1D patients are also vulnerable to other autoimmune disorders such as celiac sprue, autoimmune thyroid disease, Addison's disease, etc. An example of delayed-onset disease is latent autoimmune diabetes of adults (LADA). LADA generally presents in adults 40 years of age as a result of slowly progressive autoimmune destruction of β cells, and a slow decline in insulin secretion, with evidence of prediabetes for multiple years prior to the diagnosis of overt diabetes.

T2D Formerly known as non-insulin-dependent diabetes or adult-onset diabetes, T2D is due the combination of insulin resistance and impaired insulin secretion that is unable to compensate for the prevailing degree of insulin resistance.

Of all patients with diabetes, 90–95 % have T2D. Insulin resistance occurs early in life and may be exacerbated by the development of obesity, particularly abdominal obesity, and this places metabolic stress on β cells, which hypersecrete insulin to maintain glucose homeostasis. T2D results when insulin secretory capacity begins to fail, creating a state of relative insulin deficiency that can no longer compensate for insulin resistance. Risk factors for developing T2D include increasing age, obesity, lack of physical activity, and a positive family history indicative of a substantial genetic basis for the disease.

Three major metabolic defects generate and sustain hyperglycemia in T2D. The first is impaired β cell insulin secretion due largely to a functional defect in glucose–insulin secretion coupling and also due to a moderate decrease in β cell mass. Fasting insulin levels are usually elevated, although not to the degree that would be commensurate with the hyperglycemia (a state of relative insulin deficiency), and peak insulin responses to glucose or meals are decreased in magnitude and delayed in time. Second, rates of hepatic glucose production are elevated and correlate well with fasting glucose levels. Hepatic glucose output rates are elevated as a result of increased gluconeogenesis due in part to hepatic insulin resistance, increased flux of metabolic substrates to the liver, and high levels of glucoregulatory hormones such as glucagon. Finally, skeletal muscle, which mediates the bulk of insulin-mediated glucose uptake, is insulin resistant due to intrinsic defects in insulin action. These three major defects, present in varying degrees in essentially all patients with T2D, act in concert to produce hyperglycemia. Medical therapy for diabetes acts to reverse one or more of these metabolic abnormalities in order to achieve glycemic control. However, T2D is a progressive disease requiring intensification of therapy over time (i.e., combinations of medications), and many patients end up requiring exogenous insulin therapy to maintain glucose control.

Diabetes care optimally involves a team of professionals including a physician, nurse educator, and dietitian, all with expertise in diabetes management. The first component of diabetes treatment is modulation of lifestyle in order to optimize glucose control. This includes regular and appropriate glucose self-monitoring, diet, and increased physical activity, together with weight loss in those patients who are overweight/obese. Essentially all patients with T1D will also require insulin therapy to sustain life. The vast majority of T2D patients require oral or injectable drugs, including insulin, to control glucose values at recommended target levels that prevent the development of diabetes complications. Over the past 15 years, the number of effective diabetes medications available to health-care providers has increased. We have medications that act by: (i) enhancing insulin secretion including the sulfonylureas (glimeperide, glipizide, and glyburide), the meglitinides (nateglinide and repaglinide), and incretin axis drugs that either inhibit the degradation of glucagon-like peptide-1 (dipeptidyl peptidase-4 inhibitors such as sitagliptin, saxagliptin, linagliptin, vildagliptin, and alogliptin) or act as glucagon-like peptide-1 receptor agonists (exenatide, liraglutide, albiglutide, dulaglutide, and lixisenatide); (ii) drugs that lower hepatic glucose production (metformin, insulin); (iii) drugs that increase insulin sensitivity in muscle (the thiazolidinediones pioglitzone and rosiglitazone); (iv) drugs that act at the level of the gastrointestinal tract (pramlintide and colesevelam) including the glycosidase inhibitors (acarbose and miglitol); and (v) sodium–glucose co-transporter inhibitors that enhance glucose loss in the urine (canagliflozin, dapagliflozin, and empagliflozin).

Lifestyle Therapy: Treatment Goals

Lifestyle therapy for diabetes is designed to achieve the treatment goals shown in Table 22.2. First, lifestyle therapy is critical for chronic glycemic control in both T2D and T1D in order to prevent microvascular complications including retinopathy, nephropathy, and neuropathy. These efforts are directed at lowering A1C values to recommended levels to the degree that this can be accomplished safely in individual patients. A second objective is to prevent acute complications due to uncontrolled glucose levels, such as hyperosmolar hyperglycemic nonketotic syndrome in T2D, diabetic ketoacidosis in T1D, and infections. In addition, lifestyle therapy is directed at avoiding hypoglycemia, which is detrimental to cognitive function, can cause coma and death, and places patients at increased risk for future episodes of hypoglycemia by blunting the counter-regulatory hormonal response. All patients with diabetes are at increased risk of CVD events (myocardial infarction, stroke, and peripheral vascular disease), and therefore, improving the cardiovascular risk profile through improvements in lipids and blood

Table 22.2 Treatment goals for diabetes

Control glycemia to prevent microvascular complications
Prevent acute diabetes complications and hypoglycemia
Prevent CVD events by improving risk factors and treatment of
Dyslipidemia
Hypertension/prehypertension
Improve functionality and quality of life

pressure is another important goal of lifestyle therapy. Finally, lifestyle therapy should promote increased functionality and quality of life.

Lifestyle Therapy: Conventional Practice of Medical Nutrition Therapy and Diabetes Self-Management Education and Support

Lifestyle therapy is a cornerstone for managing patients with diabetes and includes several components: MNT, increased energy expenditure through increased physical activity, education regarding skills for self-management, and psychosocial assessment and care [2, 9]. These components of care are incorporated into two modalities, MNT and DSME&S. Standard practices for MNT and DSME&S are reviewed and updated under the authority of the ADA and other agencies, and represent the conventional approach to lifestyle therapy in diabetes [9]. MNT and DSME&S are critically important for all patients with diabetes. However, in patients who are overweight or obese, these programs lack a primary emphasis on weight loss to a degree that is commensurate with the resulting clinical benefits. Therefore, we will discuss MNT and DSME&S, together with the implementation of new tools and approaches for weight loss, in an overall approach to lifestyle therapy that optimally benefits patients with diabetes.

Medical Nutrition Therapy

MNT generally involves nutrition assessment/reassessment, nutrition diagnosis, nutrition intervention, and monitoring and evaluation intended for the prevention or management of disease [2, 9]. In T2D, MNT is instituted at the time of diagnosis. Patients sometimes want to delay the start of medication administration to determine whether an attempt at lifestyle changes, including MNT and physical activity, can improve glycemic control, and this can be considered on an individual basis. The first step in MNT for diabetes is a dietary plan, preferably developed by a registered dietitian (RD), and education provided through a DSME&S program given by a Certified Diabetes Educator (CDE). The education of patients should be followed by acquisition of self-management skills. This can prove to be extremely challenging, and most patients will need ongoing support and follow-up. The Institute of Medicine (IOM) made a recommendation in 1999 that Medicare cover individualized MNT provided by an RD as a Medicare benefit based on evidence clearly showing that MNT can improve clinical outcomes in diabetes and reduce the cost of diabetes care [23].

Nutrition therapy should be individualized taking into account personal preferences and barriers to change. Professional societies, health-care systems, and health-care insurers widely recognize the need for MNT as part of diabetes self-management education. Despite the fact that the RD and/or CDE plays a pivotal role in providing MNT, all professionals on the diabetes care team should understand the goals of MNT and play an active role in supporting patients in achieving their personal goals for meal planning and physical activity. The position statement of the ADA regarding MNT in adults with diabetes was revised in 2013 [24] and the following goals were recommended:

1. Provide education and ongoing support surrounding healthy eating practices including nutrient-dense foods and portion control;
2. Implementation of an individualized meal plan with realistic goals and expectations, which promotes beneficial outcomes while avoiding restrictive meal-planning approaches that take away the enjoyment of eating;
3. Achieve and maintain body-weight goals;
4. Achieve targets for disease management regarding glycemia, blood pressure, and lipids. Treatment goals recommended by the ADA [25, 26] are A1C≤7%, blood pressure≤140/80 mmHg, low-density lipoprotein (LDL) cholesterol <100 mg/dL, triglycerides <150 mg/dL, and high-density lipoprotein (HDL) cholesterol ≥40 mg/dL for men and ≥50 mg/dL for women. The AACE [27] recommends A1C≤6.5%, blood pressure ≤130/80 mmHg, LDL cholesterol <100 mg/dL and <70 mg/dL if high risk, and triglycerides <150 mg/dL. Both ADA and AACE acknowledge that these treatment targets may need to be modified for individual patients, depending on factors such as age, duration of diabetes, existence of hypoglycemic unawareness, severity of diabetes complications, or other possible health conditions; and
5. Delay or prevent complications of diabetes.

The provider of MNT has three major issues to consider. The first pertains to dietary carbohydrate. Carbohydrate is the primary nutrient responsible for postprandial glucose levels, and, although there is no specific amount of carbohydrate recommended for people with diabetes, the quantity and quality of the carbohydrate intake is important. Second to consider is caloric intake. All food choices affect energy balance, and weight management is a critical component in achieving glycemic control and delaying or treating other comorbidities. The third consideration is the impact of food choices related to macronutrient and micronutrient composition of the diet, which is relevant not only to glycemic control but also to other CVD risk factors such as hypertension and dyslipidemia. There is not one specific meal plan approach that works for all individuals with diabetes. Nutrition therapy needs to be individualized for the particular person and must take into account personal preferences, health literacy

(ability to use written materials in achieving health goals) and numeracy (ability to use quantitative information related to health goals), socioeconomic status, cultural preferences, readiness to change, and any barriers to implementation of the diet plan. ADA recommendations for macronutrient intake in diabetes [2] are summarized in Table 22.3. These goals for macronutrient intake can be accomplished within any one of several healthy meal plans that can be selected based on personal and cultural preferences of the patient, as discussed below.

Carbohydrate Currently, there is no compelling evidence to support a specific percentage of calories from carbohydrates in the diet for people with diabetes [2]. Carbohydrate goals should be individualized, taking into account glucose-lowering medications and physical activity. The quantity and type of carbohydrate can influence glycemic response, with simple and refined sugars producing higher glucose peaks than complex carbohydrates; however, the overall quantity of carbohydrate consumed is the primary predictor of glycemic response [28]. Therefore, managing carbohydrate intake remains an important part of the diabetes meal plan, and there are different ways to teach patients how to manage carbohydrate intake according to their personal preferences. If there are health-related literacy and numeracy issues, a simple approach such as the plate method can be taught [29]. For people on fixed dose or sliding scale insulin regimens, it is important to teach basic carbohydrate counting with the goal of consistent carbohydrate intake and timing of meals. Any person with diabetes using multiple daily injections or an insulin pump can intensify their insulin regimens and use advanced carbohydrate counting. Patients with T1D should use carbohydrate counting as the basis for determining the premeal dose of regular or rapid-acting insulin [24]. Preferred carbohydrates include those from legumes, vegetables, fruits, whole grains, and dairy products, while the consumption of carbohydrate sources with high fat, sugar, or sodium content should be reduced [30].

A more specific meal-planning approach focused on type of carbohydrate is the glycemic index (GI). GI is a measure of the glycemic response to a carbohydrate-containing food relative to white bread or glucose as a reference [31]. Using GI as the basis of a diet plan is controversial. For one thing, the glycemic load rather than the GI is most important for glucose homeostasis after a meal. The glycemic load is a function of a food's GI, and its total available carbohydrate content defined as: GI (%) × carbohydrate (g). Foods with similar GI can have markedly different glycemic loads and vice versa. An example is the comparison between watermelon, which has a high GI (=72) and low glycemic load (=5), and baked potato, which has a comparably high GI (=69) but a high glycemic load (=19). It is the baked potato that will produce a greater area under the curve in blood

Table 22.3 Highlights of the American Diabetes Association nutritional recommendations for patients with diabetes (2015). (Source: American Diabetes Association [2])

Medical nutrition therapy	Nutrition therapy recommended for all T2D and T1D patients as effective components of overall treatment plan with medications and physical activity
Macronutrient composition	The evidence does not support a recommendation for the amount of calories derived from carbohydrate, fat, or protein
Healthful meal plan	Macronutrient composition should be determined by metabolic goals within the context of healthful meal plans that are acceptable based on personal and cultural preferences, health literacy, access to foods, barriers, and willingness to change
	For adult patients who are overweight or obese, caloric reduction within the context of a healthful meal plan is recommended to promote moderate weight loss
	Meal plan should provide recommended dietary allowances for all micronutrients. No need for routine supplementation with vitamins, minerals, and antioxidants, and there is lack of sufficient evidence for recommending herbal supplements
Carbohydrates	Most important factor in determining the extent of glycemic rise after meals. Consider the amount of carbohydrate and factors influencing blood glucose response in the meal plan
	Modify the amount and timing of carbohydrate intake in synergy with medications (e.g., fixed multiple daily insulin doses) and physical activity, to improve glycemic control, minimize risk of hypoglycemia, and reduce risk of microvascular disease complications
	Carbohydrate counting as basis for premeal insulin dose is recommended in T1D
	Advise carbohydrate intake from legumes, vegetables, fruits, whole grains, and dairy products as opposed to sources with high fat, sugar, or sodium content
	Avoid sugar-sweetened beverages
	Should not displace nutrient-dense foods
Fiber	USDA recommendation for dietary fiber at 14 g fiber/1000 kcal. Majority intake of grains should be whole grains
Protein	Evidence inconclusive regarding ideal amount of protein. No need to reduce protein intake below normal in patients with chronic kidney disease
Fat	Quality of fat is more important than quantity
	Increase consumption of long-chain ω-3 fatty acids (EPA, DHA, and ALA), as obtained from fatty fish
	MUFA- and PUFA-enriched diets such as a Mediterranean diet may benefit glycemic control and CVD risk factors
Sodium	Recommended limit 2300 mg/day as for general population but less on an individual basis in patients with both diabetes and hypertension
Alcohol	Use in moderation (one drink per day for women and two drinks per day for men). May increase risk for hypoglycemia

ALA α-linolenic acid, *CVD* cardiovascular disease, *DHA* docosahexaenoic acid, *EPA* eicosapentaenoic acid, *MUFA* monounsaturated fatty acid, *PUFA* polyunsaturated fatty acid, *T1D* type-1 diabetes, *T2D* type-2 diabetes, *USDA* US Department of Agriculture

glucose following ingestion. Secondly, studies have shown varied results regarding improvements in glycemia using GI [28, 32]. It is a complicated method of meal planning to teach to patients, and it is difficult to determine if any improved glycemic effects are due to the GI or the higher fiber content of many low-GI foods [33, 34]. Similar to GI, the benefits of fiber on glycemic control are also debated. The study that showed the most significant A1C reduction with a high-fiber diet had participants consuming greater than 50 g fiber per day [35]. That is an unrealistic expectation for most people with diabetes when the average American is not meeting the current fiber recommendations of 25–30 g/day or 14 g/1000 cal [36]. Fiber has consistently been shown to improve lipid levels in studies comparing low- and high-fiber intakes [37–40]. People with diabetes should be encouraged to consume 25–30 g fiber per day with an emphasis on soluble fiber (7–13 g) for improving CVD risk factors. Insoluble fiber is largely not absorbed and does not provide calories, while soluble fiber provides calories at approximately 2 kcal/g due to their conversion to short-chain fatty acids and absorption in the gut.

Protein While recommendations for protein intake range from 10–15% to 25–30% of total calories, there is no rigorously determined standard for the percent of calories from protein in diabetes, and, as described for carbohydrate, this adds flexibility for individualization of the meal plan. However, protein is a critically important macronutrient, and the IOM recommends that adults get a minimum of 0.8 g of protein per kilogram of body weight per day [41]. For a 2000-cal diet, 10–15% calories as protein would provide 50–75 g/day, which approaches the minimum intake advocated by the IOM. A diet containing protein at 25–30% of calories provides intake of 125–150 g protein per day, which is in clear excess of minimum requirements. Therefore, an intermediate dietary prescription of 20–25% protein is reasonable in most patients. For patients following a reduced-calorie diet, there is a risk that 10–15% calories and protein would result in an absolute intake of protein that could fall below the IOM minimum. This could result in loss of lean muscle mass during weight loss. Therefore, it is important to consider that a greater percentage of calories from protein is necessary when prescribing low-calorie diets for weight loss to ensure people meet minimum protein requirements.

Results are controversial as to whether dietary protein enrichment is useful as a strategy to lower A1C values [42–44]. Proteins, specifically certain amino acids such as leucine, arginine, and lysine, can directly simulate insulin secretion independent of glucose. Therefore, patients with hypoglycemia should be instructed to treat themselves by consuming fast-acting carbohydrate sources and not foods or snacks that are highly enriched with protein. The most controversial aspect of protein in the management of diabetes is whether or not protein should be restricted in people with diabetic kidney disease. The previous recommendation to limit protein intake in order to delay the decline in kidney function is not well-founded by evidence. While one small study showed beneficial effects of a low-protein diet, this is more than counterbalanced by numerous studies of large sample size and long duration that show no effect on the glomerular filtration rate [45–49]. Since low-protein diets can cause malnutrition and hypoalbuminemia, reductions are not recommended in patients with diabetic kidney disease. Lean protein sources are generally encouraged such as poultry; fish; eggs; low-fat cheese; pork tenderloin; and lean meats such as the round, sirloin, and lean ground beef. While more studies are needed, there does not appear to be any benefit of plant protein over animal protein, independent of other factors on renal function or glycemic control in diabetes [50].

Fat There is no specific amount of fat intake recommended for people with diabetes [24]. The IOM defines an acceptable range for total fat at 20–35 % of daily calories based on perceived risk of CVD in the general population [41]. Since under isocaloric conditions, the type of fat consumed is more important than quantity [24], cardiovascular risk may be conferred by the intake of saturated fat, *trans* fat, and cholesterol as opposed to total fat. While people with diabetes have a three- to fourfold increased risk of CVD, it is recommended that patients follow the same guidelines for fat intake as that for the general population, that is, saturated fat at 10 % or less of total calories and no *trans* fats [51]. Saturated fats are found in butter, full-fat dairy products, high-fat cuts of meat, and tropical oils such as coconut and palm oil. *Trans* fats are found in some fried foods, baked goods, snack foods, and stick margarines. Any food containing partially hydrogenated oils is a source of *trans* fat. Previous recommended limits of cholesterol (i.e., 300 mg/day) have been withdrawn in the latest Dietary Guidelines for Americans since available evidence shows no appreciable relationship between consumption of dietary cholesterol and serum cholesterol [52]. In diabetes, saturated fat should be replaced with sources of unsaturated fats as opposed to replacing saturated fat with carbohydrates. Extensive research demonstrates that dietary enrichment of monounsaturated fats (MUFAs) may benefit glycemic control and cardiovascular risk factors, and, therefore, meal plans that emphasize MUFAs are healthy options for people with diabetes (see Mediterranean diet below) [53–58]. Food sources of MUFAs include olives, olive oil, nuts, nut butters, and avocados.

The benefits of polyunsaturated fats (PUFAs) are less clear than those of MUFAs, including PUFAs derived from ω-3 fatty acids are eicosapentaenoic acid (EPA), docosahexaenoic acid (DHA), and α-linolenic acid (ALA). ω-3 fatty acid supplements have not been shown to improve glycemic control but may lower triglycerides in high amounts [59]. ω-3 fatty acids are found in fatty fish such as salmon, mackerel, sardines, tuna, trout, and herring. While the basis of the recommendation is uncertain, the ADA advocates intake of fatty fish at least two times per week.

Sodium Sodium intake is recommended at ≤2300 mg/day in the general population, and in 2014, the American Heart Association (AHA) recommended the intake of sodium not exceed 1500 mg/day for people with diabetes, hypertension, and chronic kidney disease, as well as for African Americans and anyone over the age of 51 [60]. The dietary approaches to stop hypertension (DASH) diet, a meal plan approach geared towards lowering blood pressure, did lead to improvements in blood pressure in a small study in people with diabetes [61]. The DASH diet emphasizes fruits, vegetables, low-fat/nonfat dairy products, nuts, whole grains, lean meats, fish, and poultry. While a meta-analysis of randomized clinical trials indicated that lower sodium can reduce blood pressure [62], the data have not been sufficient to support lower sodium intake in diabetes. The average American is consuming greater than 4000 mg sodium per day. Challenges exist for very-low-sodium diets in Western societies due to low availability, increased costs, and reduced palatability of low-sodium foods. On balance, people with diabetes and hypertension can be prescribed diets containing less than 2300 mg/day on an individual basis [63, 64].

Nonnutritive Sweeteners Currently, there are six nonnutritive sweeteners approved by the US Food and Drug Administration (FDA), including acesulfame-K, aspartame, neotame, saccharin, sucralose, and stevia. Nonnutritive sweeteners contain zero to low calories and are alternatives to nutritive sweeteners such as table sugar. The FDA sets an acceptable daily intake for sweeteners as the level that a person can safely consume on an average every day over a lifetime without risk [65]. There are limited human studies on the effects of nonnutritive sweeteners on glycemia and weight. These studies generally show no effect on glucose, A1C, blood pressure, or body weight when comparing diets with and without nonnutritive sweeteners [66, 67]. The AHA and ADA both conclude there is insufficient evidence that nonnutritive sweeteners will lead to weight loss or improvements in glycemia, blood pressure, or lipids [68]. At the same time, nonnutritive sweeteners will not adversely affect these disease parameters, and, for this reason, people with diabetes can safely consume nonnutritive sweeteners at or below the acceptable daily intake value. It is important to educate patients that other ingredients in products containing nonnutritive sweeteners may produce a glycemic response. In theory, using nonnutritive sweeteners to replace calories consumed from nutritive sweeteners, without the addition of calories from other food sources, should help people achieve weight loss [68].

Vitamin/Mineral Supplementation There is no clear evidence that people with or without diabetes need vitamin and mineral supplementation with the exception of pregnant/lactating women, the elderly, vegetarians/vegans, people on very-low-calorie diets (VLCDs), and post bariatric surgery. A healthy, balanced diet will provide individuals with sufficient micronutrients. If vitamin or mineral deficiencies exist, then supplements should be used to correct the deficiency. Certain micronutrients and herbs are often promoted to people with diabetes such as cinnamon, vitamin D, magnesium, and chromium. The evidence is insufficient to support the contention that any of these micronutrients or herbs will improve glycemic control and should not be recommended for people with diabetes.

Alcohol People with diabetes are able to enjoy alcoholic beverages in moderation, defined as one drink per day or less for adult women and two drinks per day or less for adult men. One drink is defined as 12-ounce beer, 5-ounce wine, or 1.5-ounce distilled spirits. The biggest risk of excessive alcohol is delayed hypoglycemia, particularly in the absence of food and in patients taking insulin or insulin secretagogues [69, 70]. Symptoms of hypoglycemia can mimic symptoms that occur when drinking alcohol, and alcohol consumed at night can increase the risk for nocturnal hypoglycemia. At-risk patients should carry glucose tablets, frequently monitor blood glucose, and educate friends and family about the risks and symptoms of hypoglycemia.

Weight Management The clear majority of patients with T2D are overweight or obese, and this is becoming more of a problem in T1D as well. As is discussed below, weight loss can improve insulin resistance, glycemia, and CVD risk factors in both T2D and T1D and is recommended for people with diabetes who are overweight/obese. Achieving weight loss is best done through a lifestyle intervention program involving nutrition therapy, exercise/physical activity, and behavior modification. Despite the large number of studies showing benefits of weight loss, the conventional practice of MNT and DSME&S is generally associated with only small decreases in body weight and does not often achieve the full benefits of weight loss.

Diabetes Self-Management Education and Support

National standards for DSME&S are established by a task force of experts and stakeholder convened by the ADA and the American Association of Diabetes Educators [9]. These standards delineate self-management education strategies that are known to be effective as a guide for accredited programs and other providers. The standards also emphasize that the ongoing process of education, skill-building, and behavior change is individualized to correspond to needs, goals, and preferences of individual patients. DSME&S represents a key element of lifestyle therapy that empowers patients for better self-care behavior and has been shown to improve glucose control with lower A1C values, lower health-care costs, decrease utilization of inpatient hospital services, and enhance self-efficacy and quality of life [2].

DSME&S programs must have an internal organizational structure and allow for input and review by external experts for quality improvement [2, 9]. The providers of DSME&S must establish and construct programs that best meet the needs of local populations and communities. A coordinator must oversee planning, implementation, and evaluation of programs staffed by one or more instructors and support staff that can include physicians, nurses, dietitians, pharmacists, CDEs, sociologists, psychologists, or other health workers. Lay health counselors and trained peer advisers can also contribute to DSME&S. The program must feature a written curriculum providing information about diabetes pathophysiology and treatment options, incorporation of nutritional management and physical activity into overall lifestyle patterns, safe and proper use of medications, glucose self-monitoring, diabetes complications, psychosocial issues, and personal strategies for behavior change. The patient works in collaboration with DSME&S providers to develop an individualized plan for initial care and ongoing support. Patients are monitored for progress, and the DSME&S program is evaluated for quality improvement.

In addition to education and support, DSME&S also incorporates behavior modification interventions. Behavioral intervention is an essential aspect because it provides patients with strategies for health, such as modifying cues that lead to unwanted behaviors and self-monitoring to promote treatment adherence [2–6]. Therefore, components of a behavior program include self-monitoring of food intake and physical activity, learning to cope with negative thoughts by means other than eating, and changes in eating behavior such as portion control and consuming meals at regular times and in places where one can focus on the act of eating. Table 22.4

Table 22.4 List of applications (apps) to assist self-monitoring in patients with diabetes

App	Cost in US dollars ($)	Log blood glucose	Log food	Log exercise	Log meds/ insulin	Track weight	Email reports/ sync	Barcode scanner
MyNetDiary (for diabetes)	9.99	x	x	x	x	x	x	x
MyFitnessPal	Free		x	x		x	x	x
LoseIt!	Free		x	x		x	x	x
mySugr	Free	x	x	x	x	x	x	
Glucose Buddy	Free	x	x	x	x	x	x	
Track3	5.99	x	x	x	x	x	x	
Figwee Portion Explorer	1.99	(calculates calories and nutritional content of many foods)						

lists several applications (apps) for "smart" phones that patients with diabetes might find helpful in monitoring their diet, exercise, weight, blood glucose, and medications. A mental health professional is commonly needed to address issues such as disordered eating and depression, which, if not treated proactively, can jeopardize the effectiveness of lifestyle therapy.

Carbohydrate Counting and Insulin Dosing

An important aspect of dietary therapy in T1D, and in T2D patients taking premeal regular- or rapid-acting insulin, is carbohydrate counting. Carbohydrate is the primary nutrient affecting postprandial blood glucose. Since the carbohydrate content of meals will vary, alterations in the premeal insulin dose to accommodate greater or lesser amounts of carbohydrate provide for optimal control of postprandial glycemic excursions. There are different methods for managing carbohydrate consumption and insulin dosing. If a person is on a fixed dose or sliding scale, a consistent carbohydrate meal plan referred to as basic carbohydrate counting is the ideal approach. Patients learn to identify foods that contain carbohydrates, assess 15-g carbohydrate portions of common foods, by weighing and measuring foods and reading food labels to determine the quantity of carbohydrate per serving. Fifteen gram of carbohydrate is equal to one carb serving or one carb choice. Basic carbohydrate counting allows people with diabetes to make different food choices while keeping the total carbohydrate content (i.e., the number of 15-g carb servings) of the meal constant to correspond to the prescribed insulin dose. Another approach involves altering the insulin dose to match the quantity of ingested carbohydrate. This is termed advanced carbohydrate counting and allows people more flexibility in meal planning [71, 72]. People are able to consume smaller meals when feeling less hungry or desiring weight loss, and larger meals when feeling hungry or possibly during a celebration, and alter the insulin dose accordingly. In both basic and advanced carbohydrate counting, the patient will need to perform frequent blood glucose checks (e.g., before and 2–3 h after meals) or use a continuous glucose monitor, for optimal implementation. Also, ongoing education and support is critical to a person's

success with carbohydrate counting and achieving glycemic and weight goals.

Advanced carbohydrate counting involves matching one unit of rapid-acting insulin (aspart, lispro, and glulisine) to a certain number of carbohydrate grams, called the insulin to carbohydrate (I:C) ratio. The I:C ratio only covers the insulin demand to control the rise in glucose for the immediate planned meal, but if the premeal blood glucose level is elevated, a correction factor is used to add extra insulin to the I:C-determined insulin dose to bring the blood glucose back to goal. The correction factor reflects the absolute decrement in glucose produced by one unit of insulin. A target blood glucose is chosen, for example 100–120 mg/dL, and the correction factor determines how many units are needed to bring the elevated premeal glucose down to the blood glucose target. Since the I:C ratio is determined on an individual basis, candidates for advanced carbohydrate counting will need to meet with either an RD or a CDE to help calculate the I:C ratio and correction factor and learn how to use both the I:C ratio and correction factor to determine a premeal bolus [73]. Knowledge of simple mathematics is required as is a willingness to check glucose before meals and to count carbohydrate grams at each meal.

Formulas for calculating the I:C ratio and correction factor are:

I:C ratio using the 450 rule: 450/total daily dose (TDD) of insulin = grams of carbohydrate covered by 1 unit of rapid-acting insulin

Example: TDD = 50 units/day, 450/50 = 9, 1 unit of insulin will cover 9 g of carbohydrate

Correction factor using the 1500 rule: 1500/TDD = how many mg/dL of 1 unit of rapid-acting insulin will lower blood glucose

Example: TDD = 50 units/day, 1500/50 = 30, 1 unit of rapid-acting insulin will lower blood glucose by 30 mg/dL

By way of example, consider two lunchtime meals.

- Sample lunch one is: two slices of whole wheat bread (30-g carbohydrate or two carbohydrate servings), 4-ounce sliced turkey, two teaspoons mayonnaise, and a 4-ounce apple (15 g carbohydrate or one carbohydrate serving). This represents a total of 45-g carbohydrate or three carbohydrate servings. Using 1:15 insulin to carbohydrate ratio = 3 units for sample lunch one.

- Sample lunch two is: Foot-long sub roll (90-g carbohydrate or six carbohydrate servings), 8-ounce sliced turkey, two tablespoons mayonnaise, and 1-ounce Lays potato chips (15-g carbohydrate or one carbohydrate serving). This represents a total of 105-g carbohydrate or seven carbohydrate servings). Using 1:15 insulin to carbohydrate ratio = 7 units for sample lunch two.

It is important to note that insulin doses calculated using these formulas need to be tested in real-life situations and the I:C ratios and correction factors should be adjusted accordingly. A patient may need different I:C ratios at different meals and different correction factors for daytime and nighttime meals. Checking blood glucose premeal and 2–3 h post meal will help both patients and health professionals determine if the I:C ratio and correction factors are appropriate. Adjustments may also be needed with changes in body weight, work schedules or duties, exercise routines, and intercurrent illness.

Carbohydrate counting is challenging. Many patients will admit during education visits that they usually guess carbohydrate grams in meals and rarely measure or weigh carbohydrate-containing foods. Reference to a food label can also enhance accuracy; however, the portion or amount of the food consumed must still be quantified. In advanced carbohydrate counting, the insulin dose and consequential blood glucose response is only as good as the correctness of the carbohydrate count. A patient should be encouraged to measure and weigh foods, at least initially, and either use reference objects as cues for visual memory, as illustrated in Table 22.5, or refer to pictures of food portions saved on mobile phones. Patients can create cheat sheets with commonly eaten carbohydrate foods with portions and carbohydrate grams listed and carry the cheat sheets with them. There are multiple applications on phones and tablets available to help get carbohydrate information for foods and estimate portion sizes.

Table 22.5 Visual memory cues that can be used to estimate food volume

Item	Portion size
Palm of hand (based on an average woman's hand)	3–4 ounces
Thumb	1 tablespoon
Matchbook	1 tablespoon
Baseball	1 cup
Tennis ball	1 cup
Cupped hand	1/2 cup
Muffin or cupcake liner	1/2 cup

There are challenges that exist beyond the accuracy of carbohydrate counting. One such challenge is risk of weight gain, which is an increasing problem in patients with T1D, as is the case for society in general. Many people who have spent most of their lives with diabetes using the old exchange lists mistakenly see advanced carbohydrate counting as a newfound freedom, allowing them to eat as many carbohydrate grams as they wish. The excess calories together with higher calculated doses of rapid-acting insulin combine to promote weight gain. On the other hand, some patients may lose weight if they are no longer forced to eat more food to avoid hypoglycemia on a fixed insulin dose. Another challenge is quality of carbohydrate. If a meal contains high-GI carbohydrate choices, the postprandial blood glucose is often elevated despite an accurate carb count and insulin dose that would be effective for a lower GI meal. For rapidly digested carbohydrate-containing foods (e.g., sushi rice), it might be beneficial to take the premeal insulin dose 15–20 min prior to eating to allow more time for the insulin to peak to match the time of glucose absorption. For meals high in fat, slowing of gastric emptying causes a delayed peak for glucose absorption, in which case, it might be necessary to take the premeal insulin dose immediately before eating. If the insulin was taken earlier before a high-fat meal, the insulin peak may cause a decline in glucose and hypoglycemia before glucose absorption could occur.

Benefits of Weight Loss in Diabetes

While MNT and DSME&S recognize the importance of weight loss, the amount of weight loss that accompanies these interventions in actual practice is often minimal [74, 75]. Unless health-care professionals have been trained in weight loss therapy and advocate this to patients as a key therapeutic strategy in its own right, it is unlikely that the patients will experience clinically significant weight loss and maintenance of that weight loss. Over the past decade, research has identified effective lifestyle interventions, new medications, and bariatric surgery approaches that greatly augment both treatment options and therapeutic efficacy for weight loss [10]. *Optimal lifestyle therapy will provide for meaningful weight loss in overweight and obese patients with diabetes.* The clinical benefits of weight loss in diabetes will be summarized below followed by lifestyle interventions that can achieve these goals.

While individuals with T2D tend to have slightly more difficultly achieving and maintaining weight loss than those without diabetes [76, 77], copious data document the benefits of weight loss therapy in these patients. Weight loss in T2D lowers fasting glucose and A1C levels while reducing the need for conventional glucose-lowering medications [11–14,

78–93]. Additional benefits include reductions in blood pressure, lower triglycerides, higher HDL cholesterol, decreased levels of hepatic transaminases, and improvements in biomarkers of cardiovascular risk such as C-reactive protein, fibrinogen, and adiponectin. There is a growing awareness of the value of weight loss therapy as a primary treatment approach in T2D [14] as reflected in recent guidelines advocated by the AACE [27, 94], the Endocrine Society [95], and the American Society for Metabolic and Bariatric Surgery [96].

Weight loss as a consequence of lifestyle interventions has long been known to produce clinical benefits in T2D [11, 12], and this has most recently become apparent in the Look - AHEAD Trial [74–79]. This latter study randomized T2D patients to an intensive lifestyle intervention versus standard diabetes support and education. The intensive lifestyle intervention resulted in 4.7% weight loss after 4 years, with associated benefits of lower glycemia and A1C values with less need for diabetes medications, diabetes remission in ~10% of patients, lower diastolic and systolic blood pressures, improved lipids (higher HDL, lower triglycerides), improvements in sleep apnea as reflected by lower Apnea–Hypopnea Index scores, increased mobility, and improved quality of life [82]. However, the principal outcome measure in Look - AHEAD was CVD events, and the study was discontinued prematurely after an interim analysis showed no difference between treatment groups.

Weight loss through lifestyle changes alone is often difficult to maintain [97], and interventions such as pharmacotherapy or surgery, employed as an adjunct to lifestyle therapy, may be necessary. When the clinical decision is made to employ weight loss medications or bariatric surgery, lifestyle therapy remains a critical component of therapy for achieving and maintaining greater degrees of weight loss and for optimizing outcomes. All weight loss medications approved for chronic therapy of obesity have been studied in clinical trials enrolling T2D patients, and these data amply document the benefits of medicine-assisted weight loss. In these studies, all T2D patients are treated with a lifestyle intervention and then randomized to placebo versus weight loss medication. Weight loss in T2D patients treated with orlistat [84, 85], phentermine/topiramate extended release (ER) [86, 87], lorcaserin [88], naltrexone ER/bupropion ER [89], and high-dose liraglutide (3 mg/day) consistently led to lower A1C together with the reduced need for conventional diabetes medications in actively managed patients, when compared with patients treated with lifestyle modification alone. Medication-assisted weight loss in these studies also resulted in reductions in blood pressure and improvements in lipids. By way of example, treatment with phentermine/topiramate ER resulted in 9–10% weight loss in T2D at 1 year and A1C reduction by 0.4% in patients with mild diabetes (with value of 7.0% at baseline) and by 1.6% in patients with more severe, long-standing diabetes on multiple medications (with value of 8.6% at baseline) [86]. Importantly, these improvements were significantly greater than the lifestyle intervention alone and occurred despite greater reductions in the need for conventional diabetes drugs. The data support the conclusion that weight loss as a consequence of lifestyle therapy with or without obesity pharmacotherapy should be considered for any overweight or obese patient with overt T2D.

Bariatric surgery is the most effective and durable treatment for obesity and T2D [90–93] and, again, should be implemented in conjunction with lifestyle therapy to achieve optimal weight loss and to better maintain the weight loss over the lifetime of the patient. Bariatric surgery can be considered in patients with diabetes when the BMI is ≥ 35 kg/m^2 [96]. This approach must be balanced against the inherent risks of surgical complications and mortality, and also potential nutritional deficiencies, weight regain in some patients, and the need for lifelong lifestyle support and medical monitoring [96]. Not uncommonly, T2D patients will undergo remission defined as the ability to maintain euglycemia in the absence of any diabetes medications. A meta-analysis of 27 studies of surgical outcomes following sleeve gastrectomy demonstrated a diabetes remission rate of 66% [98]. In the Swedish Obese Subjects study, bariatric surgery produced a diabetes remission rate of 72% after 2 years, decreasing to a remission rate of 30% after 15 years, and was associated with a reduction in microvascular complications [90]. Sleeve gastrectomy and RYGB have generally been found to produce the highest diabetes remission rates followed by laparoscopic adjustable gastric banding (LAGB) and medical therapy.

One reason that weight loss attempts are often slightly less effective in diabetes is that many medications used to treat diabetes result in weight gain. The classes of drugs most likely to cause weight gain are insulin, insulin secretagogues (sulfonylureas and meglitinides), and thiazolidinediones. Insulin and insulin secretagogues also put a patient at risk for hypoglycemia. Frequent bouts of hypoglycemia can force patients to consume extra calories to treat and prevent hypoglycemia. Weight gain is the unfortunate consequence. Other glucose-lowering medications are weight neutral (dipeptidyl peptidase-4 inhibitors, alpha-glucosidase inhibitors, colesevalam, and bromocriptine) or may lead to a modest degree of weight loss (metformin, pramlintide, glucagon-like peptide-1 receptor agonists, and sodium/glucose cotransporter-2 (SGLT2) inhibitors) [27]. The medication options that are weight neutral or associated with modest weight loss are preferable in the obese T2D patient [27, 95]. Even so, clinicians should not refrain from insulin therapy when needed to achieve A1C targets, particularly in patients with long-standing disease.

Lifestyle Therapy: An Approach Emphasizing Weight Loss

In considering the diet component of lifestyle therapy in overweight/obese patients with diabetes, two important considerations in the dietary prescription for weight loss are: (i) the macronutrient composition of the diet and (ii) total daily calories. Both of these aspects of the diet should be individualized to enhance glycemic control, improve the CVD risk profile, provide for weight loss, and realize the overall goals delineated in Table 22.2. In patients with diabetes on glucose-lowering medications, the additional challenge is to coordinate these aspects of the diet with medications and physical activity for optimal overall disease management while avoiding hypoglycemia. Frequent blood glucose checks will be needed for safe implementation of weight loss therapy in patients on glucose-lowering medications.

In the initial phase of weight loss therapy, patients are prescribed a hypocaloric diet to achieve active weight loss. Over time, the weight equilibrates at a new lower level and patients convert to a chronic phase consuming an isocaloric or energy-balanced diet in an effort to maintain weight loss at the new lower level of body weight. Lifestyle therapy will require adjustments appropriate for each phase. In the initial phase, patients are prescribed a reduced-calorie diet healthy meal plan. While most studies involve nondiabetic individuals, multiple meal plans have been shown to be effective and safe in diabetes during the initial active phase of weight loss [56–59, 61, 99, 100]. However, most of these clinical trials are conducted over a year or less. There are less data addressing the energy-balanced chronic phase, which is more important considering that this phase extends over most of the lifetime of the patient. Patients with diabetes require lifelong therapy, and most of the time, patients will be energy-balanced while maintaining a reasonably stable body weight. This is true, of course, in patients with normal body weight, as well as in overweight/obese patients who are post weight loss. Given the lack of data on macronutrient composition and long-term outcomes in patients with diabetes, studies examining effects of energy-balanced (i.e., isocaloric) substitution or enrichment of various macronutrients on insulin sensitivity and CVD risk factors perhaps constitute the best data to inform the chronic diet plan.

Diet During the Initial Phase of Weight Loss (First Year)

Healthy Meal Plans

There are multiple healthy meal plans that can be delivered in a reduced-calorie format for patients with diabetes while assuring adequate intake of required nutrients [56–59, 61, 99, 100]. Furthermore, these meal plans can be constructed to adhere with the ADA recommendations for macronutrient composition shown in Table 22.3. This will usually require the participation of a dietitian. Randomized trials primarily conducted in individuals without diabetes show that any one of these diets can be equally effective in promoting long-term weight loss if patients remain compliant. Since compliance depends on a meal plan that accommodates personal and cultural food preferences [59, 101], this should be discussed with each patient and a healthy meal plan selected which best matches these preferences.

Healthy meal plans can include low-carbohydrate [100], low-fat [99, 100], "right carbohydrate" (e.g., South Beach or Zone Diets), Mediterranean [55, 56, 58], volumetrics (e.g. EatRight Diet at the University of Alabama at Birmingham) [102, 103], vegetarian [99], DASH [61], paleolithic, and raw-food diets among others (see Table 22.5 in the chapter on cardiometabolic risk and descriptions in the chapter on obesity). Any of these meal plans can be employed in the initial weight loss phase in patients with diabetes; however, patients should also be monitored for effects on fasting and postprandial glucose levels, and the need to adjust glucose-lowering medications, in order to prevent hypoglycemia or unwarranted hyperglycemia. Blood pressure and lipids should also be monitored.

There are aspects of macronutrient composition that deserve special mention in diabetes. Regarding low-carbohydrate (low-carb) diets, these patients may require a decrease in medications that act primarily to control postprandial glucose such as rapid-acting insulin and insulin secretagogues (sulfonylureas and meglitinides) due to reduced carbohydrate intake. These diets can also be termed high-fat diets since it is impractical to make up the carbohydrate caloric deficit with dietary protein alone. In patients with diabetes, the quality of dietary fat is important, and efforts should be made to minimize saturated fat in favor of MUFAs and PUFAs. On the other hand, meal plans containing more carbohydrate, such as low-fat or vegetarian diets, may require an increase in glucose-lowering medications to control postmeal glycemic excursions.

Regarding carbohydrates, patients with diabetes should minimize intake of simple or refined sugars for purposes of glycemic control, as well as any other foods found to produce high-glycemic responses on an individual basis as determined using home glucose monitoring (e.g., sushi, rice). This is conceptually relevant to the GI; however, as described above, multiple dietary and physiological factors affect GI, and its validity as a meaningful way to characterize food in the implementation of nutritional recommendations is problematic [28, 32, 104]. High dietary fiber is an important determinant of GI and may protect against weight gain [105, 106] as well as improve lipid levels in patients with diabetes [33, 34]. People with diabetes should be encouraged to consume 25–30 g fiber per day with an emphasis on soluble fiber (7–13 g) for improving CVD risk factors.

The Caloric Prescription

There must exist a caloric deficit for weight loss to occur, and caloric reduction is critical for weight loss regardless of the meal plan. During the active phase of weight loss, the health-care professional and patient can opt for: (i) a reduced calorie diet where the caloric deficit is ~500 cal a day, (ii) a VLCD defined by total daily calories of 800 or less, or (iii) a low-calorie diet in which daily calories are intermediate between reduced-calorie and VLCD. To implement reduced and low-calorie diets, daily energy expenditure are often estimated in order to calculate the caloric prescription needed for the desired caloric deficit.

Resting energy expenditure can be estimated using simple predictive equations such as 25–30 kcal/kg body weight or by more complex equations such as the Harris–Benedict equation for men and women that take into account weight, height, and age [108, 109]. Indirect calorimetry provides a more accurate measure and can be obtained in the clinic setting using hand-held, portable, self-calibrating instruments. Energy expenditure related to physical activity and the thermic effect of food can be accounted for by multiplying the resting energy expenditure by 1.2 to derive an estimate of total energy expenditure in sedentary individuals. Several recent clinical trials have targeted caloric intakes of 1200–1500 kcal/day for women and 1500–1800 kcal/day for men [78–81]. These estimates of energy expenditure provide a baseline for prescribing total daily calories that incorporate the desired caloric deficit. While these estimates may provide an acceptable starting point in formulating the caloric prescription, the patient's response to diet will need to be followed and the caloric prescription adjusted accordingly if the weight loss is suboptimal.

Meal Replacements

Meal replacements can be recommended for weight loss as an option that can provide structure to a reduced-calorie diet [110]. These products can enhance compliance for many patients due to the known caloric content that eliminates guesswork, provision of required nutrients, and convenience. Optimal products for diabetes are characterized by high protein, fiber, complex carbohydrates or modified slowly-digesting carbohydrate with no refined sugars, low saturated fat, limited sodium, and no *trans* fat. Meal replacements usually contain 175–250 kcal per serving and can be employed during the active phase of weight loss and during chronic weight loss maintenance. During active weight loss, meal replacements can be employed in VLCDs, or in low-calorie and reduced-calorie diets to comprise 1 or 2 meals/day with a third meal of portioned-controlled food. The use of meal replacements was associated with greater weight

loss over 1 year in the LookAHEAD trial [111]. The utility of highly defined dietary structure is further illustrated in studies that show that significantly greater weight loss was achieved using portion-controlled servings of conventional foods or provision of detailed menus [112, 113]. Some examples of programs that incorporate prepackaged meals or meal replacements designed for patients with diabetes are included in Table 22.6.

How Much Weight Loss Is Enough?

The weight loss goal is determined by what can be feasibly achieved in individual patients and by what is required to improve the health of the individual consistent with treatment goals (Table 22.2). Most guidelines recommend weight loss of 5–10% in diabetes. However, the question regarding how much weight loss is optimal in T2D was addressed in the LookAHEAD Trial [78–83]. This study randomized T2D patients to an intensive lifestyle intervention versus standard diabetes support and education. The intensive lifestyle intervention resulted in greater weight loss and clinical benefits than the standard intervention. Moreover, the ability of weight loss to lower A1C and fasting glucose, decrease systolic and diastolic blood pressure, increase HDL cholesterol, and decrease triglycerides was progressive over a range of weight loss from 5% to 15%. No thresholds for maximal benefits were observed, with the greater the weight loss, the greater the clinical benefits. The improvements in glycemic control were achieved despite reductions in diabetes medications, and remission of T2D was observed in ~10% of patients. Therefore, in T2D, weight loss of 15% or greater is optimal when achievable, while clinical benefits are still observed at lower levels of weight loss of (i.e., ~5%).

Diet During the Chronic Maintenance Phase of Weight Loss (Years to Decades)

After active weight loss, patients will need an energy-balanced diet prescription to maintain the new lower body weight and avoid weight regain. This can be problematic since energy expenditure decreases following weight loss [114]. Therefore, resting energy equations based on height and weight (e.g., Harris–Benedict equation) will predictably overestimate the number of calories needed for weight stabilization. For this reason, it is wise to reduce daily calories by 100 kcal/day below the calculated value and to follow the patient making further reductions in the caloric prescription based on changes in body weight. Indirect calorimetry can be helpful at this stage in providing for a more accurate estimate.

When patients are in energy balance or isocaloric, the macronutrient composition might have different effects in diabetes than during hypocaloric feeding. As discussed

Table 22.6 Options for meal replacements for patients with prediabetes and diabetes

Brand	Diabetes-specific formula or program	Characteristics	Available support
Products			
Glucerna	Specifically formulated for diabetes. Products include: Glucerna Advance, Glucerna HungerSmart and Glucerna	Shakes and bars; nutrition components include modified and slowly digesting carbohydrates, fiber, and unsaturated fat. Glucerna HungerSmart contains minimal carbohydrate, so caution needed in patients taking glucose-lowering medications	Web-based support
Boost	Boost glucose control	Shakes; nutrition components include: high protein, unsaturated fat, complex carbohydrate, and low carbohydrate, so caution needed in patients taking glucose-lowering medications	Web-based support
Slim-Fast	Slim Fast 3-2-1 plan	Shakes, bars, snacks; nutrition components include: high protein, fiber, and low carbohydrate, so caution needed in patients taking glucose-lowering medications	Web-based information
Almased	Appropriate for diabetes	Shakes; nutrition components include: Fermented soy protein, skim-milk yogurt powder, honey, high protein, and low carbohydrate, so caution needed in patients taking glucose-lowering medications	Web-based information
EAS AdvantEDGE carb control	EAS AdvantEDGE carb control	Nutrition components include: low calorie, high protein, and low carbohydrate, so caution needed in patients taking glucose-lowering medications	Web-based information
Carnation instant breakfast	Carnation breakfast essentials—no sugar added	Powder mixed with milk; nutrition components include low calorie and high fiber; when mixed with milk carbohydrates and calories are not too low	Web-based information
Programs			
OptiFast	No diabetes specific meal plan	Includes shakes, bars, soups, and powders; designed for VLCD; nutritionally complete; high protein; no fiber unless fiber powder supplement is used	Medically monitored program only available through health care professionals
Robard—New Direction and Nutrimed	No diabetes specific meal plan	Includes shakes, bars, entrées, desserts, soups, and snacks; designed for VLCD; nutritionally complete	A multidisciplinary program of behavior modification, nutrition education, physical activity, and group support to reinforce lasting lifestyle changes
Jenny Craig	Diabetes-specific meal plan available	Includes preportioned, prepared entrées and snacks coupled with fruits, vegetables, and nonfat yogurt from the grocery; food picked up at a center	Weekly meetings with a nutritional consultant; has maintenance component
Nutrisystem	Three diabetes specific meal plans available	Includes preportioned, prepared entrées and snacks coupled with fresh food from the grocery; food delivered through mail	Has a community forum and discussion boards; Nutrisystem D has support from CDEs
Medifast	Specific plan available for patients with diabetes	Most Medifast dieters use the current 5&1 plan. It provides six meals a day, five of them 100-cal Medifast products—a shake, bar, oatmeal, soup, or even cheese puffs. The sixth meal, which you can have at any time, is a lean-and-green entrée you prepare yourself, built around 5–7ounces of lean protein and three servings of non-starchy veggies. Eventually transition to more meals and fewer meal replacements	
Health Management Resources	No diabetes-specific meal plan	Includes preportioned, prepared entrées and snacks as well as shakes, bars, and soups; designed for VLCD	Medically supervised in clinics providing support and education classes or done at home using "complete diet kits"
Weight Watchers	No diabetes-specific plan	Foods are assigned a "pointsplus" value, and number of points allowed daily is individualized based on weight loss goals. "Pointsplus" values are based on protein, carb, fat, and fiber content of the food	Support provided through meetings as well as personalized coaching done online and/or phone/email/text

CDE certified diabetes educator, *VLCD* very low calorie diet

above, various healthy meal plans, which vary widely in the proportion of fat and carbohydrate content, have been relatively well studied during the active phase of weight loss. Unfortunately, little long-term data exist beyond 1 or 2 years on these diets. In particular, effects on long-term clinical outcomes, such as chronic glycemic control, CVD events, and mortality, are largely unknown. The duration of consuming an energy-balanced diet will extend over a much greater portion of the lifespan, and therefore, the impact of the various diets on cardiometabolic pathophysiology, disease biomarkers, and clinical outcomes is of great importance. The question regarding optimal diet is also relevant to normal-weight patients with diabetes who do not require weight loss.

If there is a lack of data addressing long-term outcomes, what evidence can be used to guide the dietary prescription? One consideration was highlighted in selecting the diet for active weight loss, namely, the healthy meal plan that could best accommodate personal and cultural preferences resulting in greater rates of compliance. This remains an important consideration during chronic weight maintenance. However, the second consideration is a large body of data indicating that isocaloric substitution of macronutrients can influence insulin sensitivity and cardiovascular risk factors [115]. Since insulin resistance is key to the pathophysiology and progression of diabetes and CVD risk, it is reasonable to emphasize macronutrients that enhance insulin sensitivity, and reduce nutrients that promote insulin resistance, in formulating a long-term dietary plan.

Macronutrients that favorably or adversely affect insulin sensitivity under energy-balanced conditions were described in detail in the chapter on cardiometabolic risk. Isocaloric substitution experiments indicate that diets enriched in MUFAs, PUFAs, whole grains, and high fiber result in an increase in insulin sensitivity and improvements in cardiovascular risk factors, while enrichment in saturated fat and *trans* fat, refined grains, and reduced fiber promote insulin resistance and dyslipidemia [115]. This information is relevant to the lifelong dietary prescription for patients with diabetes until data from longer-term outcome studies become available.

Several healthy meal plans are able to accommodate the nutrients that favor insulin sensitivity. However, the meal plans have relative advantages and disadvantages for patients with diabetes, and adjustments in diabetes medications will be required based on the selected diet. Low-carb diets involve increased fat consumption since protein intake cannot usually compensate for the reduction in carbohydrate calories. If the low-carb diet is to be used for chronic weight loss maintenance, it would be important to minimize saturated fat in favor of monounsaturated fat [53, 54]. Due to the limited a number of foods highly enriched in MUFAs (olive oil, avocados, and nuts), a concerted effort working with a dietitian is recommended in order to maintain a high MUFA/saturated fat ratio ($\geq 2:1$) and at the same time assure a wide range of diet choices. Furthermore, lipid panels should be followed closely for changes in LDL cholesterol, HDL cholesterol, triglycerides, and non-HDL cholesterol since there is lack of data on the long-term effects of a low-carb diet under weight maintenance conditions. As described in the chapter on cardiometabolic risk, the Mediterranean diet is a meal plan that can be effective and a diet that has been studied with respect to long-term outcomes [55–58]. This diet features MUFA-enriched olive oil as a fat source and has been associated with reduced CVD and mortality in the Lyon Diet Heart Study [116, 117]. On the other hand, low-fat diets, including volumetric, vegetarian, and DASH diets, are relatively high in carbohydrates, which could potentially have the effect to worsen glycemic control in patients with diabetes, particularly in response to meals. Complex carbohydrates and low-GI meals should be emphasized and medication regimens altered to control postprandial glycemic excursions. The patient should check glucose levels before and 2–3 h after meals and employ drugs that effectively control postprandial glucose responses (dipeptidyl peptidase-4 inhibitors, alpha-glucosidase inhibitors, glucagon-like peptide-1 receptor agonists, sulfonylureas, meglitinides, and/or rapid-acting insulin) as needed.

Physical Activity

Increased physical activity is an important component of lifestyle therapy in diabetes. Structured exercise can improve glycemic control in T2D without a change in BMI [118] and in T2D and T1D, improve fitness, muscle strength, and insulin sensitivity [119]. In the context of an overall lifestyle intervention, regular exercise can contribute to weight loss and prevention of weight regain, lower A1C values, enhance mobility, and improve cardiovascular risk factors such as lipids and blood pressure [120–121]. Studies have demonstrated beneficial effects of both aerobic and resistance exercise, and additive benefits when both forms of exercise are combined [122, 123]. Physical activity guidelines proposed by the ADA, AHA, and the American College of Sports Medicine are well aligned and advocate both aerobic and resistance exercises. A consensus recommendation would include 30 min of moderate intensity exercise 5 days/week for a total of 150 min/week, or 20–25 min of vigorous intense exercise 3 days/week for a total of 60–75 min/week, combined with resistance training involving each major muscle group 2–3 days/week [124, 125]. Reduction in sedentary behavior can be helpful, with the recommendation that sedentary periods last 90 min or less and are interrupted by periods of activity [126].

Table 22.7 Special considerations for exercise in patients with diabetes and diabetes complications

1	Foot disease/peripheral vascular disease
	Refer patient for podiatry care and prescription for optimal footwear. Educate patient regarding routine foot checks. No weight-bearing activities if active foot ulcer but can consider swimming, water aerobics, and resistance training (upper body)
2	*Orthostasis*
	Consider patient for cardiac evaluation due to high risk of underlying coronary artery disease and to exclude silent myocardial ischemia. If patient has difficulty with upright physical activity, consider recumbent chair and weight lifting, semi-recumbent cycling, and water exercise. Encourage hydration. Assess whether changes are needed in hypertension medication regimens that include vasodilatory drugs, beta-blockers, or diuretics and whether SGLT2 inhibitors diabetes may be exacerbating the orthostasis
3	*Autonomic neuropathy*
	Consider patient for cardiac evaluation due to high risk of underlying disease and to exclude silent myocardial ischemia (e.g., ECG stress test, or persantin thallium stress test). Caution needed if anhydrosis is present to avoid hyperthermia when exercising in warm environments
4	*Proliferative retinopathy*
	Avoid vigorous aerobic and resistance exercise. Consider low-impact physical activity such as stationary bicycle, swimming, stairsteppers & ellipticals, walking, and less-intense aerobics
5	*Elderly patients with diabetes*
	A combination of aerobic and resistance exercise can contribute to healthy aging by increasing fitness, insulin sensitivity, muscle strength, functional capacity, and bone health. Consider referral to an exercise professional, particularly in the setting of sarcopenia and impaired functional status. If mobility is impaired, encourage range-of-motion and movement exercises, stretching while sitting, and physical therapy referral. Resistance exercise should be emphasized in patients with sarcopenia. Special caution is needed to avoid hypoglycemia, particularly if meal schedules are irregular and if the patient is treated with insulin or insulin secretagogues

ECG electrocardiogram, *SGLT2* sodium/glucose cotransporter-2

However, many patients with diabetes cannot adhere to these optimal recommendations due to physical limitations [127–130]. It is important to individualize the prescription for physical activity to include activities and exercise regimens within the capabilities of the patient while maximizing the degree of conditioning that is possible, as delineated in Table 22.7. The activities should be enjoyable to the patient with strong support and encouragement by the health-care team and should start slow with gradual increments in intensity. Elderly patients or persons with disabilities should also try to approach levels of activity in the guidelines to the extent possible; however, even reduced activity regimens, range of motion, or flexibility exercises should be encouraged. Clearly, the health-care provider and the patient should together establish the exercise prescription with the goal for long-term compliance. Physical activity will need to be specifically designed to accommodate patients with autonomic neuropathy, retinopathy, and diabetic foot disease [127–130]. Moderate resistance and aerobic exercise is also recommended for patients with chronic kidney disease and patients on hemodialysis. While exercise can temporarily increase proteinuria, there does not appear to be any chronic effect on albuminuria or on the decline in renal function.

Patients with diabetes should be carefully evaluated by history and physical exam for CVD, and health-care professionals should use clinical judgment in selecting patients for cardiac testing prior to initiating a physical activity program [131]. High-risk patients should be encouraged to start slowly with low-intensity exercise and build gradually. While cardiac testing need not be performed on a routine basis, candidates for stress tests include: (i) established vascular disease or previous CVD events, (ii) typical or atypical chest pain, (iii) abnormal resting electrocardiogram (ECG), and (iv) patients at high risk due to chronic abnormalities in CVD risk factors. This latter category would include patients with chronic kidney disease or albuminuria. It is important to keep in mind the problem of "silent" myocardial ischemia in patients with diabetes.

In diabetes, the timing and intensity of physical activity should be integrated with meal patterns and diabetes medications to optimize glycemic control and avoid hypoglycemia [132]. Exercise itself can be used to lower plasma glucose via contraction-mediated glucose uptake into skeletal muscle in patients with diabetes; however, the response to exercise is variable among individuals. Therefore, it is important for patients to perform glucose monitoring before and after exercise to identify patterns of glucose response for future reference. In T2D, if the glucose value is elevated 300 mg/dL (16.6 mmol/L) at the beginning of exercise, the value can increase with the stress and effort of exercise in some individuals, although most patients if hydrated will not experience adverse consequences upon exercising under these conditions. T1D patients will need to take more precautions if the initial glucose is 300 mg/dL since vigorous exercise could exacerbate hyperglycemia and ketosis. T1D patients should avoid exercise when they are ketotic; however, the problem here is that urine dipsticks or capillary blood measurements for ketones may not be available. For this reason, it may be advisable for many T1D patients to postpone exercise when initial glucose values exceed 300 mg/dL. If the initial glucose is < 100 mg/dL (< 5.6 mmol/L) in patients with T2D or T1D, glucose levels could fall into the hypoglycemic range during exercise, particularly in patients treated with insulin or insulin secretagogues (sulfonylureas and meglitinides). If this is an established pattern, the patient should try eating a small mixed meal or snack containing carbohydrate prior to exercise.

Lifestyle Therapy in Patients Treated with Weight Loss Medications or Bariatric Surgery

Lifestyle therapy, while effective as a sole therapeutic approach, is also a critical component of care in combination with weight loss medications and bariatric surgery in the treatment of overweight and obese patients with diabetes. As discussed in the chapter on cardiometabolic risk, compensatory changes following weight loss promote increased hunger and energy expenditure, favoring weight regain back to the original high body weight. As sustained behavior change can be challenging, patients need help, and this can be achieved by prescribing medications as an adjunct to lifestyle modification. From 2012 to 2014, there were four new weight loss medications approved for the chronic treatment of obesity by the FDA: lorcaserin, phentermine/topiramate extended-release (ER), naltrexone ER/bupropion ER, and high-dose liraglutide (3 mg/day). Orlistat, approved in 1999, was the only preexisting medication approved for long-term pharmacotherapy and the only one currently permitted in Europe and many other countries. Orlistat is also the only approved long-term drug for obese adolescents aged ≥ 12 years. All these medications are approved in the USA as adjuncts to lifestyle modification in overweight patients with BMI 27–29.9 kg/m^2 having ≥ 1 weight-related comorbidity, generally taken to be diabetes, hypertension, or dyslipidemia, or obese patients (BMI ≥ 30 kg/m^2) whether or not comorbidities are present. With the exception of orlistat, these medications act on central mechanisms regulating appetite and satiety, and help combat the pathophysiological adaptations that are driving weight regain. This helps patients sustain weight loss and helps them comply with reduced-calorie diets. For this reason, the medications must be used as adjuncts to lifestyle therapy and reduced-calorie meal plans for optimal benefit.

In patients with T2D, all approved weight loss medications have been shown to result in greater weight loss and lower A1C values, while at the same time requiring reductions in glucose-lowering medications, when compared with patients treated with lifestyle therapy alone [14, 86, 88–91, 133, 134]. In addition to greater weight loss, the addition of pharmacotherapy to lifestyle sustains weight loss for a greater period of time than that attributable to lifestyle interventions alone. The weight loss is also generally associated with reductions in blood pressure and triglyceride levels. Thus, weight loss medications in conjunction with lifestyle therapy can be highly beneficial in the treatment of patients with diabetes [27]. This has been demonstrated in clinical trials for orlistat [84, 85, 133], phentermine/topiramate ER

[86], lorcaserin [88], naltrexone ER/bupropion ER [89], and liraglutide 3 mg/day.

Bariatric surgery can be considered in T2D when the BMI is ≥ 35 kg/m^2, especially if the diabetes or associated comorbidities are difficult to control with lifestyle and pharmacologic therapy [96]. Lifestyle therapy is critical in these patients both before and after surgery for optimal clinical outcomes and for preventing weight regain following the procedures. Bariatric surgery procedures in T2D have produced marked reductions in both A1C and diabetes medications, and can result in remission of diabetes (normal A1C values without antihyperglycemic agents) in some patients. In addition, extended follow-up demonstrated that both CVD events and mortality were reduced in patients treated by surgery [134]. In the Surgical Treatment and Medications Potentially Eradicate Diabetes Efficiently (STAMPEDE) trial, glycemic control in T2D patients following bariatric surgery was improved to a greater extent than in medically treated patients [91]. These data should be interpreted cautiously because glycemic control in the medically treated patients was not optimal and the study did not include a weight loss arm using intensive lifestyle/behavior therapy plus weight loss medications. On balance, the data support bariatric surgery as an effective therapeutic approach in T2D patients with BMI ≥ 35 kg/m^2, with uncontrolled diabetes and obesity refractory to lifestyle and pharmacotherapy. This approach must be balanced against the inherent risks of surgical complications and mortality, and also potential nutritional deficiencies, weight regain in some patients, and the need for lifelong lifestyle support and medical monitoring [96]. Nutrition therapy in these postoperative patients must guard against nutritional deficiencies and include supplementation of micronutrients including iron, calcium, vitamin D and other fat-soluble vitamins, vitamin B complex (to include thiamine, folic acid, and vitamin B$_{12}$), and minerals (copper, zinc, and selenium).

Final Summary Recommendations

1. The goals of lifestyle therapy in diabetes are: (i) control glycemia to prevent microvascular complications, (ii) prevent acute complications and hypoglycemia, (iii) prevent CVD events by improving risk factors such as dyslipidemia and hypertension, and (iv) improve functionality and quality of life.
2. MNT and DSME&S programs are critically important components of lifestyle therapy in patients with T2D and T1D. These interventions should be individualized and developed by the health-care team in collaboration with the patient.
3. Patients with diabetes should adhere to principles of macronutrient intake advocated by the ADA (Table 22.3). This can be accomplished by any one

of several healthy meal plans, which assure adequate nutrient intake and which can be selected based on personal and cultural dietary preferences.

4. Lifestyle therapy includes physical activity that optimally encompasses both aerobic and resistance exercises and a reduction in sedentary behavior. However, the prescription for physical activity must be tailored to the preferences and capabilities of patients with diabetes and take into account the presence of diabetes-related complications.

5. In diabetes, the meal plan, physical activity, and use of glucose-lowering medications are designed to work in concert with each other to synergistically enhance glycemic control and avoid hypoglycemia.

6. Patients with T1D, and those T2D patients taking premeal regular or rapid-acting insulin, can effectively manage their diabetes by practicing carbohydrate counting in concert with premeal insulin dosing for optimal control of post-meal glucose excursions.

7. Weight loss in overweight/obese patients with diabetes can dramatically benefit patients with diabetes by enhancing glycemic control with reduced need for glucose-lowering medications and by improving the CVD risk profile.

8. Despite the clear benefits of weight loss, the conventional practice of MNT and DSME&S in obese patients with diabetes does not often result in clinically meaningful weight loss. Unless health-care professionals have been trained in weight loss therapy and advocate this to patients as a key therapeutic strategy in its own right, it is unlikely that the patients will experience clinically significant weight loss and maintenance of that weight loss.

9. A new reconfigured approach to lifestyle therapy is proposed for overweight/obese patients with diabetes, which emphasizes weight loss as a primary therapeutic strategy for prevention and treatment. This approach to lifestyle therapy incorporates evidence-based practices involving diet, physical activity, behavioral interventions, and multidisciplinary care, with demonstrated effectiveness for weight loss.

10. Nutritional therapy for the active phase of weight loss (~first year) is accomplished using any one of several healthy meal plans and delivered as a very-low-calorie, low-calorie, or reduced-calorie diet.

11. During the chronic phase of weight loss maintenance (years–decades), when patients are isocaloric, there is little information on the optimal macronutrient composition with regard to safety and clinical outcomes. Given the central role of insulin resistance in diabetes and CVD risk factors, the rational choice is to emphasize nutrients shown to enhance insulin sensitivity in isocaloric substitution studies (MUFAs, fiber, whole grains, and "Mediterranean diet") and to minimize or avoid foods that promote insulin resistance (saturated fat, *trans* fat, refined grains, and "Western diet").

Case Report

A 48-year-old African American male with hypertension and T2D comes to you for care after his usual doctor retired. He was diagnosed with diabetes 7 years ago and is currently treated with metformin 2000 mg/day and glargine insulin 15 units at bedtime. He was diagnosed to have hypertension 10 years ago and is treated with atenolol 100 mg/day and hydrochlorothiazide 50 mg/day. He complains only of early morning headaches, fatigue, and forgetfulness on job, and his wife complains of his snoring.

Regarding lifestyle practices relevant to diabetes, he does not follow any particular diet and does not engage in voluntary exercise. He went through a 12-week program of diabetes education when he was diagnosed 7 years ago but otherwise has had no ongoing diabetes self-management education. He performs home glucose monitoring but only before breakfast several times a week, when values range between 120 and 180 mg/dL. He denies any episodes of hypoglycemia but was aware of symptoms that could result from hypoglycemia. He denies any past history of heart, kidney, or eye disease, although his last visit to an ophthalmologist was 2 years ago. Questions regarding weight history revealed the he began to gain weight as a young adult in his 20s after beginning to work full time in construction first in laying concrete, then as lift operator, then foreman. He no longer had time for playing sports with friends. He has been taught the meal-exchange approach for diabetes and avoids sweets but has not participated in serious attempts at weight loss. He recognizes he is overweight since this "slows him down" on the job and work around the home, and he is interested in weight loss.

Social History The patient works as foreman for a construction company. He is married with two children in high school. He drinks a few beers on weekends while watching Alabama Crimson Tide football games (or reruns) and smokes one to two cigarettes per day when the demands of his job "get the best of him." His father had T2D and renal failure requiring dialysis and passed away 2 years ago.

Physical Examination His BMI is 37 kg/m^2, waist circumference 46 in., and blood pressure 152/92 mmHg. His only other positive physical findings are 1/6 systolic flow murmur and S4 gallop, and acanthosis nigricans on posterior neck

Clinical Laboratory Findings Fasting glucose 162 mg/dL and A1C 8.2%; lipid panel with triglycerides 170 mg/dL,

LDL cholesterol 101 mg/dL, and HDL cholesterol 48 mg/dL; and serum creatinine 1.2 mg/dL and albumin/creatinine ratio 50 mg/mmol. ECG shows evidence of mild left ventricular hypertrophy.

Impression and Plan On the basis of your evaluation you conclude that he is an obese patient with hypertension and T2D, both of which are not optimally controlled, and that his lifestyle practices and diabetes self-management education are less than optimal. You note that he has microalbuminuria suggestive of early diabetic nephropathy. In addition, the presence of left ventricular hypertrophy on ECG and presence of S4 gallop indicates that his hypertension is adversely affecting his heart.

Your initial therapeutic plan is as follows. For diet, you get the history that he enjoys fruits and vegetables, although his wife cooks greens with ham hocks. Based on these dietary preferences and hypertension, you select the DASH diet as a reasonable meal plan in collaboration with the patient. You refer the patient to a dietitian (RN, CDE) for education and implementation of the DASH diet with elimination of the ham hocks. The patient also occasionally takes a walk after dinner with his wife, and you ask him to do this routinely every evening (except Saturday during the college football season) and to record the time and distance for these walks. You ask the patient to check and record his fasting glucose each day, and to check a pre-supper glucose every other day. You elect to keep his diabetes medications unchanged until he returns to the office for examination of his home glucose monitoring log and to give him some time to incorporate the diet and physical activity plan. You add benazepril 20 mg/day for hypertension and microalbuminuria. Because the review of systems suggested obstructive sleep apnea, you schedule the patient for a polysomnogram.

The patient returns to your office in 2 weeks. He has begun to walk each evening and, more recently, has added four more blocks to his normal route. He seems to like the DASH meal plan with the exception that he does not prefer dairy products. His blood pressure is 150/90 mmHg. His home glucose measurements range between 120 and 165 mg/dL in the morning and 140–190 mg/dL before supper. The polysomnogram returned with an Apnea–Hypopnea Index of 35. You conclude that he will need intensification of therapy for T2D, hypertension, and now continuous positive airway pressure (CPAP) for sleep apnea. For diabetes, you consider options that include initiation of a GLP1 receptor agonist or increasing long acting insulin glargine by five units every 3 days until fasting glucose is 100–130 mg/dL. For hypertension, you consider that he will need a higher dose of benazepril and may likely require an additional drug in the future such as a calcium-channel blocker. Alternatively, you realize that weight loss therapy reducing 10% body weight will improve glycemic control, lower blood pressure, and improve the sleep apnea Apnea–Hypopnea Index.

You discuss these treatment options with the patient. The decision is to proceed with lifestyle therapy targeting a 10% weight loss over the next 6 months. The lifestyle therapy plan includes:

1. You continue with the DASH diet as the healthy meal plan but advise the patient to emphasize fish as a protein source to substitute the dairy products he does not like. You discuss this with the dietitian and ask the dietitian to assure adequate calcium intake. For the caloric prescription, you estimate his resting metabolic rate at 2200 kcal/day based on the Harris–Benedict equation. You prescribe a 600 kcal deficit at 1600 kcal/day.

2. The physical activity plan is to continue evening walks and extending time and distance as tolerated, working towards 30 min each evening and adopting a "power walk" approach. He was asked to record these exercise episodes (date, duration, and distance). To reduce sedentary behavior, you suggest he walk around the worksites in his role as foremen instead of using a motorized golf cart.

3. You discontinue his evening dose of lantus but maintain the metformin, asking him to continue twice a day home glucose monitoring. You continue following the blood pressure on benazepril 20 mg/day and atenolol 100 mg/day but reduce the dose of hydrochlorothiazide to 12.5 mg/day. You ask that his wife take note whether there are any changes in his symptoms attributable to sleep apnea.

References

1. Rodbard HW, Jellinger PS, Davidson JA, et al. Statement by an American Association of Clinical Endocrinologists/American College of Endocrinology consensus panel on type 2 diabetes mellitus: an algorithm for glycemic control. Endocr Pract. 2009;15:540–59.
2. American Diabetes Association. Standards of medical care in diabetes–2015. Diabetes Care. 2015;38 Suppl 1:S20–30.
3. TRIAD Study Group. Health systems, patients, factors, and quality of care for diabetes: a synthesis of findings from the TRIAD study. Diabetes Care. 2010;33:940–7.
4. Duncan I, Birkmeyer C, Coughlin S, Li QE, Sherr D, Boren S. Assessing the value of diabetes education. Diabetes Educ. 2009;35:752–60.
5. Berikai P, Meyer PM, Kazlauskaite R, Savoy B, Kozik K, Fogelfeld L. Gain in patients' knowledge of diabetes management targets is associated with better glycemic control. Diabetes Care. 2007;30:1587–9.
6. Marrero DG, Ard J, Delamater AM, et al. Twenty-first century behavioral medicine: a context for empowering clinicians and patients with diabetes: a consensus report. Diabetes Care. 2013;36:463–70.

7. Norris SL, Lau J, Smith SJ, Schmid CH, Engelgau MM. Self-management education for adults with type 2 diabetes: a meta-analysis of the effect on glycemic control. Diabetes Care. 2002;25:1159–71.

8. Shah M, Kaselitz E, Heisler M. The role of community health workers in diabetes: update on current literature. Curr Diab Rep. 2013;13:163–71.

9. Haas L, Maryniuk M, Beck J, et al. National standards for diabetes self-management education and support. Diabetes Care. 2013;37 Suppl 1:S144–53.

10. Garvey WT. New tools for weight-loss therapy enable a more robust medical model for obesity treatment: rationale for a complications-centric approach. Endocr Pract. 2013;19:864–74.

11. UK Prospective Diabetes Study. 7: response of fasting plasma glucose to diet therapy in newly presenting type II diabetic patients, UKPDS Group. Metabolism. 1990;39:905–12.

12. Bosello O, Armellini F, Zamboni M, et al. The benefits of modest weight loss in type II diabetes. Int J Obes Relat Metab Disord. 1997;21(Suppl 1):S10–3.

13. Norris SL, Zhang X, Avenell A, et al. Long-term non-pharmacological weight loss interventions for adults with type 2 diabetes. Cochrane Database Syst Rev. 2005;CD005270.

14. Henry RR, Chilton R, Garvey WT. New options for the treatment of obesity and type 2 diabetes mellitus (narrative review). J Diabetes Complicat. 2013;27:508–18.

15. Garber AJ, Abrahamson MJ, Barzilay JI, et al. American association of clinical endocrinologists' comprehensive diabetes management algorithm 2013 consensus statement—executive summary. Endocr Pract. 2013;19:536–57.

16. Ogden CL, Carroll MD, Kit BK, et al. Prevalence of childhood and adult obesity in the United States, 2011–2012. JAMA. 2014;311:806–14.

17. Finkelstein EA, Trogdon JG, Cohen JW, et al. Annual medical spending attributable to obesity: payer-and-service-specific estimates. Health Aff. 2009;28:w822–31.

18. Van Gaal LF, Mentens IL, De Block CE. Mechanisms linking obesity with cardiovascular disease. Nature. 2006;444:875–80.

19. Guo F, Moellering DR, Garvey WT. The progression of cardiometabolic disease: validation of a new cardiometabolic disease staging system applicable to obesity. Obesity. 2014;22:110–8.

20. Centers for Disease Control and Prevention editor. National diabetes statistics report: estimates of diabetes and its burden in the United States, 2014. Atlanta: US Department of Health and Human Services; 2014.

21. American Diabetes Association. Economic costs of diabetes in the US in 2012. Diabetes Care. 2013;36:1033–46.

22. American Diabetes Association. Standards of medical care in diabetes–2015. Diabetes Care. 2015;38(Suppl 1):S8–16.

23. Institute of Medicine editor. The role of nutrition in maintaining health in the nation's elderly: evaluating coverage of nutrition services for the medicare population. Washington, DC: National Academies Press; 2000.

24. Evert AB, Boucher JL, Cypress M, et al. Nutrition therapy recommendations for the management of adults with diabetes. Diabetes Care. 2013;36:3821–42.

25. American Diabetes Association. Standards of medical care in diabetes–2015. Diabetes Care. 2015;38(Suppl 1):S33–40.

26. American Diabetes Association. Standards of medical care in diabetes–2015. Diabetes Care. 2015;38(Suppl 1):S49–57.

27. Handelsman Y, et al. American association of clinical endocrinologists and american college of endocrinology—clinical practice guidelines for developing a diabetes mellitus comprehensive care plan—2015. Endocr Pract. 2015;21(0):1–87.

28. Franz MJ, Powers MA, Leontos C, et al. The evidence for medical nutrition therapy for type 1 and type 2 diabetes in adults. J Am Diet Assoc. 2010;110:1852–89.

29. Camelon KM, Hådell K, Jämsén PT, Ketonen KJ, Kohtamäki HM, Mäkimatilla S, Törmälä ML, Valve RH. The plate model: a visual method of teaching meal planning. DAIS Project Group. Diabetes atherosclerosis intervention study. J Am Diet Assoc. 1998;98(10):1155–8.

30. U.S. Department of Health and Human Services and U.S. Department of Agriculture. Dietary guidelines for Americans 2010. www.health.gov/dietaryguidelines/.

31. Kirpitch A, Maryniuk M. The 3 R's of glycemic index: recommendations, research, and the real world. Clin Diabetes. 2011;29:155–9.

32. Franz MJ. Diabetes mellitus nutrition therapy: beyond the glycemic index. Arch Intern Med. 2012;172:1660–1.

33. Jenkins DJ, Kendall CW, Augustin LS, et al. Effect of legumes as part of a low glycemic index diet on glycemic control and cardiovascular risk factors in type 2 diabetes mellitus: a randomized controlled trial. Arch Intern Med. 2012;172:1653–60.

34. Thomas DE, Elliott EJ. The use of low glycaemic diets in diabetes control. Br J Nutr. 2010;104:797–802.

35. Post RE, Mainous AG 3rd, King DE, Simpson KN. Dietary fiber for the treatment of type 2 diabetes mellitus: a meta-analysis. J Am Board Fam Med. 2012;25:16–23.

36. Palmer S Fill in the fiber gaps—dietitians offer practical strategies to get clients to meet the daily requirements. Today's Dietit. 2012;14:40.

37. Riccardi G, Rivellese A, Pacioni D, Genovese S, Mastranzo P, Mancini M. Separate influence of dietary carbohydrate and fibre on the metabolic control in diabetes. Diabetologia. 1984;26:116–21.

38. Chandalia M, Garg A, Lutjohann D, von Bergmann K, Grundy SM, Brinkley LJ. Beneficial effects of high dietary fiber intakes in patients with type 2 diabetes mellitus. N Engl J Med. 2000;342:1392–8.

39. Hagander B, Asp N-G, Efendic S, Nilsson-Ehle P, Schersten B. Dietary Fiber decreases fasting blood glucose levels and plasma LDL concentration in noninsulin-dependent diabetes mellitus patients. Am J Clin Nutr. 1988;47:852–8.

40. Anderson JW, Zeigler JA, Deakins DA, Floore TL, Dillon DW, Wood CL, Oeltgen PR, Whitley RJ. Metabolic effects of high-carbohydrate high-fiber diets for insulin-dependent diabetic individuals. Am J Clin Nutr. 1991;54:936–43.

41. Institute of Medicine editor. Dietary reference intakes for energy, carbohydrate, fiber, fat, fatty acids, cholesterol, protein, and amino acids. Washington, DC: National Academies Press; 2002.

42. Brinkworth GD, Noakes M, Parker B, Foster P, Clifton PM. Long-term effects of advice to consume a high-protein, low-fat diet, rather than a conventional weight-loss diet, in obese adults with type 2 diabetes: one-year follow-up of a randomized trial. Diabetologia. 2004;47:1677–86.

43. Parker B, Noakes M, Luscombe N, Clifton P. Effect of a high-protein, high-monounsaturated fat weight loss diet on glycemic control and lipid levels in type 2 diabetes. Diabetes Care. 2002;25:425–30.

44. Gannon MC, Nuttall FQ, Saeed A, Jordan K, Hoover H. An increase in dietary protein improves the blood glucose response in persons with type 2 diabetes. Am J Clin Nutr. 2003;78:734–41.

45. Pijls LT, de Vries H, van Eijk JT, Donker AJ. Protein restriction, glomerular filtration rate and albuminuria in patients with type 2 diabetes: a randomized trial. Eur J Clin Nutr. 2002;56:1200–7.

46. Meloni C, Tatangelo P, Cipriani S, et al. Adequate protein dietary restriction in diabetic and non-diabetic patients with chronic renal failure. J Ren Nutr. 2004;14:208–13.

47. Hansen HP, Tauber-Lassen E, Jensen BR, Parving HH. Effect of dietary protein restriction on prognosis in patients with diabetic nephropathy. Kidney Int. 2002;62:220–8.

48. Dussol B, Iovanna C, Raccah D, et al. A randomized trial of low-protein diet in type 1 and in type 2 diabetes mellitus patients with incipient and overt nephropathy. J Ren Nutr. 2005;15:398–406.

49. Pan Y, Guo LL, Jin HM. Low-protein diet for diabetic nephropathy: a meta-analysis of randomized controlled trials. Am J Clin Nutr. 2008;88:660–6.

50. Wheeler ML, Gibson RG, Fineberg SE, Hackward LL, Fineberg NS. Animal versus plant protein meals in individuals with type 2 diabetes and microalbuminuria. Diabetes Care. 2002;25:1277–82.

51. Buse JB, Ginsberg HN, Barkis GL, Clark NG, Costa F, Eckel R, Fonseca V, Gerstein HC, Grundy S, Nesto RW, Pignone MP, Plutzky J, Porte D, Redberg R, Stitzel KF, Stone NJ. Primary prevention of cardiovascular disease in people with diabetes mellitus: a scientific statement from the American Heart Association and the American Diabetes Association. Diabetes Care. 2007;30:162–72.

52. http://www.health.gov/dietaryguidelines/2015-scientific-report/PDFs/Scientific-Report-of-the-2015-Dietary-Guidelines-Advisory-Committee.pdf.

53. Brehm BJ, Lattin BL, Summer SS, et al. One-year comparison of a high-monounsaturated fat diet with a high-carbohydrate diet in type 2 diabetes. Diabetes Care. 2009;32:215–20.

54. Schwingshakl L, Strasser B, Hoffmann G. Effects of monounsaturated fatty acids on glycaemic control in patients with abnormal glucose metabolism: a systematic review and meta-analysis. Ann Nutr Metab. 2011;58:290–6.

55. Itsiopoulos C, Brazionis L, Kaimakamis M, et al. Can the Mediterranean diet lower A1C in type 2 diabetes? Results from a randomized cross-over study. Nutr Metab Cardiovasc Dis. 2011;21:740–7.

56. Estruch R, Ros E, Salas-Savado J, et al. PREDIMED Study Investigators. Primary prevention of cardiovascular disease with a Mediterranean diet. N Engl J Med. 2013;368:1279–90.

57. Elhayany A, Lustman A, Abel R, Attal-Singer J, Vinker S. A low carbohydrate Mediterranean diet improves cardiovascular risk factors and diabetes control among overweight patients with type 2 diabetes mellitus: a 1-year prospective randomized intervention study. Diabetes Obes Metab. 2010;12:204–9.

58. Shai I, Schwarzfuchs D, Henkin Y, et al. Dietary intervention randomized controlled trial (DIRECT) group. Weight loss with a low-carbohydrate, Mediterranean, or low-fat diet. N Engl J Med. 2009;359:229–41.

59. Wheeler ML, Dunbar SA, Jaacks LM, et al. Macronutrients, food groups, and eating patterns in the management of diabetes. A systematic review of the literature, 2010. Diabetes Care. 2012;35:434–45.

60. http://www.heart.org/HEARTORG/GettingHealthy/Nutrition-Center/HealthyDietGoals/Sodium-Salt-or-Sodium-Chloride_UCM_303290_Article.jsp.

61. Azadbakht L, Fard NR, Karimi M, et al. Effects of the dietary approaches to stop hypertension (DASH) eating plan on cardiovascular risk among type 2 diabetic patients: a randomized cross-over clinical trial. Diabetes Care. 2011;34:55–7.

62. Suckling RJ, He FJ, Macgregor GA. Altered dietary salt intake for preventing and treating diabetic kidney disease. Cochrane Database Syst Rev. 2010;12:CD006763.

63. Thomas MC, Moran J, Forsblom C, et al. FinnDiane Study Group. The association between dietary sodium intake, ESRD, and all-cause mortality in patients with type 1 diabetes. Diabetes Care. 2011;34:861–6.

64. Ekinci E, Clarke S, Thomas MC, et al. Dietary salt intake and mortality in patients with type 2 diabetes. Diabetes Care. 2011;34:703–9.

65. Position of the American Dietetic Association. Use of nutritive and nonnutritive sweeteners. J Am Diet Assoc. 2004;104:255–75.

66. Cooper PL, Wahlquist ML, Simpson RW. Sucrose versus saccharin as an added sweetener in non-insulin dependent diabetes: short and medium-term metabolic effects. Diabetic Med. 1988;5:676–80.

67. Grotz VL, Henry RR, McGill JB, Prince MJ, Shamoon H, Trout JR, Pi-Sunyer FX. Lack of effect of sucralose on glucose homeostasis in subjects with type 2 diabetes. J Am Diet Assoc. 2003;103:1607–12.

68. Gardner C, Wylie-Rosett J, Gidding SS, et al., American Heart Association Nutrition Committee of the Council on Nutrition, Physical Activity and Metabolism, Council on Arteriosclerosis, Thrombosis and Vascular Biology, Council on Cardiovascular Disease in the Young; American Diabetes Association. Nonnutritive sweeteners: current use and health perspectives: a scientific statement from the American Heart Association and the American Diabetes Association. Diabetes Care. 2012;35:1798–808.

69. Richardson T, Weiss M, Thomas P, Kerr D. Day after the night before: influence of evening alcohol risk of hypoglycemia in patients with type 1 diabetes. Diabetes Care. 2005;28:1801–2.

70. Burge MR, Zeise TM, Sobhy TA, Rassam AG, Schade DS. Low-dose ethanol predisposes elderly fasted patients with type 2 diabetes to sulfonylurea-induced low blood glucose. Diabetes Care. 1999;22:2037–43.

71. Lowe J, Linjawi S, Mensch M, James K, Attia J. Flexible eating and flexible insulin dosing in patients with diabetes: results of an intensive self-management course. Diabetes Res Clin Pract. 2008;80(3):439–43.

72. DANFE Study Group. Training in flexible, intensive insulin management to enable dietary freedom in people with type 1 diabetes: dose adjustment for normal eating (DAFNE) randomized controlled trial. Brit Med J. 2002;325(7367):746.

73. American Association of Diabetes Educators. The art and science of diabetes self-management education desk reference, 2nd ed. Chicago: American Association of Diabetes Educators; 2011.

74. Steinsbekk A, Rygg LØ, Lisulo M, Rise MB, Fretheim A. Group based diabetes self-management education compared to routine treatment for people with type 2 diabetes mellitus. A systematic review with meta-analysis. BMC Health Serv Res. 2012;12:213.

75. Deakin TA, McShane CE, Cade JE, Williams R. Group based training for self-management strategies in people with type 2 diabetes mellitus. Cochrane Database Syst Rev. 2005;2:CD003417.

76. Guare JC, Wing RR, Grant A. Comparison of obese NIDDM and nondiabetic women: short- and long-term weight loss. Obes Res. 1995;3:329–35.

77. Wing RR, Marcus MD, Epstein LH, et al. Type II diabetic subjects lose less weight than their overweight nondiabetic spouses. Diabetes Care. 1987;10:563–6.

78. Wing RR, Lang W, Wadden TA, et al. The Look AHEAD Research Group. Benefits of modest weight loss in improving cardiovascular risk factors in overweight and obese individuals with type 2 diabetes. Diabetes Care. 2011;34:1481–6.

79. Group TLAR, Wing RR. Long-term effects of a lifestyle intervention on weight and cardiovascular risk factors in individuals with type 2 diabetes mellitus: four-year results of the Look AHEAD trial. Arch Intern Med. 2010;170:1566–75.

80. Belalcazar LM, Haffner SM, Lang W, et al. Lifestyle intervention and/or statins for the reduction of C-reactive protein in type 2 diabetes: from the look AHEAD study. Obesity. 2013;21:944–50.

81. Look AHEAD Research Group, Wing RR, Bolin P, Brancati FL, et al. Cardiovascular effects of intensive lifestyle intervention in type 2 diabetes. N Engl J Med. 2013;369:145–54.

82. Gregg EW, Chen H, Wagenknecht LE, et al. Look AHEAD Research Group. Association of an intensive lifestyle intervention with remission of type 2 diabetes. JAMA. 2012;308:2489–96.

83. Foster GD, Borradaile KE, Sanders MH, et al. Sleep AHEAD Research Group of the Look AHEAD Research Group. A randomized study on the effect of weight loss on obstructive sleep apnea among obese patients with type 2 diabetes: the Sleep AHEAD study. Arch Intern Med. 2009;169:1916–26.

84. Hollander PA, Elbein SC, Hirsch IB, et al. Role of orlistat in the treatment of obese patients with type 2 diabetes. A 1-year randomized double-blind study. Diabetes Care. 1998;21:1288–94.

85. Kelley DE, Bray GA, Pi-Sunyer FX, et al. Clinical efficacy of orlistat therapy in overweight and obese patients with insulin-treated type 2 diabetes: a 1-year randomized controlled trial. Diabetes Care. 2002;25:1033–41.

86. Garvey WT, Ryan DH, Bohannon NJ, et al. Weight-loss therapy in type 2 diabetes: effects of phentermine and topiramate extended-release. Diabetes Care. 2014;37:3309–16.

87. Gadde KM, Allison DB, Ryan DH, et al. Effects of low-dose, controlled-release, phentermine plus topiramate combination on weight and associated comorbidities in overweight and obese adults (CONQUER): a randomised, placebo-controlled, phase 3 trial. Lancet. 2011;377:1341–52.

88. O'Neil PM, Smith SR, Weissman NJ, et al. Randomized placebo-controlled clinical trial of lorcaserin for weight loss in type 2 diabetes mellitus: the BLOOM-DM study. Obesity. 2012;20:1426–36.

89. Hollander P, Gupta AK, Plodkowski R, et al. COR-Diabetes Study Group. Effects of naltrexone sustained-release/bupropion sustained-release combination therapy on body weight and glycemic parameters in overweight and obese patients with type 2 diabetes. Diabetes Care. 2013;36:4022–9.

90. Sjöström L, Peltonen M, Jacobson P, et al. Association of bariatric surgery with long-term remission of type 2 diabetes and with microvascular and macrovascular complications. JAMA. 2014;311:2297–304.

91. Schauer PR, Bhatt DL, Kirwan JP, et al. STAMPEDE Investigators. Bariatric surgery versus intensive medical therapy for diabetes—3-year outcomes. N Engl J Med. 2014;370:2002–13.

92. O'Brien PE, Macdonald L, Anderson M, et al. Long-term outcomes after bariatric surgery: fifteen-year follow-up of adjustable gastric banding and a systematic review of the bariatric surgical literature. Ann Surg. 2013;257:87–94.

93. Adams TD, Davidson LE, Litwin SE, et al. Gastrointestinal surgery: cardiovascular risk reduction and improved long-term survival in patients with obesity and diabetes. Curr Atheroscler Rep. 2012;14:606–15.

94. Garvey WT, Garber AJ, Mechanick JI, et al., On Behalf Of The AACE Obesity Scientific Committee. American association of clinical endocrinologists and American college of endocrinology position statement on the 2014 advanced framework for a new diagnosis of obesity as a chronic disease. Endocr Pract. 2014;20:977–89.

95. Apovian CM, Aronne LJ, Bessesen DH, et al. Pharmacological management of obesity: an endocrine society clinical practice guideline. J Clin Endocrinol Metab. 2015;100:342–62.

96. Mechanick JI, Youdim A, Jones DB, et al. Clinical practice guidelines for the perioperative nutritional, metabolic, and nonsurgical support of the bariatric surgery patient-2013 update: cosponsored by American association of clinical endocrinologists, the obesity society, and American society for metabolic & bariatric surgery. Endocr Pract. 2013;19:337–72.

97. Barte JC, ter Bogt NC, Bogers RP, et al. Maintenance of weight loss after lifestyle interventions for overweight and obesity, a systematic review. Obes Rev. 2010;11:899–906.

98. Gill RS, Birch DW, Shi X, et al. Sleeve gastrectomy and type 2 diabetes mellitus: a systematic review. Surg Obes Relat Dis. 2010;6:707–13.

99. Turner-McGrievy GM, Barnard ND, Cohen J, Jenkins DJA, Gloede L, Green AA. Changes in nutrient intake and dietary quality among participants with type 2 diabetes following a lowfat vegan diet or a conventional diabetes diet for 22 weeks. J Am Diet Assoc. 2008;108:1636–45.

100. Stern L, Iqbal N, Seshadri P, et al. The effects of low-carbohydrate versus conventional weight loss diets in severely obese adults: one-year follow-up of a randomized trial. Ann Intern Med. 2004;140:778–85.

101. Dansinger ML, Gleason JA, Griffith JL, Selker HP, Schaefer EJ. Comparison of the Atkins, Ornish, Weight Watchers, and Zone diets for weight loss and heart disease risk reduction: a randomized trial. JAMA. 2005;293(1):43–53.

102. Weinsier RL, Wilson NP, Morgan SL, Cornwell AR, Craig CB. EatRight lose weight: seven simple steps. Birmingham: Oxmoor House; 1997.

103. Greene LF, Malpede CZ, Henson CS, Hubbert KA, Heimburger DC, Ard JD. Weight maintenance 2 years after participation in a weight loss program promoting low-energy density foods. Obesity (Silver Spring). 2006;10:1795–801.

104. Pi-Sunyer FX. Glycemic index and disease. Am J Clin Nutr. 2002;76:290S–298S.

105. Riccardi G, Rivellese AA. Effects of dietary fiber and carbohydrate on glucose and lipoprotein metabolism in diabetic patients. Diabetes Care. 1991;14:1115–25.

106. Kiens B, Richter EA. Types of carbohydrate in an ordinary diet affect insulin action and muscle substrates in humans. Am J Clin Nutr. 1996;63:47–53.

107. Ard JD, Cox TL, Zunker C, Wingo BC, Jefferson WK, Brakhage C. A study of a culturally enhanced EatRight dietary intervention in a predominately African American workplace. J Public Health Manage Pract. 2010;16(6):E1–8.

108. Harris JA, Benedict FG. A biometric study of basal metabolism in man. Washington, DC: Carnegie Institute of Washington; 1919. (publ. no. 279).

109. Mifflin MD, Jeor ST St, Hill LA, Scott BJ, Daugherty SA, Koh YO. A new predictive equation for resting energy expenditure in healthy individuals. Am J Clin Nutr. 1990;51:251–7.

110. Heymsfield SB, van Mierlo CA, van der Knaap HC, Heo M, Frier HI. Weight management using a meal replacement strategy: meta and pooling analysis from six studies. Int J Obes Relat Metab Disord. 2003;27:537–49.

111. Wadden TA, West DS, Neiberg RH, Wing RR, Ryan DH, Johnson KC, et al. One-year weight losses in the Look AHEAD study: factors associated with success. Obesity (Silver Spring). 2009;17:713–22.

112. Finley CE, Barlow CE, Greenway FL, Rock CL, Rolls BJ, Blair SN. Retention rates and weight loss in a commercial weight loss program. Int J Obes (Lond). 2007;31:292–8.

113. Foster GD, Borradaile KE, Vander Veur SS, et al. The effects of a commercially available weight loss program among obese patients with type 2 diabetes: a randomized study. Postgrad Med. 2009;121:113–8.

114. Ochner CN, Barrios DM, Lee CD, Pi-Sunyer FX. Biological mechanisms that promote weight regain following weight loss in obese humans. Physiol Behav. 2013;120:106–13.

115. Lara-Castro C, Garvey WT. Diet, insulin resistance, and obesity: zoning in on data for Atkins dieters living in South Beach. J Clin Endocrinol Metab. 2004;89:4197–205.

116. de Lorgeril M, Salen P, Martin JL, Monjaud I, Delaye J, Mamelle N. Mediterranean diet, traditional risk factors, and the rate of cardiovascular complications after myocardial infarction: final report of the Lyon Diet Heart Study. Circulation. 1999;99(6):779–85.

117. Martinez-Gonzalez MA, Bes-Rastrollo M. Dietary patterns, Mediterranean diet, and cardiovascular disease. Curr Opin Lipidol. 2014;25(1):20–6.

118. Boulé NG, Haddad E, Kenny GP, Wells GA, Sigal RJ. Effects of exercise on glycemic control and body mass in type 2 diabetes mellitus: a meta-analysis of controlled clinical trials. JAMA. 2001;286:1218–27.

119. Colberg SR, Riddell MC. Physical activity: regulation of glucose metabolism, clinical management strategies, and weight control. In: Peters AL, Laffel LM, editors. Type1 diabetes sourcebook. Alexandria: American Diabetes Association; 2013.

120. Boulé NG, Kenny GP, Haddad E, Wells GA, Sigal RJ. Meta-analysis of the effect of structured exercise training on cardiorespiratory fitness in type 2 diabetes mellitus. Diabetologia. 2003;46:1071–81.

121. Rejeski WJ, Ip EH, Bertoni AG, et al., LookAHEAD Research Group. Lifestyle change and mobility in obese adults with type 2 diabetes. N Engl J Med. 2012;366:1209–17.

122. Sigal RJ, Kenny GP, Wasserman DH, Castaneda-Sceppa C. Physical activity/exercise and type 2 diabetes. Diabetes Care. 2004;27:2518–39.

123. Church TS, Blair SN, Cocreham S, et al. Effects of aerobic and resistance training on hemoglobin A1c levels in patients with type 2 diabetes: a randomized controlled trial. JAMA. 2010;304:2253–62.

124. Colberg SR, Sigal RJ, Fernhall B, et al. Exercise and type 2 diabetes: the American college of sports medicine and the American diabetes association: joint position statement executive summary. Diabetes Care. 2010;33:2692–6.

125. Haskell WL, Lee IM, Pate RR, Powell KE, Blair SN, Franklin BA, et al. Physical activity and public health: updated recommendation for adults from the American college of sports medicine and the American Heart Association. Circulation. 2007;116:1081–93.

126. Katzmarzyk PT, Church TS, Craig CL, Bouchard C. Sitting time and mortality from all causes, cardiovascular disease, and cancer. Med Sci Sports Exerc. 2009;41:998–1005.

127. Colberg SR. Exercise and diabetes: a clinician's guide to prescribing physical activity, 1st ed. Alexandria: American Diabetes Association; 2013.

128. Lemaster JW, Reiber GE, Smith DG, Heagerty PJ, Wallace C. Daily weight-bearing activity does not increase the risk of diabetic foot ulcers. Med Sci Sports Exerc. 2003;35:1093–9.

129. Spallone V, Ziegler D, Freeman R, et al., Toronto Consensus Panel on Diabetic Neuropathy. Cardiovascular autonomic neuropathy in diabetes: clinical impact, assessment, diagnosis, and management. Diabetes Metab Res Rev. 2011;27:639–53.

130. Pop-Busui R, Evans GW, Gerstein HC, et al., Action to control cardiovascular risk in diabetes study group. Effects of cardiac autonomic dysfunction on mortality risk in the Action to Control Cardiovascular Risk in Diabetes (ACCORD) trial. Diabetes Care. 2010;33:1578–84.

131. Bax JJ, Young LH, Frye RL, Bonow RO, Steinberg HO, Barrett EJ. Screening for coronary artery disease in patients with diabetes. Diabetes Care. 2007;30:2729–36.

132. Chu L, Hamilton J, Riddell MC. Clinical management of the physically active patient with type 1 diabetes. Phys Sports Med. 2011;39:64–77.

133. Miles JM, Leiter L, Hollander P, et al. Effect of orlistat in overweight and obese patients with type 2 diabetes treated with metformin. Diabetes Care. 2002;25:1123–8.

134. Sjostrom L, Peltonen M, Jacobson P, Sjostrom CD, Karason K, Wedel H, et al. Bariatric surgery and long-term cardiovascular events. JAMA. 2012;307:56–65.

Lifestyle Therapy in the Management of Cardiometabolic Risk: Diabetes Prevention, Hypertension, and Dyslipidemia

W. Timothy Garvey, Gillian Arathuzik, Gary D. Miller and Jamy Ard

Abbreviations

AACE	American Association of Clinical Endocrinologists
ACSM	American College of Sports Medicine
ADA	American Diabetes Association
AHA	American Heart Association
BP	Blood pressure
BMI	Body Mass Index
CBC	Complete blood count
CMDS	Cardiometabolic Disease Staging
CPA	Certified public accountant
CVD	Cardiovascular disease
DASH	Dietary Approaches to Stop Hypertension diet
DGA	Dietary Guidelines for Americans
ECG	Electrocardiogram
ER	Extended release
HCP	Health-care professionals
HDL-C	High-density lipoprotein cholesterol
IFG	Impaired fasting glucose
IGT	Impaired glucose tolerance
IDF	International Diabetes Federation
LDL	Low-density lipoprotein
LDL-C	Low-density lipoprotein cholesterol
MetS	Metabolic syndrome
PUFAs	Polyunsaturated fatty acids
RD	Registered dietitian
VLCD	Very low-calorie diets
VLDL	Very low-density lipoprotein particles
WHO	World Health Organization

W. T. Garvey (✉)
Department of Nutrition Sciences, University of Alabama at Birmingham, GRECC, Birmingham VA Medical Center, UAB

Diabetes Research Center, Birmingham, AL 35294-3360, USA
e-mail: garveyt@uab.edu

G. Arathuzik
Lahey Outpatient Center, Danvers, MA 01923, USA

Addison Gilbert Hospital, Gloucester, MA, USA

G. D. Miller
Department of Health and Exercise Science, Wake Forest University, Winston-Salem, NC 27106, USA

J. Ard
Department of Epidemiology and Prevention, Wake Forest University, Winston-Salem, NC, USA

Weight Management Center, Winston-Salem, NC 27157, USA

Introduction

Cardiometabolic risk is a process that begins early in life with relative insulin resistance, progresses to the clinically identifiable states of prediabetes and metabolic syndrome (MetS), and culminates in type-2 diabetes (T2D), cardiovascular disease (CVD) events, or both in single patients [1]. Furthermore, there is a common pathophysiological process responsible for both metabolic and vascular complications that glue together this disease spectrum. Clinical manifestations of insulin resistance include abnormal glucose tolerance, increased blood pressure, and dyslipidemia [2–6]. The relationship between obesity and insulin resistance is complex; nevertheless, weight gain can exacerbate insulin resistance and impel cardiometabolic risk progression. This chapter will focus on the application of lifestyle therapy in the management of cardiometabolic risk *prior* to the onset of T2D. The principal interventional goals in patients with insulin resistance, prediabetes, and MetS are to prevent progression to T2D and to ameliorate the CVD risk profile, which includes improvement in hypertension and dyslipidemia. In short, lifestyle therapy is highly effective in achieving these goals.

Lifestyle therapy to manage cardiometabolic risk does not involve a universal standard prescription but rather is best implemented using an individualized, patient-centric approach in collaboration with a team of health-care professionals (HCP). In addition to general principles relevant to all patients, lifestyle therapy is designed to achieve and sustain clinically meaningful weight loss as a primary objective in individuals who are overweight or obese.

© Springer International Publishing Switzerland 2016
J. I. Mechanick, R. F. Kushner (eds.), *Lifestyle Medicine*, DOI 10.1007/978-3-319-24687-1_23

Weight loss is highly effective in preventing progression to T2D, improving CVD risk factors, and treating hypertension and dyslipidemia [7–13]. Clinical algorithms and guidelines advocate diet and physical activity in prediabetes but are largely oriented to indications for glucose-lowering medications [14, 15]. In recent years, randomized clinical trials have not only demonstrated the efficacy of lifestyle therapy and the marked clinical benefits of weight loss but also those components and practices that are effective in producing and sustaining weight loss. Lifestyle therapy remains the cornerstone of weight loss therapy, alone or in combination with weight loss medications or weight loss (bariatric) surgery. Recently approved weight loss medications and refinements in bariatric surgical techniques and patient management have enabled the development of more effective strategies and medical models for management of cardiometabolic risk [16]. For example, the complications-centric approach of the American Association of Clinical Endocrinologists (AACE) emphasizes that the presence and severity of weight-related complications including prediabetes and MetS—rather than body mass index (BMI) per se—should be the primary factor used in clinical decision-making regarding weight loss treatment modality and intensity [17].

Therefore, a reconfigured approach to lifestyle therapy is proposed for patients with cardiometabolic risk, which emphasizes weight loss as a primary therapeutic strategy in patients who are overweight or obese. This approach to lifestyle therapy incorporates evidence-based practices involving diet, physical activity, behavioral change, and multidisciplinary care but also incorporates an emphasis on enhancing insulin sensitivity and managing hypertension and dyslipidemia, as needed, to counteract the underlying pathophysiology.

Cardiometabolic Risk and Prediabetes States

The increasing prevalence of T2D, together with its burden of patient suffering and social costs, underscores the importance of finding effective strategies for both treatment and prevention. Prediabetes and MetS are two clinical constructs that effectively identify individuals at high risk of future T2D [1]. Prediabetes encompasses those with increased glucose levels that are higher than the normal range but do not yet meet criteria for diabetes [18]. Prediabetes can be diagnosed on the basis of impaired fasting glucose (IFG), impaired glucose tolerance (IGT) defined by the 2-h level following as oral glucose challenge (i.e., post-oral glucose tolerance test, OGTT), or by an elevation in hemoglobin A1c (A1C) [18]. Additionally, prediabetes is part of the MetS, a condition defined by a cluster of risk factors mechanistically related to insulin resistance, including abdominal obesity, dyslipidemia, glucose intolerance, elevated blood pressure, and systemic inflammation [19].

T2D and prediabetes are not isolated entities; rather, they are manifestations of a pathophysiological process, with insulin resistance at its core, which is responsible for both metabolic and vascular disease [5, 20, 21]. Insulin sensitivity varies more than fivefold in healthy appearing individuals, and relative insulin resistance is a trait that is expressed early in life. Insulin-resistant individuals will tend to develop the MetS, which confers risk for both diabetes and CVD (e.g., myocardial infarction, stroke, and peripheral vascular disease) yielding a state of cardiometabolic risk. Hypertension and dyslipidemia are also integral manifestations of insulin resistance. Predisposition to insulin resistance and the progression of cardiometabolic risk factors to overt T2D and CVD events involves the convergence of genetic factors, behavior, and the environmental milieu, including poor diet and sedentary lifestyle. The pathophysiological process underlying cardiometabolic risk involves the accumulation of intra-abdominal fat, dysregulated secretion of adipocytokines, and systemic inflammation [22, 23]. These aspects of pathogenesis point to dysfunctional adipocytes which are insulin resistant and exhibit a diminished ability to store lipid. This causes a redistribution of fat to the intra-abdominal compartment and the accumulation of lipid within muscle cells and hepatocytes, which further exacerbates insulin resistance at the level of these organs and contributes to abnormal glucose tolerance. Generalized obesity can exacerbate insulin resistance by augmenting lipid accumulation in muscle, liver, and the visceral compartment and thus further impel progression of the cardiometabolic pathophysiological process towards the end-stage manifestations of overt T2D and CVD [24, 25]. Obesity alone, however, is not a prerequisite nor a sufficient cardiometabolic risk factor since even lean individuals can be insulin resistant and individuals with obesity can be insulin sensitive with no manifestations of MetS [1]. Nevertheless, weight loss in overweight/obese individuals with insulin resistance and cardiometabolic risk represents highly effective therapy. These principles and the spectrum of cardiometabolic risk are illustrated in Fig. 23.1.

The most common diagnostic criteria for the MetS are those advocated by the Adult Treatment Panel III of the National Cholesterol Program; other criteria have been established by the International Diabetes Federation (IDF) and the World Health Organization (WHO), as shown in Table 23.1. One of the traits used to identify MetS is IFG; thus, patients can meet criteria for both MetS and prediabetes. Patients found to exhibit MetS traits together with prediabetes on the basis of IFG and/or IGT are at particularly high risk of future T2D and should therefore be targeted for aggressive lifestyle interventions and perhaps diabetes oral agents (e.g., metformin), according to consensus statements by the American Diabetes Association (ADA) [14] and the AACE [15].

Insulin resistance is manifested by elevated fasting or postprandial insulin levels while glucose values remain nor-

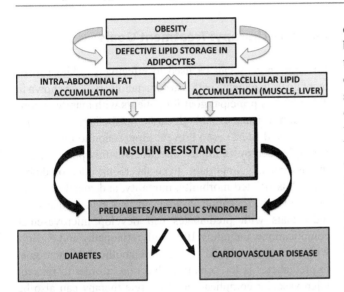

Fig. 23.1 The pathophysiology of cardiometabolic risk. Insulin resistance represents the initial lesion beginning early in life. This includes insulin resistance in adipocytes and defective capability for lipid storage, with accumulation of lipid in muscle and liver cells and in the intra-abdominal depot. There is the eventual transition to the clinically identifiable high-risk states of prediabetes and metabolic syndrome. Hypertension and dyslipidemia are common, and these individuals are then at high risk for developing type-2 diabetes, cardiovascular disease events, or both. Thus, the operant pathophysiological mechanisms give rise to both metabolic and vascular disease components. Generalized obesity is neither necessary nor sufficient as a cause for cardiometabolic disease since lean individuals can be afflicted and obese individuals can be insulin sensitive. Nevertheless, obesity can exacerbate insulin resistance and impel disease progression, and weight loss therapy represents highly effective treatment for both the prevention of diabetes and cardiovascular risk factor reduction

clinical research settings and are not commonly ascertained by primary care physicians. This presents a challenge for the identification of individuals who are insulin resistant in clinical practice and to assess the relative risk for progression to future diabetes. However, insulin resistance and risk of T2D can be clinically identified by evaluating patients for the MetS traits delineated in Table 23.1. The Cardiometabolic Disease Staging (CMDS), illustrated in Fig. 23.2, was developed and validated as a tool to assist in the clinical stratification of individuals for diabetes risk [1]. Using information readily available to the clinician, the CMDS system can be used to identify patients at greatest risk for future T2D and CVD who may benefit from more aggressive weight loss therapy [1]. The prevalence of overweight and obesity approximates 70 % of the population in the USA, and not all patients with obesity are insulin resistant with cardiometabolic risk. The presence of overweight or obesity in subjects with no MetS risk factors (termed the "metabolically healthy obese") has been well documented; these individuals exhibit lower rates of future diabetes, CVD events, and mortality [1, 26–29].

The diagnostic criteria [18] for prediabetes and T2D are shown in Table 23.2. These diagnoses have traditionally involved glucose determinations under fasting conditions, during OGTT, or random measurements. However, a criterion for the diagnostic use of HbA1C has been added, primarily to identify patients who have diabetes on the basis of elevated 2-h OGTT glucose levels who may have gone undiagnosed due to the failure of health-care professionals to perform OGTTs on a more widespread basis. The diagnosis of T2D is based on measurements of blood glucose at levels of hyperglycemia that have been shown to place patients at risk for vascular complications. The diagnostic criteria for prediabetes are generally considered to be above normal

mal (not decreased) or elevated. However, highly accurate measures of insulin resistance, such as the hyperinsulinemic euglycemic clamp procedure, are rarely assessed outside of

Table 23.1 Diagnostic criteria for metabolic syndrome

Risk factor/trait	ATP III criteria Any three out of the five risk factors	IDF criteria Abnormal waist + two risk factors	WHO criteria IFG or IGT + two risk factors
Waist circumference	≥40 in (102 cm) in males ≥35 in (85 cm) in females	Region specific, e.g., ≥90 cm in males and ≥80 cm in females among South Asians	BMI>30 Waist/hip >0.90 cm men and >0.85 cm women
Fasting triglycerides	≥150 mg/dL (>1.7 m mol/L)	≥150 mg/dL (>1.7 m mol/L)	≥150 mg/dL (>1.7 m mol/L)
HDL cholesterol	<40 mg/dL in males (<1.04 m mol/L); <50 mg/dL in females (<1.29 m mol/L)	<40 mg/dL in males (<1.04 m mol/L); <50 mg/dL in females (<1.29 m mol/L)	<35 mg/dL in males (<0.9 m mol/L); <39 mg/dL in females (<1.0 m mol/L)
Blood pressure	Systolic≥130 and/or diastolic≥85 mmHg and/or use of medication for hypertension	Systolic≥130 and/or diastolic≥85 mmHg and/or use of medication for hypertension	Systolic≥140 and/or diastolic≥90 mmHg and/or use of medication for hypertension
Fasting glucose	≥100 mg/dL (5.6 m mol/L) and/or use of medication for hyperglycemia	≥100 mg/dL (5.6 m mol/L) and/or use of medication for hyperglycemia	IFG: fasting≥100 mg/dL (5.6 m mol/L) and/or *IGT*: 2-h 140–199 mg/dL (7.8–11.0 m mol/L)
Microalbuminuria			≥20 μg/min ≥30 mg/g creatinine

ATP III Adult Treatment Panel III, *IDF* International Diabetes Federation, *WHO* World Health Organization, *BMI* Body Mass Index, *IFG* impaired fasting glucose, *IGT* Impaired glucose tolerance, *HDL* High-density lipoprotein

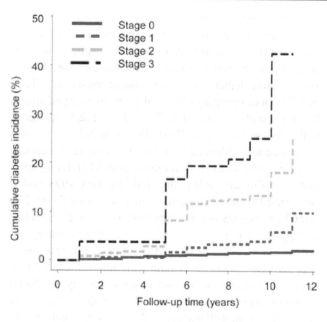

Stage 0   No risk factors; metabolically healthy obese

Stage 1   1 or 2 risk factors (waist, blood pressure, triglycerides, HDL-c)

Stage 2   Metabolic Syndrome alone or IFG alone or IGT alone

Stage 3   2 or more out of 3: Metabolic Syndrome, IFG, IGT

Fig. 23.2 Cardiometabolic Disease Staging (CMDS) quantitatively stratifies risk for future type-2 diabetes using available clinical information. The system can be used to guide aggressiveness of weight loss therapy and optimize benefit/risk ratio for interventions. *HDL-C* high-density lipoprotein cholesterol, *IFG* impaired fasting glucose, *IGT* Impaired glucose tolerance. (Data were generated from the CARDIA Study cohort. From [1])

but not high enough to qualify for T2D. Even at this level of hyperglycemia, some patients with prediabetes develop microvascular disease complications, such as background retinopathy and neuropathy [30, 31]. The use of HbA1C to diagnose prediabetes is problematic since it has acceptable specificity but low sensitivity based on fasting and 2-h glucose [32]. Furthermore, the proportion of prediabetes due to IGT rises as a function of age and the sole use of HbA1C will fail to identify many patients [33]. Thus, normal HbA1C values will not effectively exclude prediabetes, and direct measurements of fasting and 2-h glucose should be considered in high-risk individuals.

Lifestyle Therapy: Treatment Goals

Lifestyle therapy can be used to effectively achieve treatment goals in patients with cardiometabolic risk. As shown in Table 23.3, a principal goal for patients with manifestations of insulin resistance and high cardiometabolic risk (i.e., prediabetes and MetS) is to prevent progression to overt T2D. Lifestyle therapy is highly effective for this purpose, and this is critically important given the rising rates of diabetes and associated morbidity, mortality, and social costs. In the Diabetes Prevention Program, it was evident that even individuals with prediabetes can develop microvascular complications, including 10% with retinopathy and 5–10% with neuropathy [30, 31]. Therefore, another treatment goal in prediabetes is to normalize glycemia in order to prevent microvascular complications. Lifestyle therapy can also be used to treat hypertension and dyslipidemia, thus improving the cardiovascular risk profile and increase functionality and quality of life.

Benefits of Lifestyle Therapy and Weight Loss in Patients with Cardiometabolic Risk

Lifestyle therapy improves clinical outcomes in both lean and overweight/obese patients with cardiometabolic risk. In lean individuals, physical activity and a healthy meal plan with appropriate macronutrient composition can be used to achieve treatment goals. In patients who are overweight or obese, optimal lifestyle therapy should be designed to promote clinically meaningful weight loss and maintain that weight loss over time. Unless HCP have been trained in weight loss therapy and advocate this to patients as a key therapeutic strategy in its own right, it is unlikely that the patients will experience clinically significant weight loss. Over the past decade, research has identified effective lifestyle interventions that greatly augment both treatment options and therapeutic efficacy for weight loss.

Prevention of T2D

In patients who are overweight or obese, weight loss is highly effective in preventing or delaying progression to T2D, par-

Table 23.2 American Diabetes Association (ADA) diagnostic criteria for categories of glucose tolerance [18]

	Fasting glucose	2-h glucose during OGTT	HbA1C (%)	Random glucose
Diabetes	≥126 mg/dL (7.0 m mol/L)	≥200 mg/dL (11.1 m mol/L)	≥6.5	≥200 mg/dL (11.1 m mol/L) with symptoms
Prediabetes	*Impaired fasting glucose (IFG)* 100–125 mg/dL (5.6–6.9 m mol/L)	*Impaired glucose tolerance (IGT)* 140–199 mg/dL (7.8–11.0 m mol/L)	5.7–6.4	
Normoglycemic	<100 mg/dL (5.6 m mol/L)	<140 mg/dL (7.8 m mol/L)	<5.7	

OGTT oral glucose tolerance test, *HbA1C* hemoglobin A1c

Table 23.3 Treatment goals in patients with cardiometabolic risk (insulin resistance, metabolic syndrome, and prediabetes)

1. Prevent progression to T2D
2. Control glycemia to prevent microvascular complications in prediabetes
3. Prevent CVD events by improving risk factors and treatment of
a. Dyslipidemia
b. Hypertension/prehypertension
4. Improve functionality and quality of life

T2D type-2 diabetes, *CVD* cardiovascular disease

ticularly in high-risk patients with prediabetes [7–9] or MetS [12, 34, 35]. A risk-staging system, such as CMDS shown in Fig. 23.2, can be used to identify patients at greatest risk for future T2D and CVD in order to target more aggressive weight loss therapy to those individuals who will receive the greatest benefit [1]. Three major randomized clinical trials, the Diabetes Prevention Program [9, 10, 36], the Finnish Diabetes Study [8, 11, 37], and the Da Qing Study [7, 38], all demonstrated the impressive efficacy of lifestyle/behavioral therapy to prevent T2D. At the same time, weight loss also ameliorated insulin sensitivity and reduced CVD risk factors, including improvements in blood pressure, lipids, and markers of inflammation. In these studies, lifestyle modifications generally involved reductions in caloric intake (by 500–1000 cal/day), behavioral interventions, and increases in physical activity. The Diabetes Prevention Program study randomized subjects with IGT to control, metformin, and lifestyle intervention subgroups, and after 4 years, lifestyle modification reduced progression to T2D by 58% and metformin by 31%, compared with placebo. Subjects achieved approximately 6% mean weight loss at 2 years and 4% weight loss at 4 years in the lifestyle intervention arm, and in post hoc analysis, a progressive 16% reduction in T2D risk was seen with every kilogram of weight loss [9, 10]. With observational follow-up after termination of the study, there was still a significant reduction in the cumulative incidence of T2D in the lifestyle treatment group at 10 years, despite the fact that BMI levels had equalized among the three treatment arms [36]. In addition to the reductions in T2D, there was also evidence in the Da Qing Study that CVD events and mortality were reduced after 23 years when comparing the combined subgroups treated with diet and exercise with the control subgroups [38].

Weight loss through lifestyle changes alone can be difficult to maintain [39]. Therefore, interventions such as pharmacotherapy or surgery, employed as an adjunct to lifestyle therapy, may be necessary in some patients and have also been shown to be highly effective in preventing or delaying progression to T2D. When used in combination with lifestyle therapy, orlistat [13] and phentermine/topiramate extended release (ER) [12, 40] produced greater weight loss and more profound reductions in incident diabetes when compared with lifestyle alone. Furthermore, treatment with lifestyle therapy plus phentermine/topiramate ER achieved 12.1% weight loss after 2 years (compared with 2.5% weight loss in lifestyle alone) as well as a 79% reduction in the annualized T2D incidence rate in patients with MetS or prediabetes at baseline [12]. Rates of incident diabetes were reduced in patients treated with a variety of bariatric surgical procedures [41–46], which vary in their efficacy for weight loss. When the clinical decision is made to employ weight loss medications or bariatric surgery, lifestyle therapy remains a critical component of therapy for achieving and maintaining greater degrees of weight loss and for optimizing outcomes.

While lifestyle interventions, pharmacotherapy, and bariatric surgery can all produce weight loss sufficient to prevent progression to T2D, it is important to consider how much weight loss is needed for maximal efficacy in this regard. The ability to prevent T2D has been shown to be dependent on the magnitude of weight loss; however, is there a threshold for the degree of weight loss above which there is no additional benefit? In the Diabetes Prevention Program, maximal prevention of diabetes was observed at about 10% weight loss [9, 10]. This is consistent with the study employing phentermine/topiramate ER where weight loss of 10% reduced incident diabetes by 79% and any further weight loss to ≥15% did not lead to additional prevention [12]. The bariatric surgery studies produced greater weight loss than observed following lifestyle and pharmacotherapy interventions, yet, in two studies, there was a maximum of 76–80% reduction in diabetes rates [44, 46] similar to that observed in the phentermine/topiramate ER intervention despite the lesser weight loss. These combined data suggest that 10% weight loss will reduce the risk of future T2D by ~80% and represent a threshold above which further weight loss will not result in additional preventive benefits. This suggests that there is residual risk for T2D that cannot be eliminated by lifestyle therapy or weight loss. T2D is a heterogeneous disease, and some individuals may have a heavy burden of gene–environment interactions that lead inexorably to T2D regardless of weight loss. Lean individuals who are insulin resistant also develop T2D at an increased rate and are not candidates for weight loss. In any event, in high-risk patients with prediabetes and/or MetS, who are overweight or obese, a therapeutic plan producing 10% weight loss is recommended.

Management of Hypertension

Lifestyle therapy for hypertension primarily involves weight loss, reductions in dietary sodium, and exercise.

Sodium

Epidemiologic studies have suggested that populations with reduced sodium intake have lower blood pressures on average and generally tend to have less increase in blood pressure with age [47]. These populations are typically found in rural or less developed countries where much of the food supply is unprocessed. In most developed nations, a large percentage of dietary sodium is obtained from processed foods; in the USA, more than three fourths of dietary sodium intake is from processed foods [48]. The current Dietary Guidelines for Americans (DGA) suggest limiting sodium intake to less than 2300/day, or about one teaspoonful of salt [49]. Furthermore, these guidelines advocate that some groups of people, including adults 51 years and older, all African-Americans, and those with T2D, hypertension, or chronic kidney disease, limit their sodium intake to 1500 mg/day. These groups add up to about half of the US population and the majority of adults. With mean sodium intake estimated to be more than 3500 mg/day for the US population, it is not surprising that 32.6% of the population is estimated to have hypertension [50].

Because of the ubiquity of sodium in the diet and the observed relationship between sodium and blood pressure, reduction of dietary sodium intake has been widely promoted as one of the primary strategies to lower blood pressure and prevent hypertension [48]. The efficacy of sodium reduction for lowering blood pressure has been demonstrated in several well-controlled trials. One such example was the Dietary Approaches to Stop Hypertension diet (DASH)-Sodium trial that included feeding study participants fixed diets for 30-day periods at varying levels of sodium intake [51]. When sodium intake was reduced from the highest level (142 m mol/d or 3337 mg) to the intermediate level (107 m mol/d or 2438 mg), blood pressure decreased by 2.1/1.1 mmHg (systolic/diastolic) [52, 53]. Further reduction in blood pressure of 4.6/2.4 mmHg occurred when sodium was decreased to the lower level (65 m mol/d or 1495 mg). In total, reducing sodium intake from the highest level to the lower level decreased blood pressure by 6.7/3.5 mmHg.

However, challenges do exist in reducing dietary sodium. Because of its presence in the food supply, many patients will have difficulty avoiding sodium without making major changes in the way they procure and prepare food. From a practical perspective, the lower level of sodium in the DASH-Sodium trial at approximately 1500 mg is equal to less than 3/4 teaspoon of salt—a relatively small amount of salt that many Americans consume in one meal. Many fast food sandwiches contain nearly two thirds of that total amount of sodium alone. Successful implementation of dietary sodium reduction typically calls for some proficiency at label reading to identify sodium content in packaged foods and limiting restaurant meals and convenience foods. Individuals must also be able to access alternatives for higher sodium products, such as no-salt added or low-sodium versions of breads, soups, canned vegetables, and sauces or condiments. One reasonable approach to recommending sodium reduction is based on the recent Lifestyle Recommen-

dations to Reduce Cardiovascular Risk: Report of the Lifestyle Workgroup, 2013 [54]. This workgroup recommended advising patients with elevated blood pressure to consume no more than 2400 mg/day and that further blood pressure reduction can be achieved by lowering to 1500 mg/day. Even if achievement of these lower levels of sodium intake is out of reach for the individual, the workgroup recommends that blood pressure reduction can be expected if sodium intake is reduced by 1000 mg/day from the patient's baseline intake level.

DASH Dietary Pattern

The DASH dietary pattern was originally developed for blood pressure reduction in 1999 [55]. This pattern consists of a diet rich in fruits, vegetables, and low-fat dairy foods while being low in fat content (saturated fat, total fat, and cholesterol), red meat, sweets, and sugar-containing beverages. In the original DASH trial, study participants were provided the DASH dietary pattern in daily meals, and this resulted in an average blood pressure reduction of 5.5/3 mmHg at 8 weeks. Individuals who were hypertensive at baseline and/or self-identified as African-American had greater blood pressure responses to the dietary pattern. These improvements in blood pressure occurred without change in weight or sodium reduction; weight was held stable by adjusting calorie intake, and sodium was consistent with typical American intake at 3000 mg/day.

While the DASH dietary pattern is effective alone as a strategy for blood pressure reduction, it can be easily combined with other strategies to further enhance blood pressure reduction. For example, the DASH dietary pattern can be the basis of a calorie-restricted weight reduction diet. In the non-randomized phase 1 portion of the Lifestyle Interventions and Independence for Elders (LIFE) study, all study participants were instructed to adopt the DASH dietary pattern with a 500-kcal restriction, along with increasing physical activity by more than 180 min per week over a 26-week period [56]. The mean weight loss in this trial was 6.3 kg with 60% of the participants losing at least 4.5 kg. Similarly, the PRE-MIER clinical trial, which utilized the DASH dietary pattern as part of a behavioral lifestyle intervention, had weight loss of ~5 kg over a 6-month period [57]. The DASH dietary pattern can also be combined with a reduced sodium intake, resulting in greater blood pressure reduction than either strategy alone. In the DASH-Sodium trial, combining the DASH dietary pattern with 2400-mg sodium intake resulted in a blood pressure reduction of 7/4 mmHg; reducing sodium to 1500 mg while consuming the DASH dietary pattern led to blood pressure reduction of 9/5 mmHg.

Potassium

In contrast to sodium, the content of potassium in foods diminishes with food processing. In most countries, the intake of potassium is low because of frequent consumption of processed foods in conjunction with a diet low in fresh fruits and vegetables. Even though the DGA recommend a potassium intake of 120 m mol/d (4700 mg) [49], the average intake in the USA is only around 65 m mol/d (2640 mg) [58]. Fruits and vegetables contribute about 20% of total potassium intake in the typical American diet [58].

Several meta-analyses concluded that individuals with high potassium intake have lower blood pressure [59–61]. In one meta-analysis, the effect size for increased potassium intake approximated reductions of 3.5 mmHg for systolic and 2 mmHg for diastolic blood pressure [62]. The blood-pressure-lowering effect was greater for those with hypertension, with no effect found in individuals without hypertension. Aburto et al. [62] increased potassium intake to the level recommended in the DGA (up to 120 m mol/d; 4700 mg) and observed reductions in blood pressure of 7/4 mmHg. This amount of potassium intake was found to be optimal; consumption above this level did not provide additional benefit [62]. While there are no reports of adverse events resulting from high potassium intake, caution must be exercised in people with renal impairment to avoid hyperkalemia [63].

Alcohol Intake

Alcohol has a known pressor effect and increases blood pressure in a dose-dependent fashion [64]. Blood pressure begins to increase once consumption exceeds two drinks per day (a standard drink is defined as 14 g of ethanol: 12 oz of beer, 5 oz of table wine, or 1.5 oz of distilled spirits) [65]. Previous studies have shown that intake of >210 g of alcohol per week is an independent risk factor for incident hypertension [66]. As a corollary, a decrease in alcohol consumption results in lower blood pressure. In one study, when alcohol was decreased from 350 to 70 mL/week, there was a decrease in systolic blood pressure (BP) of 3.1 mmHg, independent of changes in weight that resulted from lower caloric intake [67]. In general, men should be counseled to consume ≤2 drinks per day and women ≤1 drink per day to lower blood pressure [68]. At the same time, it is important to consider that alcohol consumption is associated with morbidity and mortality (motor vehicle accidents, absenteeism from work, disrupted family, etc.).

Weight Reduction

Elevated blood pressure is an established consequence of overweight and obesity. It is therefore not surprising that one of the associated benefits of weight reduction is lowering of blood pressure. A meta-analysis of eight studies including more than 2100 participants who were randomized to either a weight-reducing diet or a control intervention demonstrated that weight loss was consistently associated with blood pressure reductions [69]. Weight loss diets led to decrements in blood pressure of 4.5/3.2 mmHg together with a

4.0 kg decrease in body weight compared with the control groups after follow-up of 6–36 months. The results of this meta-analysis are consistent with earlier analyses suggesting that blood pressure decreased by 1.2/1.0 mmHg for every kilogram of weight lost [70]. Ultimately, a weight-reducing diet based on the DASH dietary pattern with a lower sodium intake and moderate or no alcohol intake is one of the most comprehensive strategies for producing non-pharmacologic blood pressure reduction. For the motivated patient, combining these strategies can lead to synergies of treatment and pleiotropic effects that are most effectively accomplished with lifestyle therapy techniques.

Physical Activity

Physical activity is a cornerstone of the treatment of hypertension using lifestyle therapy. Many major health organizations, including the American Heart Association (AHA), the American College of Cardiology, and the Centers for Disease Control, emphasize the importance of physical activity training for lowering resting blood pressure in hypertensive and prehypertensive individuals [71]. Aerobic-based activities, such as walking, cycling, and swimming, are prescribed with the goal of achieving 30–60 min of continuous or intermittent aerobic exercise on most days of the week at 40–60% of heart rate reserve or maximal oxygen uptake [72]. The guidelines from the American College of Sports Medicine (ACSM) also promote supplementing aerobic exercise with resistance training for 2–3 days a week with at least one set of 8–12 repetitions at 60–80% of the one-repetition maximum (1-RM) targeting the major muscle groups [72]. In examining data from more than 5000 individuals in a meta-analysis, endurance training reduced blood pressures in hypertensive individuals by 8.3/5.2 mmHg (systolic/diastolic) [73]. The values were less for prehypertensive individuals at 4.2/1.7 mmHg. These conclusions are consistent with other studies testing similar physical activity interventions [74]. Several studies also suggest that the rate of developing hypertension in prehypertensive individuals is reduced in individuals engaged in more physical activity leading to greater fitness [74–76].

The modalities and intensity of the physical activity prescription should accommodate the personal preferences and capabilities of the patient, even though the ideal intensity of exercise will not be possible. Nevertheless, lower amounts of exercise can still be beneficial. Incorporating 10-min bouts of exercise at least three times a day for 5 days a week is also efficacious for blood pressure lowering [77]. This pattern of activity is associated with high adherence and is more practical in the normal daily routine of many individuals. Dynamic resistance exercise training also provides reductions in blood pressure, although the changes are smaller than with endurance exercise [78, 79]. Participating in walking groups also confers health benefits, including reducing blood pres-

Table 23.4 Healthy meal plans

Meal plan	Characteristics	Popular versions
Low carbohydrate	Restricts carbohydrates, increases dietary fat and protein	Atkin's [118]
Low fat	Restricts fat, increases carbohydrates and protein	Ornish Diet [117, 118]
"Right" carbohydrate	Low-glycemic index foods and meals; complex carbohydrates; avoid sugars; moderate restriction of fat	South Beach Diet, Zone Diet
Mediterranean	Emphasizes vegetables, legumes, fresh fruit, olive oil, and moderate amounts of fish, poultry, and red wine	[97–99]
Volumetrics diet	Low-calorie-dense foods with high water and fiber content; includes fruits, vegetables, soups, whole grains, low-fat dairy, beans, and lean meats	EatRight Diet [119–121]
Vegetarian	Avoid meat; rely on legumes, low-fat dairy, eggs, whole grains, vegetables, and fruits	[117, 122]
DASH diet	Emphasizes fruits, vegetables, and low-fat dairy products; designed to lower blood pressure	[51, 53, 55]
Paleolithic diet	Consume foods that mimic the diet of pre-agricultural, hunter–gather ancestors; high protein, low carbohydrate, high unsaturated fat	
Raw food diet	Includes foods that have not been cooked, processed, microwaved, or touched in any unnatural way; no portion limits	

DASH Dietary Approaches to Stop Hypertension

sures by 3.7/3.1 mmHg [80]. These studies demonstrate the benefits that can be achieved with less traditional exercise programs and importantly, in activities that have high adherence rates.

Treatment of Dyslipidemia

The dyslipidemia associated with insulin resistance and cardiometabolic risk is characterized by elevated triglyceride levels, as a result of an excess of large triglyceride-laden very low-density lipoprotein particles (VLDL), as well as decreased concentrations of high-density lipoprotein cholesterol (HDL-C) [81]. Levels of low-density lipoprotein cholesterol (LDL-C) may not be primarily affected; however, the cholesterol is packaged into smaller denser low-density lipoprotein (LDL) particles [81], which are more atherogenic [82–85]. High triglycerides and low HDL-C constitute two of the five diagnostic criteria for the MetS, which is associated with increased risk of CVD. While there is accumulating evidence that elevated triglycerides constitute a direct risk factor for CVD, it is uncertain whether the associations are due to indirect effects or links to other lipoprotein abnormalities and risk factors. This applies to the elevated concentrations of small dense LDL particles that confer increased risk of CVD events independent of overall LDL-C levels [83–85]. High levels of LDL-C represent a major risk factor for CVD and can occur in patients with or without insulin resistance and cardiometabolic risk. Therefore, LDL-C should be brought to recommended targets in all individuals, particularly in those patients with cardiometabolic risk who are at additional risk for CVD [86–88].

Expert panels and professional organizations have established evidence-based treatment targets for lipids and lipoproteins based on prevention of CVD [86–88]. Life-

style therapy can effectively help achieve these therapeutic targets; however, the approaches to dietary therapy require modification based on etiology. Specifically, the macronutrient composition of the diet should be modified based on the degree of hypertriglyceridemia and whether the primary abnormality being treated is elevated LDL-C [87–89].

Dyslipidemia of Insulin Resistance

The dyslipidemia of insulin resistance is responsive to lifestyle therapy including alterations in dietary macronutrient composition, weight loss in patients with overweight or obesity, physical activity, restriction of alcohol, and limited intake of sugars and refined carbohydrates. Healthy meal plans (Table 23.4) can be used effectively to treat dyslipidemia under energy-balanced conditions in patients who are normal weight, or in reduced calorie format for weight loss in patients who are overweight or obese. However, not all healthy meal patterns are appropriate for all patients with dyslipidemia. The dietary prescription will be different depending on the degree of elevation in fasting serum triglyceride [90], which reflects differences in pathophysiology as illustrated in Table 23.5.

Patients with Triglyceride Levels Below 500 mg/dL

Patients with triglyceride levels below 500 mg/dL have borderline-high or high degree of hypertriglyceridemia. These triglyceride levels typically characterize patients with insulin resistance, cardiometabolic risk, MetS, and prediabetes and are largely due to excess production of large triglyceride-enriched VLDL particles by the liver. Since carbohydrates can drive hepatic VLDL production, dietary carbohydrates, particularly sugars and refined carbohydrates, should be reduced and replaced with unsaturated fats and protein [54, 91–95]. Alcohol can also stimulate VLDL production and all patients should restrict alcohol intake (≤1 drink per day). Tri-

Table 23.5 Degrees of hypertriglyceridemia: mechanistic and therapeutic implications

NCEP ATP III criteria for severity of fasting hypertriglyceridemia [89]				
Category	Fasting triglyceride			
	mg/dL	M mol/L	Mechanisms	Aspects of treatment
Normal	<150	<1.7		
Borderline high triglycerides	150–199	1.7–2.3	Can be indicative of insulin resistance and MetS; high production of VLDL	Reduce dietary sugars and refined carbohydrates
High triglycerides	200–499	2.3–5.6	Can be indicative of insulin resistance and MetS; high production of VLDL	Reduce dietary sugars and refined carbohydrates
Very high triglycerides	≥500	≥5.6	Likely that chylomicrons are contributory; saturation of clearance mechanisms	Reduce dietary fat; consider triglyceride-lowering medications
Severe hypertriglyceridemia	≥1000	≥11.2	Risk of pancreatitis; possible genetic basis	Reduce dietary fat; medications will likely be required to lower levels to <500 mg/dL

Rule out secondary causes of hypertriglyceridemia: excess alcohol intake, untreated diabetes, renal impairment, liver disease, pregnancy, hypothyroidism, hypercortisolism, lipodystrophy, drug induced
Genetic causes include familial hypertriglyceridemia, familial combined hyperlipidemia, familial dysbetalipoproteinemia
MetS metabolic syndrome, *VLDL* very low-density lipoprotein, *NCEP ATP III* National Cholesterol Education Program Adult Treatment Panel III

glyceride levels can be markedly elevated in some patients following alcohol ingestion, and these individuals should refrain from alcohol entirely if this pattern is established.

Regarding the selection of healthy meal plans, low-fat diets should be used cautiously and modified to severely limit simple sugars, refined carbohydrates, and any foods or meals that produce a substantial hyperglycemic response. Under energy-balanced or weight-stable conditions, progressive substitution of carbohydrates by fat will produce further reductions in triglycerides and increases in HDL-C in patients with fasting triglycerides <500 mg/dL [96]. In particular, dietary intake of sugar, white flour products, fruit juices, and non-diet sodas can dramatically increase triglycerides, while restricting simple carbohydrates and increasing dietary fiber can be important adjuncts that lower triglycerides. On the other hand, low-carbohydrate diets should be modified to limit saturated fats and avoid *trans*-fat in favor of monounsaturated and polyunsaturated fat. Mediterranean diets are well suited to accommodate an optimal macronutrient composition [97–100], as can dietary prescriptions based on the DASH [55] and other meal plans, which are modified to limit refined carbohydrates and emphasize high fiber and unsaturated dietary fat.

Patients with Triglyceride Levels at 500 mg/dL or Higher

Patients with triglycerides ≥500 mg/dL have very high or severe hypertriglyceridemia. In these patients, clearance mechanisms for triglyceride-enriched lipoproteins are saturated and chylomicronemia is likely or can be rapidly induced upon consumption of fatty meals. Abnormal clearance of triglyceride-enriched lipoproteins can result from defective hydrolysis of triglycerides by lipoprotein lipase, abnormalities in hepatic uptake of chylomicron and VLDL remnants, or abnormalities in apolipoproteins regulating VLDL metabo-

lism (apoC-II, apoC-III, and apoE). These patients are at risk of pancreatitis when triglyceride levels approach 1000 mg/dL and, at higher levels, can experience eruptive xanthoma and lipemia retinalis. These patients should be placed on a low-fat diet, less that 15–25% of total calories, to reduce the release of new chylomicron particles from the gut into the circulation [101, 102]. Therefore, low-carbohydrate diets should generally be avoided since these diets cannot often accommodate the required reductions in dietary fat. Refined carbohydrates and simple sugars should also be avoided in such cases since these nutrients can accelerate hepatic production of VLDL. Thus, the Mediterranean, DASH, low-fat, volumetric, and vegetarian healthy meal plans can serve as the basis for an optimal macronutrient composition.

Omega-3 polyunsaturated fatty acids (PUFAs), derived mainly from fatty fish and some plant products (flax seed), have a unique impact to decrease triglycerides. In large amounts (2–6g/day), these fatty acids can lower triglycerides 40% or more. These doses are difficult to achieve in the diet, and purified capsules are usually necessary. Fish that contain the highest levels of omega-3 fatty acids are sardines, herring, and mackerel, and daily servings of 0.5–1 lb or more may be necessary to achieve intake levels required to predictably reduce triglycerides. In patients with very high or severe hypertriglyceridemia, it is imperative to keep triglyceride levels below 500 mg/dL to minimize the risk of pancreatitis. In fact, lifestyle therapy will often need to be combined with triglyceride-lowering medications to achieve this biochemical target.

Patients with hypertriglyceridemia should be evaluated for secondary causes. These can include pregnancy, endocrine disorders (e.g., hypothyroidism and hypercortisolism), nephrotic syndrome, lipodystrophy, and drug-induced hyperlipidemia (e.g., estrogens, alcohol, thiazide diuretics, beta-blockers, bile acid sequestrants, antihuman immunodeficiency virus medications, antipsychotics, and antidepressants). Patients with hypertriglyceridemia may have genetic defects in lipid metabolism (e.g., familial hypertriglyceridemia, familial combined hyperlipidemia, and dysbetalipoproteinemia).

Regardless of the degree of hypertriglyceridemia, weight loss is advocated for patients who are overweight or obese [94, 95]. The initial weight loss target should be 5–10% of body weight. However, greater degrees of weight loss can achieve progressive improvements in dyslipidemia. Hence, weight loss programs should be intensified when initial efforts do not achieve therapeutic targets. Healthy meal plans appropriate for patients with any degree of triglyceride elevation can be employed in a reduced calorie format. In the range of 5–10% weight loss has been shown to amplify the benefits of changes in macronutrient composition with further reductions in triglycerides, increments in HDL-C, and modest decreases in LDL-C in many studies [102, 103]. Furthermore, there are beneficial effects of weight loss on LDL subclasses characterized by reductions in small dense LDL particle concentrations and an increase in medium and large LDL particles, coupled to a mean increase in LDL particle size and reductions in total LDL particle concentration [104–

108]. In a study by Richard et al. [109], a Mediterranean diet without weight loss lowered LDL-C, apoB-100, and the percentage of small dense LDL particle associated with an increase in the fractional clearance of LDL and VLDL; additionally, lipoprotein values were further improved when this Mediterranean diet was combined with weight loss. Thus, the effects of weight loss on dyslipidemia represent a very favorable profile regarding a reduction in CVD risk.

Exercise is an integral component of lifestyle therapy independent of weight loss. The exercise prescription should be sufficient to promote cardiometabolic health (Table 23.6). The toning of large muscles groups (abdomen, back, legs, and arms) and exercise-induced improvements in insulin sensitivity augment clearance of triglyceride-rich lipoproteins via induction of lipoprotein lipase and therefore lower triglycerides [110–113]. In addition, when used together with weight loss, exercise leads to substantial and disproportionate increments in HDL-C [106].

Elevated LDL

For LDL-C lowering, the AHA recommends reductions in saturated fat intake to <7% of calories and elimination of *trans*-fat together with a healthy meal plan that emphasizes whole grains, vegetables, fruits, poultry and fish, low-fat

Table 23.6 The prescription for physical activity in patients with cardiometabolic disease

General principles
Provide the patient with an individualized prescription for increasing physical activity and decreasing sedentary behavior
Any physical activity is better than nothing. Many patients will not maintain the optimal prescription for physical activity (see below), so it is important to congratulate patients and encourage progress
Health-care team must exude positive and reenforcing attitude regarding importance of physical activity as a component of lifestyle therapy
An ideal physical activity program
Moderate or "conversational exercise"
Heart rate to 50–70% maximum (maximum heart rate=220—age in years)
150 min total per week, with exercise performed on 3–5 different days per week, and periods of non-exercise not exceeding 2 days
Maintain regular schedule over time
Resistance training 2–3 times per week if no contraindications consisting of 8–10 different single-set exercises that use the major muscle groups (arms, shoulders, chest, back, hips, and legs) with a load that permits 10–15 repetitions to a moderate level of fatigue
Reduce sedentary time such that sedentary periods do not exceed 90 min during waking hours
Individualizing the physical activity prescription
Establish an exercise schedule that starts slow and increases intensity as tolerated to minimize muscle soreness and avoid injury. Set realistic goals and schedules. The exercise prescription should accommodate any physical limitations of individual patients
The exercise prescription should accommodate the motivation, preferences, access, and life schedule of the individual patient
Consider cross-training prescriptions (walk, swim, bicycle, etc.) to add variety
Reduce sedentary behavior and incorporate more physical activity into daily lifestyle (household activities, gardening, using stairs instead of elevators, walk breaks at work, etc.)
Consider referral to an exercise professional or fitness center program for supervised exercise and periodic fitness testing
Behavioral strategies
Education regarding the benefits of exercise and how to proceed sensibly and safely
Exercise with others. The social reinforcement of others, either in a supervised setting or at home, may strengthen an exercise commitment
The physical activity program should consist of enjoyable activities or exercises to maintain motivation
Listening to music, reading, watching TV during exercise sessions may enhance compliance
Self-monitoring of physical activity; keep a chart to record exercise achievements and progress. Establish guidelines and a system for self-rewards

dairy products, legumes, nuts, and nontropical vegetable oils with limited intake of red meats, sweets, and sugar-sweetened beverages [54]. The latest DGA have withdrawn the previously recommended limits on cholesterol (i.e., <300 mg/day) due to lack of evidence that consumption of dietary cholesterol can affect serum cholesterol [114]. Nevertheless, it is prudent to avoid excessive cholesterol intake in patients with high LDL-C and CVD risk. These dietary recommendations can be adapted to meet personal and cultural food preferences in the context of healthy meal plans such as the DASH, low-fat, Mediterranean, and vegetarian diets, among others. Moderate to vigorous physical activity occurring over 3–4 sessions per week and totaling at least 150 min per week can also result in LDL-C lowering. In patients with overweight or obesity, weight loss of 5–15 % will lead to modest reductions in LDL-C; however, importantly, weight loss will also decrease the percentage of small dense LDL and overall LDL particle concentration [105–109]. Dietary adjuncts for cholesterol lowering include plant sterols and stanols (2–3 g/d), as well as viscous fibers (5–10 g/d). Dietary and other lifestyle recommendations should be reinforced in the context of a structured lifestyle intervention and referrals to a registered dietitian (RD) and exercise specialist are advisable for many patients. Given the proven cardioprotective effects of statin therapy, high-risk patients with MetS, prediabetes, hypertension, and/or dyslipidemia should be strongly considered for statin therapy in addition to lifestyle therapy, particularly if the LDL-C is ≥ 100 mg/dL [86–88]. The Jupiter study demonstrated reductions in CVD events in patients with elevated C-reactive protein, most of whom had MetS, with statin-induced lowering of LDL-C to below 70 mg/dL [115].

The dietary prescription can sometimes be a double-edged sword when treating patients with mixed hypertriglyceridemia (i.e., elevated triglycerides and LDL-C). When triglycerides are markedly elevated (>500 mg/dL), indicative of defective clearance of triglyceride-enriched lipoproteins, or when treating high LDL-C, the recommended low-fat diet will decrease the appearance of chylomicrons, circulating triglyceride concentrations, and LDL cholesterol. However, in the setting of stable weight and moderately elevated triglycerides, a low-fat diet with a de facto greater proportion of carbohydrate calories will stimulate hepatic production of VLDL, thereby increasing triglycerides and decreasing HDL-C. Therefore, in mixed hyperlipidemia, diets primarily designed to reduce LDL-C and chylomicrons can also increase triglycerides and decrease HDL-C. In such cases, the prescribed macronutrient composition may require a balanced or intermediate approach. Furthermore, a diet emphasizing healthy fat (i.e., monounsaturated and polyunsaturated fat) can be beneficial since this can promote lowering of triglycerides and increasing of HDL-C, without increments or even modest decreases in LDL-C [97–100].

Lifestyle Therapy: An Approach Emphasizing Weight Loss

In considering the diet component of lifestyle therapy with an emphasis on weight loss, both the macronutrient composition of the diet and daily calories can be individualized to achieve weight loss and the overall goals delineated in Table 23.3. There is a relative wealth of data addressing diet during the initial active phase of weight loss. Most of these clinical trials are conducted over 1 year or less with a few studies lasting 2 years. During the initial phase of active weight loss, patients are hypocaloric. Over time, the weight equilibrates at a new lower level, and patients convert to a chronic phase consuming an energy-balanced diet in an effort to maintain weight loss. Furthermore, the chronic phase extends over most of the lifetime of the patient. Patients with cardiometabolic risk require lifelong therapy, and most of the time patients will be in energy balance while maintaining a reasonably stable body weight. This is true, of course, in patients with normal body weight, as well as in patients with overweight or obesity who are post weight loss. Unfortunately, there is a dearth of rigorous data to guide diet during the chronic phase of weight loss maintenance, particularly with respect to clinical outcomes. Some of the best data to inform the chronic diet plan examine the effects of isocaloric substitution or enrichment of various macronutrients on insulin sensitivity and cardiometabolic risk factors [116]. Therefore, diets will be discussed in the context of both the initial phase of active weight loss (e.g., the first year) and the chronic phase of maintenance of weight loss over years to decades when patients are largely in energy balance.

Diet During the Initial Phase of Weight Loss (First Year)

Macronutrient Composition and Healthy Meal Plans

The notion that changes in macronutrient composition can be used to promote weight loss and enhance insulin sensitivity, independent of overall calorie ingestion, has received a great deal of attention in the popular press. Various low-carbohydrate (Atkin's Diet), "right" carbohydrate (The Zone diet, the South Beach diet), and low-fat diets (Ornish Diet) have been promulgated by best-selling books and have gained devotees. There must exist a caloric deficit for weight loss to occur, and randomized trials do not show that any one of these diets is more effective than the other in promoting long-term weight loss. Rather, success depends on the degree to which patients adhere with the meal plan based on personal and cultural food preferences [117]. Regarding treatment of insulin resistance and cardiometabolic risk, there are multiple healthy meal plans that can be delivered in a reduced calorie format while assuring adequate intake of required nutrients as shown in Table 23.4. Healthy meal plans include low-carbohydrate, low-fat, Mediterranean, volumetrics (e.g., EatRight), low-glycemic index (GI), DASH, and vegetarian diets. Any of these meal plans can generally be employed in the initial weight loss phase and will often require the participation of a dietitian, and, in some patients, monitoring of electrolytes, blood pressure, fasting glucose, and lipids.

Of the diets with variable macronutrient composition, the question remains as to which is most effective in the initial phase of weight loss. All diets can safely be used to achieve weight loss. In randomized head-to-head comparison studies, after 1 year, differences in weight loss among individual diets with varying macronutrient composition are minimal [117]. As an example, in some studies, individuals with higher initial weights, randomized to a low-carb diet, had greater weight loss at 6 months, compared with low-fat or Mediterranean diets but similar weight loss at 1 year. What is clear is that the patients who lose the most weight are those who maintain adherence with the prescribed meal plan [117]. Therefore, personal and cultural food preferences should be discussed with each patient to guide an optimal and more personalized healthy meal plan for a durable effect. Macronutrient composition can also be adjusted to include foods that match these personal and cultural preferences to assure adequate intake of required nutrients.

Low-Carb Versus Low-Fat Diets

Low-carbohydrate (low-carb) diets can also be termed high-fat diets since it is impractical to make up the carbohydrate caloric deficit with dietary protein. Low-carb high-fat diets were first described by William Banting in 1863 and were used extensively prior to the discovery of insulin by Frederick Allen and others to treat type 1 diabetes. Nevertheless, it is clear that low-carb diets can be used safely without negative effects and often with improvements in insulin sensitivity, glycemia, lipid status, blood pressure, and body weight. However, two considerations are important. First, relevant studies have generally not been extended passed 1 or 2 years such that we have little or no data on long-term outcomes. Second, these studies often ignore the composition of dietary fat, which can be clinically important.

Two landmark studies are illustrative regarding patient outcomes on a low-carb diet. Foster et al. [123] compared a low-carb "Atkins" diet against a conventional low-fat (25% of calories) reduced-calorie diet in otherwise healthy obese subjects. The low-carb diet produced a greater weight loss than the low-fat diet after six months (6.7 versus 2.7 kg) but at 1 year the amount of weight loss was not significantly different between the two groups. Of note, about 40% of the 63 randomized subjects did not finish the study. Insulin sensitivity was assessed using the quantitative insulin sensitivity check index based on fasting glucose and insulin concentrations; this showed an increase in insulin sensitivity at 6

months but no change from baseline at 1 year in both dietary subgroups, with no significant differences between the subgroups. LDL-C and total cholesterol were lower at 3 months in the low-fat diet subgroup, while HDL-C was higher and triglycerides lower at 1 year in the high-fat diet subgroup. In the second study, Samaha et al. [124] compared the effects of a low-carb versus a low-fat ($\leq$30 g/day) National Heart Lung and Blood Institute diet designed to create a caloric deficit of 500 kcal/day. Their subjects were severely obese (mean BMI 43 = kg/m^2) and most were African-Americans, hypertensive, and characterized by the presence of either T2D or the MetS. In this 6-month study, subjects on the low-carb diet lost more weight than those on the low-fat diet; however, the amount of weight loss was low and the drop-out rate was again very high, particularly in the low-carb group (47 versus 33% in the low-fat diet group), indicative of greater nonadherence. LDL-C and HDL-C were not affected by the diets although triglycerides were lowered in the high-fat diet group. The authors also emphasized that the low-carb diet led to greater improvements in insulin sensitivity than the low-fat diet group, but these effects were minimal and the authors again used a suboptimal index based on fasting glucose and insulin levels as a measure of insulin sensitivity.

The studies by Foster et al. [123] and Samaha et al. [124] did not control for the types or composition of fat or carbohydrates in the diets, which could have affected study end points. For example, Lovejoy et al. [125] used the clamp technique to show that a 3-week high-fat diet (50% fat, 35% carbohydrate, and 15% protein) did induce relative insulin resistance compared with an isocaloric low-fat diet (20% fat, 55% carbohydrate, and 15% protein); however, this could be explained by a higher proportion of saturated fatty acids in the high-fat diet. As discussed below, variations in the types of fats in the low-carb diets (e.g., amount of monounsaturated fatty acids, MUFAs) or types of carbohydrate in the low-fat diets (e.g., fiber, starch, and sugar), or other unknown factors, may have influenced study parameters and contributed to inconsistent results with respect to weight loss, insulin sensitivity, and lipid levels.

Some low-fat diets emphasize ad libitum intake of foods with low caloric density and with high fiber and water content [126]. This approach can also be used effectively to promote weight loss and benefit patients with cardiometabolic risk. As discussed above, the DASH diet is relatively enriched in carbohydrates and reduced in fat. Another example is the EatRight® program employed at the University of Alabama at Birmingham [119–121]. This program emphasizes the ingestion of large quantities of high bulk, low-energy-density foods (primarily vegetables, fruits, high-fiber grains, and cereals) and moderation in high-energy-density foods (meats, cheeses, sugars, and fats). This approach produces equal satiety at reduced energy intake compared with a high-fat diet comprising energy-dense foods. EatRight participants loose an average of 6.3–8.2 kg by the end of the 12-week program, and overall, 53 % of participants maintain their reduced weight or continue to lose weight 2 years later, while only 23 % regain all their lost weight [120].

Alterations in Dietary Carbohydrate and the GI

Dietary carbohydrate composition and distribution, as opposed to total dietary caloric content, can influence body weight and insulin sensitivity. The GI has been established to physiologically classify carbohydrates based on post-meal glycemic responses and is a measure of the degree to which a carbohydrate-containing food raises blood glucose in relationship to a reference food such as white bread or glucose. The South Beach and Zone diets advocate the "right kind" of carbohydrates characterized by a low GI. The originators of these diets purport that high GI responses are central to mechanisms promoting weight accretion; however, the data are equivocal as to whether high-GI diets promote weight gain [127]. Short-term studies indicate that consumption of high-GI carbohydrates has less of an effect to suppress appetite and a diminished ability to induce satiation and satiety than foods with lower GI [128, 129]. However, long-term controlled clinical trials assessing effects of low- versus high- GI diets on body weight are lacking. Furthermore, because multiple dietary and physiological factors affect GI, its validity as a meaningful way to characterize food has been questioned and its implementation in nutritional recommendations is problematic [130]. A recent evidence-based report from the WHO found that the only convincing dietary factor protecting against weight gain and obesity was a high dietary fiber intake [131]. Fiber has consistently been shown to improve insulin sensitivity and lipid levels in studies comparing low and high fiber intakes [132, 133]. Patients should be encouraged to consume 25–30 g fiber/day with an emphasis on soluble fiber (7–13 g) for improving cardiometabolic risk factors.

Meal Replacements

Meal replacements can be recommended for weight loss as an option that provides structure for reducing calorie consumption [134]. These products can enhance adherence for many patients due to the known caloric content that eliminates guesswork, provision of required nutrients, and convenience. Optimal products in prediabetes are characterized by high protein, fiber, complex carbohydrates or modified slowly digesting carbohydrates with no refined sugars, low saturated fat, limited sodium, and no *trans*-fat. Meal replacements usually contain 175–250 kcal per serving and can be employed during the active phase of weight loss and during chronic weight loss maintenance. During active weight loss, meal replacements can be employed in very low-calorie diets (VLCD) or in low-calorie and reduced-calorie diets to comprise one or two meals/day with a third meal of portioned-controlled food. Several studies have demonstrated greater weight loss with incorporation of meal replacements when compared with reduced-calorie diets of conventional foods or with programs using portion-controlled servings of conventional foods or provision of detailed menus.

The Caloric Prescription and Desired Degree of Weight Loss

A caloric deficit is the essential component and a sine qua non of weight loss. During the active phase of weight loss, a reduced-calorie diet where the caloric deficit is ~500 cal/day is generally recommended. However, the HCP can opt for greater degrees of caloric reduction, including VLCD defined by total daily calories of 800 or less. One strategy for developing a caloric prescription that will more predictably achieve the desired amount of weight loss is to estimate the basal metabolic rate (kcal/day) using equations based on height, weight, gender, and age [135–138] or using an indirect calorimeter. The caloric deficit is subtracted from the resting metabolic rate to determine total daily calories and can be individualized to achieve the desired rate and extent of weight loss. In patients with cardiometabolic risk, the goals include the prevention of T2D and improvements in hypertension and dyslipidemia (Table 23.3). Most guidelines for obesity recommend weight loss of 5–10 % since this is sufficient to improve multiple weight-related complications. However, as discussed above, maximal prevention of T2D was observed at 10 % weight loss which reduced incident diabetes by ~ 80 %, regardless of whether this was achieved via lifestyle therapy [9, 10], weight loss medications [12, 13], or bariatric surgery [41–43]. In contrast, no thresholds for maximal benefits were observed with the progressive weight loss from 5 to >15 % in lowering systolic and diastolic blood pressure, increasing HDL-C, and decreasing triglycerides in the LookAHEAD study [139]. For improvements in dyslipidemia and hypertension, therefore, greater weight loss provides for additional clinical benefits up to and beyond 15 % weight loss.

Diet During the Chronic Maintenance Phase of Weight Loss (Years to Decades)

A Healthy Meal Plan for the Long Term

After active weight loss, patients will need an energy-balanced prescription to maintain the new lower body weight and avoid weight regain. This can be problematic since energy expenditure decreases following weight loss. Therefore, resting energy equations based on height and weight will predictably overestimate the number of calories needed for weight stabilization. For this reason, it is wise to reduce

Table 23.7 Isocaloric dietary substitution or enrichment: impact on insulin sensitivity

Summary of conclusions from published clinical trials	
Favorable	Unfavorable
MUFAs	Saturated fat
PUFAs	*Trans*-fat
Whole grains	Refined grains
High fiber	Low fiber
Low glycemic index	High glycemic index
Mediterranean diet	"Western diet"

MUFAs monounsaturated fatty acids, *PUFAs* polyunsaturated fatty acids

daily calories by 100 kcal/day below the calculated value and then to follow the patient making further reductions in the caloric prescription based on changes in body weight. Indirect calorimetry can be helpful at this stage to provide a more accurate estimate.

Following the active weight loss (~1 year), patients will equilibrate at a lower body weight, and it is incumbent upon the patient and health-care team to maintain the weight loss. At this point, the patient will essentially be in energy balance, and the macronutrient composition might have different effects in cardiometabolic risk and T2D than during hypocaloric feeding. Various healthy meal plans have been relatively well studied during the active phase of weight loss; however, unfortunately, little long-term data exist beyond 1 or 2 years on these diets. In particular, the effects on long-term clinical outcomes, such as the progression to T2D and CVD disease events, as well as the impact of the various diets on cardiometabolic pathophysiology and disease biomarkers, are very important but largely unknown. The question regarding optimal diet is also relevant to normal-weight patients with cardiometabolic risk who do not require weight loss.

If there is a lack of data addressing long-term outcomes, what evidence can be used to guide the dietary prescription? One consideration was highlighted in selecting the diet for active weight loss, namely, the diet that could best accommodate personal and cultural preferences resulting in greater rates of compliance. This remains an important consideration during chronic weight maintenance. However, the second consideration is a large body of data indicating that isocaloric substitution of macronutrients can influence insulin sensitivity and CVD risk factors [116]. Since insulin resistance is key to the pathophysiology and progression of cardiometabolic risk, it is reasonable to augment macronutrients that enhance insulin sensitivity and reduce macronutrients that promote insulin resistance, as summarized in Table 23.7.

Saturated Versus Polyunsaturated Fat

The composition of dietary fatty acids can modulate insulin sensitivity and CVD risk factors independent of total fat or total calorie intake [140, 141]. With respect to saturated fat,

epidemiological studies show that high intake of total and saturated fat intake is associated with insulin resistance [141]. Multiple cross-sectional studies have similarly found that intake of both saturated and *trans*-fatty acids is associated with hyperinsulinemia and risk of T2D, independent of body adiposity [142, 143]. High intake of PUFAs does not appear to have the same adverse effects and may even result in an increase in insulin sensitivity [144]. For example, Summers et al. [145] studied the effect of substituting dietary saturated fat with PUFA on insulin sensitivity in healthy, obese subjects with T2D. Their findings demonstrated that an isocaloric diet enriched in PUFA resulted in both an increase in insulin sensitivity and a lowering of LDL-C, when compared with a diet rich in saturated fatty acids. However, it was not possible in this study to conclude whether it was the increase in dietary PUFA or the decrease in saturated fat that produced the relative benefits in the PUFA diet subgroup. Diets enriched in PUFA have not consistently been shown to improve insulin sensitivity [146] and long-term intervention trials have not been conducted. Discrepancies in the short-term studies are often attributable to the failure to control for dietary fatty acid and carbohydrate composition (e.g., MUFA), total calories, physical activity, and population characteristics such as age, gender, and adiposity.

Omega-6 fatty acids and omega-3 fatty acids are the two important types of dietary PUFA. While evidence suggests that omega-3 fatty acids, namely eicosapentaenoic acid, docosahexaenoic acid, and α-linolenic acid, from fish or fish oil dietary supplements may help prevent CVD [147], the effects of omega-3 and omega-6 fatty acids on glucose homeostasis are inconsistent [143, 144, 148]. However, while omega-3 fatty acids may not influence insulin sensitivity, doses of 2–6 g/day are effective in lowering circulating triglyceride levels. People are encouraged to consume whole food sources of omega-3 fatty acids, specifically fatty fish at least twice a week. Fatty fish include salmon, mackerel, sardines, tuna, trout, and herring.

Monounsaturated Fatty Acids

Beneficial effects of a high-MUFA diet on glycemic control in T2D have been demonstrated in a meta-analysis of randomized trials using isoenergetic high-MUFA diets [149]. These trials show that isocaloric substitution of MUFA for saturated fat [150], or even substituting MUFA for carbohydrates, can have positive effects on insulin sensitivity, lipids, and cardiometabolic health [151]. Accordingly, the ADA essentially places no restrictions on dietary MUFAs within the limits of the caloric prescription in diabetes.

Fiber

On balance, available data suggest that dietary fiber, rather than carbohydrate quantity or dietary GI per se, is directly responsible for any effects of carbohydrates on insulin sensitivity. In a randomized crossover study comparing isocaloric high- versus low-GI diets, there was no observed benefit of the low-GI diet on insulin sensitivity [152]. However, a low-GI diet with a greater amount of fiber and whole-grain products seemed to improve glycemic and insulin responses and lowered the risk of T2D [133], indicating that the fiber content in low-GI foods may play a metabolic role. In support of this contention, studies on the effects of dietary intake of fiber, particularly whole-grain foods, have been fairly consistent in demonstrating an effect to enhance insulin sensitivity [153–155]. Isocaloric substitution experiments indicate that diets enriched in MUFAs, PUFAs, whole grains, and high fiber result in an increase in insulin sensitivity and improvements in lipids, while enrichment in saturated and *trans*-fats, refined grains, and reduced fiber promote insulin resistance and dyslipidemia (Table 23.7). These data are relevant in the selection of a healthy meal plan during isocaloric periods in patients with cardiometabolic risk. If a low-carbohydrate diet is to be used for chronic weight loss maintenance, it would be important to minimize saturated fat in favor of MUFA, and this can be challenging given the amount of total fat consumed under energy-balanced conditions. Due to the limited number of foods highly enriched in MUFA (e.g., olive oil, avocados, and nuts), a concerted effort working with a dietitian is recommended in order to maintain a high MUFA to saturated fat ratio (≥2:1) and at the same time assure a wide range of diet choices. Furthermore, lipid panels should be followed closely for changes in LDL-C, HDL-C, and triglycerides since there is lack of data on the long-term effects of a low-carbohydrate diet under isocaloric conditions. On the other hand, low-fat diets, including volumetrics, vegetarian, and DASH diets, are relatively high in carbohydrates, which could have the effect of worsening glycemia in patients with prediabetes. Complex carbohydrates, high fiber intake, and low-GI meals should be emphasized.

Mediterranean Diets

One meal plan that can be effective in patients with cardiometabolic risk is represented by the Mediterranean diet, characterized by a reliance on olive oil as a fat source, which contains the MUFA oleic acid as ~75% of fatty acids. There are variations in the Mediterranean diet as consumed in various regions and countries; however, they are discussed here in terms of commonalities relevant to cardiometabolic risk reduction. In addition to olive oil, these diets consistently feature a high intake of vegetables, legumes, nuts, and fruits; a low intake of saturated fat; low-to-moderate consumption of dairy products; low intake of meat and poultry and relatively high intake of seafood; and regular consumption of red wine at meals in most Mediterranean cultures. This diet consists entirely of unprocessed foods and is rich in fiber, antioxidant polyphenols, vitamins and minerals, and phytochemicals. Furthermore, Mediterranean diets have been shown to have favorable clinical effects in patients with car-

diometabolic risk and insulin resistance, including long-term outcome studies demonstrating prevention of T2D and primary and secondary prevention of CVD [97–99, 156–164]. Epidemiologically, Mediterranean diets have been known to be associated with reduced CVD and mortality when compared with diets consumed in northern European countries. The Lyon Diet Heart Study is a clinical trial that assessed the efficacy of Mediterranean diets for the secondary prevention of CVD events. Patients who have had a previous myocardial infarction were randomized to a Mediterranean diet or a diet typically consumed in northern countries, such as the UK [157, 158]. After 4 years follow-up, the Mediterranean diet group had reduced rates of re-infarction and mortality. Mediterranean diets have also been shown to prevent MetS and reduce rates of progression to T2D [160–164]. Thus, Mediterranean diets are a highly rationale choice as the dietary component of long-term lifestyle therapy in patients with cardiometabolic risk.

Physical Activity

Increased physical activity is an important component of lifestyle therapy in cardiometabolic risk. Regular exercise by itself [165, 166] or as part of a comprehensive lifestyle plan [7–11] can prevent progression to T2D in high-risk individuals. Structured exercise improves fitness, muscle strength, and insulin sensitivity [167–169]. In the context of an overall lifestyle intervention, regular exercise can contribute to weight loss and prevention of weight regain, and improve CVD risk factors such as lipids and blood pressure [7–11]. Studies have demonstrated beneficial effects of both aerobic and resistance exercise and additive benefits when both forms of exercise are combined [170–172]. For cardiometabolic conditioning, the guidelines proposed by the ADA, AHA, and the ACSM are well aligned [54, 173] and are summarized in Table 23.6. Lifestyle therapy should include increased physical activity even though the patient is unable to engage in optimal physical activity. For example, studies have consistently shown that a walking program is associated with reductions in diabetes incidence [174–176]. Elderly patients or persons with disabilities should try to approach levels of activity in the guidelines to the extent possible; however, even reduced activity regimens should be encouraged. Reductions in sedentary behavior can also be helpful (e.g., duration of sedentary periods lasting less than 90 min and interrupted by periods of activity) [177]. Clearly, the HCP and the patient should together establish the exercise prescription with the goal for long-term compliance. Screening for coronary artery disease should also be performed in patients at risk [178]. Table 23.6 describes options for the exercise prescription as well as general principles and behavioral strategies to promote compliance.

Lifestyle Therapy in Patients Treated with Weight Loss Medications or Bariatric Surgery

Lifestyle therapy is also a critical component of care in combination with weight loss medications and bariatric surgery in the treatment of patients with cardiometabolic risk and obesity. Lifestyle therapy alone does not result in sustained weight loss in many patients due to pathophysiological mechanisms operative in obesity as a disease [179–185]. Weight loss medications [13, 186–189] when used as adjunctive therapy to lifestyle interventions provide for greater weight loss that might be required for optimal prevention of T2D and for improvements in hypertension and dyslipidemia [12, 13, 16]. Lifestyle therapy is also critical in bariatric surgery patients both pre- and postoperatively for optimal clinical outcomes and for preventing weight regain following the procedures. This approach must be balanced against the inherent risks of surgical complications and mortality, as well as potential nutritional deficiencies, weight regain in some patients, and the need for lifelong lifestyle support and medical monitoring [190]. Nutrition therapy in these postoperative patients must guard against nutritional deficiencies and include supplementation of micronutrients including iron, calcium, vitamin D and other fat-soluble vitamins, B vitamins (to include thiamine, folic acid, and B_{12}), and minerals (copper, zinc, selenium) [190].

Final Summary Recommendations

1. Cardiometabolic risk is represented by a spectrum of disease findings and markers with common pathophysiological mechanisms, beginning early in life with relative insulin resistance, progressing to clinically identifiable states of high risk, namely prediabetes and MetS, and culminating in T2D, CVD disease events, or both in single patients.
2. Lifestyle therapy is highly effective in achieving therapeutic goals for cardiometabolic risk: (i) prevent progression to T2D, (ii) control glycemia to prevent microvascular complications in prediabetes, (iii) improve the CVD risk factor profile and treat hypertension and dyslipidemia, and (iv) improve functionality and quality of life.
3. A new reconfigured approach to lifestyle therapy is proposed for overweight/obese patients with cardiometabolic risk, which emphasizes weight loss as a primary therapeutic strategy for prevention and treatment. This approach to lifestyle therapy incorporates evidence-based practices involving diet, physical activity, behavioral interventions, and multidisciplinary care, with demonstrated effectiveness for weight loss.

4. Weight loss in overweight/obese individuals is highly effective in preventing progression to T2D and in the treatment of hypertension and dyslipidemia. Weight loss of 10% is optimal for the prevention of T2D in high-risk patients with prediabetes or MetS.
5. Nutritional therapy for the active phase of weight loss (~first year) is accomplished using any one of several healthy meal plans, selected on the basis of personal and cultural preference, and delivered as a very low-calorie, low-calorie, or reduced-calorie diet.
6. The lifestyle therapy includes physical activity that optimally encompasses both aerobic and resistance exercise and a reduction in sedentary behavior. However, the prescription for physical activity must be tailored to the preferences and capabilities of patients with T2D and take into account the presence of diabetes-related complications.
7. During the chronic phase of weight loss maintenance (years–decades) when patients are in energy balance, there are little data indicating which macronutrient composition may be optimal with regard to long-term safety and clinical outcomes. Given the central role of insulin resistance in cardiometabolic risk, the rational choice is to emphasize nutrients shown to enhance insulin sensitivity in isocaloric substitution studies (e.g., MUFA, fiber, whole grains, and components of Mediterranean diets), and to minimize or avoid foods that promote insulin resistance (e.g., saturated fat, *trans*-fat, refined grains, and components of Western diets).
8. In overweight/obese patients with cardiometabolic risk, lifestyle therapy remains the cornerstone of treatment to optimize outcomes in patients treated with weight loss medications or bariatric surgery.

Case Report

A 48-year-old European-American female was referred to you by her family doctor for high fasting blood glucose. However, the patient offers the following as the chief complaint: "I need help with my weight. Nothing I do seems to help. I want to be a role model for my teenage daughter who also seems to be gaining weight. The whole thing makes me depressed."

Medical History

1. Gestational diabetes with birth of only child 16 years ago
2. Depression, symptoms waxing and waning over the past 10 years treated with paroxetine 40 mg/day

Social and Family History

The patient is trained as a certified public accountant (CPA) and oversees accounts of two small companies largely working from her home office. She divorced her husband 5 years ago and is a single mother of one 16-year-old daughter. She leads a sedentary lifestyle but belongs to YMCA and tries to get to the gym three times a week but averages once a week. At the gym she uses weights and walks on the treadmill. She likes a cocktail early evening and has a negative smoking history. Her family history is positive only for T2D in her mother.

Exam BMI 36 kg/m²; waist circumference 40 in.; blood pressure 148/92; trace edema in legs with varicose veins

Laboratory Fasting glucose 114 mg/dL; HbA1C 6.0%; lipid panel (mg/dL) shows total cholesterol 199, LDL-C 114, HDL-C 44, and TG 177; transaminases 1.5 times upper limits of normal; and calculated non-HDL cholesterol 155 mg/dL. Complete blood count (CBC), creatinine, and electrolytes are normal.

Weight History She had a "normal body weight" until her late twenties when she started to gain weight after "problems" began in her marriage. After the birth of her child at the age of 32, she went on several diet plans (South Beach and then Atkins) and did lose weight temporarily but had trouble staying on diet and experienced weight regain. She enrolled in Weight Watchers and the weight loss program at the YMCA in the past, but again weight loss was followed by weight regain. She has also tried *Garcinia Cambogia* and Sensa without benefit. "I need help because I get so hungry and I can't stay on diet for long. It makes me feel better to eat and less depressed in the short term but when I see my weight increasing I get even more depressed."

Assessment

The patient clearly has cardiometabolic risk factors as evidenced by the fact that she meets criteria for both prediabetes due to IFG (114 mg/dL) and MetS (elevated waist circumference, low HDL-C, high triglycerides, high fasting glucose, and high blood pressures). Risk stratification using the Cardiometabolic Disease Staging System (CMDS) [1] indicates that she is in the highest risk category for future T2D and CVD mortality. The positive family history for T2D and gestational diabetes during her pregnancy 16 years ago further compound the risk for progression to overt diabetes. Based on the single, sitting blood pressure in your office you conclude that she likely has hypertension, another cardiometabolic risk factor, which you will confirm on a

subsequent visit. She also displays the dyslipidemia associated with insulin resistance and cardiometabolic risk with elevated triglycerides and low HDL levels for a female. The non-HDL cholesterol is 155 mg/dL (treatment goal should be <130 mg/dL). The fact that the non-HDL cholesterol is greater than 30 units above the level of LDL-C indicates that she has high concentrations of small dense LDL particles. Finally, her insulin resistance and obesity put her at risk of nonalcoholic fatty liver disease, and this is suspected as the explanation for the elevated transaminases.

In summary, this patient has multiple manifestations of cardiometabolic risk and is at particularly high risk of future diabetes and CVD. You could recommend medications for IGT, hypertension, and dyslipidemia, but you elect to discuss lifestyle therapy with an emphasis on weight loss with the patient since this will result in improvements in glycemia, blood pressure, and lipids.

Plan

The patient has dietary preferences for fish, poultry, and salads and tends to cook with olive oil. At home, while working as a CPA, she does snack frequently between meals, sometimes with chips and popcorn. You place her on a Mediterranean diet healthy meal plan, with 500 kcal/day energy deficit diet. You ask her to avoid between-meal snacks except that you recommend celery or cucumbers if she gets hungry between meals. You refer her to a dietitian for instructions, implementation, and follow-up. Because the patient has experienced weight regain on several dietary interventions in the past, you discuss the addition of a weight loss medication to help her adhere to the reduced-calorie meal plan and because you want to assure the achievement and maintenance of at least 10% weight loss, which will maximize your efforts to prevent diabetes in this high-risk patient. For physical activity, you recommend taking a break at lunch and going to the YMCA three times a week and once on weekends for 40 min of brisk walking on the treadmill and support her suggestion to engage a trainer at the facility. You place her on atorvastatin 40 mg/day. You schedule her for return visit in 2 weeks.

Additional Testing Two-hour OGTT glucose value 182 mg/dL indicative of IGT; electrocardiogram (ECG) normal; apoB-100 value of 110 mg/dL consistent with an elevated LDL particle concentration; spot urine showing normal albumin to creatinine ratio

Two Weeks Later Patient has lost 3 lb and is excited about the meal plan, the physical activity prescription, and contact with the dietitian. Her daughter wants to join her for "work-outs" at the YMCA on Saturdays. Blood pressure remains elevated at 145/92 mmHg. You add an oral weight loss medication known to suppress appetite as an adjunct to lifestyle therapy. You encourage the patient and discuss the plan to follow fasting glucose, hepatic transaminases, blood pressure, and lipids as the indicators of success for lifestyle therapy. You schedule monthly visits for the next 3 months alternating every 2 weeks with monthly visits to the dietitian.

Acknowledgments We acknowledge the support of the Diabetes Research Center at the University of Alabama at Birmingham funded by an award from the National Institutes of Health (DK-079626).

References

1. Guo F, Moellering DR, Garvey WT. The progression of cardio-metabolic disease: validation of a new cardiometabolic disease staging system applicable to obesity. Obesity. 2014;22:110–8.
2. Reaven GM. Pathophysiology of insulin resistance in human disease. Physiol Rev. 1995;75:473–86.
3. Liao Y, Kwon S, Shaughnessy S, Wallace P, Hutto A, Jenkins AJ, Klein RL, Garvey WT. Critical evaluation of adult treatment panel III criteria in identifying insulin resistance with dyslipidemia. Diabetes Care. 2004;27:978–83.
4. Reaven GM. Insulin resistance: the link between obesity and cardiovascular disease. Med Clin North Am. 2011;95:875–92.
5. Eckel RH, Grundy SM, Zimmet PZ. The metabolic syndrome. Lancet. 2005;365:1415–28.
6. Lorenzo C, Okoloise M, Williams K, Stern MP, Haffner SM, San Antonio Heart Study. The metabolic syndrome as predictor of type 2 diabetes: the San Antonio heart study. Diabetes Care. 2003;26:3153–9.
7. Pan XR, Li GW, Hu YH, et al. Effects of diet and exercise in preventing NIDDM in people with impaired glucose tolerance. The Da Qing IGT and Diabetes Study. Diabetes Care. 1997;20:537–44.
8. Tuomilehto J, Lindstrom J, Eriksson JG, et al. Prevention of type 2 diabetes mellitus by changes in lifestyle among subjects with impaired glucose tolerance. N Engl J Med. 2001;344:1343–50.
9. Knowler WC, Barrett-Connor E, Fowler SE, et al. Reduction in the incidence of type 2 diabetes with lifestyle intervention or metformin. N Engl J Med. 2002;346:393–403.
10. Hamman RF, Wing RR, Edelstein SL, et al. Effect of weight loss with lifestyle intervention on risk of diabetes. Diabetes Care. 2006;29:2102–7.
11. Laaksonen DE, Lindstrom J, Lakka TA, et al. Physical activity in the prevention of type 2 diabetes: the Finnish diabetes prevention study. Diabetes. 2005;54:158–65.
12. Garvey WT, Ryan DH, Henry R, Bohannon NJ, Toplak H, Schwiers M, et al. Prevention of type 2 diabetes in subjects with prediabetes and metabolic syndrome treated with phentermine and topiramate extended release. Diabetes Care. 2014;37:912–21.
13. Torgerson JS, Hauptman J, Boldrin MN, Sjostrom L. XENical in the prevention of diabetes in obese subjects (XENDOS) study: a randomized study of orlistat as an adjunct to lifestyle changes for the prevention of type 2 diabetes in obese patients. Diabetes Care. 2004;27:155–61. Erratum in Diabetes Care. 2004;27:856.
14. Nathan DM, Davidson MB, DeFronzo RA, et al. Impaired fasting glucose and impaired glucose tolerance: implications for care. Diabetes Care. 2007;30:753–9.
15. Garber AJ, Handelsman Y, Einhorn D, Bergman DA, Bloomgarden ZT, Fonseca V, Garvey WT, Gavin JR 3rd, Grunberger G, Horton ES, Jellinger PS, Jones KL, Lebovitz H, Levy P, McGuire DK, Moghissi ES, Nesto RW. Diagnosis and management of prediabetes in the continuum of hyperglycemia: when do the risks of diabetes begin? A consensus statement from the American College of Endocrinology and the American Association of Clinical Endocrinologists. Endocr Pract. 2008;14:933–46.
16. Garvey WT. New tools for weight loss therapy enable a more robust medical model for obesity treatment: rationale for a complications-centric approach. Endocr Pract. 2013;19:864–74.
17. Garvey WT, Garber AJ, Mechanick JI, Bray GA, Dagogo-Jack S, Einhorn D, Grunberger G, Handelsman Y, Hennekens CH, Hurley DL, McGill J, Palumbo P, Umpierrez G. On behalf of the AACE Obesity Scientific Committee. American Association of Clinical Endocrinologists and American College of Endocrinology position statement on the 2014 advanced framework for a new diagnosis of obesity as a chronic disease. Endocr Pract. 2014;20:977–89.
18. American Diabetes Association. Standards of medical care in diabetes—2015. Diabetes Care. 2015;38 Suppl 1:S8–16.
19. Grundy SM, Brewer Jr HB, Cleeman JI, American Heart A. Definition of metabolic syndrome: report of the National Heart, Lung, and Blood Institute/American Heart Association conference on scientific issues related to definition. Circulation. 2004;109:433–8.
20. Milicevic Z, Raz J, Beattie SD, et al. Natural history of cardiovascular disease in patients with diabetes: role of hyperglycemia. Diabetes Care. 2008;31(2):155–60.
21. Van Gaal LF, Mentens IL, De Block CE. Mechanisms linking obesity with cardiovascular disease. Nature. 2006;444:875–80.
22. Nigro J, Osman N, Dart AM, Little PJ. Insulin resistance and atherosclerosis. Endocr Rev. 2006;27:242–59.
23. Olefsky JM, Glass CK. Macrophages, inflammation, and insulin resistance. Annu Rev Physiol. 2010;72:219–46.
24. Després J-P, Lemieux I. Abdominal obesity and metabolic syndrome. Nature. 2006;444:881–7.
25. Lara-Castro C, Garvey WT. Intracellular lipid accumulation in liver and muscle and the insulin resistance syndrome. Endocrinol Metab Clin North Am. 2008;37:841–56.
26. Stefan N, Kantartzis K, Machann J, et al. Identification and characterization of metabolically benign obesity in humans. Arch Intern Med. 2008;168:1609–16.
27. Wildman RP, Muntner P, Reynolds K, et al. The obese without cardiometabolic risk factor clustering and the normal weight with cardiometabolic risk factor clustering: prevalence and correlates of 2 phenotypes among the US population (NHANES 1999–2004). Arch Intern Med. 2008;1 68:1617–24.
28. Meigs JB, Wilson PW, Fox CS, et al. Body mass index, metabolic syndrome, and risk of type 2 diabetes or cardiovascular disease. J Clin Endocrinol Metab. 2006;91:2906–12.
29. Yusuf S, Hawken S, Ounpuu S, et al. Obesity and the risk of myocardial infarction in 27,000 participants from 52 countries: a case-control study. Lancet. 2005;366:1640–9.
30. Ratner R, Goldberg R, Haffner S, et al. Diabetes Prevention Program Research Group. Impact of intensive lifestyle and metformin therapy on cardiovascular disease risk factors in the diabetes prevention program. Diabetes Care. 2005;28:888–94.
31. Carnethon MR, Prineas RJ, Temprosa M, et al. Diabetes Prevention Program Research Group. The association among autonomic nervous system function, incident diabetes, and intervention arm in the Diabetes Prevention Program. Diabetes Care. 2006;29:914–9.
32. Guo F, Moellering DR, Garvey WT. Use of HbA1c for diagnoses of diabetes and prediabetes: comparison with diagnoses based on fasting and 2-hour glucose values and effects of gender, race, and age. Metab Syndr Relat Disord. 2014;12:258–68.
33. DECODE Study Group. Age- and sex-specific prevalences of diabetes and impaired glucose regulation in 13 European cohorts. Diabetes Care. 2003;26(1):61–9.
34. Deedwania PC, Volkova N. Current treatment options for the metabolic syndrome. Curr Treat Options Cardiovasc Med. 2005;7:61–74.
35. Grundy SM, Cleeman JI, Daniels SR, et al. Diagnosis and management of the metabolic syndrome: an American Heart Associa-

tion/National Heart, Lung, and Blood Institute Scientific Statement. Circulation. 2005;112:2735–52.

36. Diabetes Prevention Program Research Group, Knowler WC,
Fowler SE, Hamman RF, et al. 10-year follow-up of diabetes incidence and weight loss in the Diabetes Prevention Program Outcomes Study. Lancet. 2009;374:1677–86.

37. Lindström J, Ilanne-Parikka P, Peltonen M, et al. Finnish Diabetes
Prevention Study Group. Sustained reduction in the incidence of
type 2 diabetes by lifestyle intervention: follow-up of the Finnish
Diabetes Prevention Study. Lancet. 2006;368:1673–9.

38. Li G, Zhang P, Wang J, et al. Cardiovascular mortality, all-cause
mortality, and diabetes incidence after lifestyle intervention for
people with impaired glucose tolerance in the Da Qing Diabetes
Prevention Study: a 23-year follow-up study. Lancet Diabetes Endocrinol. 2014;2:474–80.

39. Barte JC, ter Bogt NC, Bogers RP, et al. Maintenance of weight
loss after lifestyle interventions for overweight and obesity, a systematic review. Obes Rev. 2010;11:899–906.

40. Garvey WT, Ryan DH, Look M, et al. Two-year sustained weight
loss and metabolic benefits with controlled-release phentermine/
topiramate in obese and overweight adults (SEQUEL): a randomized, placebo-controlled, phase 3 extension study. Am J Clin Nutr.
2012;95:297–308.

41. Wentworth JM, Hensman T, Playfair J, et al. Laparoscopic adjustable gastric banding and progression from impaired fasting glucose to diabetes. Diabetologia. 2014;57:463–8.

42. Sjöholm K, Anveden A, Peltonen M, et al. Evaluation of current
eligibility criteria for bariatric surgery: diabetes prevention and
risk factor changes in the Swedish obese subjects (SOS) study.
Diabetes Care. 2013;36:1335–40.

43. Carlsson LM, Peltonen M, Ahlin S, et al. Bariatric surgery and
prevention of type 2 diabetes in Swedish obese subjects. N Engl J
Med. 2012;367:695–704.

44. Magliano DJ, Barr EL, Zimmet PZ, et al. Glucose indices, health
behaviors, and incidence of diabetes in Australia: the Australian Diabetes, Obesity and Lifestyle Study. Diabetes Care.
2008;31:267–72.

45. Sjöström L, Peltonen M, Jacobson P, et al. Bariatric surgery
and long-term cardiovascular events. J Amer Med Assoc.
2012;307:56–65.

46. Booth H, Khan O, Prevost T, et al. Incidence of type 2 diabetes
after bariatric surgery: population-based matched cohort study.
Lancet Diabetes Endocrinol. 2014;2:963–8.

47. Institute of Medicine (U.S.). Committee on the Consequences of
Sodium Reduction in Populations, et al. Sodium intake in popu-
lations: assessment of evidence. xiv. Washington, DC: National
Academies Press; 2013. 209 p.

48. Institute of Medicine (U.S.). Committee on Strategies to Reduce
Sodium Intake, et al. Strategies to reduce sodium intake in the
United States. xii. Washington, DC: National Academies Press;
2010. 493 p.

49. Report of the Dietary Guidelines Advisory Committee on the Dietary Guidelines for Americans. U.D.o.H.a.H.S. U.S. Department
of Agriculture, Editors. Washington, DC: U.S. Department of Agriculture, US Department of Health and Human Services; 2010.

50. Mozaffarian D, et al. Heart disease and stroke statistics-2015 update: a report from the American Heart Association. Circulation.
2015;131(4):e29–322.

51. Svetkey LP, et al. The DASH diet, sodium intake and blood pres-
sure trial (DASH-sodium): rationale and design. DASH-Sodium
Collaborative Research Group. J Am Diet Assoc. 1999;99(8
Suppl):S96–104.

52. Vollmer WM, et al. Effects of diet and sodium intake on blood
pressure: subgroup analysis of the DASH-sodium trial. Ann Intern
Med. 2001;135(12):1019–28.

53. Sacks FM, et al. Effects on blood pressure of reduced dietary sodium and the dietary approaches to stop hypertension (DASH)
diet. DASH-Sodium Collaborative Research Group. N Engl J
Med. 2001;344(1):3–10.

54. Eckel RH, et al. 2013 AHA/ACC guideline on lifestyle management to reduce cardiovascular risk: a report of the American College of Cardiology/American Heart Association Task Force on
Practice Guidelines. Circulation. 2014;129(25 Suppl 2):S76–99.

55. Svetkey LP, et al. Effects of dietary patterns on blood pressure: subgroup analysis of the dietary approaches to stop hypertension (DASH) randomized clinical trial. Arch Intern Med.
1999;159(3):285–93.

56. Elder CR, et al. Impact of sleep, screen time, depression and stress
on weight change in the intensive weight loss phase of the LIFE
study. Int J Obes. 2012;36(1):86–92.

57. Appel LJ, et al. Effects of comprehensive lifestyle modification
on blood pressure control: main results of the PREMIER clinical
trial. JAMA. 2003;289(16):2083–93.

58. Hoy MK, Goldman JD. Potassium intake of the US population:
what we eat in America, NHANES 2009–1010. Food Surveys Research Group Dietary Data Brief No. 10; 2012. 10.

59. Cappuccio FP, MacGregor GA. Does potassium supplementation
lower blood pressure? A meta-analysis of published trials. J Hypertens. 1991;9(5):465–73.

60. Geleijnse JM, Kok FJ, Grobbee DE. Blood pressure response to
changes in sodium and potassium intake: a metaregression analysis of randomised trials. J Hum Hypertens. 2003;17(7):471–80.

61. Whelton PK, et al. Effects of oral potassium on blood pressure.
Meta-analysis of randomized controlled clinical trials. JAMA.
1997;277(20):1624–32.

62. Aburto NJ, et al. Effect of increased potassium intake on cardiovascular risk factors and disease: systematic review and meta-
analyses. BMJ. 2013;346:f1378.

63. Medicine, I.o., Dietary Reference Intakes for Water, Potassium,
Sodium, Chloride, and Sulfate. 2005: National Academies Press.

64. Puddey IB, Vandongen R, Beilin LJ. Pressor effect of alcohol.
Lancet. 1985;2(8464):1119–20.

65. Klatsky AL, et al. Alcohol consumption and blood pressure Kai-
ser-Permanente multiphasic health examination data. N Engl J
Med. 1977;296(21):1194–200.

66. Fuchs FD, et al. Alcohol consumption and the incidence of hypertension: The Atherosclerosis Risk in Communities Study. Hypertension. 2001;37(5):1242–50.

67. Puddey IB, et al. A randomized controlled trial of the effect of
alcohol consumption on blood pressure. Clin Exp Pharmacol
Physiol. 1985;12(3):257–61.

68. Chobanian AV, et al. The seventh report of the Joint National Committee on prevention, detection, evaluation, and treatment of high
blood pressure: the JNC 7 report. JAMA. 2003;289(19):2560–72.

69. Siebenhofer A, et al. Long-term effects of weight-reducing
diets in hypertensive patients. Cochrane Database Syst Rev.
2011;(9):CD008274.

70. Staessen J, Fagard R, Amery A. The relationship between body
weight and blood pressure. J Hum Hypertens. 1988;2(4):207–17.

71. Bushman B. Promoting exercise as medicine for prediabetes and
prehypertension. Curr Sports Med Rep. 2014;13(4):233–9.

72. Medicine, A.C.o.S., ACSM's Guidelines for Exercise Testing and
Prescription. 9th ed. 2014, Philadelphia: Lippincott Williams and
Wilkins.

73. Cornelissen VA, Smart NA. Exercise training for blood pressure: a systematic review and meta-analysis. J Am Heart Assoc.
2013;2(1):e004473.

74. Kokkinos P. Cardiorespiratory fitness, exercise, and blood pressure. Hypertension. 2014;64(6):1160–4.

75. Barlow CE, et al. Cardiorespiratory fitness is an independent predictor of hypertension incidence among initially normotensive
healthy women. Am J Epidemiol. 2006;163(2):142–50.

76. Huai P, et al. Physical activity and risk of hypertension: a meta-analysis of prospective cohort studies. Hypertension. 2013;62(6):1021–6.

77. Staffileno BA, et al. Blood pressure responses to lifestyle physical activity among young, hypertension-prone African-American women. J Cardiovasc Nurs. 2007;22(2):107–17.

78. Cornelissen VA, Buys R, Smart NA. Endurance exercise beneficially affects ambulatory blood pressure: a systematic review and meta-analysis. J Hypertens. 2013;31(4):639–48.

79. Cornelissen VA, et al. Impact of resistance training on blood pressure and other cardiovascular risk factors: a meta-analysis of randomized, controlled trials. Hypertension. 2011;58(5):950–8.

80. Hanson S, Jones A. Is there evidence that walking groups have health benefits? A systematic review and meta-analysis. Br J Sports Med, 2015.

81. Garvey WT, Kwon S, Zheng D, Shaughnessy S, Wallace P, Pugh K, Jenkins AJ, Klein RL, Liao Y. The effects of insulin resistance and type 2 diabetes mellitus on lipoprotein subclass particle size and concentration determined by nuclear magnetic resonance. Diabetes. 2003;52:453–62.

82. Zambon A, Hokanson JE, Brown BG, Brunzell JD. Evidence for a new pathophysiological mechanism for coronary artery regression: hepatic lipase-mediated changes in LDL density. Circulation. 1999;99:1959–64.

83. St-Pierre AC, Cantin B, Dagenais GR, Mauriege P, Bernard PM, Despres JP, Lamarche B. Low density lipoprotein subfractions and the long term risk of ischemic heart disease in men: 13-year follow up data from the Quebec Cardiovascular Study. Arterioscler Thronmb Vasc Biol. 2005;25:553–9.

84. Ip S, Lichtenstein AH, Chung M, Lau J, Balk EM. Systematic review: Association of low-density lipoprotein subfractions with cardiovascular outcomes. Ann Intern Med. 2009;150:474–84.

85. Mora S, Szklo M, Otvos JD, Greenland P, Psaty BM, Goff JDC, O'Leary DH, Saad MF, Tsai MY, Sharrett AR. LDL particle subclasses, LDL particle size, and carotid atherosclerosis in the Multi-Ethnic Study of Atherosclerosis (MESA). Atherosclerosis. 2007;192:211–7.

86. Jellinger PS, Smith DA, Mehta AE, Ganda O, Handelsman Y, Rodbard HW, Shepherd MD, Seibel JA. AACE Task Force for Management of Dyslipidemia and Prevention of Atherosclerosis. American Association of Clinical Endocrinologists' Guidelines for Management of Dyslipidemia and Prevention of Atherosclerosis. Endocr Pract. 2012;18 Suppl 1:1–78.

87. Garber AJ, Abrahamson MJ, Barzilay JI, Blonde L, Bloomgarden ZT, Bush MA, Dagogo-Jack S, Davidson MB, Einhorn D, Garber JR, Garvey WT, Grunberger G, Handelsman Y, Hirsch IB, Jellinger PS, McGill JB, Mechanick JI, Rosenblit PD, Umpierrez G, Davidson MH. Aace/ace comprehensive diabetes management algorithm 2015. Endocr Pract. 2015;21(4):438–47.

88. Jacobson TA, Ito MK, Maki KC, et al. National Lipid Association recommendations for patient-centered management of dyslipidemia: part 1-executive summary. J Clin Lipidol. 2014;8(5):473–88.

89. Ewald N, Hardt PD, Kloer HU. Severe hypertriglyceridemia and pancreatitis: presentation and management. Curr Opin Lipidol. 2009; 20:497–504.

90. National Cholesterol Education Program (NCEP) Expert Panel on Detection, Evaluation, and Treatment of High Blood Cholesterol in Adults (Adult Treatment Panel III). Third Report of the National Cholesterol Education Program (NCEP) Expert Panel on Detection, Evaluation, and Treatment of High Blood Cholesterol in Adults (Adult Treatment Panel III) final report. Circulation. 2002. 17; 106(25):3143–3421.

91. Johnson RK, Appel LJ, Brands M, Howard BV, Lefevre M, Lustig RH, Sacks F, Steffen LM, Wylie-Rosett J, American Heart Association Nutrition Committee of the Council on Nutrition, Physical Activity, and Metabolism and the Council on Epidemiology and Prevention. Dietary sugars intake and cardiovascular health: a scientific statement from the American Heart Association. Circulation. 2009;120(11):1011–20.

92. Appel LJ, Sacks FM, Carey VJ, Obarzanek E, Swain JF, Miller ER 3rd, Conlin PR, Erlinger TP, Rosner BA, Laranjo NM, Charleston J, McCarron P, Bishop LM, OmniHeart Collaborative Research Group. Effects of protein, monounsaturated fat, and carbohydrate intake on blood pressure and serum lipids: results of the Omni-Heart randomized trial. JAMA. 2005;294(19):2455–64.

93. de Souza RJ, Swain JF, Appel LJ, Sacks FM. Alternatives for macronutrient intake and chronic disease: a comparison of the OmniHeart diets with popular diets and with dietary recommendations. Am J Clin Nutr. 2008;88(1):1–11.

94. Miller M, Stone NJ, Ballantyne C, et al., American Heart Association Clinical Lipidology, Thrombosis, and Prevention Committee of the Council on Nutrition, Physical Activity, and Metabolism; Council on Arteriosclerosis, Thrombosis and Vascular Biology; Council on Cardiovascular Nursing; Council on the Kidney in Cardiovascular Disease. Triglycerides and cardiovascular disease: a scientific statement from the American Heart Association. Circulation. 2011;123:2292–333.

95. Bays HE, Toth PP, Kris-Etherton PM, et al. Obesity, adiposity, and dyslipidemia: a consensus statement from the National Lipid Association. J Clin Lipidol. 2013;7:304–83.

96. Mensink RP, Zock PL, Kester AD, Katan MB. Effects of dietary fatty acids and carbohydrates on the ratio of serum total to HDL cholesterol and on serum lipids and apolipoproteins: a meta-analysis of 60 controlled trials. Am J Clin Nutr. 2003;77:1146–55.

97. Itsiopoulos C, Brazionis L, Kaimakamis M, et al. Can the Mediterranean diet lower HbA1c in type 2 diabetes? Results from a randomized cross-over study. Nutr Metab Cardiovasc Dis. 2011;21:740–7.

98. Estruch R, Ros E, Salas-Savado J, et al. PREDIMED Study Investigators. Primary prevention of cardiovascular disease with a Mediterranean diet. N Engl J Med. 2013;368:1279–90.

99. Elhayany A, Lustman A, Abel R, Attal-Singer J, Vinker S. A low carbohydrate Mediterranean diet improves cardiovascular risk factors and diabetes control among overweight patients with type 2 diabetes mellitus: a 1-year prospective randomized intervention study. Diabetes Obes Metab. 2010;12:204–9.

100. Shai I, Schwarzfuchs D, Henkin Y, et al., Dietary Intervention Randomized Controlled Trial (DIRECT) Group. Weight loss with a low-carbohydrate, Mediterranean, or low-fat diet. N Engl J Med. 2009;359:229–41.

101. Kjems L, Filozof C, Wright M, Keefe D. Association between fasting triglycerides and presence of fasting chylomicrons in patients with severe hypertriglyceridemia. J Clin Lipidol. 2014;8:312. (Abstract 121).

102. Viljoen A, Wierzbicki AS. Diagnosis and treatment of severe hypertriglyceridemia. Expert Rev Cardiovasc Ther. 2012;10:505–14.

103. Nordmann AJ, Nordmann A, Briel M, Keller U, Yancy WS Jr, Brehm BJ, Bucher HC. Effects of low-carbohydrate vs low-fat diets on weight loss and cardiovascular risk factors: a meta-analysis of randomized controlled trials. JAMA Intern Med. 2006;166(3):285–93. Erratum in: JAMA Intern Med. 2006;166(8):932.

104. Morgan LM, Griffin BA, Millward DJ, DeLooy A, Fox KR, Baic S, Bonham MP, Wallace JM, MacDonald I, Taylor MA, Truby H. Comparison of the effects of four commercially available weight-loss programmes on lipid-based cardiovascular risk factors. Public Health Nutr. 2009;12(6):799–807.

105. Varady KA, Bhutani S, Klempel MC, Lamarche B. Improvements in LDL particle size and distribution by short-term alternate day modified fasting in obese adults. Br J Nutr. 2011;105(4):580–3.

106. Varady KA, Bhutani S, Klempel MC, Kroeger CM. Comparison of effects of diet versus exercise weight loss regimens on LDL and HDL particle size in obese adults. Lipids Health Dis. 2011;10:119.

107. Krauss RM, Blanche PJ, Rawlings RS, Fernstrom HS, Williams PT. Separate effects of reduced carbohydrate intake and weight loss on atherogenic dyslipidemia. Am J Clin Nutr. 2006;83(5):1025–31.

108. Wood RJ, Volek JS, Liu Y, Shachter NS, Contois JH, Fernandez ML. Carbohydrate restriction alters lipoprotein metabolism by modifying VLDL, LDL, and HDL subfraction distribution and size in overweight men. J Nutr. 2006;136(2):384–9.

109. Richard C, Couture P, Ooi EM, Tremblay AJ, Desroches S, Charest A, Lichtenstein AH, Lamarche B. Effect of Mediterranean diet with and without weight loss on apolipoprotein B100 metabolism in men with metabolic syndrome. Arterioscler Thromb Vasc Biol. 2014;34(2):433–8.

110. Graham TE. Exercise, postprandial triacylgyceridemia, and cardiovascular disease risk. Can J Appl Physiol. 2004;29:781–99.

111. Dekker MJ, Graham TE, Ooi TC, Robinson LE. Exercise prior to fat ingestion lowers fasting and postprandial VLDL and decreases adipose tissue IL-6 and GIP receptor mRNA in hypertriacylglycerolemic men. J Nutr Biochem. 2010;21(10):983–90.

112. Tambalis K, Panagiotakos DB, Kavouras SA, Sidossis LS. Responses of blood lipids to aerobic, resistance, and combined aerobic with resistance exercise training: a systematic review of current evidence. Angiology. 2009;60(5):614–32.

113. Pitsavos C, Panagiotakos DB, Tambalis KD, Chrysohoou C, Sidossis LS, Skoumas J, Stefanadis C. Resistance exercise plus to aerobic activities is associated with better lipids' profile among healthy individuals: the ATTICA study. Q J Med. 2009;102(9):609–16.

114. http://www.health.gov/dietaryguidelines/2015-scientific-report/PDFs/Scientific-Report-of-the-2015-Dietary-Guidelines-Advisory-Committee.pdf.

115. Ridker PM, Danielson E, Fonseca FA, Genest J, Gotto AM Jr, Kastelein JJ, Koenig W, Libby P, Lorenzatti AJ, MacFadyen JG, Nordestgaard BG, Shepherd J, Willerson JT, Glynn RJ, JUPITER Study Group. Rosuvastatin to prevent vascular events in men and women with elevated C-reactive protein. N Engl J Med. 2008;359(21):2195–207.

116. Lara-Castro C, Garvey WT. Diet, insulin resistance, and obesity: zoning in on data for Atkins dieters living in South Beach. J Clin Endocrinol Metab. 2004;89:4197–205.

117. Dansinger ML, Gleason JA, Griffith JL, Selker HP, Schaefer EJ. Comparison of the Atkins, Ornish, Weight Watchers, and Zone diets for weight loss and heart disease risk reduction: a randomized trial. J Amer Med Assoc. 2005;293(1):43–53.

118. Stern L, Iqbal N, Seshadri P, et al. The effects of low-carbohydrate versus conventional weight loss diets in severely obese adults: one-year follow-up of a randomized trial. Ann Intern Med. 2004;140:778–85.

119. Weinsier RL, Wilson NP, Morgan SL, Cornwell AR, Craig CB. EatRight lose weight: seven simple steps. Birmingham: Oxmoor House; 1997.

120. Greene LF, Malpede CZ, Henson CS, Hubbert KA, Heimburger DC, Ard JD. Weight maintenance 2 years after participation in a weight loss program promoting low-energy density foods. Obesity. 2006;10:1795–801.

121. Ard JD, Cox TL, Zunker C, Wingo BC, Jefferson WK, Brakhage C. A study of a culturally enhanced EatRight dietary intervention in a predominately African American workplace. J Public Health Manag Pract. 2010;16(6):E1–8.

122. Turner-McGrievy GM, Barnard ND, Cohen J, Jenkins DJA, Gloede L, Green AA. Changes in nutrient intake and dietary quality among participants with type 2 diabetes following a lowfat vegan diet or a conventional diabetes diet for 22 weeks. J Am Diet Assoc. 2008;108:1636–45.

123. Foster GD, Wyatt HR, Hill JO, McGuckin BG, Brill C, Mohammed BS, Szapary PO, Rader DJ, Edman JS, Klein S. A randomized trial of a low-carbohydrate diet for obesity. N Engl J Med. 2003;348:2082–90.

124. Samaha FF, Iqbal N, Seshadri P, Chicano KL, Daily DA, McGrory J, Williams T, Williams M, Gracely EJ, Stern L. A low-carbohydrate as compared with a low-fat diet in severe obesity. N Engl J Med. 2003;348:2074–81.

125. Lovejoy JC, Windhauser MM, Rood JC, de la Bretonne JA. Effect of a controlled high-fat versus low-fat diet on insulin sensitivity and leptin levels in African-American and Caucasian women. Metabolism. 1998;47:1520–4.

126. Astrup A, Astrup A, Buemann B, Flint A, Raben A. Low-fat diets and energy balance: how does the evidence stand in 2002? Proc Nutr Soc. 2002;61:299–309.

127. Schwartz MW, Figlewicz DP, Baskin DG, Woods SC, Porte D Jr. Insulin in the brain: a hormonal regulator of energy balance. Endocr Rev. 1992;13:387–414.

128. Ludwig DS. Dietary glycemic index and obesity. J Nutr. 2000;130:280S–3.

129. Roberts SB. High-glycemic index foods, hunger, and obesity: is there a connection? Nutr Rev. 2000;58:163–9.

130. Pi-Sunyer FX. Glycemic index and disease. Am J Clin Nutr. 2002;76:290S–8.

131. World Health Organization. Diet, nutrition and the prevention of chronic diseases. 916. Geneva: WHO Technical Report Series; 2003.

132. Pereira MA, Jacobs DR Jr, Pins JJ, Raatz SK, Gross MD, Slavin JL, Seaquist ER. Effect of whole grains on insulin sensitivity in overweight hyperinsulinemic adults. Am J Clin Nutr. 2002;75:848–55.

133. Hu FB, van Dam RM, Liu S. Diet and risk of type II diabetes: the role of types of fat and carbohydrate. Diabetologia. 2001;44(7):805–17.

134. Heymsfield SB, van Mierlo CA, van der Knaap HC, Heo M, Frier HI. Weight management using a meal replacement strategy: meta and pooling analysis from six studies. Int J Obes Relat Metab Disord. 2003;27:537–49.

135. Harris JA, Benedict FG. A biometric study of basal metabolism in man. Washington, DC: Carnegie Institute of Washington; 1919 (publ. no. 279).

136. Mifflin MD, St. Jeor ST, Hill LA, Scott BJ, Daugherty SA, Koh YO. A new predictive equation for resting energy expenditure in healthy individuals. Am J Clin Nutr. 1990;51:251–7.

137. Martin K, Wallace P, Rust PF, Garvey WT. Estimation of resting energy expenditure considering effects of race and diabetes status. Diabetes Care. 2004;27:1405–11.

138. Hipskind P, Glass C, Charlton D, Nowak D, Dasarathy S. Do handheld calorimeters have a role in assessment of nutrition needs in hospitalized patients? A systematic review of literature. Nutr Clin Pract. 2011;26(4):426–33.

139. Wing RR, Lang W, Wadden TA, et al. The Look AHEAD Research Group. Benefits of modest weight loss in improving cardiovascular risk factors in overweight and obese individuals with type 2 diabetes. Diabetes Care. 2011;34:1481–6.

140. Rivellese AA, De Natale C, Lilli S. Type of dietary fat and insulin resistance. Ann N Y Acad Sci. 2002;967:329–35.

141. Mayer-Davis EJ, Monaco JH, Hoen HM, Carmichael S, Vitolins MZ, Rewers MJ, Haffner SM, Ayad MF, Bergman RN, Karter AJ. Dietary fat and insulin sensitivity in a triethnic population: the role of obesity. The Insulin Resistance Atherosclerosis Study (IRAS). Am J Clin Nutr. 1997;65:79–87.

142. Maron DJ, Fair JM, Haskell WL. Saturated fat intake and insulin resistance in men with coronary artery disease. The Stanford Coronary Risk Intervention Project Investigators and Staff. Circulation. 1991;84:2020–7.

143. Marshall JA, Bessesen DH, Hamman RF. High saturated fat and low starch and fibre are associated with hyperinsulinaemia in a non-diabetic population: the San Luis Valley Diabetes Study. Diabetologia. 1997;40:430–8.

144. Salmeron J, Hu FB, Manson JE, Stampfer MJ, Colditz GA, Rimm EB, Willett WC. Dietary fat intake and risk of Type 2 Diabetes in women. Am J Clin Nutr. 2001;73:1019–26.

145. Summers LK, Fielding BA, Bradshaw HA, Ilic V, Beysen C, Clark ML, Moore NR, Frayn KN. Substituting dietary saturated fat with polyunsaturated fat changes abdominal fat distribution and improves insulin sensitivity. Diabetologia. 2002;45:369–77.

146. Mayer EJ, Newman B, Quesenberry CP Jr, Selby JV. Usual dietary fat intake and insulin concentrations in healthy women twins. Diabetes Care. 1993;16:1459–69.

147. Simopoulos AP. Omega-3 fatty acids in the prevention-management of cardiovascular disease. Can J Physiol Pharmacol. 1997;75:234–9.

148. Vessby B, Aro A, Skarfors E, Berglund L, Salminen I, Lithell H. The risk to develop NIDDM is related to the fatty acid composition of the serum cholesterol esters. Diabetes. 1994;43:1353–7.

149. Garg A. High-monounsaturated-fat diets for patients with diabetes mellitus: a meta-analysis. Am J Clin Nutr. 1998;67:577S–82.

150. Perez-Jimenez F, Lopez-Miranda J, Pinillos MD, Gomez P, Paz-Rojas E, Montilla P, Marin C, Velasco MJ, Blanco-Molina A, Jimenez Pereperez JA, Ordovas JM. A Mediterranean and a high-carbohydrate diet improve glucose metabolism in healthy young persons. Diabetologia. 2001;44:2038–43.

151. Thomsen C, Rasmussen O, Christiansen C, Pedersen E, Vesterlund M, Storm H, Ingerslev J, Hermansen K. Comparison of the effects of a monounsaturated fat diet and a high carbohydrate diet on cardiovascular risk factors in first degree relatives to Type-2 diabetic subjects. Eur J Clin Nutr. 1999;53:818–23.

152. Kiens B, Richter EA. Types of carbohydrate in an ordinary diet affect insulin action and muscle substrates in humans. Am J Clin Nutr. 1996;63:47–53.

153. Liese AD, Roach AK, Sparks KC, Marquart L, D'Agostino RB Jr, Mayer-Davis EJ. Whole-grain intake and insulin sensitivity: the Insulin Resistance Atherosclerosis Study. Am J Clin Nutr. 2003;78:965–71.

154. McKeown NM, Meigs JB, Liu S, Saltzman E, Wilson PW, Jacques PF. Carbohydrate nutrition, insulin resistance, and the prevalence of the metabolic syndrome in the Framingham Offspring Cohort. Diabetes Care. 2004;27:538–46.

155. Pereira MA, Jacobs DR Jr, Pins JJ, Raatz SK, Gross MD, Slavin JL, Seaquist ER. Effect of whole grains on insulin sensitivity in overweight hyperinsulinemic adults. Am J Clin Nutr. 2002;75:848–55.

156. Shai I, Schwarzfuchs D, Henkin Y, et al. Dietary Intervention Randomized Controlled Trial (DIRECT) Group. Weight loss with a low-carbohydrate, Mediterranean, or low-fat diet. N Engl J Med. 2009;359:229–41.

157. de Lorgeril M, Salen P, Martin JL, Monjaud I, Delaye J, Mamelle N. Mediterranean diet, traditional risk factors, and the rate of cardiovascular complications after myocardial infarction: final report of the Lyon Diet Heart Study. Circulation. 1999;99(6):779–85.

158. Martinez-Gonzalez MA, Bes-Rastrollo M. Dietary patterns, Mediterranean diet, and cardiovascular disease. Curr Opin Lipidol. 2014;25(1):20–6.

159. Hoevenaar-Blom MP, Nooyens AC, Kromhout D, Spijkerman AM, Beulens JW, van der Schouw YT, Bueno-de-Mesquita B, Verschuren WM. Mediterranean style diet and 12-year incidence of cardiovascular diseases: the EPIC-NL cohort study. PLoS ONE. 2012;7(9):e45458.

160. Kastorini CM, Milionis HJ, Esposito K, Giugliano D, Goudevenos JA, Panagiotakos DB. The effect of Mediterranean diet on metabolic syndrome and its components: a meta-analysis of 50 studies and 534,906 individuals. J Am Coll Cardiol. 2011;57:1299–313.

161. Esposito K, Maiorino MI, Ceriello A, Giugliano D. Prevention and control of type 2 diabetes by Mediterranean diet: a systematic review. Diabetes Res Clin Pract. 2010;89:97–102.

162. Salas-Salvadó J, Bulló M, Babio N, et al. Reduction in the incidence of type 2 diabetes with the Mediterranean diet: results of the PREDIMED-Reus nutrition intervention randomized trial. Diabetes Care. 2011;34:14–9.

163. Martínez-González MA, de la Fuente-Arrillaga C, Nuñez-Córdoba JM, et al. Adherence to Mediterranean diet and risk of developing diabetes: prospective cohort study. Brit Med J. 2008;336:1348–51.

164. Salas-Salvadó J, Fernández-Ballart J, Ros E, et al. Effect of a Mediterranean diet supplemented with nuts on metabolic syndrome status: one-year results of the PREDIMED randomized trial. Arch Intern Med. 2008;168:2449–58.

165. Jeon CY, Lokken RP, Hu FB, van Dam RM. Physical activity of moderate intensity and risk of type 2 diabetes: a systematic review. Diabetes Care. 2007;30(3):744–52.

166. Duncan GE, Perri MG, Theriaque DW, Hutson AD, Eckel RH, Stacpoole PW. Exercise training, without weight loss, increases insulin sensitivity and postheparin plasma lipase activity in previously sedentary adults. Diabetes Care. 2003;26(3):557–62.

167. Houmard JA, Tanner CJ, Slentz CA, Duscha BD, McCartney JS, Kraus WE. Effect of the volume and intensity of exercise training on insulin sensitivity. J Appl Physiol. 2004;96(1):101–6.

168. Bajpeyi S, Tanner CJ, Slentz CA, et al. Effect of exercise intensity and volume on persistence of insulin sensitivity during training cessation. J Appl Physiol. 2009;106(4):1079–85.

169. Myers VH, McVay MA, Brashear MM, Johannsen NM, Swift DL, Kramer K, Harris MN, Johnson WD, Earnest CP, Church TS. Exercise training and quality of life in individuals with type 2 diabetes: a randomized controlled trial. Diabetes Care. 2013;36(7):1884–90.

170. Johannsen NM, Swift DL, Lavie CJ, Earnest CP, Blair SN, Church TS. Categorical analysis of the impact of aerobic and resistance exercise training, alone and in combination, on cardiorespiratory fitness levels in patients with type 2 diabetes: results from the HART-D study. Diabetes Care. 2013;36(10):3305–12.

171. Snowling NJ, Hopkins WG. Effects of different modes of exercise training on glucose control and risk factors for complications in type 2 diabetic patients: a meta-analysis. Diabetes Care. 2006;29(11):2518–27.

172. Sigal RJ, Kenny GP, Boule NG, Wells GA, Prud'homme D, Fortier M, et al. Effects of aerobic training, resistance training, or both on glycemic control in type 2 diabetes: a randomized trial. Ann Intern Med. 2007;147:357–69.

173. American College of Sports Medicine and the American Diabetes Association. Joint position statement: exercise and type 2 diabetes. Med Sci Sports Exerc. 2010;42:2282–303.

174. Katzmarzyk PT, Church TS, Craig CL, Bouchard C. Sitting time and mortality from all causes, cardiovascular disease, and cancer. Med Sci Sports Exerc. 2009;41(5):998–1005.

175. Helmrich SP, Ragland DR, Leung RW, Paffenbarger RS Jr. Physical activity and reduced occurrence of non-insulin-dependent diabetes mellitus. N Engl J Med. 1991;325(3):147–52.

176. Hu FB, Sigal RJ, Rich-Edwards JW, et al. Walking compared with vigorous physical activity and risk of type 2 diabetes in women: a prospective study. JAMA. 1999;282(15):1433–9.

177. Manson JE, Rimm EB, Stampfer MJ, et al. Physical activity and incidence of non-insulin-dependent diabetes mellitus in women. Lancet. 1991;338(8770):774–8.

178. Bax JJ, Young LH, Frye RL, Bonow RO, Steinberg HO, Barrett EJ. Screening for coronary artery disease in patients with diabetes. Diabetes Care. 2007;30:2729–36.

179. Maclean PS, Bergouignan A, Cornier MA, Jackman MR. Biology's response to dieting: the impetus for weight regain. Am J Physiol Regul Integr Comp Physiol. 2011;301:R581–R600.

180. Leibel RL, Rosenbaum M, Hirsch J. Changes in energy expenditure resulting from altered body weight. N Engl J Med. 1995;332:621–8.

181. Ebbeling CB, Swain JF, Feldman HA, et al. Effects of dietary composition on energy expenditure during weight-loss maintenance. JAMA. 2012;307:2627–34.

182. Sumithran P, Prendergast LA, Delbridge E, et al. Long-term persistence of hormonal adaptations to weight loss. N Engl J Med. 2011;365:1597–604.

183. Sumithran P, Proietto J. The defence of body weight: a physiological basis for weight regain after weight loss. Clin Sci. 2013;124:231–41.

184. Doucet E, Imbeault P, St-Pierre S, et al. Appetite after weight loss by energy restriction and a low-fat diet-exercise follow-up. Int J Obes Relat Metab Disord. 2000;24:906–14.

185. Ochner CN, Barrios DM, Lee CD, Pi-Sunyer FX. Biological mechanisms that promote weight regain following weight loss in obese humans. Physiol Behav. 2013;120:106–13.

186. Fidler MC, Sanchez M, Raether B, et al. A one-year randomized trial of lorcaserin for weight loss in obese and overweight adults: the BLOSSOM trial. J Clin Endocrinol Metab. 2011;96:3067–77.

187. Wadden TA, Foreyt JP, Foster GD, et al. Weight loss with naltrexone SR/bupropion SR combination therapy as an adjunct to behavior modification: the COR-BMOD trial. Obesity. 2011;19:110–20.

188. Wadden TA, Hollander P, Klein S, et al. Weight maintenance and additional weight loss with liraglutide after low-calorie-diet-induced weight loss: the SCALE Maintenance randomized study. Int J Obes. 2013;37:1514.

189. Wadden TA, Berkowitz RI, Sarwer DB, Prus-Wisniewski R, Steinberg C. Benefits of lifestyle modification in the pharmacologic treatment of obesity: a randomized trial. Arch Intern Med. 2001;161(2):218–27.

190. Mechanick JI, Youdim A, Jones DB, et al. Clinical practice guidelines for the perioperative nutritional, metabolic, and nonsurgical support of the bariatric surgery patient-2013 update: cosponsored by American Association of Clinical Endocrinologists, the Obesity Society, and American Society for Metabolic & Bariatric Surgery. Endocr Pract. 2013;19:337–72.

Cancer

24

Elaine Trujillo, Barbara K. Dunn and Peter Greenwald

Abbreviations

BMI	Body Mass Index
FDA	Food and Drug Administration
IL-1	Interleukin-1
IL-6	Interleukin-6
PA	Physical activity
SELECT	Selenium and Vitamin E Cancer Prevention Trial
SNP	Singlenucleotide polymorphisms
TNF-α	Tumor necrosis factor-α
WCRF/AICR	World Cancer Research Fund/American Institute for Cancer Research
WHEL	Women's Healthy Eating and Living
WINS	Women's Intervention Nutrition Study

Introduction

A number of lifestyle factors affect cancer risk and survival in individuals diagnosed with cancer. Key among these is nutrition, along with the related factors of overweight/obesity and energy balance, physical activity (PA), alcohol, and tobacco. These risk factors are "exogenous" in that they generally reflect voluntary exposures, that is, they are based on lifestyle choices. Since they are not innate to the individual, exposure to such adverse cancer-associated factors can be, in theory, avoided. However, "endogenous" factors—innate

E. Trujillo (✉)
Bethesda, MD, USA
e-mail: trujille@mail.nih.gov

P. Greenwald
Division of Cancer Prevention at the National Cancer Institute (NCI), Bethesda, MD, USA

B. K. Dunn
NIH/National Cancer Institute/Division of Cancer Prevention/ Chemopreventive Agent Development Research Group, NIH Clinical Center, 9609 Medical Center Drive, Bethesda, MD 20892, USA
e-mail: dunnb@mail.nih.gov

characteristics of the individual that are not voluntary—can both promote the exposure and influence the effects of exposure of various lifestyle factors in cancer. Specifically, inherited genetic variation among individuals can influence tendencies toward harmful lifestyle exposures. For example, certain inherited genetic variants, including specific single-nucleotide polymorphisms (SNP), are associated with higher levels of craving nicotine, thereby enhancing the level of addiction to tobacco [1]. Similarly, genetic variants have been identified that retard or enhance the carcinogenic effects of these exposures. Not all heavy smokers develop lung cancer, despite long-term exposure to the carcinogens in tobacco. Variability in genes involved in metabolizing tobacco carcinogens and in modulating other tobacco-related carcinogenic mechanisms contributes to determining who actually develops cancer when exposed.

In addition, epigenetic processes influence the adverse or beneficial effects of lifestyle exposures. Unlike genetic variants, which are inherited and involve alterations in the DNA sequence, epigenetic mechanisms comprise several processes that influence whether a gene is expressed in a given cell. In some cases, epigenetic changes can also be inherited and, hence, are considered to be "metastable." The three basic molecular mechanisms that contribute to epigenetic changes in the cell include methylation of DNA, histone modifications, and expression of microRNAs. These mechanisms work together to up- or downregulate gene expression. The epigenetic modifications in cancer cells often diverge from those in the normal cells of the same tissue type, with the differential modifications presumably contributing to carcinogenesis. Importantly, lifestyle factors influence epigenetic modifications and ultimately the profile of expressed genes. In this manner, epigenetic processes serve as a venue through which exogenous lifestyle exposures are funneled mechanistically into the molecular pathways that regulate gene expression. Dietary components, often referred to as bioactive food components, are known to modify methylation of DNA in a manner that can increase or decrease carcinogenesis [2]. As

J. I. Mechanick, R. F. Kushner (eds.), *Lifestyle Medicine*, DOI 10.1007/978-3-319-24687-1_24

an example, epigallocatechin-3-gallate, a key constituent of green tea, inhibits the procarcinogenic DNA methylation that is observed in a number of cancers, including esophageal, colon, prostate, and mammary cancers. Diet–epigenome interactions are believed to occur in utero, yielding an early-life impact of nutrition on carcinogenesis later in life.

Nutrition

In 1981, Doll and Peto [3] estimated that approximately 30% of cancers are associated with diet (see Fig. 24.1). Diet, a person's genetic makeup, and the cancer type are key components in the diet–cancer relationship. The term "diet" is often used broadly when applied to cancer research. Diet may imply a dietary pattern, such as a vegetarian diet, or the Mediterranean-style eating pattern. Diet may also refer to specific foods, nutrients, and bioactive food compounds, of which there are thousands, many of which are thought to play a role in cancer prevention.

Public health guidelines for cancer prevention from the World Cancer Research Fund/American Institute for Cancer Research (WCRF/AICR) [4], the World Health Organization [5], and the American Cancer Society [6] recommend a plant-based diet (Table 24.1). Although the specific recommendations of these organizations vary, the basis of the recommendations includes a diet rich in a variety of vegetables and fruits, legumes, nuts, whole grains, minimally processed staple foods, limited red and processed meat, limited fats, especially saturated fats, limited refined starchy foods (such as sugars and sweets), limited salt, and limited alcohol intake. In 2007, the WCRF/AICR compiled a comprehensive evidence-based report on the role of food, nutrition, and can-

cer prevention [4] and it continues to update the information through the Continuous Update Project [7–11].

In addition to a plant-based diet, many nutrients and bioactive food components from plant and animal products continue to be studied for their potential anticancer properties (see Table 24.2). Although the evidence varies and is sometimes unclear, the weight of evidence suggests that diet plays a role in cancer development and risk.

Large Nutrition and Cancer Clinical Trials

Although general dietary patterns are usually emphasized for cancer prevention, few clinical trials have proven cancer reduction related to diet modification. The Women's Health Initiative Dietary Modification Trial [12] was the largest and longest randomized controlled study of the effect of dietary change on disease outcomes in postmenopausal women. Diet modification aimed at reducing fat intake to 20% of energy and increasing consumption of vegetables, fruits, and grains failed to significantly reduce the risk of colorectal or breast cancer during 8 years of follow-up, although breast cancer was nonsignificantly reduced by 9% [12]. Another component of the trial found that taking 1000 mg/day of calcium plus 400 international units of vitamin D3 had no effect on colorectal cancer risk [12].

Because of the high rates of esophageal/gastric cardia cancer and low intakes of several nutrients in Linxian, China, a large randomized, double-blind placebo trial was conducted in this region [13]. In this trial, 4 different combinations of 9 vitamins and minerals were provided to approximately 30,000 adults who were followed for about 5 years [13]. Those who received a combination of selenium, beta-carotene, and vitamin E had reduced total mortality, total cancer mortality, and total gastric cancer mortality, and the beneficial effects were still seen up to 10 years after ending supplementation [13].

The Selenium and Vitamin E Cancer Prevention Trial (SELECT) [14] found that selenium and vitamin E, taken alone or together for an average of 5.5 years, did not prevent prostate cancer. In fact, the men taking vitamin E had a 17% increased risk of prostate cancer compared to men taking the placebo; men who started the trial with high levels of selenium doubled their risk of developing a high-grade prostate cancer by taking selenium supplements and men who had low levels of selenium at the start of the trial doubled their risk of high-grade prostate cancer by taking vitamin E [14].

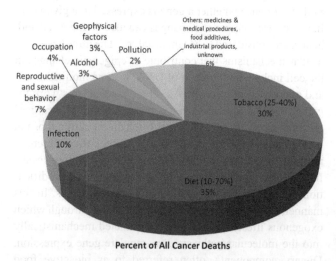

Percent of All Cancer Deaths

Fig. 24.1 Proportions of cancer deaths attributed to various factors [3]. Data represent the best estimate of percent of all cancer deaths. The range of acceptable estimates is shown for diet and tobacco in *parentheses*

Fruits and Vegetables

A plant-based diet including fruits and non-starchy vegetables is associated with reduced risk of developing several cancers, in particular, cancers of the mouth, pharynx, larynx,

Table 24.1 Lifestyle guidelines for cancer prevention. (Adapted from: Appendix 1: Public Health Guidelines for Cancer Prevention and Survivorship. In: Leser M, Ledesma N, Bergerson S, Trujillo E, eds. Oncology Nutrition for Clinical Practice. Chicago, IL: Oncology Nutrition Dietetic Practice Group; 2013:249–250)

	World Cancer Research Fund American Institute for Cancer Research	World Health Organization
Plant-based diet	Choose a plant-based diet rich in a variety of vegetables and fruits, legumes, and minimally processed starchy staple foods	Increase consumption of fruits and vegetables, legumes and whole grains, and nuts
Vegetable and fruit	Eat five or more portions (14 oz or 400 g) of a variety of non-starchy vegetables and of fruits daily	Increase consumption of fruits and vegetables, legumes and whole grains, and nuts. Consume at least 400 g of total fruits and vegetables per day
Breads, grains and cereals	Eat relatively unprocessed cereals (grains) and/or legumes with every meal	Increase consumption of fruits and vegetables, legumes and whole grains, and nuts
Animal products	People who eat red meat should limit intake to less than 18 oz per week, very little, if any, to be processed	Moderate consumption of preserved meat (sausage, salami, bacon, and ham) and red meat (beef, pork, and lamb). Poultry and fish are preferable
Dietary fat	Consume energy-dense foods sparingly. Certain plant oils, nuts, and seeds are important sources of fat and nutrients and should not be avoided	Limit energy intake from fat and shift fat consumption away from saturated fats to unsaturated fats. Eliminate *trans* fat consumption
Processed foods and refined sugar	Eat relatively unprocessed cereals (grains) and/or legumes with every meal. Limit refined starchy foods. Avoid sugary drinks	Limit the intake of free sugars
Salt and sodium	Limit consumption of processed foods with added salt to ensure an intake of less than 6 g (2.4 g sodium) per day	Limit salt (sodium) consumption from all sources and ensure that salt is iodized
Alcohol	If consumed at all, limit alcoholic drinks to no more than two drinks a day for men and one for women	Consumption of alcoholic beverages is not recommended. If consumed, do not exceed 20 g per day
Dietary supplements	For those who follow the above recommendations, dietary supplements are not recommended for reducing cancer risk. Aim to meet nutrient needs through diet alone. Talk with your health care team about supplements for other specific health reasons	No recommendations provided
Body weight	Be as lean as possible within the normal range of body weight. Maintain body weight within the normal range from age 21. Avoid weight gain and increases in waist circumference throughout adulthood	Achieve energy balance and a healthy weight. Maintain weight such that BMI is in the range of 18.5–25 kg/m^2 and avoid weight gain during adulthood
Physical activity	Be moderately physically active for at least 30 min every day. As fitness improves, aim for 60 min or more of moderate, or 30 min or more of vigorous physical activity every day. Limit sedentary habits like watching television	Engage in regular physical activity. Adults aged 18–64 should accumulate at least 150 min of moderate intensity aerobic activity or at least 75 min of vigorous aerobic activity throughout the week. Strength training should be done at least 2 days per week

esophagus, stomach, and lung [4]. Nutrients, bioactive food components, and fiber contained in fruits and vegetables are also associated with a decreased risk of several cancers. Public guidelines for cancer prevention recommend a diet high in fruits and vegetables, at least two and half cups daily [6].

Cruciferous vegetables are part of the *Brassica* genus of plants, which includes arugula, broccoli, Brussels sprouts, cabbage, cauliflower, collard greens, kale, radishes, and turnips. They are rich in carotenoids, particularly beta-carotene, lutein, zeaxanthin, as well as vitamins C, E, and K, folate, and minerals. Cruciferous vegetables are also a good source of fiber and a rich source of glucosinolates, which are sulfur-containing compounds responsible for their pungent aroma and bitter taste. Glucosinolates are broken down to form biologically active compounds, such as indole, indole-3-carbinol, and the isothiocyanate, sulforaphane, which in preclinical studies has been found to inhibit the development of cancer of the bladder, breast, colon, liver, lung, and stomach [15]. Studies in humans have shown mixed results and no clear association has emerged. There exists a possibility that genetic variants influence the response to these food components. For example, a glutathione S-transferase genotype has been found to influence the relationship between cruciferous vegetable intake and lung and colorectal cancer risk [16].

Lycopene is the predominant carotenoid in blood and tissues; it is the pigment that gives some fruits and vegetables

Table 24.2 Selected foods, bioactive compounds and mechanisms for cancer prevention

Food	Bioactive compound	Mechanism for protection
Cruciferous vegetables	Indoles and isothiocyanates	DNA damage
		Antiviral and antibacterial effects
		Anti-inflammatory effects
		Induce apoptosis
		Inhibit angiogenesis and tumor cell migration
Dark green leafy vegetables	Folate	DNA damage
		Prevents tumor initiation
		Facilitates progression of precancerous lesions (not protective)
Soy	Isoflavones (genistein, daidzein)	Reduce estradiol exposure
		Modify estrogen metabolites
		Inhibit angiogenesis
		Inhibit growth factors
		Modify genotoxic compounds
Tomato	Carotenoids (lycopene)	Prevent oxidations of DNA, proteins, lipids
		Induce phase II detoxification enzymes
		Suppress carcinogen-induced phosphorylation of regulatory proteins
		Inhibit cell division
Garlic	Allyl sulfur compounds	Block nitrosamine formation
		Suppresses of bioactivation of carcinogens
		Enhance DNA repair
		Reduce cell proliferation
		Induce apoptosis
Fish	Omega-3 fatty acids	Reduce eicosanoid biosynthesis
		Inhibit cyclooxygenase-2
Oats	β (beta)-glucan	Enhance cytotoxicity against tumors

their red coloring. These foods include tomatoes, watermelon, pink grapefruits, apricots, and others. Most of the US dietary lycopene comes from processed tomato products such as sauces, juices, and ketchup. Lycopene in fresh fruits and vegetables is poorly absorbed. Heat processing into tomato paste, juice, and other foods improves lycopene bioavailability. Lycopene seems to reduce plasma prostate-specific antigen levels in men with prostate cancer [17]; epidemiological studies suggest that consuming foods containing lycopene decreases prostate cancer risk [4]. However, interventional study data do not consistently confirm this chemopreventive effect [18].

The vegetable garlic is part of the *Allium* class of bulb-shaped plants that also includes onions, chives, and leeks. Garlic has been used for centuries for its antimicrobial and anticarcinogenic effects, and for protective effects from cardiovascular disease. Garlic contains sulfur, arginine, selenium, potassium, calcium, magnesium, phosphorus, vitamin C, and folate. The allyl sulfur compounds in garlic may block the formation and activation of carcinogens, enhance DNA repair, reduce cell proliferation, and/or induce apoptosis [19]. Preclinical studies provide strong evidence that garlic and its associated sulfur components can suppress tumor incidence in the breast, colon, skin, uterus, esophagus, and lung. Epidemiological studies suggest that garlic intake is associated with a reduced risk of cancers of the gastrointestinal tract, such as the stomach and colon [4]. A dose–response relation-

ship has been identified for colorectal cancer; as garlic intake increased, the risk of colorectal cancer decreased. Although compounds in garlic demonstrate anticancer activity, there is insufficient evidence for recommending garlic supplements.

Folate, an essential B vitamin, is found in fruits and vegetables, especially dark green leafy vegetables. There is some evidence that foods containing folate protect against esophageal cancer [4, 8, 9]. Folate is important for DNA synthesis and DNA repair; folate deficiency may increase the risk of DNA damage. Folate is a good example of a nutrient that may play different roles in different stages of carcinogenesis. Once carcinogenesis in initiated, folate provides substrates for DNA synthesis and accelerates cancer cell proliferation and tumor expansion. The anti-folate chemotherapeutic agent, methotrexate, inhibits folate-mediated DNA synthesis to decrease cell proliferation. Folate in the form of calcium leucovorin may be used to rescue patients suffering from methotrexate toxicity [19].

Folic acid is the supplemental form of folate and is used in vitamin supplements, and, since 1998, has been added to bread and other grain products in order to decrease the occurrence of neural tube defects in newborns. In 2007, the Aspirin and Folic Acid Polyp Prevention Study found unexpected increases in advanced colorectal adenomas and prostate cancer after 7 years of treatment with folic acid. However, a meta-analysis found that folic acid supplementation does not affect cancer incidence [20]. Pharmacologic doses of folic acid supplementation are not warranted for cancer prevention. Eating foods rich in folate has not been associated with cancer risk. Yet, a diet high in folate-rich foods, such as fruits and vegetables, is considered part of a healthy diet.

Meat and Protein

The WCRF/AICR recommends to limit the intake of red meat to less than 500 g (18 ounces) a week and avoid processed meat. Red meat refers to beef, lamb, pork, and goat; processed meat refers to meats preserved by smoking, curing, or salting, or by the addition of chemical preservatives. Processed meats are usually red meats and include ham, bacon, hot dogs, pastrami, salami, and other sausages. These recommendations are based on convincing evidence that red meat and processed meat are causes of colorectal cancer [4, 8].

There are several potential mechanisms that underlie the observed positive association of red meat consumption with colorectal cancer. Red meat contains heme iron, which promotes the formation of potentially carcinogenic N-nitroso compounds. N-nitroso compounds also form when nitrites used to preserve meat combine with amines from amino acids, and also can be created during the curing process. Cooking red meat at high temperatures results in the production of heterocyclic amines and polycyclic aromatic hydrocarbons that can cause colon cancer in people with a genetic predisposition due to specific SNP [8].

Not all animal foods are associated with an increased cancer risk. Poultry, fish, and eggs are not associated with an increased or decreased cancer risk.

Fats

Dietary fat intake has been tied most closely to breast cancer risk, in particular postmenopausal breast cancer. Data from preclinical studies suggest that polyunsaturated fatty acids (PUFA) of the omega-6 class promote cancers at various sites, including the mammary gland. However, epidemiological evidence regarding these fats has been inconsistent and, overall, limited evidence suggests that consumption of total fat is a cause of postmenopausal breast cancer [7].

Two clinical trials looked at the effect of dietary fat reduction and breast cancer outcome. The Women's Healthy Eating and Living (WHEL) trial found that a low-fat intake, with 15–20 % of total calories in the form of fat, along with higher fruit, vegetable, and fiber intake, in breast cancer survivors did not reduce additional breast cancer events [21]. However, the Women's Intervention Nutrition Study (WINS) found that a reduced dietary fat intake, with 20 % of calories coming from fat, resulted in a 24 % reduction in relative risk of breast cancer recurrence with modest weight loss [22]. Sub-

set analyses suggested that the largest risk reduction (42 %) was among women with estrogen receptor-negative disease.

Omega-3 PUFA, both from marine (eicosapentaenoic acid and docosahexaenoic acid) and plant (α-linolenic acid) sources, are recognized to have anticancer activity. The antineoplastic mechanisms of omega-3 PUFA include modulation of cyclooxygenase activity, alteration of membrane dynamics and cell surface receptor function, and suppression of increased cellular oxidative stress. Although studies in animals fed omega-3 PUFA show reduced colorectal tumor incidence, epidemiological studies are inconsistent and do not show a relationship between omega-3 PUFA intakes and colorectal cancer [8]. Studies also suggest that marine omega-3 PUFA may prevent telomere shortening and, thus, may play a role in antagonizing cell aging [23].

Milk, Dairy, and Calcium

As milk and dairy products are good sources of calcium, they are often intertwined. However, the associations appear to be quite different and how milk, cheese, and other dairy products affect cancer risk is difficult to interpret. While milk (from cows) and calcium (from supplements at a dose of 1200 mg/day) probably decrease colorectal cancer risk, limited evidence suggests that cheese may increase colorectal cancer risk [8]. There is more consistency with regard to prostate cancer. Diets high in calcium (around 1.5 g/day) probably increase the risk, and limited evidence suggests that milk and dairy products also increase prostate cancer risk [4]; cheese does not seem to be related to risk.

Calcium and vitamin D act synergistically and evidence suggests that people with lower than average vitamin D levels do not benefit from calcium supplements. Vitamin D is often fortified in dairy products, and small amounts can be found in eggs, mushrooms, and fish. The best source of vitamin D is sunlight exposure. The cancer–vitamin D connection, suggestive of suppression of cancer by vitamin D, originates from the observation that colon cancer mortality rates were lower in the southwestern parts, that is, the sunnier parts of the USA, compared to the northeastern parts of the country. Furthermore, some studies suggest that lower serum 25-hydroxyvitamin D levels are associated with increased risk of breast, prostate, and colorectal cancers. Despite these observations, the weight of the evidence is inconclusive [7, 8]. In a meta-analysis from the US Preventive Services Task Force that examined the benefits and harms of vitamin D with or without calcium supplementation on clinical outcomes, including cancer and fractures in adults, no conclusions could be drawn regarding the benefits or harms of vitamin D supplementation for the prevention of cancer [24]. Vitamin D supplementation is guided by serum 25-hydroxyvitamin D [25(OH)D] levels and there are no guidelines providing optimal levels for cancer prevention. According to the Endocrine Society Clinical Practice Guidelines, a 25(OH)D level below 20 ng/ml is considered vitamin D deficiency and between 21 and 29 ng/ml is considered vitamin D insufficiency [25]. The most widely accepted guidelines are from the Institute of Medicine for bone health, which are for serum levels to be greater than 20 ng/ml.

Grains

Whole grains, such as wheat, oat, barley, brown rice, and rye, contain the cereal germ, endosperm, as well as bran. In contrast, refined grains retain only the endosperm. Whole grains are a good source of dietary fiber. Convincing evidence from epidemiological studies suggests that foods containing dietary fiber reduce colorectal cancer risk [4, 8]. Although the protective role of dietary fiber has not been firmly established, it increases fecal weight and decreases transit time, leading to fewer carcinogen interactions within the colonic mucosa. This decreased transit time may also enhance the removal of secondary bile acids, which is thought to be tumor promoters. In preclinical studies, dietary fermentation products in the colon, such as short-chain fatty acids, induce apoptosis, cell cycle arrest, and differentiation [4].

β-glucans (beta-glucans) are polysaccharides commonly found in oats and other grains, barley, yeast, bacteria, algae, and mushrooms. β-glucans are thought to act as biological response modifiers that restore or enhance humoral and cell-mediated immune responses. They increase macrophage phagocytosis of tumor cells, increase the cytotoxicity of natural killer cells, and stimulate the release of interleukin-1 (IL-1) and tumor necrosis factor-α (TNFα). Most of the anticancer effects of β-glucan have been shown in in vitro and in vivo experimental studies, although preliminary clinical trials in patients with gastric, ovarian, cervical, and head and neck cancers have shown a positive effect on patient survival and quality of life using β-glucans in the adjuvant setting [26].

Legumes

Soy is a legume that has been a staple food in Asia for thousands of years. The low rates of cancer in Asian countries spurred research investigating a possible soy and cancer connection. Soybeans are used to make tofu, flours, and sauces, and pure soy protein, or soy isolate, is used in a variety of meat substitutes. Soy foods contain a variety of compounds that may have anticancer effects, including protease inhibitors, saponins, phenolic acids, and isoflavones.

Soy's isoflavones (genistein and daidzein) resemble weak forms of natural hormones; for this reason, soy research has focused on hormone-related cancers of the breast and prostate. Despite numerous laboratory studies, population-based studies, and clinical trials, the evidence is inconclusive as to whether soy isoflavones reduce the risk of breast or prostate cancer, although no studies have demonstrated an increase in cancer risk from eating whole soy foods. Because genistein has been shown to stimulate the growth of estrogen-dependent human tumor cells that were injected into animals, women receiving anti-estrogen treatments, such as tamoxifen, should avoid consumption of high-dose purified forms of isoflavones, such as those found in dietary supplements [27]. Some evidence suggests that the timing of soy exposure may affect cancer risk. For example, animal and human studies show that soy consumed in childhood may be protective against breast cancer in adulthood.

Obesity and Energy Balance

Obesity accounts for approximately 20% of all cancer cases and is the cause of 15% of all cancer deaths in men and 20% of cancer deaths in women. Overweight, obesity, and body fatness have been associated with increased risk of cancers of the esophagus, breast (postmenopausal), endometrium, ovary, colon, kidney, pancreas, gallbladder, and possibly others [4, 7–11]. Unlike postmenopausal breast cancer, premenopausal breast cancer risk is inversely associated with body fatness.

The causal relationship of body fatness and obesity to cancer risk is unclear. Obesity influences the levels of hormones and growth factors. Insulin and leptin can promote the growth of cancer cells; both these hormones are elevated in people with obesity. Hyperinsulinemia increases the risk of cancers of the colon, endometrium, and possibly pancreas and kidney. Having increased adipose stores is thought to increase the conversion of androgens to estrogens; increased estrogen levels are strongly associated with the risk of endometrial and postmenopausal breast cancers [11].

Excess adipose tissue is a source of low-grade inflammation. Adipocytes produce pro-inflammatory factors, such as TNFα, interleukin-6 (IL-6), and C-reactive protein. Patients with obesity have higher circulating levels of these factors than patients who are lean. Importantly, chronic inflammation is a known risk factor for cancer development [11].

Worldwide, 35% of adults are overweight or obese. In the USA, 69% of Americans are overweight or obese, which is double the amount in the 1980s. Americans consumed an average of 2586 calories a day in 2010 compared with 2109 calories a day in 1970 [28]. Not surprisingly, in this time period, the average body weight of adults in the USA increased by nearly 20 pounds. Genetic, environmental, behavioral, and socioeconomic factors are thought to play a role in this increase in obesity.

Body mass index (BMI), defined as weight (kg)/height $(m)^2$, serves as an indirect measurement of adipose tissue and is currently used to define overweight and obesity. BMI is not a direct measurement of body fat, but has been shown to correlate with direct body fat measures such as underwater weight. BMI may be overestimated in athletes and those who have a muscular build; BMI may be underestimated in older persons or those who have muscle loss or wasting.

Distribution of body fat may be an important factor in the association of obesity with cancer risk. Specifically, abdominal obesity, which can be measured by waist circumference, has been shown to be associated with increased colon cancer risk and may be an important factor in the association of overweight and obesity with pancreatic cancer, endometrial cancer, and postmenopausal breast cancer [4]. Waist circumference is an important measurement to obtain when screening for obesity. Waist circumference is measured at the level of the top of the iliac crest with the measuring tape snug against the skin. According to the AICR, a waist measurement of ≥31.5 in. (80 cm) for women and ≥37 in. (94 cm) for men is associated with elevated cancer risk [4].

Health guidelines for cancer prevention advise the public to be as lean as possible with a normal range of body weight without becoming underweight and specifically to have a median adult BMI between 21 and 23. Maintenance of a healthy weight throughout life may be one of the most important ways to protect against cancer [4]. Achieving weight loss and maintaining a healthy weight can be difficult. Clinical practice guidelines from various professional medical societies have outlined management strategies and frameworks for overweight and obesity [29, 30].

Physical Activity and Sedentary Behavior

Physical activity (PA) may protect against cancer in general, improve long-term health of cancer survivors, and possibly reduce the risk of cancer recurrence. Convincing evidence suggests that PA is protective for colorectal cancer, probable evidence exists for an association between PA and reduced risk of postmenopausal breast cancer and endometrial cancer, and PA may prevent lung and pancreatic cancers [4, 7–10].

PA includes walking, doing laundry, grocery shopping, or any activity that involves moving around. Exercise is structured recreational PA and includes aerobic activity such as swimming, jogging, cycling, or dancing. The current guidelines for PA as defined by the Guidelines for Physical Activity [31] are:

Adults (> 18 years of age):

- Adults should perform an equivalent of 150 min of moderate intensity activity per week with the goal of achieving and maintaining a healthy body weight. This equates to approximately 22 min of moderate intensity PA each day.
- Alternately, adults can complete 75 min of vigorous activity per week.
- Adults should also include muscle-strengthening activities that involve all major muscle groups 2 or more days per week into their routine.
- The 2010 Dietary Guidelines for Americans [32] suggest that some adults will need more exercise, possibly more than 300 min per week to achieve and maintain a healthy body weight. This equates to approximately 43 min or more each day.

Sedentary behavior is defined as low energy expenditure, generally exemplified by prolonged sitting or lying down and the absence of whole-body movement. "Screen time" (watching television, working at a computer, or playing video games) and driving or sitting in an automobile typify sedentary behavior. Sedentary behavior and physical inactivity are not necessarily equivalent. An individual may engage in 150 min of moderate intensity activity per week, yet be sedentary for the remaining time. On the other hand, physical inactivity is the absence of health-enhancing PA in everyday life. It is physical inactivity that is associated with an increased incidence of cancer mortality [33]. Preliminary evidence suggests a likely metabolic health benefit from regular interruptions to sitting time and overall reduction in sedentary time [34].

Alcohol

More than one half of American adults consume alcohol in the form of ethanol each year, with 88,000 excess deaths associated with its use, a majority of which are due to traffic accidents and binge drinking (8 drinks per binge). The economic cost of alcohol abuse on lost workplace productivity, health care expenses, and crime is estimated to be $223.5 billion per year [35]. Considerable evidence from large prospective observational trials has confirmed the association between drinking alcohol and cancers of the mouth, pharynx, larynx, esophagus, liver, colon and rectum, and breast [36]. This increased risk of cancer is observed regardless of the form in which alcohol is consumed: beer, whiskey, vodka, or mixed drinks. Alcohol acts in various ways to increase cancer risk, including acting as an irritant to damage tissue, producing acetaldehyde (a known carcinogen) in the intestines, inflaming and scarring the liver, lowering the body's ability to absorb folate, raising the levels of estrogen, and increasing the risk of weight gain. Each of these carcinogenic mechanisms increases over time in direct relationship to the amount of alcohol consumed. In addition, alcohol acts as a solvent that allows harmful chemicals, such as those in tobacco, to enter the lining of the upper digestive tract; this may be one reason why simultaneous tobacco and alcohol use produces a higher risk of mouth and throat cancers than the use of either alone [36].

A recent meta-analysis of 222 studies on alcohol and cancer found that light (≤ 1 drink/day) consumption increases the risk of oropharyngeal cancer (70%), esophageal squamous cell carcinoma (30%), and breast cancer (5%), but found no association with colorectal, liver, or laryngeal cancers [37]. A recent analysis of the prospective observational Nurses' Health Study confirmed that light consumption of alcohol was associated with a 15% increase in breast cancer risk, with cumulative consumption throughout adult life as the most important measure [38]. A review of heavy (≥ 4 drinks/day) alcohol consumption resulted in an approximate five-fold increase for oropharyngeal cancer and esophageal squamous cell carcinoma, a 2.5-fold increase for laryngeal cancer, 50% increases for colorectal and breast cancers, and a 30% increase for pancreatic cancer [39]. Confounding factors in studies on heavy drinkers include poor diet, lack of exercise, and maintaining an unhealthy weight, each of which contributes to increments of the increased risk for these cancers.

Although alcohol use by adolescents has been decreasing for the past decade, this still is a societal problem due to the negative impact on individuals, such as drunk driving. In 2013, the number of adolescents who reported drinking in the past 30 days by school grade was 10% for 8th graders, 26% for 10th graders, and 39% for 12th graders [40]. By the end of high school, 68% of students report they have used alcohol, including 52% of 12th graders and 12% of 8th graders who said they had been drunk at least once. A recent study found that adolescent exposure to alcohol may result in adolescent-typical phenotypes into adulthood, including those associated with behavioral, cognitive, electrophysiological, and neuroanatomical characteristics not seen in those who begin consuming alcohol in adulthood [41]. Little data exist as to whether adolescent drinking leads to higher rates of alcohol-related cancers in adulthood. There are, however, data from a population-based study of Finnish twins that found that adolescents with identified drinking problems have a 74% chance of becoming adult alcoholics, especially if they have been binge drinkers as adolescents [42]. The strong association between alcohol and increased cancer risk at many sites should prompt future research.

Since any level of alcohol consumption has the potential to increase cancer risk at various sites, formal recommendations generally take a very conservative approach [4]. The American Cancer Society recommends that individuals drink no more than 1 drink/day for women and 2 drinks/day for men [6]. The lower recommendation for women is due to their smaller size and the fact that they tend to break down alcohol more slowly than men, thus experiencing a greater negative impact on the body at the same alcohol intake level

as men. For clinical practice, asking the patient about his/her history of and current alcohol consumption and informing him/her of the health consequences should be a regular part of each office visit. The decision to drink responsibly or abstain should be based on the individual's risk factors in addition to cultural and social norms.

Tobacco

Fifty Years of Progress Against Tobacco Use

The release of the 1964 Surgeon General's report on *The Health Consequences of Smoking* [43] initiated a concerted effort by government agencies at all levels, public health officials, and medical professionals to reduce the unequivocally harmful consequences of tobacco use. Although the 1964 report focused on tobacco's association with dramatic increases in lung cancers and other respiratory conditions, the ensuing 50 years have provided a vast array of research findings that show tobacco use in any form is associated with diseases of practically all organs in the human body, including multiple cancers, cardiovascular diseases, reproductive disorders, and diabetes (Fig. 24.2). The recently released Surgeon General's report on *Health Consequences of Smoking—50 Years of Progress* [44] shows that significant progress has been made to alleviate the societal and personal health burden of tobacco use, but cautions that the next 50 years will have major challenges for continuing that progress. This is especially true, given new smoking hazards on the horizon, including electronic tobacco delivery systems, other smokeless tobacco products, and the steps toward decriminalizing marijuana in various states.

Although US smoking rates have decreased considerably in the past 50 years, one in five deaths per year is still attributable to smoking. Of special concern is the significant increase in worldwide tobacco use, which is likely to become the greatest health risk worldwide by 2030. Deaths from smoking killed more than 100 million people in the twentieth century and are projected to be the cause of death of one of every two smokers, a billion people, in the twenty-first century. In the USA, tobacco use accounts for approximately 30% of all cancer deaths, including 87% of lung cancer deaths among men and 70% of lung cancer deaths among women [45]. In spite of the proven health risks from tobacco use, 22% of American men and 17% of women still smoke.

Strategies for Tobacco Control

Strategies for tobacco control have matured in the past 50 years to include both population and individual initiatives. Population-directed strategies have been quite effective in

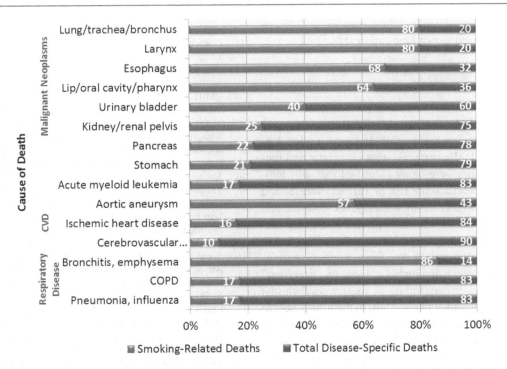

Fig. 24.2 Tobacco-related mortality by disease or condition [51]. Data were adapted from estimates from the Centers for Disease Control and Prevention 2000–2004, National Health Interview Survey responses, and the 2000–2004 National Center for Health Statistics death certificate data. Smoking-related deaths are represented as percentages of total number of deaths

translating research findings into patient and public information campaigns. An ongoing wave of initiatives for tobacco control has included federal and local restrictions on where tobacco can be consumed, taxation strategies to make tobacco products less available, restrictions on tobacco advertising, and community research projects targeting specific populations, such as young people. Medical approaches and strategies have included the use of oral drugs (e.g., bupropion and varenicline), nicotine replacement therapy (e.g., gums and patches), and nicotine vaccines [1]. In addition, a better understanding of behaviors that lead individuals to start smoking or continue to smoke has led to an array of behavioral programs to address this aspect of tobacco use. Although neither medical nor behavioral strategies guarantee smoking cessation, an impressive number of people have quit smoking using these diverse cessation strategies.

Future Challenges

Although conventional tobacco use is likely to continue to decline in the USA as societal pressures and regulations are increased, challenges still remain ahead. Of immediate concern is the increasing sale and use of electronic nicotine delivery devices, such as electronic cigarettes (e-cigarettes). E-cigarettes, both sale and use, presently are unregulated

by the US Food and Drug Administration (FDA) except for those marketed for therapeutic usage. The FDA currently is developing regulations to control personal use. Recent reports indicate that e-cigarette use has doubled from 2011 to 2012 among US middle and high school students [46], and furthermore, that calls to poison control centers for e-cigarette nicotine overdose increased from 1 in September 2010 to 215 in February 2014 [47]. The most common adverse health effects in e-cigarette exposure calls were vomiting, nausea, and eye irritation.

A significant future challenge in the smoking milieu is the spread of legislation allowing personal marijuana use. Twenty four states and the District of Columbia have passed legislation to allow medical use of marijuana, with Colorado and Washington allowing full decriminalization. It is unknown what the medical and societal consequences will be of these loosened regulations. The association of marijuana use with an increase in cancer is sparse. A recent review of 34 epidemiological studies found little evidence of an association [48]. A recent review of cellular, tissue, and animal studies found that marijuana smoke may increase the risk of lung cancer because it contains a higher concentration of polycyclic aromatic hydrocarbons and other carcinogens than found in tobacco smoke [49]. A pooled case-control analysis of human studies by the International Lung Cancer Consortium that investigated the risk of lung cancer among those who smoke cannabis habitually or long term found little evidence for an increased risk of lung cancer [50].

Conclusion

Current research will bring more attention to cancer prevention and lifestyle factors that contribute to cancer development (see Fig. 24.1). Biomarkers—that is, genetic and molecular characteristics—are being identified that will indicate with greater precision the risk of various diseases and molecular pathways contributing to these risks. Furthermore, knowledge of genetic associations with risk-conferring lifestyles will inform the targeting of interventions intended to alter detrimental behaviors and/or their carcinogenic outcomes to appropriate individuals—a form of "precision" medicine. A deeper understanding of dietary mechanisms will contribute to this knowledge. Thus, in the future, people in their 30s or 40s, or even younger, will learn about their risks for developing common and rare diseases and potential lifestyle factors contributing to their risk. These scientific developments will lead to increased attention to cancer-preventive strategies involving eating patterns, PA, alcohol limitations, and tobacco avoidance.

References

1. Greenwald P, Dunn BK. Smoking. In: Rose MD, DeVita VT, Lawrence TS, Rosenberg SA, editors. Oncology in primary care. Philadelphia: Lippincott Williams & Wilkins; 2013. p. 30–5.
2. Ong TP, Moreno FS, Ross SA. Targeting the epigenome with bioactive food components for cancer prevention. J Nutrigenet Nutrigenomics. 2011;4(5):275–92. PMID:22353664.
3. Doll R, Peto R. The causes of cancer: quantitative estimates of avoidable risks of cancer in the United States today. J Natl Cancer Inst. 1981;66(6):1191–308. PMID:7017215.
4. Koya DL, Egede LE. Association between length of residence and cardiovascular disease risk factors among an ethnically diverse group of United States immigrants. J Gen Intern Med. 2007;22(6):841–6. PMID:17503110. http://www.ncbi.nlm.nih.gov/pubmed/17503110.
5. Key TJ, Schatzkin A, Willett WC, Allen NE, Spencer EA, Travis RC. Diet, nutrition and the prevention of cancer. Public Health Nutr. 2004;7(1A):187–200. PMID:14972060.
6. Rock CL, Doyle C, Demark-Wahnefried W, Meyerhardt J, Courneya KS, Schwartz AL, et al. Nutrition and physical activity guidelines for cancer survivors. CA Cancer J Clin. 2012;62(4):243–74. PMID:22539238.
7. Continuous Update Project Report. Food, nutrition, physical activity, and the prevention of breast cancer. 2010.
8. Continuous Update Project Report. Food, nutrition, physical activity, and the prevention of colorectal cancer. 2011.
9. van Rompay MI, McKeown NM, Castaneda-Sceppa C, Falcon LM, Ordovas JM, Tucker KL. Acculturation and sociocultural influences on dietary intake and health status among Puerto Rican adults in Massachusetts. J Acad Nutr Diet. 2012;112(1):64–74. PMID:22389874. http://www.ncbi.nlm.nih.gov/pubmed/22389874.
10. Continuous Update Project Report. Food, nutrition, physical activity and the prevention of endometrial cancer. 2013.
11. Continuous Update Project Report. Food, nutrition, physical activity, and the prevention of ovarian cancer. 2014.
12. Prentice RL, Anderson GL. The women's health initiative: lessons learned. Annu Rev Public Health. 2008;29:131–50. PMID:18348708.
13. Blot WJ, Li JY, Taylor PR, Guo W, Dawsey S, Wang GQ, et al. Nutrition intervention trials in Linxian, China: supplementation with specific vitamin/mineral combinations, cancer incidence, and disease-specific mortality in the general population. J Natl Cancer Inst. 1993;85(18):1483–92. PMID:8360931.
14. Kristal AR, Darke AK, Morris JS, Tangen CM, Goodman PJ, Thompson IM, et al. Baseline selenium status and effects of selenium and vitamin E supplementation on prostate cancer risk. J Natl Cancer Inst. 2014;106(3):djt456. PMID:24563519.
15. Murillo G, Mehta RG. Cruciferous vegetables and cancer prevention. Nutr Cancer. 2001;41(1–2):17–28. PMID:12094621.
16. Seow A, Vainio H, Yu MC. Effect of glutathione-S-transferase polymorphisms on the cancer preventive potential of isothiocyanates: an epidemiological perspective. Mutat Res. 2005;592(1–2):58–67. PMID:16019037.
17. Kucuk O, Sarkar FH, Sakr W, Djuric Z, Pollak MN, Khachik F, et al. Phase II randomized clinical trial of lycopene supplementation before radical prostatectomy. Cancer Epidemiol Biomarkers Prev. 2001;10(8):861–8. PMID:11489752.
18. Kristal AR, Arnold KB, Neuhouser ML, Goodman P, Platz EA, Albanes D, et al. Diet, supplement use, and prostate cancer risk: results from the prostate cancer prevention trial. Am J Epidemiol. 2010;172(5):566–77. PMID:20693267.
19. Inoue-Choi M, Robien K. Cancer and nutrition: significance and background. In: Leser M, Ledesma N, Bergerson S, Trujillo E, editors. Oncology nutrition for clinical practice. Chicago: Oncology Nutrition Dietetic Practice Group; 2013. p. 9–14.
20. Vollset SE, Clarke R, Lewington S, Ebbing M, Halsey J, Lonn E, et al. Effects of folic acid supplementation on overall and site-specific cancer incidence during the randomised trials: meta-analyses of data on 50,000 individuals. Lancet. 2013;381(9871):1029–36. PMID:23352552.
21. Pierce JP, Natarajan L, Caan BJ, Parker BA, Greenberg ER, Flatt SW, et al. Influence of a diet very high in vegetables, fruit, and fiber and low in fat on prognosis following treatment for breast cancer: the Women's Healthy Eating and Living (WHEL) randomized trial. JAMA. 2007;298(3):289–98. PMID:17635889.
22. Chlebowski RT, Blackburn GL, Thomson CA, Nixon DW, Shapiro A, Hoy MK, et al. Dietary fat reduction and breast cancer outcome: interim efficacy results from the Women's Intervention Nutrition Study. J Natl Cancer Inst. 2006;98(24):1767–76. PMID:17179478.
23. Farzaneh-Far R, Lin J, Epel ES, Harris WS, Blackburn EH, Whooley MA. Association of marine omega-3 fatty acid levels with telomeric aging in patients with coronary heart disease. JAMA. 2010;303(3):250–7. PMID:20085953.
24. Chung M, Lee J, Terasawa T, Lau J, Trikalinos TA. Vitamin D with or without calcium supplementation for prevention of cancer and fractures: an updated meta-analysis for the U.S. Preventive Services Task Force. Ann Intern Med. 2011;155(12):827–38. PMID: 22184690.
25. Holick MF, Binkley NC, Bischoff-Ferrari HA, Gordon CM, Hanley DA, Heaney RP, et al. Evaluation, treatment, and prevention of vitamin D deficiency: an Endocrine Society clinical practice guideline. J Clin Endocrinol Metab. 2011;96(7):1911–30. PMID:21646368.
26. Aleem E. β-Glucans and their applications in cancer therapy: focus on human studies. Anticancer Agents Med Chem. 2013;13(5):709–19. PMID:23140353.

27. Villaseca P. Non-estrogen conventional and phytochemical treatments for vasomotor symptoms: what needs to be known for practice. Climacteric. 2012;15(2):115–24. PMID:22148909.

28. Go AS, Mozaffarian D, Roger VL, Benjamin EJ, Berry JD, Blaha MJ, et al. Heart disease and stroke statistics–2014 update: a report from the American Heart Association. Circulation. 2014;129(3):e28–292. PMID:24352519.

29. Jensen MD, Ryan DH, Apovian CM, Ard JD, Comuzzie AG, Donato KA, et al. 2013 AHA/ACC/TOS guideline for the management of overweight and obesity in adults: a report of the American College of Cardiology/American Heart Association Task Force on Practice Guidelines and The Obesity Society. Circulation. 2014;129(25 Suppl 2):S102–38. PMID:24222017.

30. Gonzalez-Campoy JM, St Jeor ST, Castorino K, Ebrahim A, Hurley D, Jovanovic L, et al. Clinical practice guidelines for healthy eating for the prevention and treatment of metabolic and endocrine diseases in adults: cosponsored by the American Association of Clinical Endocrinologists/the American College of Endocrinology and the Obesity Society. Endocr Pract. 2013;19(Suppl 3):1–82. PMID:24129260.

31. United States Department of Health and Human Services. 2008 physical activity guidelines for Americans: be active, healthy, and happy! Washington, DC: U.S. Department of Health and Human Services; 2008. ix, 61 p.

32. United States Department of Agriculture. Human Nutrition Information Service. Dietary Guidelines Advisory Committee., United States. Agricultural Research Service. Report of the Dietary Guidelines Advisory Committee on the dietary guidelines for Americans, 2010: to the Secretary of Agriculture and the Secretary of Health and Human Services. Washington, D.C.: United States Department of Agriculture: United States Department of Health and Human Services; 2010. vi, 445 p.

33. Lee IM, Shiroma EJ, Lobelo F, Puska P, Blair SN, Katzmarzyk PT. Effect of physical inactivity on major non-communicable diseases worldwide: an analysis of burden of disease and life expectancy. Lancet. 2012;380(9838):219–29. PMID:22818936. http://www.ncbi.nlm.nih.gov/pubmed/22818936.

34. Healy GN, Dunstan DW, Salmon J, Cerin E, Shaw JE, Zimmet PZ, et al. Breaks in sedentary time: beneficial associations with metabolic risk. Diabetes Care. 2008;31(4):661–6. PMID:18252901.

35. Bouchery EE, Harwood HJ, Sacks JJ, Simon CJ, Brewer RD. Economic costs of excessive alcohol consumption in the U.S., 2006. Am J Prev Med. 2011;41(5):516–24. PMID:22011424.

36. Matias SL, Stoecklin-Marois MT, Tancredi DJ, Schenker MB. Adherence to dietary recommendations is associated with acculturation among Latino farm workers. J Nutr. 2013;143(9):1451–8. PMID:23864507. http://www.ncbi.nlm.nih.gov/pubmed/23864507.

37. Bagnardi V, Rota M, Botteri E, Tramacere I, Islami F, Fedirko V, et al. Light alcohol drinking and cancer: a meta-analysis. Ann Oncol. 2013;24(2):301–8. PMID:22910838.

38. Chen WY, Rosner B, Hankinson SE, Colditz GA, Willett WC. Moderate alcohol consumption during adult life, drinking patterns, and breast cancer risk. JAMA. 2011;306(17):1884–90. PMID:22045766.

39. Pelucchi C, Tramacere I, Boffetta P, Negri E, La Vecchia C. Alcohol consumption and cancer risk. Nutr Cancer. 2011;63(7):983–90. PMID:21864055.

40. Johnston LD, O'Malley PM, Miech RA, Bachman JG, Schulenberg JE. Monitoring the future national results on drug use: 1975–2013: overview, key findings on adolescent drug use. Ann Arbor: Institute for Social Research, The University of Michigan; 2014.

41. Spear LP, Swartzwelder HS. Adolescent alcohol exposure and persistence of adolescent-typical phenotypes into adulthood: a mini-review. Neurosci Biobehav Rev. 2014;45C:1–8. PMID:24813805.

42. Dick DM, Aliev F, Viken R, Kaprio J, Rose RJ. Rutgers alcohol problem index scores at age 18 predict alcohol dependence diagnoses 7 years later. Alcohol Clin Exp Res. 2011;35(5):1011–4. PMID:21323682.

43. Smoking and health: report of the Advisory Committee to the Surgeon General of the Public Health Service. Washington, DC: Public Health Service, Office of the Surgeon General; 1964.

44. The health consequences of smoking—50 years of progress: a report of the Surgeon General. Atlanta GA; 2014.

45. Cancer Facts & Figures. Atlanta: American Cancer Society, 2014.

46. Notes from the field: electronic cigarette use among middle and high school students—United States, 2011–2012. MMWR Morb Mortal Wkly Rep. 2013;62(35):729–30. PMID:24005229.

47. Chatham-Stephens K, Law R, Taylor E, Melstrom P, Bunnell R, Wang B, et al. Notes from the field: calls to poison centers for exposures to electronic cigarettes—United States, September 2010–February 2014. MMWR Morb Mortal Wkly Rep. 2014;63(13):292–3. PMID:24699766.

48. Huang YH, Zhang ZF, Tashkin DP, Feng B, Straif K, Hashibe M. An epidemiologic review of marijuana and cancer: an update. Cancer Epidemiol Biomarkers Prev. 2015;24(1):15–31. PMID:25587109.

49. Underner M, Urban T, Perriot J, de Chazeron I, Meurice JC. Cannabis smoking and lung cancer. Rev Mal Respir. 2014;31(6):488–98. PMID:25012035.

50. Zhang LR, Morgenstern H, Greenland S, Chang SC, Lazarus P, Teare MD, et al. Cannabis smoking and lung cancer risk: pooled analysis in the International Lung Cancer Consortium. Int J Cancer. 2015;136(4):894–903. PMID:24947688.

51. Smoking-attributable mortality, years of potential life lost, and productivity losses—United States, 2000–2004. MMWR Morb Mortal Wkly Rep. 2008;57(45):1226–8. PMID:19008791.

Lifestyle Medicine for the Prevention and Treatment of Depression

Jerome Sarris and Adrienne O'Neil

Abbreviations

BMI	Body Mass Index
NCDs	Noncommunicable diseases
NESDA	Netherlands Study of Depression and Anxiety
PA	Physical activity
PFC	Prefrontal cortex
PREDIMED	Prevención con Dieta Mediterránea
RCTs	Randomized controlled trials
T2D	Type-2 diabetes
5-HT	5-hydroxytryptamine
UPBEAT	Understanding the Prognostic Benefits of Exercise and Antidepressant Therapy

Background

The number of people affected by depression has increased in recent decades. While this is partially due to diagnostic practices, urbanization and factors associated with the modern Western environment are undoubtedly contributing to such a trend. For example, in Western society, individuals are becoming increasingly sedentary and consuming poorer-quality diets when compared with previous generations. In conjunction with disruptions to the sleep/wake cycle, substance misuse, and psychosocial stressors including time pressures and social isolation, this type of lifestyle may compromise mental health. Nevertheless, the association between "Westernization" and mental health is complex and

not linear. For example, stress, fatigue, physical inactivity, and sleep deficiency can lead to obesity, and then indirectly exacerbate sedentary behaviour, all culminating in a depressed state. Obesogenic environments and the interaction of factors modulating deleterious effects on mental health warrant the use of a "Lifestyle Medicine" approach for the prevention, promotion, and management of depression. Such a model offers a potentially safe and cost-effective adjunctive treatment option for management of the condition. To date, however, there remains a dearth of evidence around the utility of Lifestyle Medicine in psychiatry. In this chapter, we will consider the role of lifestyle and environmental factors as forming the basis for practical interventions for the management of depression.

Lifestyle Medicine in the Context of Mental Health

"Lifestyle Medicine", particularly in the context of mental health, is a relatively new field. While the idea has been recognised by practitioners for centuries as a means by which to improve health outcomes, little attention has been given to its application for mental health and in particular depression. This is despite its high disability burden and it being arguably one of the prevalent noncommunicable diseases (NCDs), with similar pathways to that of the more commonly recognised "lifestyle" disorders including cardiovascular disease and type-2 diabetes (T2D). In addition to some evidence that patients with mild depression respond well to lifestyle strategies (though improvements in depression may not directly improve adherence to healthy diet [1]), there is indeed a bio-behavioural framework that helps explain the way in which the modern lifestyle impacts mental health that extends beyond the putative assumption that the presence of depression precipitates an unhealthy diet via low motivation or lack of pleasure. Obesity, poor diet, poor/decreased sleep, exposure to chemicals and pollutants, and high stress levels have all been shown to increase low-grade systemic inflam-

A. O'Neil (✉)
IMPACT Strategic Research Centre, Deakin University, Ryrie St, Geelong, VIC 3220, Australia
e-mail: aoneil@barwonhealth.org.au

J. Sarris
Department of Psychiatry & The Melbourne Clinic, University of Melbourne, Parkville, VIC, Australia

Centre for Human Psychopharmacology, Swinburne University of Technology, Hawthorn, VIC, Australia

© Springer International Publishing Switzerland 2016
J. I. Mechanick, R. F. Kushner (eds.), *Lifestyle Medicine*, DOI 10.1007/978-3-319-24687-1_25

mation and oxidative stress—the same pathways at play in the pathogenesis of other NCDs—as well as disruptions to the hypothalamic–pituitary–adrenal axis and cortisol secretion that characterise depression [2]. Specifically, increased levels of pro-inflammatory cytokines, interferon gamma, neopterin, reactive oxygen and nitrogen species, and resultant damage by oxidative and nitrosative stress, in combination with lowered levels of antioxidants, may potentially damage mitochondria and mitochondrial DNA [2]. These events culminate in neurodegeneration and reduced neurogenesis [2] and provide context to nutritional mechanisms in the prevention and management of depression.

Lifestyle Elements with Supportive Data

Diet

The past century has seen the occurrence of dietary changes across the globe, whereby there has been a major shift in the common dietary patterns of Western societies. Diets are typically characterised by low nutrient and energy-dense foods, processed carbohydrates and refined sugar. In fact, the former now contribute to one third of the daily intakes by Americans [3]. Evidence suggests that unhealthy eating patterns may even be important in the pathogenesis of depression. While the strength and nature of this relationship remains unclear [4], both cross-sectional and longitudinal data show a significant relationship between unhealthy eating patterns and depressed mood and anxiety [5]. Moreover, there is potential for healthy eating patterns to be protective against depression. A recent prospective study of Australian adolescents found that better diet quality was associated with improved adolescent mental health both cross-sectionally and prospectively [6]. Importantly, improvements in mental health were also mirrored by improvements in diet quality. The first randomised trial to determine whether a dietary pattern prescription can prevent the onset of depression has shown promising results. Nested within the larger trial examining the effects of the Mediterranean diet in the prevention of cardiovascular events, the *Prevención con Dieta Mediter-ránea* (PREDIMED) investigators found that adherence to the diet supplemented by nuts was protective against depression, particularly in those with T2D [7]. These data support findings from other trials conducted within T2D showing that intensive lifestyle interventions can prevent symptoms of depression (relative risk, RR=0.66; 95 % confidence interval, 95 % CI=0.5–0.8; $P<0.001$) when compared with a control group [8].

Though poorly understood, there are a range of pathways to explain the pathophysiology underpinning the relationship between diet and mental health, including brain plasticity and function, the stress response system, mitochondrial function, inflammation, and oxidative processes [9]. There

is also increasing evidence that some diets, particularly the Western dietary pattern, may be pro-inflammatory, whereby certain foods and food groups are associated with increased markers of systemic inflammation [10]. In fact, high levels of serum high-sensitivity C-reactive protein (a general marker of systemic inflammation) have been shown to be an independent risk factor for depression [11]. Similarly, particular dietary patterns (e.g. whole foods and Mediterranean diets) have been defined as anti-inflammatory, providing protein, flavonoids, essential fatty acids as well as micronutrients crucial to neurochemical function, such as magnesium, B-complex vitamins, vitamin C, and zinc.

To date, there remains a dearth of evidence from randomised controlled trials (RCTs) about the potential for diets to be utilised as a therapeutic target in the management of depression. A pilot RCT [12] was enacted to elucidate the effects of a 10-day nutrient-rich diet on the mood of healthy female adults. Compared with controls, those receiving the intervention yielded significant improvements in self-rated vigour, alertness, and contentment. Others have observed the benefits of supplements (omega-3 polyunsaturated fatty acid, PUFA) in depressed populations; meta-analyses [13] have highlighted the benefits of eicosapentaenoic acid particularly for those with greater symptom intensity. The first clinical trial to evaluate the effect of a modified Mediterranean diet in those with clinical depression is currently underway [14]. Regardless of limited empirical evidence for dietary modification as a therapeutic target for the treatment of major depression, the past decade has witnessed the advent of evidence demonstrating its contribution to the pathogenesis of the condition. As diet has a major impact on co-morbid medical conditions that are increasingly common in people diagnosed with depression, including cardiovascular disease and metabolic disorders, it is likely to be a source of untapped potential. However, at this stage, the precautionary principle should guide practice.

Physical Activity and Exercise

Modern lifestyles are becoming increasingly sedentary. Sedentary behaviour is not only a key driver of the obesity epidemic but may now be a risk factor for the development of depression [15] and other inflammatory conditions. It has long been known that increased physical activity (PA) is associated with decreased depressive symptoms. Indeed, PA may exert protective effects against mental disorders, with regular PA in childhood related to reduced risk of adult onset depression. In addition to the benefits of PA for primary prevention, exercise has been shown to be an effective mood elevator [16] for those with symptomatic depression. For example, Dunn et al. [17] found that aerobic exercise (conducted in a laboratory setting) at a dose consistent with public health recommendations (17.5 kcal/kg/week) is effective for depression of mild to moderate severity as measured by the Hamilton Depression Rating Scale. Lower doses (7.0 kcal/kg/week) were comparable to placebo effect (3 days/week flexibility exercise).

The beneficial effects of exercise result from a host of biological pathways including: inflammatory cytokines, oxidative stress, neurotrophins (e.g. brain-derived neurotropic factor, BDNF [18]), and enhanced neurogenesis [19]. Others have explained the apparent antidepressant effects of exercise as a modulation of monoamine systems. PA has also been shown to increase the expression of serotonin (5-HT) in animal models [20]. There are sustained beneficial effects of PA on these systems via the neuroendocrine axis, normalization of cortisol levels, and circulating beta-endorphins. PA is an attractive option for depression management for those with mild to moderate symptomology because it is feasible, safe, and cost-effective and is thought to yield cognitive and psychosocial benefits, promote self-efficacy, self-esteem and social engagement, and enhance body image. Of all the components of lifestyle medicine, the evidence base for the application of exercise in depression management is arguably the most extensive.

A recent Cochrane review comprising 28 RCTs ($n=1101$) revealed moderate to large effects in favour of exercise over standard treatment or control [21]. When the data from seven trials ($n=373$) with long-term follow-up data were pooled, a more modest clinical effect was observed in favor of exercise. However, only four trials ($n=326$) with adequate allocation concealment, blinding, and intent-to-treat analysis were located, resulting in a more modest effect size in favour of exercise of -0.31 (95% CI$=-0.63$ to 0.01). Pooled data from seven trials ($n=373$) with long-term follow-up data also found a small clinical effect in favor of exercise of -0.39 (95% CI$=-0.69$ to -0.09). Further to this finding, Krogh et al. [22] found no significant long-term effect in a meta-analysis of five pooled studies. However, they did find an association between exercise intensity, exercise duration, and improved clinical effect, thus it is possible that participants in longer-term studies may lack the motivation of shorter-term interventions.

Clinical practice guidelines for exercise recommend physician and/or exercise physiologist assessment before commencing a new regime, which should consist of moderate (150 min per week) to vigorous (75 min per week) aerobic physical activity, in addition to anaerobic weight-bearing exercises twice weekly. Exposure to social interaction and nature when exercising may also be advised. In summary, the balance of evidence supports the use of exercise of adequate intensity and duration to improve mood and reduce depressive symptoms, with stronger effects being seen in clinical depression. This effect appears to be comparable to conventional antidepressants.

Mindfulness Meditation

The advent of yoga, mindfulness, and meditation has led to the evaluation of these practices on mental health outcomes. A systematic review of 12 RCTs [23] found moderate evidence of beneficial short-term effects of yoga compared to "usual care". Like more traditional forms of cardiovascular exercise, there are physiological and cognitive benefits of yoga. For example, yoga may quell rumination, a symptom common in depression. Notwithstanding these benefits, while yoga is regarded as generally safe, significant adverse events from its practice have been documented, including those affecting the musculoskeletal system, the nervous system, and the eyes [24]. Thus, yoga should be practised carefully under the guidance of a qualified instructor.

Meditative practices, often categorized into "open monitoring" or "focused" forms, may also have an application in mood management and relapse prevention. A key constituent aspect is mindfulness: "paying attention in a particular way: on purpose, in the present moment, and non-judgmentally" [25]. When the neurological effects of meditation have been observed using neuroimaging studies, biological changes including alterations in gray matter morphology, increased cortical thickness in the prefrontal cortex (PFC) and right anterior insula, increased oxygenated hemoglobin in the anterior PFC, and elevations in whole blood 5-hydroxytryptamine (5-HT) levels have been noted [26]. To date, the quality of studies supporting the efficacy of mindfulness therapy is poor. However, the evidence base is growing. Meta-analyses of controlled studies examining anxiety and mood-related endpoints have yielded large effect sizes [27]. Nevertheless, it remains unclear which types of meditation are best for differing depressive symptomatologies.

Management of Recreational Substances

Evidence suggests that there is a shared genetic vulnerability to both smoking and depression. Smoking cigarettes is a potential risk factor for depression—for example, adolescent smokers are at increased risk of subsequent depression later in life [28]. Conversely, depressed individuals generally smoke at an increase rate, which is particularly problematic given that smoking can interfere with treatment response. Smoking is often used as a form of self-medication for acute dysphoric symptom reduction [29]. In fact, regular smokers can be viewed as being in a persistent dysphoric withdrawal state, interspersed with intoxication when consuming nicotine. There are two key biological processes thought to link smoking to depression: (1) the dopaminergic system, which is responsible for regulating both mood and addiction and (2) the immune system, whereby smoking aggravates inflammation and provokes oxidative stress.

Similarly, there exists a well-documented bidirectional relationship between alcohol consumption and affective disorders. The presence of either an alcohol or affective disorder doubles the risk of having the other [30]. Compared with the general population, the prevalence of alcohol abuse and dependence is overrepresented in populations with affective disorders. Conversely, there is a two- to threefold increased lifetime risk for depression and anxiety in those with alcohol dependence/abuse [31]. This is a trend that has been observed in adolescents and young adults, where alcohol use in adolescence predicts later onset of depression. While the actual mechanisms underpinning this association remain unclear, acute alcohol consumption has been shown to increase monoamine release [32], with withdrawal precipitating the dysregulation of monoamine and neuroendocrine pathways which can initiate anxiety or dysphoria [32]. Studies have demonstrated that depressed mood can be substantially alleviated within a short time after abstaining from alcohol, with a brief education intervention (the provision of safe drinking guidance and homework tasks) effective in reducing symptoms when compared to control participants [33].

Sleep

A common symptom of depression relates to sleep hygiene: difficulty falling or staying asleep, waking earlier than desired, and/or general disruption to the circadian rhythm. Sleep difficulties, in particularly insomnia, can be both an outcome and predictor of depression, with poor sleeping patterns predictive of subsequent depression relapse. Of the former, data form the Netherlands Study of Depression and Anxiety (NESDA) revealed that people with a depressive or anxiety disorder or remittent depression had significant sleep disturbance, independent of other factors that may interfere with sleep patterns such as sociodemographic factors and psychotropic medication use [34]. Of the latter, a review of 21 prospective studies [35] found that insomnia doubled the risk for depression. Moreover, almost half of insomniacs experience another comorbid psychiatric disorder [36] and are therefore at heightened risk of other somatic conditions, including cardiovascular disease, metabolic disorders, and obesity [37]. A systematic review also provides some evidence of a mutual relationship between obstructive sleep apnea and depression; however, the nature of this relationship remains unclear [38].

Many present-day treatment strategies incorporate sleep hygiene techniques into traditional therapeutic models like cognitive behavioural therapy [39]. Lifestyle modification programs that target sedentary behaviours, poor diet, caffeine use, and alcohol use have the capacity to extend beyond their immediate benefits to improve sleep hygiene. An uncontrolled study comprising 2624 individuals aged 30–80 years [40], assessed at baseline and four weeks following a 40-h program focusing on nutrition, physical activity, and sleep, found that of the 10 % of participants experiencing insomnia, two thirds reported reduced sleep disturbance at study completion. While increased PA, reduced body mass index (BMI), and caffeine consumption were linked to better sleep quality, reduced alcohol and tobacco consumption were not.

Caffeine is a psychoactive substance that increases cognition, mood, attention, and state of alertness. There is some evidence that those with dysphoric mood are predisposed to increased caffeine use because of its mood-elevating potential which acts via the noradrenergic and dopaminergic pathways [41]. Caffeine also modulates the adenosine system, and its anxiogenic potential is influenced by A2A receptor polymorphisms [42]. Patterns of caffeine use appear to differ by disorder. For example, there is evidence to support the avoidance of caffeine in anxiety disorders [43], which may be due to its effects on the central nervous system. Thus, caffeine use (e.g. from coffee consumption) could be protective against depression as a result of adenosine system dysregulation in depression [44]. A longitudinal study comprising over 50,000 US women (mean age, 63 years) free of depressive symptoms demonstrated that those consuming two to three cups of coffee per day were at reduced risk of diagnosed depression at follow-up when compared with those consuming one or fewer cups per week [45], an effect that was even stronger for those consuming more than four cups daily and one not observed for decaffeinated coffee. While such findings suggest the benefits of moderate intake of caffeine, high caffeine affects insomnia, which can incite depressed mood [46].

Social Interaction and Support

Positive, supportive, and intimate relationships with family, friends, or other relationships have long been known to have beneficial effects on general health, specifically for maintaining psychological health [47]. Ibarra-Rovillard and Kuiper [47] propose that the extent to which social relationship partners are perceived to fulfill (or undermine) basic psychological needs serves to explain both the positive and negative effects on the well-being of depressed individuals. The English Longitudinal Study of Aging [48] found that negative, but not positive, exchanges with family and friends were associated with greater occurrence of depression, after adjusting for confounding factors. Positive relationships can promote self-efficacy in achieving or maintaining health-promoting activities. For example, a prospective cohort study of 5395 middle-aged adults in the UK found that recommended levels of leisure-time PA were more likely to persist when accompanied by high levels of emotional support [49].

Lifestyle Elements with Emerging Data

Recreation and Relaxation Activities

Identification and enactment of pleasurable activities is often incorporated into therapeutic treatments for clinical depression. However, the effects of recreational activities per se have not been evaluated extensively. When the role of organized physical recreation is investigated as a strategy for improving mental health in the USA and Australia [50], results suggest that participants are more resilient against stressors and show a clear reduction in depressed mood (although directionality was unclear). Formalized relaxation techniques have also proven beneficial. A meta-analysis comprising 11 trials using relaxation techniques (progressive muscle relaxation, relaxation imagery, and autogenic training) versus control comparators found that although clinician-rated outcomes were nonsignificant, self-rated depressive symptoms were reduced [51]. However, these effects are inferior to those of psychological interventions on self-reported depression [52].

Environmental Factors

External factors affecting health are often classified as (1) *environmental*: nature/greenspace, climate, season, and pollution (noise, air, and water quality; chemical exposure) and *social*: interaction with relationships, family, friends, animals, or pets. While there is strong evidence that social isolation is a risk factor for depression, and that social support can be potentially protective in depression, there remains only weak evidence for other elements. Intuitively, exposure to nature may provide theoretical benefits for general health. Studies have confirmed this association even when considered independent of PA [52], though exercising in nature may synergistically increase well-being beyond that observed in an urban setting [53]. Evidence around "nature-assisted" therapy, for example, nature hikes, suggests a therapeutic effect. A review [54] found health improvements in 26 out of 29 studies. Of course, it is possible that the mechanisms underpinning such effects may be related to exposure to fresh air and sunlight. However, there remains an inconsistent relationship between seasonal variations and depression [55, 56]. Benefits of sunlight on mental health may be mediated, in part, by vitamin D [57]. On the other hand, when this has been studied in multiple sclerosis populations, greater exposure to sunshine was shown to decrease depression in the absence of a correlation with vitamin D levels [58]. Overall, when the use of vitamin D supplements for the treatment of depression has been evaluated, conflicting evidence has been observed [9, 57, 59].

Other emerging environmental factors range from exposure to noise pollution to technological devices. Indeed, continual hyperstimulation is a theoretical concern for both cognitive and mental health. Environmental toxins have a potential adverse effect on the central nervous system [60], inducing neuro-inflammation, oxidative stress, cerebrovascular dysfunction, and microglial activation, and potentially altering the blood–brain barrier [60]. Animal studies investigating exposure to ambient fine airborne particulate matter (compared with filtered air), demonstrated effects on both cognitive and affective responses of mice [61]. In fact, long-term air pollution led to more depressive-like responses and impairments in spatial learning and memory compared to exposure with filtered air. A longitudinal study of 537 elderly Koreans revealed that exposure to air pollution was associated with an increase in depressive symptoms [62]. Nevertheless, there is still inconsistency in the literature and more research is required. In respect to pet "ownership", a recent Scandinavian cross-sectional study was conducted of 12,093 older adults (65 years of age) who were non-pet owners, cat owners, and dog owners to determine any relationship between animal ownership and depression/anxiety levels. Results revealed no interactions were recognized between pet ownership and subjective general health status, loneliness, or marital status, while no data was present supporting lower depression or anxiety in cat or dog owners versus non-pet owners [63].

Review of Clinical Considerations

The associated benefits of lifestyle medicine largely relate to the long-term sustainability of self-management and treatment effects. Whilst this is particularly true for those with mild to moderate depression symptoms for whom lifestyle intervention alone can be particularly effective, exercise, for example, has been show to produce small effect sizes between 0.2–0.5 [22] in those with clinically diagnosed depression. For those with symptoms of greater intensity, lifestyle interventions are rarely prescribed as first-line treatment but rather in conjunction with pharmacotherapy. Indeed, the benefits of adjunctive treatments can go beyond self-reported improvements in symptomatology. The Understanding the Prognostic Benefits of Exercise and Antidepressant Therapy (UPBEAT) trial demonstrated that a combined exercise/pharmacotherapy intervention for coronary patients provided the additional benefit of improving cardiac biomarkers including heart rate variability [64]. Regardless, while it is currently unknown whether lifestyle modifications in general are augmenting beyond the effect of antidepressants, these interventions can be safely combined with medication, and thus represent a benign adjunctive approach.

However, there are a range of barriers preventing people from implementing lifestyle change, including motivational issues, time restrictions, financial limitations, perspective around the source of difficulties, and treatment priorities.

Ownership over one's own self-management and a sense of shared partnership in the development and planning of treatment could be of benefit. Collectively, the weight of evidence supports different aspects of lifestyle medicine in the management of depression, favoring a personalized and step-wise approach. Readiness to change is the foundation of lifestyle modification and is concordant with the *trans*-theoretical model [65]. Embarking on this strategy is appropriate for patients who are beyond pre-contemplation [65].

Clinicians should understand the importance of nutrients that are critical for healthy neurological function (e.g. magnesium, folate, zinc, and essential fatty acids) and, from a dietary intake perspective, the foods in which they are predominantly found, such as leafy green vegetables, legumes, whole grains, lean red meat, and fish. Polyphenol-rich foods (e.g. berries, tea, dark chocolate, wine, and certain herbs) have also been shown to promote cognitive and cardiovascular function [66, 67]. In concordance with dietary recommendations for other common inflammatory based disorders, whole foods intake should be augmented and processed food intake reduced. Indeed, the potential benefits of the Mediterranean diet in potentially preventing mental health symptoms, as observed in the PREDIMED study, should be remembered [7]. There is also burgeoning epigenetic and other evidence identifying the role of preconception and antenatal maternal eating patterns as a key component of early programming of offspring, whereby poor antenatal dietary intake can result in mental health problems in offspring [68], or perhaps even more astoundingly, result in permanent phenotypic changes in offspring [69].

Clinical guidelines for exercise recommend physician assessment (or referral to an exercise physiologist) before commencing a new regime, which should consist of moderate to vigorous aerobic exercise (30–60 min) in addition to anaerobic weight-bearing exercises approximately 4–6 days per week [70, 71]. Regarding the dosage and type of exercise for recommendation, the evidence suggests that regular moderate to strong intensity exercise elicits the most positive effects in improving mood [72, 73]. Exercise within the context of nature and a socially rich environment may be useful on theoretical grounds.

The integration of meditative practices can be readily incorporated into most people's lifestyle, in a formal way (e.g. yoga) or employing unstructured mindfulness techniques (mindful walking or eating, breathing exercises). For the former, it is advised that individuals practise under a qualified instructor, proceeding in a graded manner (it is recommended that patients with comorbidities such as glaucoma or osteoporosis proceed with caution).

Due to its impact upon depression risk and treatment [74, 75], routine clinical assessment around alcohol consumption is appropriate, differentiating and managing problem drinking and psychoeducation around modest alcohol consumption and prevention of heavy and/or binge drinking. Clinicians should be cognizant of potential interactions between alcohol and medications. Like many targets for behaviour change, techniques that combine motivational interviewing and cognitive behavioural therapy may be beneficial for dual diagnoses [76, 77]. Similarly, evidence-based smoking cessation interventions should be employed for smokers [78]; the adjunctive use of PA has been shown to be a protective strategy against relapse in quitters [79]. While the act of cessation is commonly associated with withdrawal symptoms including aggravation of the depression itself [80], symptoms are likely to dissipate once the neurochemical set point has readapted to the absence of nicotine. Despite an absence of data from smoking cessation trials examining changes in depression risk, other data suggest that quitting is related to better social functioning and self-perceived health status [81].

There is a range of sleep hygiene techniques that can be used to counteract poor sleep or insomnia. Augmenting caffeine use, limiting exposure to sunlight [82] and/or the bed, and adherence to strict sleep/wake times [83] each help to promote regulation of the circadian rhythm [84]. Other sleep hygiene advice includes reducing stimulants or caloric intake close to sleep to avoid rebound hypoglycaemia. Other lifestyle targets of interest to clinicians may be promoting adequate exposure to sunlight for vitamin D enhancement and serotonin turnover ([85]; notwithstanding skin cancer risks, including time of day, season, and skin pigmentation/complexion). Despite a paucity of data with respect to its association with depression, limiting exposure to environmental toxins, chemicals pollutants [60], and noise pollution [86] is also recommended. In the future, the moderation of excessive technological interface (e.g. mobile phones, computers, and television) may also emerge as a clinical recommendation in the context of lifestyle medicine [87].

Case Study

Overview

SG is a 29-year-old female who reports a 4-week history of episodic low mood, general fatigue, and apathy. She has no suicidal ideation. SG has limited desire to commence antidepressant medication and is interested in changing some aspects of her lifestyle to improve her mood and overall health. Her diet has been poor of late, and she reports slipping into a pattern of late nights on the Internet, with no physical activity, and smoking (half pack of cigarettes per day) and drinking alcohol excessively (15–20 units of alcohol per week). SG has been recently diagnosed with an episode of minor depression.

Suggested Initial Prescription

After thorough case taking, diagnostic screening, and charting of mood level and suicidality risk, SG is provided some options about various elements of her lifestyle that can be modified to improve her general mental and physical health.

It is collaboratively decided that for the next 2 weeks she will focus on three main areas:

1. To get to bed between 10.30 pm–11.30 pm and initiate sleep hygiene measures (e.g. low evening light, reduced computer use, and reduced stimulants)
2. To walk to work 2–3 times per week (3 miles) and swim on the weekend
3. To make an attempt to reduce refined sugars and processed foods, and increase lean protein, fruits and vegetables with color, nuts, and omega-3 rich foods

Follow-up Prescription

After reporting an increase in mood and energy, SG is interested in some further advice to improve her health and wellbeing. It is decided she will now:

1. Take a slightly longer route walking to work via the local park (green space time)
2. Spend more time socializing in person and less time on the Internet
3. Attempt to reduce cigarette and alcohol consumption

Prescriptive Considerations

It is important that the clinician develops a working plan in concert with the patient to promote change that is achievable in a graded manner. The use of an actual written "prescription" of these proposed lifestyle modifications is helpful as a formalized medical intervention as opposed to being regarded as general advice. The description of specific aspects to change can be detailed in the prescription, for example which foods to introduce or reduce, type/duration/intensity/modality of exercise, and sleep hygiene elements. If mood significantly worsens then medication and/or psychological intervention is advised, although the lifestyle modifcations should be maintained.

Summary

While many factors, including genetics, personality, cognition, and environmental stressors, contribute to the etiology of depression, lifestyle plays an important role in the disorder's pathogenesis. Targets for lifestyle modification exist and have application in front-line clinical care alongside pharmacotherapies and psychological techniques. These targets can promote responsiveness to treatment as well as better self-management of depression. While preliminary data in this area of research are promising, rigorous research is required to address the long-term application of lifestyle medicine for depression prevention and management. Studies exploring lifestyle modification involving multiple lifestyle

elements are needed, though often difficult to enact, in order to elucidate effects. In any case, there is wide agreement that a more integrative approach for depression is required, and the evidence suggests that lifestyle modification be a routine part of treatment and considered for preventive efforts.

References

1. Kronish IM, et al. The effect of enhanced depression care on adherence to risk-reducing behaviors after acute coronary syndromes: findings from the COPES trial. Am Heart J. 2012;164(4):524–9.
2. Maes M, Fišar Z, Medina M, et al. New drug targets in depression: inflammatory, cell-mediated immune, oxidative and nitrosative stress, mitochondrial, antioxidant, and neuroprogressive pathways. And new drug candidates-Nrf2 activators and GSK-3 inhibitors. Inflammopharmacology. 2012;20(3):127–50.
3. Kant AK. Consumption of energy-dense, nutrient-poor foods by adult Americans: nutritional and health implications. The third National Health and Nutrition Examination Survey, 1988–1994. Am J Clin Nutr. 2000;72(4):929–36.
4. Quirk S, et al. The association between diet quality, dietary patterns and depression in adults: a systematic review. BMC Psychiatry. 2013;13(1):175.
5. Jacka FN, et al. Associations between diet quality and depressed mood in adolescents: results from the Australian Healthy Neighbourhoods study. Aust N Z J Psychiatry. 2010;44(5):435–42.
6. Jacka F, et al. A prospective study of diet quality and mental health in adolescents. PLoS ONE. 2011;6(9):e24805.
7. Sanchez-Villegas A, et al. Mediterranean dietary pattern and depression: the PREDIMED randomized trial. BMC Med. 2013;11(1):208.
8. Faulconbridge LF, et al. One-year changes in symptoms of depression and weight in overweight/obese individuals with type 2 diabetes in the Look AHEAD study. Obesity. 2012;20(4):783–93.
9. Berk M, Jacka F. Preventive strategies in depression: gathering evidence for risk factors and potential interventions. Br J Psychiatry. 2012;201:339–41.
10. Nettleton J, et al. Associations between dietary patterns and flow cytometry-measured biomarkers of inflammation and cellular activation in the Atherosclerosis Risk in Communities (ARIC) Carotid Artery MRI Study. Atherosclerosis. 2010;212(1):260–7.
11. Pasco JA, et al. Association of high-sensitivity C-reactive protein with de novo major depression. Br J Psychiatry. 2010;197(5):372–7.
12. McMillan L, Owen L, Kras M, Scholey A. Behavioural effects of a 10-day Mediterranean diet. Results from a pilot study evaluating mood and cognitive performance. Appetite. 2011;56(1):143–7.
13. Sarris J, Mischoulon D, Schweitzer I. Adjunctive nutraceuticals with standard pharmacotherapies in bipolar disorder: a systematic review of clinical trials. Bipolar Disord. 2011;13(5–6):454–65.
14. O'Neil A, et al. A randomised, controlled trial of a dietary intervention for adults with major depression (the "SMILES" trial): study protocol. BMC Psychiatry. 2013;13:114.
15. Brown WJ, et al. Prospective study of physical activity and depressive symptoms in middle-aged women. Am J Prev Med. 2005;29(4):265–72.
16. Chaouloff F. Effects of acute physical exercise on central serotonergic systems. Med Sci Sports Exerc. 1997;29(1):58–62.
17. Dunn AL, Trivedi MH, Kampert JB, Clark CG, Chambliss HO. Exercise treatment for depression: efficacy and dose response. Am J Prev Med. 2005;28(1):1–8.
18. Erickson KI, Miller DL, Roecklein KA. The aging hippocampus: interactions between exercise, depression, and BDNF. Neuroscientist. 2012;18(1):82–97.

19. Ernst C, et al. Antidepressant effects of exercise: evidence for an adult-neurogenesis hypothesis? J Psychiatry Neurosci. 2006;31(2):84–92.

20. Dey S, Singh RH, Dey PK. Exercise training: significance of regional alterations in serotonin metabolism of rat brain in relation to antidepressant effect of exercise. Physiol Behav. 1992;52(6):1095–9.

21. Rimer J, Dwan K, Lawlor DA, et al. Exercise for depression. Cochrane Database Syst Rev. 2012;7:CD004366. doi:10.1002/14651858. CD004366.pub5.

22. Krogh J, et al. The effect of exercise in clinically depressed adults: systematic review and meta-analysis of randomized controlled trials. J Clin Psychiatry. 2011;72(4):529.

23. Cramer H, Lauche R, Langhorst J, Dobos G. Yoga for depression: a systematic review and meta-analysis. Depress Anxiety. 2013;30(11):1068–83.

24. Cramer H, Krucoff C, Dobos G. Adverse events associated with yoga: a systematic review of published case reports and case series. PLoS ONE. 2013;8(10):e75515.

25. Kabat-Zinn J. Wherever you go, there you are: mindfulness meditation in everyday life. New York: Hyperion; 1994.

26. Yu X, et al. Activation of the anterior prefrontal cortex and serotonergic system is associated with improvements in mood and EEG changes induced by Zen meditation practice in novices. Int J Psychophysiol. 2011;80(2):103–11.

27. Hofmann SG, et al. The effect of mindfulness-based therapy on anxiety and depression: a meta-analytic review. J Consult Clin Psychol. 2010;78(2):169–83.

28. Steuber TL, Danner F. Adolescent smoking and depression: which comes first? Addict Behav. 2006;31(1):133–6.

29. Glynn SM, Sussman S. Why patients smoke. Hosp Community Psychiatry. 1990;41(9):1027–8.

30. Boden JM, Fergusson DM. Alcohol and depression. Addiction. 2012;106(5):906–14.

31. Swendsen JD, et al. The comorbidity of alcoholism with anxiety and depressive disorders in four geographic communities. Compr Psychiatry. 1998;39(4):176–84.

32. Clapp P, Bhave SV, Hoffman PL. How adaptation of the brain to alcohol leads to dependence: a pharmacological perspective. Alcohol Res Health. 2008;31(4):310–39.

33. Wilton G, Moberg DP, Fleming MF. The effect of brief alcohol intervention on postpartum depression. MCN Am J Matern Child Nurs. 2009;34(5):297–302.

34. van Mill JG, et al. Insomnia and sleep duration in a large cohort of patients with major depressive disorder and anxiety disorders. J Clin Psychiatry. 2010;71(3):239–46.

35. Baglioni C, et al. Insomnia as a predictor of depression: a meta-analytic evaluation of longitudinal epidemiological studies. J Affect Disord. 2011;135(1–3):10–9.

36. Roth T. Insomnia as a risk factor for depression. Int J Neuropsychopharmacolog. 2004;7:S34–S5.

37. Grandner MA, et al. Sleep disturbance is associated with cardiovascular and metabolic disorders. J Sleep Res. 2012;21(4):427–33.

38. Ejaz SM, et al. Obstructive sleep apnea and depression: a review. Innov Clin Neurosci. 2011;8(8):17–25.

39. Riemann D, et al. Chronic insomnia: clinical and research challenges—an agenda. Pharmacopsychiatry. 2011;44(1):1–14.

40. Merrill RM, et al. The effects of an intensive lifestyle modification program on sleep and stress disorders. J Nutr Health Aging. 2007;11(3):242–8.

41. Nehlig A, Daval JL, Debry G. Caffeine and the central nervous system: mechanisms of action, biochemical, metabolic and psychostimulant effects. Brain Res Brain Res Rev. 1992;17(2):139–70.

42. Lara DR. Caffeine, mental health, and psychiatric disorders. J Alzheimers Dis. 2010;20(Suppl 1):S239–48.

43. Vilarim MM, Rocha Araujo DM, Nardi AE. Caffeine challenge test and panic disorder: a systematic literature review. Expert Rev Neurother. 2011;11(8):1185–95.

44. Berk M, et al. Blunted adenosine A2a receptor function in platelets in patients with major depression. Eur Neuropsychopharmacol. 2001;11(2):183–6.

45. Lucas M, et al. Coffee, caffeine, and risk of depression among women. Arch Intern Med. 2011;171(17):1571–8.

46. Broderick P, Benjamin AB. Caffeine and psychiatric symptoms: a review. J Okla State Med Assoc. 2004;97(12):538–42.

47. Ibarra-Rovillard MS, Kuiper NA. Social support and social negativity findings in depression: perceived responsiveness to basic psychological needs. Clin Psychol Rev. 2011;31(3):342–52.

48. Stafford M, et al. Positive and negative exchanges in social relationships as predictors of depression: evidence from the English Longitudinal Study of Aging. J Aging Health. 2011;23(4):607–28.

49. Kouvonen A, et al. Social support and the likelihood of maintaining and improving levels of physical activity: the Whitehall II Study. Eur J Public Health. 2012;22(4):514–8.

50. Street G, James R, Cutt H. The relationship between organised physical recreation and mental health. Health Promot J Austr. 2007;18(3):236–9.

51. Jorm AF, Morgan AJ, Hetrick SE. Relaxation for depression. Cochrane Database Syst Rev. 2008;4:CD007142.

52. Lee AC, Maheswaran R. The health benefits of urban green spaces: a review of the evidence. J Public Health (Oxf). 2011;33(2):212–22.

53. Barton J, Pretty J. What is the best dose of nature and green exercise for improving mental health? A multi-study analysis. Environ Sci Technol. 2010;44(10):3947–55.

54. Annerstedt M, Wahrborg P. Nature-assisted therapy: systematic review of controlled and observational studies. Scand J Public Health. 2011;39(4):371–88.

55. Hahn IH, et al. Does outdoor work during the winter season protect against depression and mood difficulties? Scand J Work Environ Health. 2011;37(5):446–9.

56. Radua J, Pertusa A, Cardoner N. Climatic relationships with specific clinical subtypes of depression. Psychiatry Res. 2010;175(3):217–20.

57. Berk M, et al. Vitamin D deficiency may play a role in depression. Med Hypotheses. 2007;69(6):1316–9.

58. Knippenberg S, Damoiseaux J, Bol Y, Hupperts R, et al. Higher levels of reported sun exposure, and not vitamin D status, are associated with less depressive symptoms and fatigue in multiple sclerosis. Acta Neurol Scand. 2014;129(2):123–31.

59. Sanders KM, et al. Annual high-dose vitamin D3 and mental well-being: randomised controlled trial. Br J Psychiatry. 2011;198(5):357–64.

60. Genc S, et al. The adverse effects of air pollution on the nervous system. J Toxicol. 2012;2012:782462.

61. Fonken LK, et al. Air pollution impairs cognition, provokes depressive-like behaviors and alters hippocampal cytokine expression and morphology. Mol Psychiatry, 2011;16(10):987–95, 973.

62. Lim YH, et al. Air pollution and symptoms of depression in elderly adults. Environ Health Perspect. 2012;120(7):1023–8.

63. Enmarker I, et al. Health in older cat and dog owners: the Nord-Trondelag Health Study (HUNT)-3 study. Scand J Public Health. 2012;40(8):718–24.

64. Blumenthal JA, et al. Exercise and pharmacological treatment of depressive symptoms in patients with coronary heart disease: results from the UPBEAT (Understanding the Prognostic Benefits of Exercise and Antidepressant Therapy) study. J Am Coll Cardiol. 2012;60(12):1053–63.

65. Prochaska J, et al. Initial efficacy of MI, TTM tailoring and HRI's with multiple behaviors for employee health promotion. Prev Med. 2008;46(3):226–31.

66. Ross JA, Kasum CM. Dietary flavonoids: bioavailability, metabolic effects, and safety. Annu Rev Nutr. 2002;22:19–34.

67. Howes MJ, Perry E. The role of phytochemicals in the treatment and prevention of dementia. Drugs Aging. 2011;28(6):439–68.

68. Jacka FN, Ystrom E, Brantsaeter AL, et al. Maternal and early postnatal nutrition and mental health of offspring by age 5 years:

a prospective cohort study. J Am Acad Child Adolesc Psychiatry. 2013;52(10):1038–47.

69. Dominguez-Salas P, et al. Maternal nutrition at conception modulates DNA methylation of human metastable epialleles. Nat Commun. 2014;5:3746. doi:10.1038/ncomms4746.

70. Khan NA, et al. The 2009 Canadian Hypertension Education Program recommendations for the management of hypertension: part 2–therapy. Can J Cardiol. 2009;25(5):287–98.

71. Daley A. Exercise and depression: a review of reviews. J Clin Psychol Med Settings. 2008;15(2):140–7.

72. Dunn AL, et al. Exercise treatment for depression: efficacy and dose response. Am J Prev Med. 2005;28(1):1–8.

73. Singh NA, et al. A randomized controlled trial of high versus low intensity weight training versus general practitioner care for clinical depression in older adults. J Gerontol A: Biol Sci Med Sci. 2005;60 A(6):768–76.

74. Worthington J, et al. Consumption of alcohol, nicotine, and caffeine among depressed outpatients. Relationship with response to treatment. Psychosomatics. 1996;37(6):518–22.

75. Rae AM, et al. The effect of a history of alcohol dependence in adult major depression. J Affect Disord. 2002;70(3):281–90.

76. Baker AL, et al. Psychological interventions for alcohol misuse among people with co-occurring depression or anxiety disorders: a systematic review. J Affect Disord. 2012;139(3):217–29.

77. Baker AL, et al. Randomized controlled trial of cognitive-behavioural therapy for coexisting depression and alcohol problems: short-term outcome. Addiction. 2010;105(1):87–99.

78. Berk M. Should we be targeting smoking as a routine intervention? Acta Neuropsychiatrica. 2007;19:131–2.

79. Bernard P, et al. Physical activity as a protective factor in relapse following smoking cessation in participants with a depressive disorder. Am J Addict. 2012;21(4):348–55.

80. Hughes JR. Depression during tobacco abstinence. Nicotine Tob Res. 2007;9(4):443–6.

81. Aversa LH, et al. PTSD and depression as predictors of physical health-related quality of life in tobacco-dependent veterans. J Psychosom Res. 2012;73(3):185–90.

82. Coogan AN, Thome J. Chronotherapeutics and psychiatry: setting the clock to relieve the symptoms. World J Biol Psychiatry. 2011;12(Suppl 1):40–3.

83. Stepanski EJ, Wyatt JK. Use of sleep hygiene in the treatment of insomnia. Sleep Med Rev. 2003;7(3):215–25.

84. Monteleone P, Martiadis V, Maj M. Circadian rhythms and treatment implications in depression. Prog Neuropsychopharmacol Biol Psychiatry. 2011;35(7):1569–74.

85. Lambert GW, et al. Effect of sunlight and season on serotonin turnover in the brain. Lancet. 2002;360(9348):1840–2.

86. Riediker M, Koren HS. The importance of environmental exposures to physical, mental and social well-being. Int J Hyg Environ Health. 2004;207(3):193–201.

87. Walsh R. Lifestyle and mental health. Am Psychol. 2011;66(7): 579–92.

Patricia Robinson, David Bauman and Bridget Beachy

Introduction

Persistent pain presents a substantial challenge for patients with regard to continuing or adopting healthy lifestyle behaviors; health-care providers need to address this challenge with a coordinated, continuous approach informed by psychological research. In this chapter, evidence is reviewed about conditions associated with persistent pain and their interactions with lifestyle behaviors. Additionally, specific interventions are described that promote psychological acceptance and improved engagement in daily activities, even among patients with chronic pain. Acceptance and commitment therapy (ACT) (pronounced as the word "act") is an evidence-based approach to treating chronic pain [1–6] and can be adapted to various primary care and specialty care settings [7, 8]. ACT interventions include values clarification and values connection exercises, mindfulness practices, and activities that promote commitment to change.

Many pain management specialists believe the term "persistent pain" is useful in describing chronic pain conditions because it promotes attention to the ways pain may interrupt functioning, well-being, and quality of life. Here, chronic pain and persistent pain are used interchangeably in discussions focusing on interactions among the experience of pain and smoking, reduced physical activity, and depressive behaviors, such as lack of engagement in social activities.

The International Association for the Study of Pain defines pain as an "unpleasant emotional and sensory experience associated with actual or potential tissue damage…" [9]. Acute pain generally results in tissue damage from a sudden injury or from surgery and is often accompanied by emotional discomfort [10]. While unpleasant, acute pain is useful in conveying to the person that there is something wrong. Without this signal or warning, the person might experience further bodily harm. In the case of acute pain, the source of the pain is usually clear, and once treated, the pain resolves [10]. Chronic pain is pain that is pervasive, usually lasting for at least 3–6 months or lasting longer (than what is a reasonably expected time frame for the injury to heal). It often occurs in the absence of a clear organic etiology; however, this does not diminish the perception of pain in the patient [10]. A patient's experience of pain maps closely with physiological, emotional, behavioral, and psychological states. Environmental or psychosocial stressors may combine with these states and amplify the pain experience. Whatever the source of the pain, injury, or illness, pain that does not resolve with medical treatment may have a pervasive impact on lifestyle and general quality of life.

Conditions Associated with Persistent Pain

Musculoskeletal Disorders

One of the most common causes of chronic pain is musculoskeletal pain, which affects the muscles, ligaments and tendons, bones, and nerves. It may be acute or chronic, or it may be generalized or localized. Common causes of musculoskeletal pain include injury, overuse, poor posture, and immobilization [11]. Chronic low back pain and myalgia are two common musculoskeletal disorders. People with these

P. Robinson (✉)
Mountainview Consulting Group, Inc., Zillah, USA
e-mail: patti1510@msn.com

D. Bauman · B. Beachy
Central Washington Family Medicine Residency Program, Yakima, WA, USA

© Springer International Publishing Switzerland 2016
J. I. Mechanick, R. F. Kushner (eds.), *Lifestyle Medicine,* DOI 10.1007/978-3-319-24687-1_26

conditions experience aching or stiffness, fatigue, twitching muscles, burning in muscles, and sleep disturbances. While symptoms can vary greatly among patients and according to the area affected, most patients report increased pain with movement [12]. This has a pronounced impact on patient engagement in various healthy lifestyle behaviors, such as regular exercise and even engaging in social activities outside the home.

Low Back Pain

Low back pain is the most common chronic pain problem resulting in disability [12]. Lumbar degenerative disc disease (DDD), a syndrome consisting of a compromised disc in the lumbar spine, is one of the most common causes of low back pain [13]. The exact cause of lumbar DDD is unknown; however, lumbar DDD is likely multifaceted and includes genetic components, wear and tear, and in some cases, an impact injury that worsens over time. Lumbar DDD is actually a fairly common condition, with some disc space degeneration present in at least 30 % of people between 30 and 50 years of age [13]. After the age of 60, lumbar DDD is common [13]. Lumbar DDD may be of limited concern to many adults, as many have these structural abnormalities without any associated pain. Interestingly, some people will experience lumbar pain and have no structural abnormalities [13]. This incongruence is one of the challenges in treating low back pain. Patients without a loss in disc space often struggle to accept that the assessment did not reveal structural damage, given their experience of pain and the toll it has had on their lives over time.

Joint Disease

Joints are another common area identified by patients reporting chronic pain. Joints connect two or more bones, such as the knee, hip, elbow, and shoulder [14]. Joint damage may occur through injury or disease. Another well-known cause of chronic pain is arthritis, a condition associated with joint inflammation, pain, stiffness, and swelling. The most common type of arthritis is osteoarthritis, which is related to aging and may develop from an injury. Rheumatoid arthritis is an autoimmune disease, and is often diagnosed in people under 45 years of age and may occur in children. Bursitis, or the inflammation of the fluid-filled sac that provides cushioning for joints, muscles, tendons, or skin, is another painful joint condition and may be brought on by either overuse or injury [14].

In addition to musculoskeletal problems, low back pain, and joint disease, there are many other pain syndromes, including chronic fatigue syndrome, endometriosis, fibromy-algia, systemic lupus erythematosis, inflammatory bowel disease, interstitial cystitis, temporomandibular joint dysfunction, headaches, migraines, and vulvodynia, among others. Medical debilitation and frailty—the loss of strength and vigor—can accompany most of these conditions. Concomitant with debilitation, patients often experience problems with occupational functioning which can lead to financial problems. While losing their usual income, patients often also experience high medical costs. The result is limited resources—financial and emotional—to care for themselves and their families.

Lifestyle Factors and Debilitation

The level of debilitation patients with various medical problems associated with chronic pain experience may be exacerbated by numerous lifestyle factors. For example, tobacco use can worsen chronic pain, subjective patients' levels of pain, and overall functioning [15]. Specifically, individuals who smoked reported not only higher overall levels of pain but also greater impairment in physical activity, mood, work, social relationships, sleep, and overall life enjoyment. Furthermore, higher levels of nicotine dependence were associated with greater impairment in work, overall life enjoyment, and self-reported pain levels [15]. Tobacco use among patients with chronic pain is also associated with greater use of opioids [16]. All in all, when treating individuals for chronic pain, tobacco use needs to be addressed.

Symptoms of depression are common among patients with chronic pain. While available data do not address causation, patients diagnosed with major depressive disorder have been found to be four times more likely to have disabling chronic pain than those without this diagnosis [17]. Patients with chronic pain who experience significant symptoms of depression also report greater pain intensity [16]. Along with higher levels of depression, primary care patients with chronic pain report lower levels of perceived health [18]. Poorer quality of life has been found to be associated with lack of sleep and emotional difficulties among patients with musculoskeletal pain [19]. Research has also found alcohol habits to be associated with a poorer quality of life in patients with chronic pain [19].

Being overweight or obese is a factor that may not only complicate the treatment of chronic pain but also impair quality of life. While data assessing the directional relationship between obesity and chronic pain are not available, the relationship between weight and chronic pain is documented in a number of disorders, including low back pain and osteoarthritis [20]. Janke and colleagues hypothesize that as an individual gains weight, there is increased structural demand, which may result in bone and joint pain [20]. Obesity is related to metabolic problems (e.g., diabetes), which may also result in neuropathy and other pain-related complaints.

Weight gain may additionally cause or increase pain as a result of decreased mobility and reduced activity level [20].

Acceptance and Commitment Therapy

General Remarks

The American Psychological Association (APA) provides a list of evidence-based interventions for chronic pain that includes ACT [21]. ACT is one of several new cognitive and behavior therapies referred to as the "third wave" of behavior therapy [22]. As its name suggests, ACT seeks to promote acceptance of unwanted private experiences (e.g., "This pain is killing me") through the application of various mindfulness strategies (e.g., "I have a dull ache in my back and I am sitting in a room listening to my child play the piano"). These strategies include moving from a participant perspective ("I hate this pain and I can't make it go away") to an observer perspective ("I have pain and an emotional response of sadness and frustration to it; I don't deserve this pain; I just have it; I can have love and enjoyment in my life, along with pain; I can make choices in this moment about my lifestyle behaviors; healthy lifestyle behavior will help me pursue more of what matters to me in life"). They also include methods to help the patient contact the present moment. For example, by momentarily connecting with a sensory experience (such as what it is like to have a tongue). ACT interventions help patients disconnect from the literal aspects of private experience (including thoughts, feelings, memories, sensations, images, etc.).

As the "C" in ACT suggests, the overarching goal of ACT is to help the patient develop skills for "committing" to healthy lifestyle behaviors in a psychologically flexible manner. As the patient with chronic pain makes gains in healthy lifestyle behaviors, he or she is more able to pursue directions in life consistent with vitality, purpose, and meaning. Because it is not possible to "get rid" of pain or thoughts about pain (e.g., "I must get rid of this pain"; "There must be another treatment"), the patient with chronic pain needs extraordinary skills for accepting and acting with pain.

Central to the ACT view is that suffering and loss of vitality occur when a patient over-relies on avoiding or eliminating distressing thoughts, feelings, memories, or sensations related to pain. This pain avoidance agenda leads to progressively more behavioral and experiential avoidance strategies over time, such as taking more pain medications, increasingly restricting physical and social activities, using nicotine for a short-term lift in mood, and overeating comfort or favorite foods. The result is an escalation of unhealthy lifestyle behaviors and ongoing loss of meaning. Healthy lifestyle behaviors and pursuit of a meaningful life are inextricably intertwined.

Evidence Supporting ACT Treatment of Chronic Pain

Support of the use of ACT with chronic pain includes six randomized controlled trials [1–6]. Additionally, a number of partially controlled trials [23–25] and several effectiveness studies [26, 27] suggest that ACT is a useful approach for helping patients with chronic pain. In these studies, average effect sizes across outcome domains are large in early follow-up (0.85–0.89) and moderate 3 years posttreatment (0.57) [28]. Consistent positive effects associated with ACT interventions include increased physical and social functioning (measured by the Sickness Impact Profile) and decreased pain-related medical visits (even 3 years following treatment).

In addition to outcomes, most ACT trials concerning chronic pain have investigated treatment processes. Results indicate that increases in acceptance of pain correlated with improvements during treatment in the form of reduced anxiety, depression, and disability [24, 26]. Additionally, increases in consistency between daily behaviors and values correlated with reductions in anxiety, depression, and disability at 3-month follow-up [26]. Finally, increases in acceptance of pain, general psychological acceptance, mindfulness, and value-consistent behaviors during the active phase of treatment significantly correlated with improvements in anxiety, depression, and disability, at a 3-month follow-up, independent of changes in pain [27].

Intervening: Open, Aware, and Engaged

Patients with chronic pain need to learn new skills in order to reverse the lifestyle-harming cycle of pain avoidance and move toward adoption of healthy lifestyle behaviors. These skills include those that (1) help patients open up to the experience of pain, (2) promote a better awareness of present-moment experience and differing perspectives on the pain experience, and (3) engender better engagement in life activities reflective of their values. Some patients will have strengths in one or more of these central areas and the health-care professional can determine this through the results of the clinical interview. Figure 26.1 provides a graphic representation of the six processes involved in the ACT approach to persistent pain. Figure 26.2 offers a flexibility grid (open, aware, and engaged) for health-care professionals to use in assessing relative strengths and weaknesses of individual patients in these areas.

Patients who are weak in the first area (open) tend to be fearful of pain and to see it as dangerous; they may report anxiety and depression. To help them make gains in this area, health-care professionals can suggest "noticing and naming" strategies [29]. Noticing involves watching for thoughts, feelings, and sensations, and allowing them to come and go (as

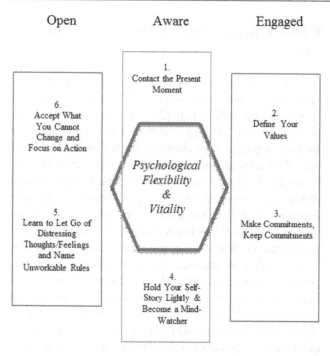

Fig. 26.1 The acceptance and commitment therapy approach to persistent pain

	Weak					Strong	
Open	0	1	2	3	4	5	6
Aware	0	1	2	3	4	5	6
Engaged	0	1	2	3	4	5	6

Intervention Plan: What to Strengthen and How

Open:

Aware:

Engaged:

Fig. 26.2 The flexibility grid

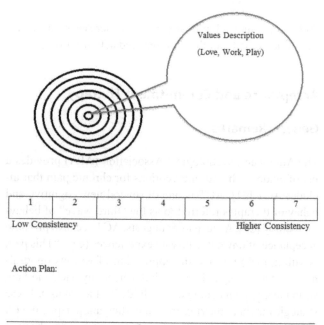

Fig. 26.3 The Bull's-Eye Plan

A second core skill area is that of awareness (aware). Pain is a commanding experience and it can easily rob a patient of attention, ability to sustain focus, and the capacity to shift flexibly among perspectives. When weak in this skill area, the patient may seem distracted by pain sensations (e.g., shifting uncomfortably in his seat), experience difficulties with receiving medical information and instructions, and tell a repeated story about his initial injury (or diagnosis) and failed medical procedures. There is a feeling of nothing new, fresh, or immediate in these stories. Interventions that help the patient become more aware include those that help the patient tune in to immediate sensory experience (such as the sensation on his legs created by contact with the chair he is sitting on, the rise and fall of his chest when he breathes, or the sounds in the room or clinic where more behavioral choice is possible). Learning to shift awareness from internal experience to external experience helps a patient learn to experience pain in a larger context where it is less compelling and where more choice and less automatic responding are possible.

Another intervention that may help patients with deficits in this area is introducing the idea of how all humans have stories that they tell about themselves. Some of the stories (e.g., "I am a hard worker... I did this...") are helpful when they are told in the right context, such as a job interview. However, some stories (e.g., "I am damaged... I can't go for a walk... I'll pay for it!") may not promote behavioral choices (e.g., going for a walk) that would be a step toward the start of a healthier lifestyle and, in some cases, a different story (e.g., "I have back pain and I walk for my health"). Even in brief visits, providers can help patients better hear their stories, evaluate their stories' impact or workability, and identify them with brief nicknames.

they quite naturally do). Naming involves giving thoughts, feelings, and sensations a name. The name may simply be a frame, such as "I am having the thought that I can't do anything I want to do because of this pain." Alternatively, naming may be a simple descriptive term, such as "feeling," "thinking," "sensing," or "starting to tell an old familiar story about pain." The key component of interventions that promote openness is that they promote acceptance. Acceptance is not the same as "liking something" or "giving up," but is more akin to "allowing" or "making room" for what is already there.

1. Ask the patient to choose Love, Work, or Play as a focus for a short discussion about values. Ask the patient to explain what is important to him or her in each area of life.

2. Listen closely, reflect what you heard and then write a statement on the Bull's-Eye Plan using the words (global, abstract) the patient used in talking about the value.

3. Explain that the Bull's-Eye on the target represents the patient's hitting her / his value target on a daily basis (and explain that most of us fall far short of that on a day to day basis, but knowing the targets helps us making choices, set goals, and implement plans).

4. Ask patient to choose a number to represent how close to the Bull's-Eye value statement her/his behavior has come over the past 2 weeks.

5. Ask patient to plan 2 specific behavior experiments for the next 2 weeks that patient believes will make her / his behavior more value consistent (closer to the Bull's-Eye target).

6. At follow-up, ask patient to re-rate and identify barriers to engaging in planned behaviors.

7. If time allows, rate the patient's current functioning level in one core area on the Flexibility Grid (see Figure 2). This will provide a baseline against which you can judge the impact of the Bull's-Eye Plan.

8. If time allows in an initial or follow-up visit, teach a skill to help the patient improve skills for accepting distressing thoughts about pain (OPEN), being more skillful in finding the present moment and taking an observer perspective on pain (AWARE), or clarifying and connecting with important life values and lifestyle behaviors consistent with those values (ENGAGED).

Fig. 26.4 Guide for using the Bull's-Eye Plan

The third skill area that many patients with persistent pain are in need of remediating is that of clarifying and connecting with their values (engage). When pain becomes chronic, patients often spend more and more time trying to control or avoid it. As a consequence, they tend to drop out of valued activities, such as being a leader in their family or a worker drawing an income for delivering a useful service. As disconnection from valued activities progresses, many patients with chronic pain experience symptoms of depression. They may try to avoid this by, for example, taking medications or using alcohol that helps numb their emotional experience, or by withdrawing from social activities in an effort to hide their feelings from others. Health-care professionals can help patients connect with their values by discussing them with the patient. The Bull's-Eye Plan (Fig. 26.3) is a great intervention for identifying patient values in the three basic areas of life: love (or relationships with family, friends, or pets), work (paid or volunteer) or study, and play (including spiritual and other restorative activities) [30]. Figure 26.4 provides directions for health-care professional use of the Bull's-Eye Plan in initial and follow-up visits. The Bull's-Eye Plan is a great method for filling in gaps in health-care services, as it may start in specialty or primary care contexts and be supported as the patient steps up and steps down in levels of care. Robinson, Gould, and Strosahl provide more information about the use of the Bull's-Eye Plan with ongoing care of primary care patients with chronic pain [7]. Strosahl, Robinson, and Gustavsson [29] provide extensive instruction for use of the open–aware–engaged approach as an approach to both assessment and intervention.

Lifestyle Change in Patients with Chronic Pain: The NEEDS Approach

As patients learn to be more psychologically flexible in addressing the difficult problems associated with persistent pain, they gain confidence in approaching lifestyle changes. The nutrition, exercise, enjoyment, don't smoke or drink, and sleep (NEEDS) approach supports providers and patients in their

Table 26.1 The NEEDS approach to changing lifestyle behaviors in patients with persistent pain

Nutrition	Encourage fresh foods, four light meals per day, avoid eating while watching television
Exercise	Short walks throughout the day, on a regular basis; gentle stretching exercises twice daily
Enjoyment	Encourage social activities, exploration of hobbies, participation in activities that provide a sense of accomplishment
Don't smoke or drink	Avoid, reduce, or stop use of tobacco and alcohol; cultivate other relaxation activities
Sleep	Learn to relax intermittently throughout the day and prior to bed; keep a regular wake and sleep time; learn to soften/relax when experiencing pain in bed

efforts to systematically address lifestyle behavior change. Table 26.1 provides an explanation of the NEEDS approach.

The NEEDS approach may be useful as a tip sheet for patients with chronic pain. Additionally, it can serve as a starting point for health-care professional and patient conversations about lifestyle change. Ideally, the health-care professional can help a patient identify a priority area from the patient's perspective. It is best to start with one area and only discuss other areas when the patient is making progress in the initial area of interest.

Assessing Outcomes

In assessing outcomes, providers need to look at patient gains in lifestyle goals, individually and collectively. The NEEDS approach can be built into the electronic health record (EHR) and providers can use a rating scale of 1–10 (1 = weak lifestyle behavior and 10 = strong lifestyle behavior) to assess progress. The Bull's-Eye consistency score may also be built into the EHR. Finally, a quality-of-life measure is recommended at all visits such as the Duke Health Profile [31]. These functional approaches are far superior to pain intensity ratings, as this measure likely reflects a great deal of variation that is generally not under the patient's or the provider's control. Furthermore, most patients would prefer to have a meaningful life—a high quality of life (even with pain)—to a life disconnected from their values and free of pain.

Case Example: Anne

Anne is a 45-year-old woman with rheumatoid arthritis. She works as a reading specialist in an elementary school. In order to function at work, she added opioids to her long list of medications several years prior to her consultation with her new rheumatologist. Anne's husband had died suddenly a year earlier and she had steadily increased her opioid dose and started medications for anxiety and depression. She had stopped her daily walks, was eating more at night and less in the morning, had gained 18 lb in the past year, and admitted to having a drink or two every evening before dinner. Dr. Anderson introduced the Bull's-Eye Plan in her initial consultation with Anne. They talked about her values in regard to relationships, particularly her relationships with her two children (one in high school and one in college). Anne

did not feel her behavior was consistent with her values as a parent and wanted to improve on the model she was providing for her children. Anne set initial goals of taking a morning walk on weekends and avoiding alcohol on work nights. Additionally, she agreed to explore relaxation apps on the Internet and to practice exercises from one she found to be of interest. Dr. Anderson made adjustments to Anne's medications and sent a summary of the consult to Dr. Meyer, Anne's primary care provider. Anne followed up with Dr. Meyer 2 weeks later and reported (when asked) that she was working on her Bull's-Eye Plan. Specifically, she was now walking on several afternoons as well as on weekends. She had significantly reduced alcohol consumption. She had found a relaxation app that she liked and some meditation music as well. She and a woman friend were now making a couple of meals on the weekend together, so that they would have food prepared for healthy lunches during the work week. A behavioral health consultant (BHC) had recently joined Dr. Meyer's primary care practice and offered a monthly class on behavioral strategies for managing chronic pain (for more information on BHC services, see Robinson and Reiter [32]). When Dr. Meyer suggested that Anne consult with the BHC about strategies for reducing her dose of opioids and begin attending the class, she readily agreed. In the class, Anne received consistent support on making value-based behavior changes and continuing to improve her lifestyle goals. When barriers arose, she discussed them in the class and learned new strategies for addressing them (including how to be more open, aware, and engaged).

References

1. Buhrman M, Skoglund A, Hussell J, Bergstrom K, Gordh T, Hursti T, et al. Guided internet-delivered Acceptance and Commitment Therapy for chronic pain patients: a randomized controlled trial. Behav Res Ther. 2013;51:307–15.
2. Dahl J, Wilson KG, Nilsson A. Acceptance and Commitment Therapy and the treatment of persons at risk for long-term disability resulting from stress and pain symptoms: a preliminary randomized trial. Behav Res Ther. 2004;35:785–802.
3. Thorsell J, Finnes A, Dahl J, Lundgren T, Gybrant M, Gordh T, et al. A comparative study of 2 manual-based self-help interventions, Acceptance and Commitment Therapy and Applied Relaxation, for persons with chronic pain. Clin J Pain. 2011;27(8):716–23.
4. Wetherell JL, Afari N, Rutledge T, Sorrell JT, Stoddard JA, Petkus AJ, et al. A randomized, controlled trial of acceptance and commitment therapy and cognitive-behavioral therapy for chronic pain. Pain. 2011;152:2098–107.

5. Wicksell RK, Ahlgvist J, Bring A, Melin L, Olsson GL. Can exposure and acceptance strategies improve functioning and life satisfaction in people with chronic pain and whiplash-associated disorders (WAD)? Cogn Behav Ther. 2008;37(3):1–14.

6. Wicksell RK, Kemani M, Jensen K, Kosek E, Kadetoff D, Sorionen K, et al. Acceptance and Commitment Therapy for fibromyalgia: a randomized controlled trial. Eur J Pain. 2013;17:599–611.

7. Robinson PJ, Gould D, Strosahl KD. Real behavior change in primary care. Strategies and tools for improving outcomes and increasing job satisfaction. Oakland: New Harbinger; 2011.

8. Robinson P, Wicksell R, Olsson GL. Act with chronic pain patients. In: Hayes S, Storsahl K, editors. A practical guide to acceptance and commitment therapy. New York: Springer; 2005.

9. Merskey H, Bogduk N. Part III: pain terms, a current list with definitions and notes on usage. In: Merskey H, Bogduk N, editors. Title: classification of chronic pain. 2nd ed. Seattle: IASP Press; 1994.

10. National Institute of Neurological Disorders and Stroke. Pain: hope through research. http://www.ninds.nih.gov/disorders/chronic_pain/detail_chronic_pain.htm. Accessed 15 Aug 2014.

11. Cherney K. Musculoskeletal disorders. http://www.healthline.com/health/musculoskeletal-disorders#Definition1. Accessed 15 Aug 2014.

12. Clinic C. Musculoskeletal pain. http://my.clevelandclinic.org/disorders/musculoskeletal_pain/hic_musculoskeletal_pain.aspx. Accessed 15 Aug 2014.

13. Ullrich PF Jr. Lumbar degenerative disc disease. http://www.spine-health.com/conditions/degenerative-disc-disease/lumbar-degenerative-disc-disease-ddd. Accessed 15 Aug 2014.

14. NIH. Joint disorder. http://www.nlm.nih.gov/medlineplus/joint-disorders.html. Accessed 15 Aug 2014.

15. Weingarten TN, Moeschler SM, Ptasynski AE, Hooten WM, Beeebe TJ, Warner DO. An assessment of the association between smoking status, pain intensity, and functional interference in patients with chronic pain. Pain Physician. 2008;11:643–53.

16. Hooten WM, Shi Y, Gazelka HM, Warner DO. The effects of depression and smoking on pain severity and opioid use in patients with chronic pain. Pain. 2011;151(1):223–9.

17. Arnow BA, Hunkeler EM, Blasey CM, Lee J, Constantino MJ, Fireman B, et al. Comorbid depression, chronic pain, and disability in primary care. Psychosom Med. 2006;86(2):262–8.

18. Gureje O, Von Korff M, Simon GE, Gater R. Persistent pain and well-being: a World Health Organization study in primary care. JAMA. 1998;280(2):147–51.

19. Arvidsson S, Arvidsson B, Fridlund B, Bergman S. Health predicting factors in a general population over an eight-year period in subjects with and without chronic musculoskeletal pain. Health Qual Life Outcomes. 2008;6:98.

20. Janke EA, Collins A, Kozak AT. Overview of the relationship between pain and obesity: what do we know? Where do we go next? J Rehabil Res Dev. 2007;44(2):245–62.

21. Society of Clinical Psychology. Acceptance and Commitment Therapy for chronic pain. http://www.div12.org/Psychological-Treatments/disorders/pain_general.php. Accessed 15 Aug 2014.

22. Hayes SC, Strosahl KD, Wilson KG. Acceptance and Commitment Therapy: the process and practice of mindful change. 2nd ed. New York: Guilford Press; 2012.

23. Johnston M, Foster M, Shennan NJ, Johnson A. The effectiveness of an Acceptance and Commitment Therapy self-help intervention for chronic pain. Clin J Pain. 2010;26:393–402.

24. McCraken LM, Vowles KE, Eccleston C. Acceptance-based treatment for persons with complex, long standing chronic pain: a preliminary analysis of treatment outcome in comparison to a waiting phase. Behav Res Ther. 2005;43:1335–46.

25. Vowles KE, Wetherell JL, Sorrell JT. Targeting acceptance, mindfulness, and values-based action in chronic pain: findings of two preliminary trials of an outpatient group-based intervention. Cognit Behav Pract. 2009;16:49–58.

26. Vowles KE, McCracken LM. Acceptance and values-based action in chronic pain: a study of treatment effectiveness and process. J Consult Clin Psychol. 2008;76:397–407.

27. McCraken LM, Gutierrez-Martinez O. Processes of change in psychological flexibility in an interdisciplinary group-based treatment for chronic pain based on Acceptance and Commitment Therapy. Behav Res Ther. 2011;49(4):267–74.

28. Vowles KE, McCracken LM, Zhao-O'Brien J. Acceptance and values-based action in chronic pain: a three year follow-up analysis of treatment effectiveness and process. Behav Res Ther. 2011;49:748–55.

29. Strosahl KD, Robinson PJ, Gustavsson T. Brief interventions for radical change: principles and practice of focused acceptance and commitment therapy. Oakland: New Harbinger; 2012.

30. Lundgren T, Luoma JB, Dahl J, Strosahl K, Robinson P, Melin L. The Bull's-Eye Values Survey: a psychometric evaluation. Cogn Behav Pract. 2012;19:518–26.

31. Parkerson GF Jr, Broadhead WE, Tse CK, Tse CK. The Duke Health Profile. A 17-item measure of health and dysfunction. Med Care. 1990;28(11):1056–72.

32. Robinson PJ, Reiter JT. Behavioral consultation and primary care: a guide to integrating services. 2nd ed. New York: Springer; 2015.

Forestalling Age-Related Brain Disorders

Mark P. Mattson

Abbreviations

AD	Alzheimer's disease
AMP	Adenosine monophosphate
ANS	Autonomic nervous system
APP	Amyloid precursor protein
BDNF	Brain-derived neurotrophic factor
CERAD	Consortium to establish a registry for Alzheimer's disease
CSF	Cerebrospinal fluid
CVD	Cardiovascular disease
HRV	Heart rate variability
HDL	High-density lipoprotein
IER	Intermittent energy restriction
LDL	Low-density lipoprotein
PD	Parkinson's disease
T2D	Type-2 diabetes

Introduction

Emerging findings suggest that optimal brain health is promoted by a healthy lifestyle that includes intermittent physical and intellectual challenges. Four such challenges to brain cells are intermittent fasting, exercise, cognitive stimulation, and phytochemicals in fruits and vegetables. Detailed reviews of the scientific literature on these topics have recently been published [1–5]. One major reason that these different challenges benefit brain function is that they impose a mild stress on brain cells, similar in many ways to the stress that occurs in muscles and the cardiovascular system during vigorous exercise. The (good) stress the neurons experience includes metabolic (reduced energy availability and/or increased energy demand), oxidative, and ionic (resulting from increased electrical activity/membrane depolarization)

stress. As described below, neurons respond adaptively to the mild stress of intermittent challenges by engaging signaling pathways that boost cellular energy metabolism, increase stress resistance, and enhance repair or removal of damaged molecules and mitochondria. These adaptive response mechanisms are examples of hormesis and have presumably been selected for during evolution because they provide a survival advantage [6–8]. For example, when food availability is limited, individuals most likely to survive and produce offspring are those whose brains function optimally so that they can outwit their competitors to acquire food. This evolutionary perspective is consistent with the evidence that food deprivation (fasting) and running (e.g., to catch prey) improve cognitive function [2].

In modern industrialized societies, inexpensive high-calorie-density processed food is omnipresent, and for many occupations, the need for vigorous physical activity is nonexistent. As a result of this lifestyle, cells, tissues, and organ systems experience a chronic state of metabolic complacency resulting in an increased susceptibility to dysfunction and disease. While being overweight and sedentary has long been known to promote cardiovascular disease (CVD), type-2 diabetes (T2D), and some cancers, only recently has it become clear that a "couch potato" lifestyle can also endanger the brain, rendering it vulnerable to Alzheimer's disease (AD), Parkinson's disease (PD), and ischemic stroke [2, 9]. The ability of brain cells to respond adaptively to stress is reduced during normal aging, with age being the major risk factor for AD, PD, and stroke [10]. While there remains much to learn about why an overindulgent sedentary lifestyle promotes deterioration of the brain, the evidence described below suggests that an important factor is a decline in the brain's cellular and molecular defenses against stress. It is therefore likely that regular intermittent challenges throughout adult life will reduce the risk of age-related brain diseases.

M. P. Mattson (✉)
Laboratory of Neurosciences, National Institute on Aging Intramural Research Program, Baltimore, MD, USA
e-mail: mattsonm@grc.nia.nih.gov

© Springer International Publishing Switzerland 2016
J. I. Mechanick, R. F. Kushner (eds.), *Lifestyle Medicine*, DOI 10.1007/978-3-319-24687-1_27

Table 27.1 Cognitive tests used to evaluate patients for mild cognitive impairment and Alzheimer's disease

Cognitive test	Domains
CERAD Word List Recall	Memory
CERAD Word List Recognition	Memory
Memory of three phrases	Memory
Recall of drawings	Memory
Mini-Mental State Examination	Memory, attention, and language ability
CERAD Boston Naming Test	Language ability
Categorical verbal fluency	Language ability
Wisconsin Card Sorting Test	Executive function
Phonological Verbal Fluency Test	Executive function
Trail-Making Test	Attention
Clock-Drawing Test	Visuospatial abilities

CERAD consortium to establish a registry for Alzheimer's disease

Evaluation of Cognitive Domains in the Clinical Setting

There are four major cognitive domains that should be evaluated in patients referred for evaluation for the insidious development of symptoms of mild cognitive impairment and AD: (1) short-term memory related to hippocampal function, (2) language related to function of neuronal circuits in the region where the parietal and temporal lobes abut in the dominant hemisphere, (3) visual—spatial function, and (4) executive functions (e.g., working memory, problem-solving, reasoning) mediated by the frontal lobes [11]. Ideally, the interview and testing is done in the presence of a spouse or other person who regularly spends time with the patient and who can provide insight into problems in daily functioning of the patient. Before administering specific tests of each domain, it is important to interview the patient and their family member regarding daily functioning of the patient and specific instances where the patient has demonstrated difficulties that may be related to cognitive impairment.

There are several well-established and validated tests for each of the four cognitive domains (Table 27.1). Because a deficit in short-term memory is a hallmark of cognitive impairment in AD that is associated with neuronal degeneration in the hippocampus, this domain should be tested rigorously. A delayed recall test is used to evaluate short-term memory. The patient is typically asked to remember three unrelated words. The subject is then asked to perform an "interference task" such as counting backwards from 100 by 8s, or drawing a picture of a clock or building to distract their attention from the three words. If the patient has difficulty in recalling the three words, then they should be given a second chance to memorize the words and a second interference task administered. Difficulty in recalling the three words a second time suggests a deficit in short-term memory. Two general methods for evaluating language capabilities are to ask the patient to follow a series of at least three commands; for example, stand up, hold your right hand over your head, and touch your nose with the index finger on your left hand. Patients in the early stages of AD patients will often have difficulty in remembering all three commands. Even when language comprehension and the ability to carry on conversations appear relatively normal, testing semantic fluency can be informative. The patient is given 1 min to name as many words in a designated category (e.g., words beginning with the letter s or names of animals). Eleven words or more in 1 min is normal. Visuospatial ability is tested by asking the patient to draw a three-dimensional cube, for example. Executive functions involving complex pattern processing are mediated by the highly evolved frontal lobes [12]. Commonly used tests of executive functioning include asking the patient to perform a sequence of movements that you demonstrate to them; a "Trails B" test in which the subject is asked to draw a continuous line connecting numbers and letters randomly distributed on a sheet of paper (1-A-2-B-3-C, etc.); the clock-drawing test in which the subject is asked to draw a clock with the hours (1–12) in their proper location and with the hands on the clock set to a specific time (e.g., 11:45).

Because performance on any of the cognitive tests can be influenced by factors such as stress, recent illness, etc., it is important to repeat testing periodically over a period of several years to solidify conclusions regarding the probability of the patient being affected by AD or other age-related dementias.

Intermittent Energy Restriction Promotes Optimal Brain Function and May Forestall Neurodegenerative Diseases

The phenotypes of modern humans were molded during evolution in environments where food was less abundant and obesity was likely absent. As with many other species, humans are therefore genetically programmed to thrive in environments in which meals are eaten sporadically (e.g., 3–6 meals/week) and physical activity is required to obtain sustenance and avoid hazards. The latter type of conditions can be modeled in laboratory animals by intermittent energy restriction (IER) diets such as alternate-day food deprivation [1] and by provision of running wheels on which mice and rats often run over 5 km/day [13]. In this section and the next section, study findings are summarized concerning the effects of IER and exercise, respectively, on the brain in relation to vulnerability of neurons to dysfunction and degeneration.

Before describing the evidence that IER diets benefit the brain, it is important to provide examples of studies in human subjects that have demonstrated the feasibility of IER diets and their effects on general health indicators. When asthma patients followed a diet in which they consumed only 600 calories on alternate days (while eating normally on the intervening days) their asthma symptoms and airway resistance improved, and markers of inflammation and oxidative stress were significantly reduced during the course of 2 months [14]. Using a similar IER diet, Varady et al. found that markers of risk for CVD (low-density lipoprotein (LDL) and high-density lipoprotein (HDL) cholesterol and triglycerides) improved significantly [15]. A randomized controlled trial of a more practical IER diet was performed in women at risk for breast cancer. Over 100 women were divided into two groups with the IER group consuming only 500 calories 2 days/week while eating normally the other 5 days, and a second calorie restriction group reducing their daily calorie intake by 25% [16]. During the course of this 6-month study women in both diet groups lost weight and had improvements in various metabolic parameters. However, the women in the 5:2 IER group had a significantly greater reduction in abdominal fat, and a significantly greater improvement in insulin sensitivity compared to the daily caloric restriction group. Over 80% of the subjects on the IER diet completed the 6-month study suggesting that such an IER diet may be doable for many people [16].

IER diets have been shown to protect the brain against dysfunction and degeneration in animal models relevant to AD, PD, and stroke. In mice that develop age-related accumulation of amyloid outside of cells, and neurofibrillary tangle-like aggregates of the protein Tau inside of neurons, both IER and daily calorie restriction diets ameliorate learning and memory deficits [17]. The daily calorie restriction reduces the amount of pathological accumulation of amyloid and Tau, whereas IER may not, suggesting that IER can protect neurons against the potentially neurotoxic effects of amyloid and Tau. In an animal model of PD in which mice produce a mutated human protein (α-synuclein) that causes inherited PD, an alternate-day fasting diet protected the autonomic nervous system against dysfunction, whereas a high-fat diet exacerbated the dysfunction [18]. Being overweight, sedentary, and having hypertension and insulin resistance are risk factors for stroke. When rats or mice are maintained on an IER diet they suffer less brain damage and have a better functional outcome after an experimental stroke [19].

Consistent with the results of experiments using animal models, there is increasing evidence from studies of human subjects that eating patterns can determine whether or not an individual develops a neurodegenerative disorder or suffers a stroke [20]. Epidemiological studies of human populations are consistent with the possibility that moderation in energy intake can promote healthy brain aging [9]. Being overweight and having T2D during midlife increases the risk of AD [21]. It is estimated that approximately 30% of AD cases are attributable to modifiable risk factors, with midlife obesity, physical inactivity, and T2D being prominent risk factors [22]. Metabolic morbidity resulting from overeating and a sedentary lifestyle adversely affects brain cells by many of the same mechanisms responsible for its disease-promoting effects on the cardiovascular, renal, and other organ systems, including inflammation, mitochondria dysfunction, and increased oxidative damage to cellular macromolecules [23]. While it was long thought that overeating promotes oxidative damage by simply increasing the production of free radicals in mitochondria, recent findings suggest that an impaired ability of cells to respond adaptively to oxidative and metabolic stress is also an important factor. Thus, animals fed a high-calorie diet exhibit reduced levels of antioxidant defenses and neurotrophic factors in their brain cells [24, 25].

IER stimulates responses of brain cells and peripheral organs that together enhance the ability of the individual to cope with stress and resist diseases, including neurodegenerative disorders and stroke. In the brain, these responses may include production of nerve cell growth and survival factors such as brain-derived neurotrophic factor (BDNF), increased ability of cells to repair damaged DNA, increased numbers of mitochondria in neurons, and production of protein chaperones that prevent accumulation of misfolded/damaged proteins in neurons (Fig. 27.1) [26–28]. These adaptive responses of neurons result, in part, from increased excitatory synaptic activity in neurons involved in cognition and food-seeking behaviors. Calcium-activated kinases and the transcription factor cyclic adenosine monophosphate (AMP) response element-binding protein (CREB) appear to play important roles in bolstering neuronal bioenergetics and intrinsic defenses against oxidative stress [2]. Signals from peripheral tissues may also mediate neuroprotective effects of IER. One such factor is the ketone body β-hydroxybutyrate, which is generated in liver cells from fatty acids released from adipose cells during fasting periods of 12–16 h or greater. β-hydroxybutyrate can protect neurons against excitotoxic injury and has also been reported to ameliorate cognitive deficits and attenuate neuropathological abnormalities in a mouse model of AD [29]. Several neuroactive hormones produced during fasting (e.g., ghrelin) may also contribute to the beneficial effects of IER on brain function and disease resistance [30].

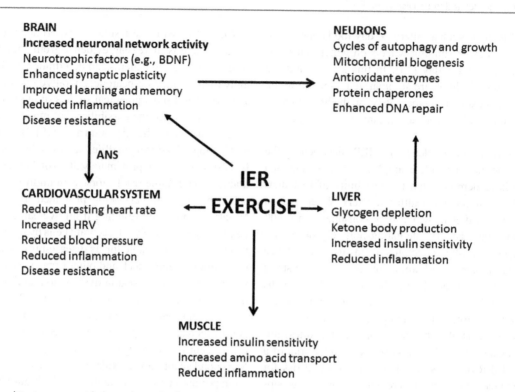

Fig. 27.1 Intermittent energy restriction and exercise improve brain health and disease resistance by direct and indirect effects on neurons. *ANS* autonomic nervous system, *BDNF* brain-derived neurotrophic factor, *HRV* heart rate variability, *IER* intermittent energy restriction

Regular Exercise Bolsters Brain Function and Resilience

Beneficial effects of aerobic exercise on mood and cognitive function are widely experienced and well established in human research studies [3, 31]. Epidemiological studies have revealed strong associations between regular exercise and maintenance of cognitive function during aging; individuals who exercise regularly during middle age and beyond may have a reduced risk for AD [32, 33]. The results of numerous exercise intervention trials have provided direct compelling evidence that aerobic exercise can improve cognitive performance acutely in the minutes and hours following the exercise. For example, school children perform better on tests of verbal memory when they engage in vigorous exercise prior to the testing [34]. In addition, mild aerobic exercise in young adults improves executive function, which is associated with increased activation of neuronal circuits in the prefrontal cortex [35]. Regular vigorous aerobic exercise has also been shown to improve cognitive performance in subjects when compared to either their own pre-exercise program performance or to control groups that perform stretching exercises. For example, the results of a 1-year randomized controlled trial of aerobic exercise (40 min of brisk walking, several days each week) versus 40 min of light stretching in healthy older adults showed significant improvement in cognitive function (measured using a computerized spatial memory task) and, remarkably, a significant increase in the size of

the hippocampus measured by MRI compared to subjects in the stretching control group [36]. Moreover, a study of monkeys showed that daily treadmill running for 1 h resulted in significant improvements in cognitive performance during a 5-month period compared to sedentary control monkeys; however, the beneficial effects of running were reversed during a 3-month sedentary period indicating the importance of continued regular exercise for optimal brain function [37].

Regular exercise may improve brain function in subjects with age-related brain disorders, including those with mild cognitive impairment, AD, PD, and stroke. In a study of elderly subjects with mild cognitive impairment, a multimodal supervised exercise program including aerobic exercises (walking, marching, running) and strength training resulted in improved learning and memory during a 4-month period compared to baseline and to a control sedentary group [38]. Older adults with insulin resistance (a risk factor for AD) who participated in an aerobic exercise program (treadmill, stationary bicycle, and elliptical trainer at 75–85% of maximum heart rate) 45–60 min/day, 4 days/week for 6 months exhibited improved cognitive (executive) function compared with a stretching-only control group [39]. Another study showed that aerobic fitness is associated with the size of the hippocampus, a brain region critical for learning and memory in elderly human subjects [40], suggesting that regular aerobic exercise may protect the brain against age-related atrophy. Patients with AD may also benefit from exercise. In a population-based prospective study, individuals with

AD who engaged in more physical activity lived longer than those who did not [41]. In a study of the interactive effects of high-intensity exercise (running, biking, and/or aerobic exercise classes) with diet (high-fat/high-glycemic index or low-fat/low-glycemic index diets) on cerebrospinal fluid (CSF) markers associated with AD brain neuropathology in normal subjects and patients with mild cognitive impairment, it was found that exercise counteracts AD-related changes in CSF Tau and amyloid-β in normal subjects and that the combination of exercise and the low-fat/low-glycemic index diet reverses AD-related CSF biomarkers [42]. In the case of PD, numerous studies have reported beneficial effects of exercise on mobility [43]. Exercise protocols that specifically target the neuronal circuits most affected by a stroke (the limbs on the side of the body opposite the damaged brain hemisphere) can enhance functional recovery of stroke patients [44].

Animal studies have provided evidence that regular aerobic exercise (voluntary running in rats and mice) can protect neurons against dysfunction and degeneration in models of AD, PD, and stroke. In transgenic mice that express a mutated form of human amyloid precursor protein (APP) and exhibit age-related amyloid accumulation and cognitive impairment, running lessens the amyloid accumulation and ameliorates the cognitive deficits [45]. In another mouse model of AD, running-wheel exercise prevented memory deficits and also ameliorated the heightened anxiety state of the mice [46]. When APP mutant mice are maintained on a high-fat diet, amyloid deposition and memory deficits are accelerated; these adverse effects of the high-fat diet can be reversed by maintaining the mice in an enriched environment that includes running wheels [47]. Exercise may reduce the amount of amyloid in the brain by stimulating its degradation and/or removal by immune cells [48]. Exercise can also increase the resistance of dopamine-producing neurons to degeneration in animals exposed to toxins that cause PD-like symptoms [49, 50]. When initiated during and after toxin-induced damage to dopaminergic neurons, running-wheel exercise can enhance recovery of motor function in mice [51]. Moreover, when initiated only after neurotoxin-induced dopaminergic neuron damage in rats, running reverses motor deficits and restores neuronal circuit activity alterations in several brain regions involved in motor control [52]. In both rat and mouse models of focal ischemic stroke, running-wheel exercise reduces the extent of brain damage and lessens functional deficits [53–55].

The mechanisms by which exercise can promote optimal brain function and resistance to neurodegenerative disorders are being elucidated. Exercise induces the expression of BDNF in multiple brain regions, and BDNF may mediate several beneficial effects of exercise, including enhanced hippocampal neurogenesis and synaptic plasticity, and improved learning and memory [2, 3]. BDNF can protect neurons against dysfunction and degeneration in experimental models of AD, PD, and stroke, consistent with the possibility that increased production of BDNF plays an important role in the neuroprotective effects of exercise [56–58]. BDNF can also increase the number of mitochondria in neurons and thereby enables the neurons to form new synapses and to maintain existing synapses [26]. The latter findings suggest that, similar to its effects on muscle cells, exercise can enhance the energy-generating capability of neurons. Because a cellular energy deficit is a major factor contributing to the degeneration of neurons in AD, PD, and stroke [10, 59, 60], exercise may protect against these disorders by sustaining neuronal bioenergetics. Unrepaired damage to DNA occurs in brain cells during normal aging and to a much greater extent in AD, PD, and stroke [61]. Running-wheel exercise and BDNF enhance the ability of neurons to repair damaged DNA [62], suggesting that regular exercise can prevent the accumulation of damaged DNA in neurons. Finally, animal studies have shown that running can promote the growth of cerebral blood vessels (angiogenesis), increase cerebral blood flow, and thereby counteract any reduction in cerebral blood flow occurring with aging and neurodegenerative disorders [63].

Interestingly, recent findings suggest the possibility that, in addition to its actions on neurons in brain regions involved in cognition, BDNF plays an important role in beneficial effects of exercise on the cardiovascular system. Regular exercise results in a reduction in resting heart rate and an increase in heart rate variability (an indicator of heart health) by increasing parasympathetic tone, which involves increased activity of cholinergic neurons in the brainstem that innervate the heart [64]. A study in which heart rate was monitored continuously in mice with reduced or increased BDNF levels showed that BDNF acts on brainstem cardio-vagal (parasympathetic) neurons to increase their activity and slow heart rate [65]. Moreover, transgenic mice expressing a mutational form of α-synuclein that causes an inherited form of PD exhibit an elevated resting heart rate as a result of reduced function of brainstem cardio-vagal neurons [16]. It is therefore likely that regular exercise can counteract dysfunction of the autonomic nervous system that occurs in PD.

Intellectual Challenges Strengthen the Brain

Epidemiological studies have provided evidence that individuals who attain a higher educational status and who are socially engaged throughout their life are less likely to develop AD late in life [66]. In a study of approximately 2000 subjects, higher education/occupation scores and higher levels of cognitive challenges in midlife and late life were associated with higher levels of cognitive performance in late life [67]. A study of nuns found that low linguistic ability in early adulthood was associated with increased probability of cognitive impairment, greater cerebral atrophy, neurofibrillary brain pathology, and AD late in life [68]. Interestingly, many individuals whose brains continue to function well late in life exhibit considerable AD-like amyloid pathology upon autopsy, suggesting that they have a greater level of cognitive reserve, possible because they developed more synaptic connections as a result of greater intellectual engagement [69]. Brain-imaging studies have documented that educational attainment is positively associated with hippocampal volume (i.e., more highly educated individuals have a larger hippocampus) [70], which may reflect increased cognitive reserve and decreased risk for AD.

Laboratory rodents are normally housed in groups of four in small cages that lack any objects for play, nest building, or other cognitive challenges. When rodents live in larger cages with more cage mates and with numerous objects to explore and climb on, or hide and build nests in, their brains change so as to improve their cognitive function, sensory–motor function, and resistance to dysfunction and degeneration [71]. Environmental enrichment during midlife can forestall age-related cognitive deficits in mice [72], suggesting that intellectual challenges during middle age can protect the brain against the adversities of aging. When transgenic mice that express mutated human genes that cause AD in humans are maintained in enriched environments, they exhibit a slowing of age-related cognitive deficits, which is associated with maintenance of hippocampal neurogenesis, synaptic plasticity, and cerebrovascular function [73, 74]. Environmental enrichment can also counteract amyloid accumulation and cognitive impairment in AD mice fed a high-fat diet [75]. The increased cognitive stimulation, over and above the increased physical activity, is believed to play an important role in counteracting neuronal dysfunction in AD mice [76]. In rat or mouse models of PD, in which the animals are administered dopaminergic neurotoxins, environmental enrichment reduces the degeneration of the dopaminergic neurons and improves motor function compared to animals maintained in the usual lab cage environment [77–79]. Recovery from a stroke is also improved by environmental enrichment in animal models [80, 81].

What are the cellular and molecular mechanisms by which intellectual challenges bolster brain function and resilience throughout the life course? Studies of environmental enrichment in animal models suggest the following sequence of events: (1) There is increased activation of excitatory glutamatergic synapses in neuronal circuits involved in cognitive processing; (2) Ca^{2+} influx through plasma membrane glutamate receptor channels and voltage-dependent channels occurs in dendrites; (3) Ca^{2+} activates kinases such as $Ca^{2+}/$calmodulin-dependent protein kinase II and protein kinase C; (4) the kinases activate transcription factors with CREB being a prominent example; (5) the transcription factor induces the expression of genes encoding neurotrophic factors (e.g., BDNF), DNA repair enzymes, and peroxisome proliferator-activated receptor gamma coactivator 1α (PGC-1α), among others; BDNF and CREB have been shown to play key roles in the improvements of synaptic plasticity, and learning and memory that occur in response to envi-

ronmental enrichment; and (6) BDNF signaling stimulates mitochondrial biogenesis, promotes synapse formation, and promotes neurogenesis [82–84]. There is also evidence that intellectual challenges can stimulate angiogenesis of cerebral blood vessels resulting in increased energy and nutrient supply to neurons [85]. Collectively, the effects of regular intellectual challenges on brain structure and function are robust, can help counteract age-related declines in brain function, and may reduce the risk of neurodegenerative disorders.

Dietary Phytochemicals May Benefit the Brain by Hormesis-Based Mechanisms

Emerging findings suggest a fourth lifestyle approach that may promote optimal brain function and resistance to disease. Population-based studies suggest that people who consume a diet replete with vegetables, fruits, and whole grains, including vegetarian diets and the Mediterranean diet, are at a reduced risk of age-related cognitive deficits and AD [86, 87]. Prospective epidemiological studies support the notion that consumption of vegetable-rich diets in midlife can protect against cognitive decline in late life [88]. Vegetarian diets have also been associated with improved mood (fewer symptoms of depression) in a cross-sectional study [89]. The results of a small randomized controlled trial of a vegetarian diet in subjects that previously consumed meat suggest that mood can be improved relatively rapidly by eliminating meat from the diet [90].

Studies in which rats or mice are fed diets supplemented with fruits (blueberries, strawberries, apples, grapes, and others) or vegetables (broccoli, spinach, garlic, onions, and others) have provided evidence that chemicals in fruits and vegetables can enhance brain function and counteract the adverse effects of aging and neurodegenerative disorders. Young rats that consumed food enriched with blueberries performed better in a test of spatial memory than did those not consuming blueberries [91]. Old rats fed a diet containing spinach exhibited reduced levels of the pro-inflammatory cytokine tumor necrosis factor (TNF)-α and pro-inflammatory TNF-β in their cerebellum and improved learning and memory in a cerebellum-mediated eyeblink-conditioning test [92]. Similarly, feeding old rats a diet supplemented with walnuts reduced inflammation and accumulation of damaged and polyubiquitinated proteins in their brains [93]. Other studies have shown that dietary grape juice can improve cognitive function in old rats [94]. A study of a mouse model of AD showed that a diet rich in fruits and cocoa ameliorate behavioral deficits and stimulate proliferation of stem cells in the subventricular zone [95].

Some of the specific phytochemicals in vegetables and fruits that may be beneficial for the brain are being elucidated. Three such phytochemicals that have been particularly well studied are curcumin, sulforaphane, and resveratrol. Studies in animal models of age-related neurodegenerative disorders have provided evidence that curcumin, a phytochemical present in high amounts in turmeric root and commonly used as a spice in Indian cooking, can protect neurons against dysfunction and degeneration. Using a mouse model of AD, Frautschy et al. [96] found that curcumin administration can reverse cognitive deficits, enhance synaptic integrity, and reduce the amount of amyloid-β accumulation in the brain. In a mitochondrial neurotoxin-based rat PD model, curcumin treatment reduced damage to dopaminergic neurons and reduced motor deficits [97]. When rats were treated with curcumin 4 h after cerebral ischemia (experimental stroke), the amounts of brain tissue damage and oxidative stress were reduced, and the neurological deficits caused by the stroke were lessened [98]. Rats fed a high-fat diet exhibited increased brain damage and associated cognitive deficits caused by a traumatic blow to the head; however, when the high-fat diet was supplemented with curcumin, the brain damage and cognitive deficits were reduced indicating that curcumin can counteract the adverse effects of high-fat diet on the vulnerability of the brain to injury [99]. Sulforaphane is a phytochemical present in high amounts in cruciferous vegetables such as broccoli. In a mouse model of cholinergic dysfunction-induced cognitive impairment, administration of sulforaphane ameliorated the memory impairment [100]. Sulforaphane also protected dopaminergic neurons in a mouse model of PD [101] and was beneficial in animal models of stroke [102] and traumatic brain injury [103]. Resveratrol, which is present in red grapes, cocoa, and peanuts, has been reported to have beneficial effects in animal models of relevance to AD, amyotrophic lateral sclerosis, and traumatic brain injury [104, 105].

Until recently, it was dogma that vegetables and fruits are good for general health (and brain health) because they contain chemicals that are antioxidants that directly neutralize free radicals and thereby protect cells [106]. However, emerging findings point to a quite different mechanism whereby phytochemicals can improve health and prevent or reverse disease processes. Plants produce many chemicals that are noxious to insects and other organisms; these chemicals are natural pesticides [107, 108]. When we eat fruits and vegetables, the noxious chemicals they contain activate adaptive stress responses in cells throughout our body and brain, thereby increasing the resistance of the cells to injury and disease [5]. This "neurohormetic phytochemical" hypothesis for the mechanism by which chemicals in plants promote brain health and disease resistance was proposed in 2006 [109]. Several prominent adaptive response cellular signaling pathways that are activated by phytochemicals have been identified including those involving histone deacetylases and the transcription factors nuclear factor erythroid 2 related factor (NRF)-2, CREB, and forkhead box (FOXO)-3 (5). Activation of these pathways results in increased production of neurotrophic factors, antioxidant enzymes, and phase 2 detoxification enzymes, which can bolster neuronal stress resistance (Fig. 27.2).

PLANTS
Fruits, Vegetables
Nuts, Herbs

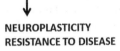

HORMETIC PHYTOCHEMICALS
curcumin, sulforaphane,
resveratrol, epicatechins,
and many others

NEURONAL STRESS RESPONSES
Antioxidant enzymes
Detoxification enzymes
Enhanced autophagy
Neurotrophic factor production

**NEUROPLASTICITY
RESISTANCE TO DISEASE**

Fig. 27.2 Model for the mechanisms by which neurohormetic phytochemicals enhance neuroplasticity and may protect the brain against injury and disease

A Pressing Need to Meet the Brain Health Challenge

The brain can now be added to the list of organ systems adversely affected by the kinds of unchallenging lifestyles that have rapidly become commonplace in modern societies. These "brain-wasting lifestyles" are characterized by lack of exercise, lack of dietary challenges, such as fasting and consumption of hormetic phytochemicals, and in some cases few intellectual challenges. Advances in early diagnosis and effective treatments for CVD and some cancers have contributed to the recent robust increase in the number of individuals between the ages of 65 and 90, the danger zone for AD, PD, and stroke. Because many such elderly individuals did not challenge themselves with vigorous exercise, fasting, or cognitive endeavors during their earlier years, their risks for AD, PD, and stroke are increased [2]. Unfortunately, there are many factors that have converged to facilitate obesogenic lifestyles, including the processed and fast food industries, which market high-energy-density low-cost foods, and drinks replete with sugar and fat, and devoid of hormetic phytochemicals [20, 110]. Advertisements for processed foods and beverages, and for drugs to treat disease symptoms, are omnipresent. Processed foods and drinks are made to be addictive by inclusion of specially designed blends of ingredients [110, 111]. Conversely, fruits, vegetables, and nuts are relatively expensive and not advertised to the extent of processed foods. The challenge of regular vigorous exercise has become unnecessary for most occupations, and door-to-door transportation and elevators are widely used, making a sedentary lifestyle common. It should also be noted that medical training and practice deemphasizes, and even discounts, implementation of compliable prescriptions for diet and exercise interventions. Instead, the emphasis is on treating the symptoms of diseases with drugs promoted by the pharmaceutical industry. The mentality of a major proportion of the US population has therefore become that diseases cannot be avoided and so are dealt with by drugs and surgery once they become manifest. Unfortunately for them and their relatives, there are no effective treatments for AD, PD, and stroke.

The widespread adoption of intermittent challenge-based diets (intermittent fasting, consumption of fruits and vegetables) and lifestyles would require the concerted efforts of government agencies, primary and secondary education, the entire health-care system, employers, and parents. Doable intermittent fasting and exercise regimens are available and can be effectively implemented if there is rigorous follow-up during the first month of the intervention [20, 112, 113]. Community planning that facilitates exercise (bike paths, parks, etc.), and work environments that promote exercise, must proliferate. These living and working environments should also include readily available healthy foods at a low cost. Importantly, education from K–12 should emphasize the importance of diet and exercise for brain health. The take-home message here is that attaining and maintaining optimal brain health and disease resistance throughout life requires that individuals challenge themselves in four major ways: regular vigorous exercise, intermittent fasting, eating fruits and vegetables, and engaging in intellectually challenging endeavors. To become commonplace, this will require the commitment of parents, schools, communities, and the entire health-care system.

Case Studies

Two case studies illustrate the evidence that the risk of AD is influenced by environmental factors, on the one hand, and that interventions that challenge the brain can ameliorate cognitive deficits in AD patients, at least in the early stages of the disease, on the other hand. While there are genetic factors that can either cause AD (mutations in the beta-APP or presenilin 1) or affect the risk of AD (apolipoprotein E4 allele), environmental factors including lifestyle and diet may influence the age of onset and risk of AD. Case studies of monozygotic (identical) twins support important roles for lifestyle and environmental factors in AD. In a case study of British monozygotic female twins, one sister developed dementia which was first evident at age 52 and progressively worsened until she became completely debilitated and died at the age of 64 [114]. During the disease course, her cognitive function progressively worsened, and postmortem histological analysis of her brain revealed extensive neuronal loss, and neurofibrillary tangles and plaques, consistent with a diagnosis of AD. The unaffected twin was evaluated in the clinic at age 64, and her cognitive function was deemed to be within the normal range. While many aspects of the lives of the twin sisters were similar, three clear differences were noted; the unaffected sister was married, whereas the sister with AD was not married; the unaffected sister was more physically and socially active during her midlife; and the affected sister had experienced a concussion when she was 39 years old. Altogether, this case study is consistent with the possibilities that a more cognitively stimulating lifestyle may have protected one sister against AD, while head trauma in midlife may have hastened the onset of AD in the affected sister.

It may be possible to improve the cognitive abilities of AD patients who are in the early stage of the disease by challenging them with exercise or intellectual enrichment. One example is a case study of a 66-year-old man, retired from a teaching career and recently diagnosed with probable AD [115]. He had been experiencing a progressive worsening of his ability to remember names of members of his social group, which was disconcerting to him. He had been taking a cholinesterase inhibitor (rivastigmine), which was apparently of little or no benefit for his difficulty putting names to faces. An intervention was developed aimed at improving the patient's ability to recognize/name his friends; this intervention consisted of mnemonic plus expanding rehearsal or repeated presentation. Photographs of 13 friends were used in sessions in which the patient was presented with a friend's picture, repeated their name together with a mnemonic, and then after a 30-s delay the patient was asked to recall the person's name. The patient was also asked to practice at home. During the first 3 months, the subject focused on five pictures/names, and during the subsequent 3 months the subject focused on the other eight pictures/names. The patient's performance improved dramatically and was maintained at a 6-month follow-up evaluation. This case study provides evidence that the neuronal circuits in the brain of an individual in the early stages of AD are capable of responding adaptively to cognitive challenges suggesting that, with considerable effort, a patient with AD is capable of improving their functioning within their social group.

References

1. Longo VD, Mattson MP. Fasting: molecular mechanisms and clinical applications. Cell Metab. 2014;19:181–92.
2. Mattson MP. Energy intake and exercise as determinants of brain health and vulnerability to injury and disease. Cell Metab. 2012;16:706–22.
3. Voss MW, Vivar C, Kramer AF, van Praag H. Bridging animal and human models of exercise-induced brain plasticity. Trends Cogn Sci. 2013;17:525–44.
4. Barulli D, Stern Y. Efficiency, capacity, compensation, maintenance, plasticity: emerging concepts in cognitive reserve. Trends Cogn Sci. 2013;17:502–9.
5. Lee J, Jo DG, Park D, Chung HY, Mattson MP. Adaptive cellular stress pathways as therapeutic targets of dietary phytochemicals: focus on the nervous system. Pharmacol Rev. 2014;66:815–68.

6. Calabrese EJ, Bachmann KA, Bailer AJ, Bolger PM, Borak J, Cai L, Cedergreen N, et al. Biological stress response terminology: integrating the concepts of adaptive response and preconditioning stress within a hormetic dose-response framework. Toxicol Appl Pharmacol. 2007;222:122–8.

7. Rattan SI. Hormesis in aging. Ageing Res Rev. 2008;7:63–78.

8. Mattson MP. Evolutionary aspects of human exercise–born to run purposefully. Ageing Res Rev. 2012;11:347–52.

9. Lee EB, Mattson MP. The neuropathology of obesity: insights from human disease. Acta Neuropathol. 2014;127:3–28.

10. Mattson MP, Magnus T. Ageing and neuronal vulnerability. Nat Rev Neurosci. 2006;7:278–94.

11. McCarten JR. Clinical evaluation of early cognitive symptoms. Clin Geriatr Med. 2013;29:791–807.

12. Mattson MP. Superior pattern processing is the essence of the evolved human brain. Front Neurosci. 2014;8:265.

13. van Praag H, Christie BR, Sejnowski TJ, Gage FH. Running enhances neurogenesis, learning, and long-term potentiation in mice. Proc Natl Acad Sci U S A. 1999;96:13427–31.

14. Johnson JB, Summer W, Cutler RG, Martin B, Hyun DH, Dixit VD, Pearson M, Nassar M, Telljohann R, Maudsley S, Carlson O, John S, Laub DR, Mattson MP. Alternate day calorie restriction improves clinical findings and reduces markers of oxidative stress and inflammation in overweight adults with moderate asthma. Free Radic Biol Med. 2007;42:665–74.

15. Klempel MC, Kroeger CM, Varady KA. Alternate day fasting (ADF) with a high-fat diet produces similar weight loss and cardio-protection as ADF with a low-fat diet. Metabolism. 2013;62:137–43.

16. Harvie MN, Pegington M, Mattson MP, Frystyk J, Dillon B, Evans G, Cuzick J, Jebb SA, Martin B, Cutler RG, Son TG, Maudsley S, Carlson OD, Egan JM, Flyvbjerg A, Howell A. The effects of intermittent or continuous energy restriction on weight loss and metabolic disease risk markers: a randomized trial in young overweight women. Int J Obes (Lond). 2011;35:714–27.

17. Halagappa VK, Guo Z, Pearson M, Matsuoka Y, Cutler RG, Laferla FM, Mattson MP. Intermittent fasting and caloric restriction ameliorate age-related behavioral deficits in the triple-transgenic mouse model of Alzheimer's disease. Neurobiol Dis. 2007;26:212–20.

18. Griffioen KJ, Rothman SM, Ladenheim B, Wan R, Vranis N, Hutchison E, Okun E, Cadet JL, Mattson MP. Dietary energy intake modifies brainstem autonomic dysfunction caused by mutant α-synuclein. Neurobiol Aging. 2013;34:928–35.

19. Arumugam TV, Phillips TM, Cheng A, Morrell CH, Mattson MP, Wan R. Age and energy intake interact to modify cell stress pathways and stroke outcome. Ann Neurol. 2010;67:41–52.

20. Mattson MP, Allison DB, Fontana L, Harvie M, Longo VD, Malaisse WJ, Mosley M, Notterpek L, Ravussin E, Scheer FAJL, Seyfried T, Varady K, Panda S. Meal frequency and timing in health and disease. Proc Natl Acad Sci U S A. 2014;111:16647–53.

21. Tolppanen AM, Solomon A, Soininen H, Kivipelto M. Midlife vascular risk factors and Alzheimer's disease: evidence from epidemiological studies. J Alzheimers Dis. 2012;32:531–40.

22. Norton S, Matthews FE, Barnes DE, Yaffe K, Brayne C. Potential for primary prevention of Alzheimer's disease: an analysis of population-based data. Lancet Neurol. 2014;13:788–94.

23. Prolla TA, Mattson MP. Molecular mechanisms of brain aging and neurodegenerative disorders: lessons from dietary restriction. Trends Neurosci. 2001;24:S21–S31.

24. Stranahan AM, Norman ED, Lee K, Cutler RG, Telljohann RS, Egan JM, Mattson MP. Diet-induced insulin resistance impairs hippocampal synaptic plasticity and cognition in middle-aged rats. Hippocampus. 2008;18:1085–8.

25. Morrison CD, Pistell PJ, Ingram DK, Johnson WD, Liu Y, Fernandez-Kim SO, White CL, Purpera MN, Uranga RM, Bruce-Keller AJ, Keller JN. High fat diet increases hippocampal oxidative stress and cognitive impairment in aged mice: implications for decreased Nrf2 signaling. J Neurochem. 2010;114:1581–9.

26. Cheng A, Wan R, Yang JL, Kamimura N, Son TG, Ouyang X, Luo Y, Okun E, Mattson MP. Involvement of PGC-1α in the formation and maintenance of neuronal dendritic spines. Nat Commun. 2012;3:1250.

27. Yang JL, Lin YT, Chuang PC, Bohr VA, Mattson MP. BDNF and exercise enhance neuronal DNA repair by stimulating CREB-mediated production of apurinic/apyrimidinic endonuclease 1. Neuromolecular Med. 2014;16:161–74.

28. Qiu G, Spangler EL, Wan R, Miller M, Mattson MP, So KF, de Cabo R, Zou S, Ingram DK. Neuroprotection provided by dietary restriction in rats is further enhanced by reducing glucocorticoids. Neurobiol Aging. 2012;33:2398–410.

29. Kashiwaya Y, Bergman C, Lee JH, Wan R, King MT, Mughal MR, Okun E, Clarke K, Mattson MP, Veech RL. A ketone ester diet exhibits anxiolytic and cognition-sparing properties, and lessens amyloid and tau pathologies in a mouse model of Alzheimer's disease. Neurobiol Aging. 2013;34:1530–9.

30. Andrews ZB. The extra-hypothalamic actions of ghrelin on neuronal function. Trends Neurosci. 2011;34:31–40.

31. Loprinzi PD, Herod SM, Cardinal BJ, Noakes TD. Physical activity and the brain: a review of this dynamic, bi-directional relationship. Brain Res. 2013;1539:95–104.

32. Ahlskog JE, Geda YE, Graff-Radford NR, Petersen RC. Physical exercise as a preventive or disease-modifying treatment of dementia and brain aging. Mayo Clin Proc. 2011;86:876–84.

33. Gregory MA, Gill DP, Petrella RJ. Brain health and exercise in older adults. Curr Sports Med Rep. 2013;12:256–71.

34. Etnier J, Labban JD, Piepmeier AT, Davis ME, Henning DA. Effects of an acute bout of exercise on memory in 6th grade children. Pediatr Exerc Sci. 2014;26:250–8.

35. Byun K, Hyodo K, Suwabe K, Ochi G, Sakairi Y, Kato M, Dan I, Soya H. Positive effect of acute mild exercise on executive function via arousal-related prefrontal activations: an fNIRS study. Neuroimage. 2014;98:336–45.

36. Erickson KI, Voss MW, Prakash RS, Basak C, Szabo A, Chaddock L, Kim JS, Heo S, Alves H, White SM, Wojcicki TR, Mailey E, Vieira VJ, Martin SA, Pence BD, Woods JA, McAuley E, Kramer AF. Exercise training increases size of hippocampus and improves memory. Proc Natl Acad Sci U S A. 2011;108:3017–22.

37. Rhyu IJ, Bytheway JA, Kohler SJ, Lange H, Lee KJ, Boklewski J, McCormick K, Williams NI, Stanton GB, Greenough WT, Cameron JL. Effects of aerobic exercise training on cognitive function and cortical vascularity in monkeys. Neuroscience. 2010;167:1239–48.

38. Nascimento CM, Pereira JR, Pires de Andrade L, Garuffi M, Ayan C, Kerr DS, Talib LL, Cominetti MR, Stella F. Physical exercise improves peripheral BDNF levels and cognitive functions in elderly mild cognitive impairment individuals with different BDNF Val-66Met genotypes. J Alzheimers Dis. 2014. [Epub ahead of print].

39. Baker LD, Frank LL, Foster-Schubert K, Green PS, Wilkinson CW, McTiernan A, Cholerton BA, Plymate SR, Fishel MA, Watson GS, Duncan GE, Mehta PD, Craft S. Aerobic exercise improves cognition for older adults with glucose intolerance, a risk factor for Alzheimer's disease. J Alzheimers Dis. 2010;22:569–79.

40. Erickson KI, Prakash RS, Voss MW, Chaddock L, Hu L, Morris KS, White SM, Wójcicki TR, McAuley E, Kramer AF. Aerobic fitness is associated with hippocampal volume in elderly humans. Hippocampus. 2009;19:1030–9.

41. Scarmeas N, Luchsinger JA, Brickman AM, Cosentino S, Schupf N, Xin-Tang M, Gu Y, Stern Y. Physical activity and Alzheimer disease course. Am J Geriatr Psychiatry. 2011;19:471–81.

42. Baker LD, Bayer-Carter JL, Skinner J, Montine TJ, Cholerton BA, Callaghan M, Leverenz JB, Walter BK, Tsai E, Postupna N, Lampe J, Craft S. High-intensity physical activity modulates diet effects on cerebrospinal amyloid-β levels in normal aging and mild cognitive impairment. J Alzheimers Dis. 2012;28:137–46.

43. van der Kolk NM, King LA. Effects of exercise on mobility in people with Parkinson's disease. Mov Disord. 2013;28:1587–96.

44. Quaney BM, Boyd LA, McDowd JM, Zahner LH, He J, Mayo MS, Macko RF. Aerobic exercise improves cognition and motor function poststroke. Neurorehabil Neural Repair. 2009;23:879–85.

45. Adlard PA, Perreau VM, Pop V, Cotman CW. Voluntary exercise decreases amyloid load in a transgenic model of Alzheimer's disease. J Neurosci. 2005;25:4217–21.

46. García-Mesa Y, López-Ramos JC, Giménez-Llort L, Revilla S, Guerra R, Gruart A, Laferla FM, Cristòfol R, Delgado-García JM, Sanfeliu C. Physical exercise protects against Alzheimer's disease in 3xTg-AD mice. J Alzheimers Dis. 2011;24:421–54.

47. Maesako M, Uemura K, Kubota M, Kuzuya A, Sasaki K, Asada M, Watanabe K, Hayashida N, Ihara M, Ito H, Shimohama S, Kihara T, Kinoshita A. Environmental enrichment ameliorated high-fat diet-induced Aβ deposition and memory deficit in APP transgenic mice. Neurobiol Aging. 2012;33(5):1011.e11–23.

48. Nichol KE, Poon WW, Parachikova AI, Cribbs DH, Glabe CG, Cotman CW. Exercise alters the immune profile in Tg2576 Alzheimer mice toward a response coincident with improved cognitive performance and decreased amyloid. J Neuroinflammation. 2008;5:13.

49. Lau YS, Patki G, Das-Panja K, Le WD, Ahmad SO. Neuroprotective effects and mechanisms of exercise in a chronic mouse model of Parkinson's disease with moderate neurodegeneration. Eur J Neurosci. 2011;33:1264–74.

50. Tillerson JL, Caudle WM, Reverón ME, Miller GW. Exercise induces behavioral recovery and attenuates neurochemical deficits in rodent models of Parkinson's disease. Neuroscience. 2003;119:899–911.

51. Fredriksson A, Stigsdotter IM, Hurtig A, Ewalds-Kvist B, Archer T. Running wheel activity restores MPTP-induced functional deficits. J Neural Transm. 2011;118:407–20.

52. Wang Z, Myers KG, Guo Y, Ocampo MA, Pang RD, Jakowec MW, Holschneider DP. Functional reorganization of motor and limbic circuits after exercise training in a rat model of bilateral parkinsonism. PLoS ONE. 2013;8(11):e80058.

53. Ding Y, Li J, Luan X, Ding YH, Lai Q, Rafols JA, Phillis JW, Clark JC, Diaz FG. Exercise pre-conditioning reduces brain damage in ischemic rats that may be associated with regional angiogenesis and cellular overexpression of neurotrophin. Neuroscience. 2004;124:583–91.

54. Ploughman M, Attwood Z, White N, Doré JJ, Corbett D. Endurance exercise facilitates relearning of forelimb motor skill after focal ischemia. Eur J Neurosci. 2007;25:3453–60.

55. Gertz K, Priller J, Kronenberg G, Fink KB, Winter B, Schröck H, Ji S, Milosevic M, Harms C, Böhm M, Dirnagl U, Laufs U, Endres M. Physical activity improves long-term stroke outcome via endothelial nitric oxide synthase-dependent augmentation of neovascularization and cerebral blood flow. Circ Res. 2006;99:1132–40.

56. Han J, Pollak J, Yang T, Siddiqui MR, Doyle KP, Taravosh-Lahn K, Cekanaviciute E, Han A, Goodman JZ, Jones B, Jing D, Massa SM, Longo FM, Buckwalter MS. Delayed administration of a small molecule tropomyosin-related kinase B ligand promotes recovery after hypoxic-ischemic stroke. Stroke. 2012;43:1918–24.

57. Caccamo A, Maldonado MA, Bokov AF, Majumder S, Oddo S. CBP gene transfer increases BDNF levels and ameliorates learning and memory deficits in a mouse model of Alzheimer's disease. Proc Natl Acad Sci U S A. 2010;107:22687–92.

58. Real CC, Ferreira AF, Chaves-Kirsten GP, Torrão AS, Pires RS, Britto LR. BDNF receptor blockade hinders the beneficial effects of exercise in a rat model of Parkinson's disease. Neuroscience. 2013;237:118–29.

59. Kapogiannis D, Mattson MP. Disrupted energy metabolism and neuronal circuit dysfunction in cognitive impairment and Alzheimer's disease. Lancet Neurol. 2011;10:187–98.

60. Reddy PH. Mitochondrial medicine for aging and neurodegenerative diseases. Neuromolecular Med. 2008;10:291–315.

61. Canugovi C, Misiak M, Ferrarelli LK, Croteau DL, Bohr VA. The role of DNA repair in brain related disease pathology. 2013;12:578–87.

62. Yang JL, Lin YT, Chuang PC, Bohr VA, Mattson MP. BDNF and exercise enhance neuronal DNA repair by stimulating CREB-mediated production of apurinic/apyrimidinic endonuclease 1. Neuromolecular Med. 2014;16:161–74.

63. Swain RA, Harris AB, Wiener EC, Dutka MV, Morris HD, Theien BE, Konda S, Engberg K, Lauterbur PC, Greenough WT. Prolonged exercise induces angiogenesis and increases cerebral blood volume in primary motor cortex of the rat. Neuroscience. 2003;117:1037–46.

64. Cantwell JD. Cardiovascular aspects of running. Clin Sports Med. 1985;4:627–40.

65. Wan R, Weigand LA, Bateman R, Griffioen K, Mendelowitz D, Mattson MP. Evidence that BDNF regulates heart rate by a mechanism involving increased brainstem parasympathetic neuron excitability. J Neurochem. 2014;129:573–80.

66. Bennett DA, Arnold SE, Valenzuela MJ, Brayne C, Schneider JA. Cognitive and social lifestyle: links with neuropathology and cognition in late life. Acta Neuropathol. 2014;127:137–50.

67. Vemuri P, Lesnick TG, Przybelski SA, Machulda M, Knopman DS, Mielke MM, Roberts RO, Geda YE, Rocca WA, Petersen RC, Jack CR Jr. Association of lifetime intellectual enrichment with cognitive decline in the older population. JAMA Neurol. 2014;71:1017–24.

68. Riley KP, Snowdon DA, Desrosiers MF, Markesbery WR. Early life linguistic ability, late life cognitive function, and neuropathology: findings from the Nun Study. Neurobiol Aging. 2005;26:341–7.

69. Stern Y. Cognitive reserve and Alzheimer disease. Alzheimer Dis Assoc Disord. 2006;20:112–7.

70. Shpanskaya KS, Choudhury KR, Hostage C Jr, Murphy KR, Petrella JR, Doraiswamy PM, Alzheimer's Disease Neuroimaging Initiative. Educational attainment and hippocampal atrophy in the Alzheimer's disease neuroimaging initiative cohort. J Neuroradiol. 2014. pii: S0150-9861(13)00128-4.

71. Nithianantharajah J, Hannan AJ. Enriched environments, experience-dependent plasticity and disorders of the nervous system. Nat Rev Neurosci. 2006;7:697–709.

72. Freret T, Billard JM, Schumann-Bard P, Dutar P, Dauphin F, Boulouard M, Bouet V. Rescue of cognitive aging by long-lasting environmental enrichment exposure initiated before median lifespan. Neurobiol Aging 2012;33:1005.e1–10.

73. Herring A, Yasin H, Ambrée O, Sachser N, Paulus W, Keyvani K. Environmental enrichment counteracts Alzheimer's neurovascular dysfunction in TgCRND8 mice. Brain Pathol. 2008;18:32–9.

74. Veeraraghavalu K, Choi SH, Zhang X, Sisodia SS. Endogenous expression of FAD-linked PS1 impairs proliferation, neuronal differentiation and survival of adult hippocampal progenitors. Mol Neurodegener. 2013;8:41.

75. Maesako M, Uemura K, Kubota M, Kuzuya A, Sasaki K, Asada M, Watanabe K, Hayashida N, Ihara M, Ito H, Shimohama S, Kihara T, Kinoshita A. Environmental enrichment ameliorated high-fat diet-induced Aβ deposition and memory deficit in APP transgenic mice. Neurobiol Aging. 2012;33(5):1011.e11–23.

76. Cracchiolo JR, Mori T, Nazian SJ, Tan J, Potter H, Arendash GW. Enhanced cognitive activity—over and above social or physical activity—is required to protect Alzheimer's mice against cognitive impairment, reduce Abeta deposition, and increase synaptic immunoreactivity. Neurobiol Learn Mem. 2007;88:277–94.

77. Faherty CJ, Raviie Shepherd K, Herasimtschuk A, Smeyne RJ. Environmental enrichment in adulthood eliminates neuronal death in experimental Parkinsonism. Brain Res Mol Brain Res. 2005;134:170–9.

78. Jadavji NM, Kolb B, Metz GA. Enriched environment improves motor function in intact and unilateral dopamine-depleted rats. Neuroscience. 2006;140:1127–38.

79. Goldberg NR, Fields V, Pflibsen L, Salvatore MF, Meshul CK. Social enrichment attenuates nigrostriatal lesioning and reverses motor impairment in a progressive 1-methyl-2-phenyl-1,2,3,6-tetrahydropyridine (MPTP) mouse model of Parkinson's disease. Neurobiol Dis. 2012;45:1051–67.

80. Biernaskie J, Corbett D. Enriched rehabilitative training promotes improved forelimb motor function and enhanced dendritic growth after focal ischemic injury. J Neurosci. 2001;21:5272–80.

81. Johansson BB, Belichenko PV. Neuronal plasticity and dendritic spines: effect of environmental enrichment on intact and postischemic rat brain. J Cereb Blood Flow Metab. 2002;22:89–96.

82. Donato F, Rompani SB, Caroni P. Parvalbumin-expressing basket-cell network plasticity induced by experience regulates adult learning. Nature. 2013;504:272–6.

83. Hu YS, Long N, Pigino G, Brady ST, Lazarov O. Molecular mechanisms of environmental enrichment: impairments in Akt/GSK3β, neurotrophin-3 and CREB signaling. PLoS ONE. 2013;8(5):e64460.

84. Novkovic T, Mittmann T, Manahan-Vaughan D. BDNF contributes to the facilitation of hippocampal synaptic plasticity and learning enabled by environmental enrichment. Hippocampus. 2014. doi:10.1002/hipo.22342. [Epub ahead of print].

85. Ekstrand J, Hellsten J, Tingström A. Environmental enrichment, exercise and corticosterone affect endothelial cell proliferation in adult rat hippocampus and prefrontal cortex. Neurosci Lett. 2008;442:203–7.

86. Frisardi V, Panza F, Seripa D, Imbimbo BP, Vendemiale G, Pilotto A, Solfrizzi V. Nutraceutical properties of Mediterranean diet and cognitive decline: possible underlying mechanisms. J Alzheimers Dis. 2010;22:715–40.

87. Gu Y, Scarmeas N. Dietary patterns in Alzheimer's disease and cognitive aging. Curr Alzheimer Res. 2011;8:510–9.

88. Kesse-Guyot E, Andreeva VA, Ducros V, Jeandel C, Julia C, Hercberg S, Galan P. Carotenoid-rich dietary patterns during midlife and subsequent cognitive function. Br J Nutr. 2014;111:915–23.

89. Beezhold BL, Johnston CS, Daigle DR. Vegetarian diets are associated with healthy mood states: a cross-sectional study in seventh day adventist adults. Nutr J. 2010;9:26. doi:10.1186/1475-2891-9-26.

90. Beezhold BL, Johnston CS. Restriction of meat, fish, and poultry in omnivores improves mood: a pilot randomized controlled trial. Nutr J. 2012;11:9.

91. Rendeiro C, Vauzour D, Kean RJ, Butler LT, Rattray M, Spencer JP, Williams CM. Blueberry supplementation induces spatial memory improvements and region-specific regulation of hippocampal BDNF mRNA expression in young rats. 2012;223:319–30.

92. Cartford MC, Gemma C, Bickford PC. Eighteen-month-old Fischer 344 rats fed a spinach-enriched diet show improved delay classical eyeblink conditioning and reduced expression of tumor necrosis factor alpha (TNFalpha) and TNFbeta in the cerebellum. J Neurosci. 2002;22:5813–6.

93. Poulose SM, Bielinski DF, Shukitt-Hale B. Walnut diet reduces accumulation of polyubiquitinated proteins and inflammation in the brain of aged rats. J Nutr Biochem. 2013;24:912–9.

94. Joseph JA, Shukitt-Hale B, Willis LM. Grape juice, berries, and walnuts affect brain aging and behavior. J Nutr. 2009;139:1813 S–7 S.

95. Fernández-Fernández L, Comes G, Bolea I, Valente T, Ruiz J, Murtra P, Ramirez B, Anglés N, Reguant J, Morelló JR, Boada M, Hidalgo J, Escorihuela RM, Unzeta M. LMN diet, rich in polyphenols and polyunsaturated fatty acids, improves mouse cognitive decline associated with aging and Alzheimer's disease. Behav Brain Res. 2012;228:261–71.

96. Frautschy SA, Hu W, Kim P, Miller SA, Chu T, Harris-White ME, Cole GM. Phenolic anti-inflammatory antioxidant reversal of Abeta-induced cognitive deficits and neuropathology. Neurobiol Aging. 2001;22:993–1005.

97. Zbarsky V, Datla KP, Parkar S, Rai DK, Aruoma OI, Dexter DT. Neuroprotective properties of the natural phenolic antioxidants curcumin and naringenin but not quercetin and fisetin in a 6-OHDA model of Parkinson's disease. Free Radic Res. 2005;39:1119–25.

98. Dohare P, Garg P, Jain V, Nath C, Ray M. Dose dependence and therapeutic window for the neuroprotective effects of curcumin in thromboembolic model of rat. Behav Brain Res. 2008;193:289–97.

99. Wu A, Ying Z, Gomez-Pinilla F. Dietary curcumin counteracts the outcome of traumatic brain injury on oxidative stress, synaptic plasticity, and cognition. Exp Neurol. 2006;197:309–17.

100. Lee S, Kim J, Seo SG, Choi BR, Han JS, Lee KW, Kim J. Sulforaphane alleviates scopolamine-induced memory impairment in mice. Pharmacol Res. 2014;85:23–32.

101. Morroni F, Tarozzi A, Sita G, Bolondi C, Zolezzi Moraga JM, Cantelli-Forti G, Hrelia P. Neuroprotective effect of sulforaphane in 6-hydroxydopamine-lesioned mouse model of Parkinson's disease. Neurotoxicology. 2013;36:63–71.

102. Zhao J, Kobori N, Aronowski J, Dash PK. Sulforaphane reduces infarct volume following focal cerebral ischemia in rodents. Neurosci Lett. 2006;393:108–12.

103. Dash PK, Zhao J, Orsi SA, Zhang M, Moore AN. Sulforaphane improves cognitive function administered following traumatic brain injury. Neurosci Lett. 2009;460:103–7.

104. Kim D, Nguyen MD, Dobbin MM, Fischer A, Sananbenesi F, Rodgers JT, Delalle I, Baur JA, Sui G, Armour SM, Puigserver P, Sinclair DA, Tsai LH. SIRT1 deacetylase protects against neurodegeneration in models for Alzheimer's disease and amyotrophic lateral sclerosis. EMBO J. 2007;26:3169–79.

105. Singleton RH, Yan HQ, Fellows-Mayle W, Dixon CE. Resveratrol attenuates behavioral impairments and reduces cortical and hippocampal loss in a rat controlled cortical impact model of traumatic brain injury. J Neurotrauma. 2010;27:1091–9.

106. Ames BN, Shigenaga MK, Hagen TM. Oxidants, antioxidants, and the degenerative diseases of aging. Proc Natl Acad Sci U S A. 1993;90:7915–22.

107. Futuyma DJ, Agrawal AA. Macroevolution and the biological diversity of plants and herbivores. Proc Natl Acad Sci U S A. 2009;106:18054–61.

108. Isman MB. Botanical insecticides, deterrents, and repellents in modern agriculture and an increasingly regulated world. Annu Rev Entomol. 2006;51:45–66.

109. Mattson MP, Cheng A. Neurohormetic phytochemicals: low-dose toxins that induce adaptive neuronal stress responses. Trends Neurosci. 2006;29:632–9.

110. Moubarac JC, Martins AP, Claro RM, Levy RB, Cannon G, Monteiro CA. Consumption of ultra-processed foods and likely impact on human health. Evidence from Canada. Public Health Nutr. 2013;16:2240–8.

111. Volkow ND, Wang GJ, Tomasi D, Baler RD. The addictive dimensionality of obesity. Biol Psychiatry. 2013;73:811–8.

112. Harvie M, Wright C, Pegington M, McMullan D, Mitchell E, Martin B, Cutler RG, Evans G, Whiteside S, Maudsley S, Camandola S, Wang R, Carlson OD, Egan JM, Mattson MP, Howell A. The effect of intermittent energy and carbohydrate restriction v. daily energy restriction on weight loss and metabolic disease risk markers in overweight women. Br J Nutr. 2013;110:1534–47.

113. Mosley M, Spencer M. The fast diet. New York: atria books; 2013. p. 208.

114. Hunter R, Dayan AD, Wilson J. Alzheimer's disease in one monozygotic twin. J Neurol Neurosurg Psychiatry. 1972;35:707–10.

115. Clare L, Wilson BA, Carter G, Hodges JR. Cognitive rehabilitation as a component of early intervention in Alzheimer's disease: a single case study. Aging Ment Health. 2010;7:15–21.

Chronic Kidney Disease

28

Girish N. Nadkarni and Joseph A. Vassalotti

Abbreviations

ACE	Angiotensin-converting enzyme
ADA	American Diabetes Association
AKI	Acute kidney injury
ARBs	Angiotensin receptor blockers
BP	Blood pressure
BV	Biological value
BUN	Blood urea nitrogen
CKD	Chronic kidney disease
eGFR	Estimated glomerular filtration rate
ESRD	End-stage renal disease
GFR	Gomerular filtration rate
HD	Hemodialysis
HEI	Healthy Eating Index
KDOQI	Kidney disease quality outcomes initiative
MNT	Medical Nutrition Therapy
OSA	Obstructive sleep apnea
PD	Peritoneal dialysis
PSQI	Pittsburgh Sleep Quality Index
PUFA	Polyunsaturated fatty acids
RAPA	Rapid assessment of physical activity
RD	Registered dietitian
T	Teaspoonful
T2D	Type-2 diabetes
UACR	Urine albumin/creatinine ratio

Introduction

Chronic kidney disease (CKD) affects 10–15 % of individuals in the USA, Europe, and Asia [1]. CKD is largely an asymptomatic condition associated with kidney failure, premature cardiovascular mortality, complications, decreased quality of life, and increased health-care expenditures. Approximately two thirds of CKD cases are attributable to diabetes (40 %) and hypertension (28 %; [2]). CKD is defined by loss of kidney function as estimated glomerular filtration rate (eGFR) below 60 ml/min/1.73 m^2 and/or persistent increased urinary albumin–creatinine ratio lasting 90 or more days or other markers of kidney damage (glomerular hematuria, imaging abnormalities, and kidney biopsy findings). Loss of kidney function can progress to kidney failure or end-stage renal disease (ESRD) requiring dialysis or kidney transplantation. CKD is now classified into six "G" stages based on the eGFR and three "A" stages based on the amount of albumin in the urine, with higher stages conferring worse prognosis (G stage 3 now includes both 3A and 3B, see Fig. 28.1; [2]). CKD is also a major independent risk factor for cardiovascular disease, all-cause mortality, and cardiovascular mortality [1, 2]. Other CKD complications are acute kidney injury, anemia, bone and mineral disorders (abnormal biochemical parameters, bone abnormalities, and vascular calcification), and metabolic acidosis. However, this common condition is under-diagnosed, even in those at risk with type-2 diabetes (T2D) and/or hypertension.

Although medications such as angiotensin-converting enzyme (ACE) inhibitors or angiotensin receptor blockers (ARBs) retard progression of CKD with albuminuria and hypertension, there currently exist no specific medications to treat most etiologies of CKD. In the absence of definitive drug therapy for this common disease, prevention of both the development and progression of CKD are essential. CKD is a complex multiplier of comorbidities, risk conditions, and complications. Since many of the comorbidities associated with CKD are modifiable by changes in health behaviors, lifestyle modification is a promising, potentially impactful therapeutic area that may be easy for the busy clinician to overlook. There are currently limited trial data on optimal utilization of lifestyle modification in CKD, making additional research important. In this chapter, key lifestyle medicine recommendations for primary, secondary, and tertiary prevention of kidney disease are reviewed (Table 28.1).

G. N. Nadkarni (✉) · J. A. Vassalotti
Division of Nephrology, Department of Medicine, Icahn School of Medicine at Mount Sinai, New York, NY, USA
e-mail: girish.nadkarni@mountsinai.org

J. A. Vassalotti
National Kidney Foundation, Inc., New York, NY, USA

© Springer International Publishing Switzerland 2016
J. I. Mechanick, R. F. Kushner (eds.), *Lifestyle Medicine,* DOI 10.1007/978-3-319-24687-1_28

Guide to Frequency of Monitoring (number of times per year) by GFR and Albuminuria category

				Albuminuria categories Description and range		
				A1	A2	A3
				Normal to mildly increased	Moderately increased	Severely increased
				<30 mg/g <3 mg/mmol	30-299 mg/g 3-29 mg/mmol	≥300 mg/g ≥30 mg/mmol
GFR categories (ml/min/1.73 m² Description and range	G1	Normal or high	≥90	1 if CKD	1	2
	G2	Mildly decreased	60-90	1 if CKD	1	2
	G3a	Mildly to moderately decreased	45-59	1	2	3
	G3b	Moderately to severely decreased	30-44	2	3	3
	G3	Severely decreased	15-29	3	3	4+
	G5	Kidney failure	<15	4+	4+	4+

Fig. 28.1 Recent staging and grading of chronic kidney disease (CKD) based on estimated glomerular filtration rate and albuminuria. The colors above show the relative risk of morbidity and mortality in CKD. (*Green*: low risk (if no other markers of kidney disease, no CKD), *yellow*: moderate risk, *orange*: high risk, and *red*: very high risk). The frequency of recommended follow-up appointments annually is shown in each box. *GFR* glomerular filtration rate. (Modified with permission from Macmillan Publishers Ltd: Kidney International. KDIGO. Summary of recommendation statements. Kidney Inc 2013; 3(Suppl):5. Copyright © 2013)

Table 28.1 Definition of prevention levels in chronic kidney disease (CKD)

Level of prevention	Definition
Primary	Prevent the development of CKD in the population at risk with diabetes and/or hypertension
Secondary	Prevent the progression of CKD (loss of kidney function over time) and prevent or delay CKD complications
Tertiary	Prevent adverse outcomes in those with CKD treated with renal replacement therapy (dialysis or kidney transplantation) by optimizing care

Primary Prevention of Kidney Disease

There are limited data regarding lifestyle interventions and development of CKD. Improvement in blood pressure (BP) and glycemic control are the focus of primary prevention of CKD caused by hypertension and/or T2D, respectively. Approximately 30% of incident CKD cases are due to immune-mediated diseases (glomerulonephritis) and adverse drug events that are not likely to be directly amendable to lifestyle intervention. Therefore, the next section reviews lifestyle modifications for the optimal management of hypertension and T2D.

Primary Prevention of CKD in Hypertension

Hypertension has a strong, graded association with CKD development in several prospective studies [3]. The recent Joint National Committee-8 (JNC-8) guidelines recommend a BP goal ≤140/90 for age ≤60 years and ≤150/90 for age >60 years (both in mmHg) in the T2D, CKD, and general populations [4]. Lifestyle modifications are crucial for both attaining and sustaining goal BP with or without antihypertensive medications.

Physical Activity in Hypertension

Meta-analyses of studies including a large number of participants with sedentary lifestyles have found significant reductions in BP (approximately 5 systolic and 3 diastolic mmHg)

Table 28.2 Commonly used terms on food labels and their corresponding sodium content

Terminology	Sodium content of food
Sodium free	Trivial amount of sodium per serving
Very low sodium	35 mg or less per serving
Low sodium	140 mg or less per serving
Reduced sodium	Foods in which the level of sodium is reduced by 25%
Light or lite in sodium	Foods in which the sodium is reduced by at least 50%

with both aerobic (30 min/day at least 3 times/week for a minimum for 12 weeks) and resistance training (dynamic or isometric for 20 min/day at least 3 times/week for a minimum of 12 weeks). Also, trials of yoga (60 min/day at least 2–3 times/week for a minimum of 20 weeks) and transcendental meditation (30 min/day at least 3 times/week for a minimum of 8 weeks) in pre-hypertensive and hypertensive subjects showed sustained, significant decreases in BP (approximately 7 systolic and 3 diastolic mmHg). Thus, physical activity incorporating aerobic and resistance training with yoga and meditation as adjuncts is effective in lowering BP and theoretically should prevent CKD, although direct data are lacking to support this conclusion.

Healthy Diet and Weight Loss in Hypertension

A number of studies have established the direct relationship between reduced sodium intake, BP reduction, and hypertension prevention. The recommended dietary sodium intake is 1500–2300 mg/day [5]. Since most dietary sodium comes from processed and canned foods, consumers should be aware of sodium content in specific food items. Table 28.2 shows the common terms used in food labels with the corresponding sodium content in milligrams. A recent study also found a significant decrease in the development of CKD in patients with hypertension who were adherent to a low sodium (1500 mg/day) Mediterranean diet [6]. This 7-year observational study assessed the eating habits of a prospective cohort of 900 patients and found that patients with hypertension consuming a fruit-and-vegetable-rich, low-saturated-fat diet had a 50% decrease in incident CKD compared to a standard American diet. With respect to weight loss, a meta-analysis showed that an average weight loss of 5.1 kg led to mean systolic and diastolic BP reductions of 4.4 and 3.6 mmHg, respectively [7].

In summary, lifestyle modification, including physical activity that incorporates aerobic and resistance training and weight loss, with yoga and meditation as adjuncts, along with a low-sodium, fruit-and-vegetable-rich, low-saturated-fat diet, demonstrates benefit in terms of decreased BP in patients with hypertension, which should reduce the risk of incident CKD accordingly.

Primary Prevention of CKD in T2D

The American Diabetes Association (ADA) recommends a hemoglobin A1C (A1C) target <7% for most nonpregnant adults with diabetes [8]. Achieving this target A1C has been shown to reduce the onset of albuminuria in the randomized trial of intensive insulin therapy (Diabetes Control and Complications Trial) [9], providing a rationale for improved glycemic control reducing the incidence of CKD. This section will focus on lifestyle interventions specific to glycemic control.

Physical Activity in T2D

Cohort studies that demonstrate A1C reductions of 0.5–1% with aerobic exercise support recommendations for moderate intensity exercise in sedentary individuals and increasing exercise intensity in those who are already physically active [10]. Yoga and meditation also have salutary effects on A1C and thus are effective adjunctive measures, although large-scale trials are still needed to establish degree of benefit.

Healthy Diet in T2D

A prospective study involving a large cohort of 6000 patients with T2D found that a low-sodium, high-potassium, high-quality diet incorporating higher fruit and green leafy vegetable intake and moderate alcohol intake were associated with reduced risk of developing CKD [11]. There are evidence-based guidelines for optimal diet management [12, 13], but fewer than half of T2D patients achieve the recommendations. There are recent studies that show training in mindful eating to increase awareness of internal experience, reduce automatic eating patterns, and interrupt stress-related eating behaviors could potentially improve fruit and vegetable consumption. Thus, training in mindful eating should be considered as an option by both clinicians and patients to improve healthy diet adherence [14].

In conclusion, increased physical activity, particularly aerobic exercise, along with a fruit-and-vegetable-rich, low-saturated-fat diet implemented with training in mindful eating comprise a comprehensive lifestyle approach to glycemic control to prevent CKD.

Secondary Prevention of Kidney Disease

Physical Fitness in CKD

Impaired physical fitness is common in CKD, with exercise capacity in early stages being 70% of expected and then declining further as CKD progresses. Poor physical activity in CKD patients is significantly associated with adverse clinical outcomes, including cardiovascular morbidity and mortality [15]. A Cochrane meta-analysis showed that aerobic and/or resistance training showed improved objective and subjective parameters in CKD stages G1–4 including assessments of physical fitness and BP control [16]. This analysis selected studies with a minimum of 3-times/week physical activity for at least 3-months follow-up. No studies included hard outcomes such as cardiovascular mortality or worsening of kidney function. Since exercise caused improvement in surrogate endpoints, there may be significant benefit from a combination of cardiovascular and resistance training in CKD patients [16]. Not included in the Cochrane analysis is an interesting Chinese observational study of over 6000 patients with CKD G3–5 that showed an association of increased self-reported walking with lower risk of ESRD and mortality [17]. Walking is an attractive low-risk physical activity that is inexpensive and relatively easy to implement, in contrast to alternatives such as gym membership and participation in exercise classes. Assessment of physical activity can be performed quickly using validated surveys such as the rapid assessment of physical activity (RAPA) [18], but a practical assessment integrates low-intensity physical activities, such as walking, aerobic exercise, stretching, and strengthening.

Meditation and CKD

A proof of concept study in 13 patients with CKD stage G3 showed that mindfulness meditation lowered BP and sympathetic nerve activity [19]. Since CKD is characterized by chronic sympathetic overactivity, this reduction could potentially lead to slower progression.

Diet and CKD

Sodium Intake

Modification of dietary sodium intake is a valuable target for reducing CKD progression and cardiovascular risk in CKD. A recent randomized controlled trial of dietary sodium in CKD (4600 mg/day in controls vs. 1800 mg/day in the intervention group with potassium controlled in both groups) showed a reduction of 10 and 4 mmHg in systolic and diastolic BP, respectively [20]. The recommended daily intake for CKD stages G1–4 is 2000 g/day, a challenging level to achieve in the context of the average American intake of over 3000 mg [5], emphasizing the importance of the awareness of sodium content in foods. The 24-h urine collection for sodium is a reliable estimate of intake in stable outpatients that is subject to day-to-day variability. Dietary recall collection tools are also useful, generally requiring Medical Nutrition Therapy (MNT) with a registered dietitian (RD).

Potassium Intake

The Kidney Disease Quality Outcomes Initiative (KDOQI) guidelines generally recommend a 2000–4000 mg/day potassium intake for individuals with CKD at risk for hyperkalemia [21]. The restriction in the later stages is to reduce risk of hyperkalemia which can be life threatening. This is especially of concern in patients who are on ACE inhibitors or ARBs and in those with low eGFR. Several recent randomized controlled trials have demonstrated hyperkalemia and acute kidney injury (AKI) safety signals with the combination of ACE inhibitors and ARB in hypertension with or without T2D, making it important to use monotherapy only in routine practice [2]. Also, in the CKD population with and at risk for hyperkalemia, salt substitutes, containing potassium chloride, should be avoided. Table 28.3 presents the potassium content in selected foods.

Phosphorus Intake

Homeostatic mechanisms to counter-regulate phosphorus retention typically occur in CKD stage G3b and higher. Hence, dietary phosphorus restriction may not be necessary in the earlier stages. Recommendations in stages G3–5 are to reduce intake to 800–1000 mg/day [21]. Phosphorus binders may be necessary to maintain the serum phosphorus at desirable levels in the normal laboratory range. Another concern is that inorganic phosphorus is present ubiquitously in processed foods, but inconsistently disclosed on the nutrition facts panel, complicating estimates of and interventions in phosphorus intake. Therefore, patients with CKD stage G3–5 should restrict their consumption of processed food and increase intake of fruits and green leafy vegetables.

Table 28.3 Potassium content of selected foods[a]

Food group	Low potassium foods	Potassium content in mg	High potassium foods	Potassium content in mg
Dairy	Cottage cheese	103	Milk (250 ml)	400
Eggs	Egg (one)	63	–	–
Grain	White bread (two slices)	70	Bran cereal (one cup)	253
Vegetables	Lettuce (one cup)	82	Beets	274
	Carrot (one raw)	97	Cooked broccoli	241
Fruit	Apple	148	Banana	422
Meat	Chicken (75 g)	179	Beef (75 g)	300
Fish	Cod (75 g)	183	Canned salmon (75 g)	255
Legumes	Peanut butter (T)	122	Lentils	385

[a] *T* Teaspoonful

Table 28.4 Biological value of common protein-containing foods

Food	Biological Value (BV)
Poultry/fish/meat	
Egg (reference)	100
Chicken	79
Fish	76
Beef	74
Vegetables and grains	
Soy bean	96
Whole bean	96
Rice (brown, unpolished)	83
Rice (polished)	64
Corn	60
Kidney bean	49
White flour	41
Dairy	
Milk (cow)	90
Cheese	84

Protein Intake

Dietary protein restriction may protect against CKD progression by several mechanisms including reduction in intraglomerular hypertension, modulation of cytokine expression and matrix synthesis, or reduced kidney fibrosis. However, whether these translate into a clinically relevant protective effect in CKD is controversial. One of the challenges is the independent assessment of the benefit of dietary protein restriction in the context of an association of high-protein diets with other deleterious components such as high sodium and enriched phosphorus. Moreover, the risks of excessively low-protein diets are catabolism and malnutrition, making protein restriction appropriate only for stable outpatients. Current data suggest that there may be a small but significant attenuation in eGFR decline with a low-protein diet without significant detriment. Thus, in stable outpatients with CKD stage G3 or higher, the recommended protein intake is 0.8 g/kg/day of which at least 50% is high biological value (BV) [2]. This is the same level of recommended intake for all Americans by the US Department of Agriculture in the context of high protein intake in the general population. BV is not only a measure of the proportion of absorbed protein that is incorporated into the proteins of the body, but also an indirect measure of essential amino acid content, which affects the efficiency of protein synthesis. Egg protein, containing all of the essential amino acids, is considered to have a BV of 100 as the reference standard. Table 28.4 shows the BV of common protein-containing foods. A 24-h urine collection for urea nitrogen can be used to calculate adherence to the 0.8 g/kg/day protein diet as follows [22].

- Protein intake = protein excretion
- Protein intake = UUN (24-h urine urea nitrogen) + NUN (non-urea nitrogen or fecal excretion)
- Protein intake = UUN + 0.031 g nitrogen × kg body weight.

MNT with an RD is most likely to be successful in developing an individualized meal plan incorporating safe protein restriction.

Other Beneficial Dietary Approaches

The impact of saturated dietary fat on CKD progression is well documented. In a meta-analysis of randomized controlled trials, CKD patients consuming n-3 polyunsaturated fatty acids (PUFA) in fish oil were more likely to have a reduction in urine protein and eGFR stabilization [23]. Fish oil may have an advantage over fish servings, since daily intake of the latter may not be palatable or available and certain fish (salmon and sardines canned with bones) are high in phosphorus. In a number of randomized controlled trials, a higher intake of fruits and green leafy vegetables decreased progression in CKD stage G2 and significantly reduced metabolic acidosis in CKD stage G3 [24, 25]. High-fiber diets were associated with reduced inflammation and decreased mortality in two important studies: the Uppsala Longitudinal Study of elderly Swedish men and the National Health and Nutrition Examination Survey III, a stratified random sample of the US adult ambulatory population [26, 27]. For every 10 g/day increase in total dietary fiber in subjects with CKD as defined by an eGFR <60 ml/min/1.73 m^2, there were associations with 42 and 19% reductions in all-cause mortality, respectively [26, 27]. Both studies also showed significantly reduced hazard ratios for serum C-reactive protein >3 mg/L associated with a high-fiber diet. Although as yet unproven in randomized trials, the high-fiber diet could also play a role in reducing progression of loss of kidney function in CKD by increasing fecal bacteria and in turn nitrogen excretion [26]. This speculation is supported by a pilot investigation of 13 patients with CKD stage G3–4 demonstrating that dietary supplementation with probiotics conferred a significant reduction in the blood urea nitrogen (BUN) and serum uric acid over 6 months [28]. High soda consumption has been linked to both incidence and progression of CKD and should be assiduously avoided [29]. Recent data show that a Mediterranean diet may have a beneficial effect in retarding CKD progression [30]. Lastly, clinicians should consider MNT with an RD for precise assessment of diet quality and design of an individualized meal plan. RDs use validated assessments of diet such as the Healthy Eating Index (HEI) [31].

Smoking and CKD Progression

A large population-based study involving 65,193 individuals has demonstrated a significant, dose-dependent increase in risk of developing CKD stage G3b or higher for cumulative lifetime cigarette exposure (adjusted relative risk, RR 1.42 for 25–49 pack-years and 2.05 for >50 pack-years, respectively) especially in individuals who were obese and sedentary [32]. Thus, a comprehensive tobacco cessation plan is an important consideration and should include psychological support, smoking cessation aids, and referral to a specialized clinic if necessary.

Sleep and CKD Progression

The prevalence of obstructive sleep apnea (OSA) is 30–73 % in patients with CKD stages G4 and G5 and those treated with dialysis compared to 2–4 % in the general population [33, 34]. Heterogeneity in the definition of OSA across studies contributes to the range in reported prevalence rates. OSA can contribute to CKD progression in two ways. First, sympathetic hyperactivity is often present in patients with CKD, and exacerbation due to OSA may cause progression. This is demonstrated in a study including patients with advanced CKD who were unable to increase vagal tone during the transition to sleep [35]. Secondly, OSA prevents the normal nighttime dipping of BP by causing persistent nocturnal elevation of renin, aldosterone, and catecholamines. Loss of diurnal variation in renin–angiotensin–aldosterone system activity could play a role in progression of CKD, arterial stiffness, and atherosclerosis. There are no prospective investigations of OSA and kidney function decline, but cross-sectional trials associate OSA severity with increased proteinuria [36] and cardiovascular mortality. Sleep disturbances are a novel risk factor for the progression of CKD and early treatment may have a therapeutic benefit. Thus, sleep duration and quality should be part of the initial and follow-up assessment of the CKD patient. One of the most widely used research instruments to evaluate sleep quality is the Pittsburgh Sleep Quality Index (PSQI) [37]. A practical simplification of the PSQI for clinical use would include an assessment of the duration of sleep, including typical bedtime and wake-up time, and specific sleeping problems (difficulty falling asleep, interruptions due to cough, trouble breathing, nocturia, and early awakenings). If there is a roommate or bed partner, additional questions should be asked regarding snoring, breath pauses, and leg twitching. Patients should also be informed about lifestyle interventions that may be beneficial in sleep disturbances, including sleep posture (sleeping on the side instead of the back), sleep hygiene (avoiding alcohol and caffeine 4 h before bedtime, sleeping at the same time every day, and maintaining at least 7 h of sleep per night), smoking cessation, and maintaining a healthy weight.

Hence, lifestyle modifications for secondary prevention of CKD include:

1. Physical activity including aerobic/resistance training and yoga/meditation
2. Healthy diet incorporating fiber-containing fruits and vegetables, low sodium and phosphorus content, approximately 0.8 g/kg/day protein of which at least 50 % is high BV, and utilizing the lowest possible amount of processed food

3. Smoking cessation
4. Assessment of sleep duration and quality, sleep hygiene, and early identification and treatment for sleep disturbances, particularly OSA

Tertiary Prevention of CKD

Exercise in Patients Treated with Renal Replacement Therapy

There is a large body of evidence that suggests significant and sustained benefits of exercise in patients undergoing intermittent hemodialysis. A 2011 Cochrane review found substantial evidence that aerobic and/or weight training exercise (moderate intensity for at least 30 min daily/3 times a week) significantly improved surrogate markers in dialysis patients including measures of physical fitness, cardiovascular and nutritional parameters, and patient-related outcomes such as depression measures and quality of life scales [16]. The duration of physical activity required was at least 3 months for significant improvement in most parameters. Similarly, a combination of cardiovascular and resistance training showed more significant improvement in all parameters as compared to either exercise modality alone. This benefit was constant irrespective of the modality of renal replacement therapy (hemodialysis, peritoneal dialysis, or kidney transplant) and whether exercise was supervised or not. A significant limitation of all of these studies was short follow-up ranging from 3–12 months, limiting the accrual of hard endpoints for cardiovascular mortality or morbidity.

Future studies should address long-term outcomes by potentially increasing follow-up and/or utilizing national registries of patients undergoing dialysis. Also, some experts have concerns about the potential risks of exercise in this population, particularly given the high cardiovascular morbidity and mortality. Two studies showed no significant difference in exercise-induced injuries or complications compared to controls, including arteriovenous (AV) fistula infections, angina, incidence of falls, acute illness, and number of healthcare professional visits [16]. Thus, most patients on renal replacement therapy should have a combination of aerobic and resistance training at least 3 times a week.

Yoga in Patients on Renal Replacement Therapy

Several uncontrolled case series show yoga improves both subjective and objective parameters in dialysis patients. One randomized controlled trial of a 30-min, twice-weekly yoga regimen in 37 hemodialysis patients showed improvements in both patient-reported symptoms (pain, fatigue, and sleep disturbance) and biochemical parameters (cholesterol and hematocrit) [38]. Yoga appears to be a safe and effective clinical exercise modality in patients on hemodialysis, although larger studies with longer follow-up are lacking.

Meditation in Patients on Renal Replacement Therapy

There are currently no randomized controlled trials of meditation in ESRD patients. However, the previously reviewed mindfulness meditation in CKD stage 3 suggests potential benefit. There is currently a trial testing the efficacy of meditation in dialysis patients. Thus, meditation should be considered as a reasonable and safe lifestyle modification of yet unproven efficacy.

Diet in Patients on Renal Replacement Therapy

Sodium Intake
Volume overload is a common problem in chronic dialysis patients and is associated with adverse cardiac outcomes including hypertension and mortality [39]. Most of the studies of dietary sodium restriction (<2000 mg/day) in dialysis patients had limited sample size with short follow-up and did not assess mortality risk. However, they uniformly showed a decrease in weight gain between hemodialysis sessions, improved BP control, and reduction in antihypertensive drug utilization [40, 41]. These studies justify an increased effort in hemodialysis patients for dietary sodium restriction especially in those with cardiac conditions. One retrospective study showed higher all-cause mortality in peritoneal dialysis patients with low dietary sodium intake independent of caloric intake. Reverse causality or comorbidities associated with poor intake such as cardiomyopathy could have confounded this association [42]. In the absence of more data, dietary sodium intake in peritoneal dialysis patients should be individualized, depending on the BP and comorbidities.

Potassium Intake
Hyperkalemia is the most common electrolyte abnormality in chronic dialysis patients, associated with significant mortality risk. In a 3-year study of more than 70,000 hemodialysis patients, serum potassium >6 mEq/L before dialysis was significantly associated with a 1.5 times all-cause mortality risk [43]. Since dietary intake is the major source of excess potassium, KDOQI guidelines suggest limiting potassium intake to 2000–3000 mg in hemodialysis and 3000–4000 mg in peritoneal dialysis patients [21]. Since most fruits and vegetables are rich sources of potassium and even modest potassium-containing foods can cause hyperkalemia if taken in excess, this presents a nutritional challenge for the dialysis patient. Examples of foods that contain a high amount of potassium (≥200 mg per serving) and a low amount of potassium (<200 mg per serving) are shown in Table 28.3. Also,

the potassium content of packaged foods are not routinely listed on the Nutrition Facts Panel, presenting a particular challenge for dialysis patients [44]. Potassium additives may be present in foods that appear to be less processed, misleading patients about the actual content [45]. An approach to remove potassium from foods during preparation includes leaching or double cooking.

Phosphorus and Protein Intake
These two nutrients are discussed together, since protein-rich foods are usually high in phosphorus. Protein-energy malnutrition is a serious complication in maintenance dialysis with 20–70% of patients affected, associated with significantly increased mortality. Etiologies include inadequate dietary intake, catabolism, and decreased nutrient absorption. However, balancing sufficient protein intake and limiting phosphorus content in foods is challenging [46]. Several studies have demonstrated a strong, direct, and graded relationship between elevated serum phosphorus levels and adverse outcomes in maintenance dialysis patients [47]. Dietary phosphorus restriction and oral phosphate binders are effective in lowering serum phosphorus [48]. However, there are specific foods that might have high protein content without the accompanying phosphorus. Humans lack the intestinal enzyme phytase and thus the bioavailability of phosphorus from plant foods is half that of animal foods [49]. Also, most of the phosphorus is concentrated in the egg yolk, making the egg white a phosphorus-free protein of high BV [50]. Specific cooking techniques using prolonged soaking and boiling allow a greater reduction in phosphorus while preserving protein content. Lastly, the high bioavailability of inorganic phosphorus in processed foods provides an additional rationale for limiting intake.

Other Beneficial Dietary Approaches
There are data demonstrating that replacing saturated fat with PUFA including linoleic acid in patients on hemodialysis has a beneficial effect on mortality [51]. A cohort study of 100 patients with sudden cardiac death in the first year after starting hemodialysis versus 300 patients who survived the first year of treatment in the USA showed that serum levels of long-chain n-3 fatty acids displayed an inverse relationship with sudden cardiac death [52].

Smoking Cessation in Patients on Renal Replacement Therapy

Multiple observational trials found that active smoking in dialysis patients is associated with increased all-cause mortality [53]. The patient and physician should make a concerted effort for smoking cessation, including referral to a specialized clinic and utilization of smoking cessation aids if necessary.

Table 28.5 Nutritional therapy for each CKD stage

Nutrient	Stage 1	Stage 2	Stage 3	Stages 4–5	Dialysis
Sodium (mg/day)	2000	2000	2000	2000	2000
Energy (kcal/kg/day)	35 under age 60 and 30–35 age 60 and older				
Fat	<30% of total nonprotein caloric intake, replace saturated fats with mono or polyunsaturated fats				
Protein (g/kg/day)[a]	0.8	0.8	0.8	0.8	0.8–1.2(HD)/1.3 (PD)
Potassium (mg/day)	V^+	V^+	V^+	V^+	2000–3000 (HD) 3000–4000 (PD)
Phosphate (mg/day)	None	None	800–1000	800–1000	800–1000

V^+ variable depending on the presence and risk of hyperkalemia, *PD* peritoneal dialysis, *HD* hemodialysis
[a] At least 50% of protein intake should be of high biologic value (BV)

Lifestyle modifications for tertiary prevention in CKD should include:

1. Physical activity incoporating aerobic exercise with progressive resistance training and perhaps yoga and meditation
2. Healthy-eating patterns that are low in sodium, potassium, and phosphorus content with protein intake according to dialysis modality (see Table 28.5), of which 50% is high BV, and also implementing expert guidance from a nutritionist or RD
3. Smoking cessation

Case Study

A 54-year-old Caucasian male with a history of T2D (last A1C of 8%) and hypertension for 12 years presents for routine follow-up. Current medications are lisinopril 20 mg, aspirin 81 mg, and glipizide 10 mg (all daily). Vital signs are BP 148/90 mmHg, heart rate 78 beats per minute and regular, and body mass index (BMI) 33 kg/m². Physical examination is remarkable for trace pitting ankle edema and decreased monofilament sensation in his soles. An assessment of his lifestyle reveals a diet rich in saturated fat and refined carbohydrates (including eating out at fast food restaurants several times a week), sugar sweetened soda consumption at least three 12 oz. cans a day, limited physical activity (minimal walking, no aerobic exercise, and no stretching or strengthening), disturbed sleep patterns (feeling tired in the morning), and half a pack per day tobacco use for 10 year). His wife notes loud snoring but no breath pauses, or irregular breathing. Laboratory assessment reveals a creatinine of 1.5 mg/dL with a CKD-EPI eGFR of 52 ml/min/1.73 m²; the urine studies reveal an unremarkable urinalysis, and a urine albumin/creatinine ratio (UACR) of 900 mg/g of creatinine. This is stage G3a, A3 CKD caused by diabetic nephropathy. The lisinopril dose is intensified to 40 mg for albuminuria with high BP, and lifestyle medicine counseling is provided using a multidisciplinary team consisting of the physician, a nutritionist, and a physical therapist. The interventions consist of:

1. A graded exercise regimen with cardiovascular/isometric handgrip resistance exercises three times a week
2. A 2000 mg sodium diet with the saturated fatty acids replaced by PUFAs and rich in plant protein of high BV (Table 28.5)
3. Counseling with an RD to eliminate sodas/sugary drinks, consume at least five helpings of fruit/green leafy vegetables per day, and incorporate a gradual weight loss program to a goal BMI <30 kg/m² in 3 months
4. Referral to a smoking cessation clinic

The physician reinforced understanding by using the "teach-back" technique in which the patient repeats his understanding of the lifestyle interventions. At this point, additional interventions could include cardiology consultation to assess cardiovascular disease given multiple risk conditions as well as a sleep study.

At follow-up 8 weeks later, he has been adherent with his new diet and exercise regimen along with quitting smoking with the aid of a nicotine patch and intensive counseling. He reports having more energy and has lost a significant amount of weight with a decrease in BMI to 31 kg/m² and improved BP at 140/85 mmHg. The team further reinforces the importance of lifestyle interventions by emphasizing the success the patient has had but underlining that this is an ongoing stepwise process.

On his next follow-up appointment 8 weeks later, the patient is continuing to be adherent with diet and exercise and is still tobacco free. He has lost even more weight and now his BMI is 29.5 kg/m² with BP at goal of 130/80 mmHg. His repeat comprehensive metabolic panel reveals stable serum creatinine 1.4 mg/dL and some improvement in UACR 500 mg/g of creatinine.

Conclusions

The above case study illustrates how lifestyle medicine can be applied in CKD. See Fig. 28.2 for a flow map of the CKD lifestyle interventions with the domains of diet, sleep, physical activity, and tobacco use. A multidisciplinary approach

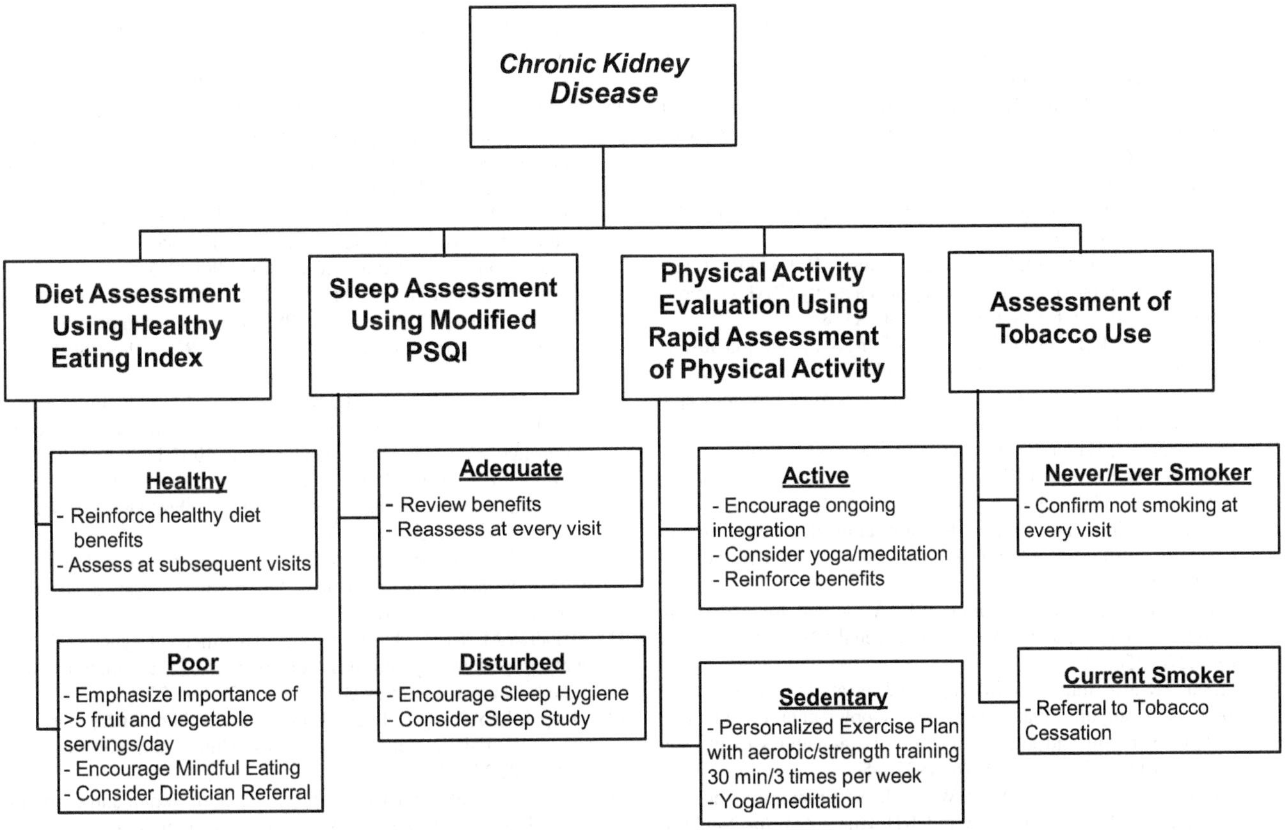

Fig. 28.2 Recommended flow sheet for primary care practitioners to assess lifestyle in CKD patients, *PSQI* Pittsburgh Sleep Quality Index

including, at minimum, an RD for MNT is most likely to be successful to implement lifestyle modification for CKD patients in a busy clinical practice.

References

1. Levey AS, Stevens LA, Coresh J. Conceptual model of CKD: applications and implications. Am J Kidney Dis. 2009;53(3 Suppl 3):S4–16.
2. Inker LA, Astor BC, Fox CH, et al. KDOQI US commentary on the 2012 KDIGO clinical practice guideline for the evaluation and management of CKD. Am J Kidney Dis. 2014;63(5):713–35.
3. Botdorf J, Chaudhary K, Whaley-Connell A. Hypertension in cardiovascular and kidney disease. Cardiorenal Med. 2011;1(3):183–92.
4. James PA, Oparil S, Carter BL, et al. Evidence-based guideline for the management of high blood pressure in adults: report from the panel members appointed to the Eighth Joint National Committee (JNC 8). JAMA. 2014;311(5):507–20.
5. Centers for Disease Control and Prevention (CDC). Application of lower sodium intake recommendations to adults–United States, 1999–2006. MMWR Morb Mortal Wkly Rep. 2009;58(11):281–3.
6. Khatri M, Moon YP, Scarmeas N, Gu Y, et al. The association between a Mediterranean-style diet and kidney function in the Northern Manhattan Study cohort. Clin J Am Soc Nephrol. 2014;9(11):1868–75.
7. Neter JE, Stam BE, Kok FJ, Grobbee DE, Geleijnse JM. Influence of weight loss on blood pressure: a meta-analysis of randomized controlled trials. Hypertension. 2003;42(5):878–84.
8. American Diabetes Association. Glycemic targets. Sec. 6. In standards of medical care in diabetes—2015. Diabetes Care. 2015;38(Suppl 1):S33–40.
9. The Diabetes Control and Complications Trial Research Group. The effect of intensive treatment of diabetes on the development and progression of long-term complications in insulin-dependent diabetes mellitus. N Engl J Med. 1993;329(14):977–86.
10. Colberg SR, Sigal RJ, Fernhall B, American College of Sports Medicine, American Diabetes Association, et al. Exercise and type 2 diabetes: the American College of Sports Medicine and the American Diabetes Association: joint position statement. Diabetes Care. 2010;33(12):2692–6.
11. Dunkler D, Dehghan M, Teo KK, ONTARGET Investigators, et al. Diet and kidney disease in high-risk individuals with type 2 diabetes mellitus. JAMA Intern Med. 2013;173(18):1682–92.
12. Handelsman Y, Mechanick JI, Blonde L, American Association of Clinical Endocrinologists, et al. American Association of Clinical Endocrinologists Medical Guidelines for clinical practice for developing a diabetes mellitus comprehensive care plan. Endocr Pract. 2011;17(Suppl 2):1–53.
13. Gonzalez-Campoy JM, Jeor ST St, Castorino K, American Association of Clinical Endocrinologists, American College of Endocrinology and the Obesity Society, et al. Clinical practice guidelines for healthy eating for the prevention and treatment of metabolic and endocrine diseases in adults: cosponsored by the American Association of Clinical Endocrinologists/the American College of Endocrinology and the Obesity Society. Endocr Pract. 2013;19(Suppl 3):1–82.
14. Miller CK, Kristeller JL, Headings A, Nagaraja H. Comparison of a mindful eating intervention to a diabetes self-management intervention among adults with type 2 diabetes: a randomized controlled trial. Health Educ Behav. 2014;41(2):145–54.

15. Painter P, Roshanravan B. The association of physical activity and physical function with clinical outcomes in adults with chronic kidney disease. Curr Opin Nephrol Hypertens. 2013;22(6):615–23.

16. Heiwe S, Jacobson SH. Exercise training for adults with chronic kidney disease. Cochrane Database Syst Rev. 2011;5(10):CD003236.

17. Chen IR, Wang SM, Liang CC, et al. Association of walking with survival and RRT among patients with CKD stages 3–5. Clin J Am Soc Nephrol. 2014;9(7):1183–9.

18. Topolski TD, LoGerfo J, Patrick DL, Williams B, Walwick J, Patrick MB. The rapid assessment of physical activity (RAPA) among older adults. Prev Chronic Dis. 2006;3(4):A118.

19. Park J, Lyles RH, Bauer-Wu S. Mindfulness meditation lowers muscle sympathetic nerve activity and blood pressure in African-American males with chronic kidney disease. Am J Physiol Regul Integr Comp Physiol. 2014;307(1):R93–101.

20. McMahon EJ, Bauer JD, Hawley CM, Isbel NM, Stowasser M, Johnson DW, Campbell KL. A randomized trial of dietary sodium restriction in CKD. J Am Soc Nephrol. 2013;24(12):2096–103.

21. National Kidney Foundation. KDOQI clinical practice guidelines for nutrition in chronic renal failure. Am J Kidney Dis. 2000;35(Suppl 2):S1–136.

22. Maroni BJ, Steinman TI, Mitch WE. A method for estimating nitrogen intake of patients with chronic renal failure. Kidney Int. 1985;27(1):58–65.

23. Miller ER 3rd, Juraschek SP, Appel LJ, et al. The effect of n-3 long-chain polyunsaturated fatty acid supplementation on urine protein excretion and kidney function: meta-analysis of clinical trials. Am J Clin Nutr. 2009;89(6):1937–45.

24. Ricardo AC, Madero M, Yang W, et al. Adherence to a healthy lifestyle and all-cause mortality in CKD. Clin J Am Soc Nephrol. 2013;8(4):602–9.

25. Goraya N, Simoni J, Jo CH, Wesson DE. Treatment of metabolic acidosis in patients with stage 3 chronic kidney disease with fruits and vegetables or oral bicarbonate reduces urine angiotensinogen and preserves glomerular filtration rate. Kidney Int. 2014;86(5):1031–8.

26. Xu H, Huang X, Risérus U, et al. Dietary fiber, kidney function, inflammation, and mortality risk. Clin J Am Soc Nephrol. 2014;9(12):2104–10.

27. Krishnamurthy VM, Wei G, Baird BC, et al. High dietary fiber intake is associated with decreased inflammation and all-cause mortality in patients with chronic kidney disease. Kidney Int. 2012;81(3):300–6.

28. Ranganathan N, Friedman EA, Tam P, Rao V, Ranganathan P, Dheer R. Probiotic dietary supplementation in patients with stage 3 and 4 chronic kidney disease: a 6-month pilot scale trial in Canada. Curr Med Res Opin. 2009;25(8):1919–30.

29. Bomback AS, Katz R, He K, Shoham DA, Burke GL, Klemmer PJ. Sugar-sweetened beverage consumption and the progression of chronic kidney disease in the Multi-Ethnic Study of Atherosclerosis (MESA). Am J Clin Nutr. 2009;90(5):1172–8.

30. Huang X, Jimenez-Moleon JJ, Lindholm B, et al. Mediterranean diet, kidney function, and mortality in men with CKD. Clin J Am Soc Nephrol. 2013;8(9):1548–55.

31. Guenther PM, Kirkpatrick SI, Reedy J, et al. The Healthy Eating Index-2010 is a valid and reliable measure of diet quality according to the 2010 Dietary Guidelines for Americans. J Nutr. 2014;144(3):399–407.

32. Hallan S, de Mutsert R, Carlsen S, Dekker FW, Aasarød K, Holmen J. Obesity, smoking, and physical inactivity as risk factors for CKD: are men more vulnerable? Am J Kidney Dis. 2006;47(3):396–405.

33. Sim JJ, Rasgon SA, Kujubu DA, et al. Sleep apnea in early and advanced chronic kidney disease: Kaiser Permanente Southern California cohort. Chest. 2009;135(3):710–6.

34. Kang EW, Abdel-Kader K, Yabes J, Glover K, Unruh M. Association of sleep-disordered breathing with cognitive dysfunction in CKD stages 4–5. Am J Kidney Dis. 2012;60(6):949–58.

35. Roumelioti ME, Ranpuria R, Hall M, et al. Abnormal nocturnal heart rate variability response among chronic kidney disease and dialysis patients during wakefulness and sleep. Nephrol Dial Transplant. 2010;25(11):3733–41.

36. Faulx MD, Storfer-Isser A, Kirchner HL, Jenny NS, Tracy RP, Redline S. Obstructive sleep apnea is associated with increased urinary albumin excretion. Sleep. 2007;30(7):923–9.

37. Buysse DJ, Reynolds CF, Monk TH, Berman SR, Kupfer DJ. The Pittsburgh Sleep Quality Index (PSQI): a new instrument for psychiatric research and practice. Psychiatry Res. 1989;28(2):193–213.

38. Yurtkuran M, Alp A, Yurtkuran M, Dilek K. A modified yoga-based exercise program in hemodialysis patients: a randomized controlled study. Complement Ther Med. 2007;15(3):164–71.

39. Wizemann V, Wabel P, Chamney P, et al. The mortality risk of overhydration in haemodialysis patients. Nephrol Dial Transplant. 2009;24(5):1574–9.

40. Chazot C. Can chronic volume overload be recognized and prevented in hemodialysis patients? Use of a restricted-salt diet. Semin Dial. 2009;22(5):482–6.

41. Ozkahya M, Toz H, Unsal A, et al. Treatment of hypertension in dialysis patients by ultrafiltration: role of cardiac dilatation and time factor. Am J Kidney Dis. 1999;34(2):218–21.

42. Dong J, Li Y, Yang Z, Luo J. Low dietary sodium intake increases the death risk in peritoneal dialysis. Clin J Am Soc Nephrol. 2010;5(2):240–7.

43. Kovesdy CP, Regidor DL, Mehrotra R, et al. Serum and dialysate potassium concentrations and survival in hemodialysis patients. Clin J Am Soc Nephrol. 2007;2(5):999–1007.

44. Curtis CJ, Niederman SA, Kansagra SM. Availability of potassium on the nutrition facts panel of US packaged foods. JAMA Intern Med. 2013;173(9):828–9.

45. Sherman RA, Mehta O. Potassium in food additives: something else to consider. J Ren Nutr. 2009;19(6):441–2.

46. Cupisti A, Gallieni M, Rizzo MA, Caria S, Meola M, Bolasco P. Phosphate control in dialysis. Int J Nephrol Renovasc Dis. 2013;6:193–205.

47. Kestenbaum B, Sampson JN, Rudser KD, et al. Serum phosphate levels and mortality risk among people with chronic kidney disease. J Am Soc Nephrol. 2005;16(2):520–8.

48. Sullivan C, Sayre SS, Leon JB, et al. Effect of food additives on hyperphosphatemia among patients with end-stage renal disease: a randomized controlled trial. JAMA. 2009;301(6):629–35.

49. Bohn L, Meyer AS, Rasmussen SK. Phytate: impact on environment and human nutrition. A challenge for molecular breeding. J Zhejiang Univ Sci B. 2008;9(3):165–91.

50. Cupisti A, Morelli E, D'Alessandro C, Lupetti S, Barsotti G. Phosphate control in chronic uremia: don't forget diet. J Nephrol. 2003;16(1):29–33.

51. Huang X, Stenvinkel P, Qureshi AR, et al. Clinical determinants and mortality predictability of stearoyl-CoA desaturase-1 activity indices in dialysis patients. J Intern Med. 2013;273(3):263–72.

52. Friedman AN, Yu Z, Tabbey R, et al. Inverse relationship between long-chain n-3 fatty acids and risk of sudden cardiac death in patients starting hemodialysis. Kidney Int. 2013;83(6):1130–5.

53. Liebman SE, Lamontagne SP, Huang LS, Messing S, Bushinsky DA. Smoking in dialysis patients: a systematic review and meta-analysis of mortality and cardiovascular morbidity. Am J Kidney Dis. 2011;58(2):257–65.

Nonalcoholic Fatty Liver Disease and Steatohepatitis

29

Erin M. McCarthy and Mary E. Rinella

Abbreviations

AA	Arachidonic acid
ACSM	American College of Sports Medicine
AGB	Adjustable gastric band
ALA	α-linolenic acid
ALB	Albumin
ALKPHOS	Alkaline phosphatase
ALT	Alanine aminotransferase
AST	Aspartate aminotransferase
BMI	Body Mass Index
CAD	Coronary artery disease
CBT	Cognitive behavioral therapy
CHD	Coronary heart disease
CHO	Carbohydrates
CVD	Cardiovascular disease
DHA	Docosahexaenoic acid
DNL	De novo lipogenesis
EPA	Eicosapentaenoic acid
FA	Fatty acid
GI	Gastrointestinal
HCC	Hepatocellular carcinoma
HDL	High-density lipoprotein
HFCS	High-fructose corn syrup
IL-6	Interleukin-6
IHS	Isolated hepatic steatosis
LA	Linoleic acid
LDL-cholesterol	Low-density lipoprotein cholesterol
MUFA	Monounsaturated fatty acid
NAFLD	Nonalcoholic Fatty Liver Disease
NASH	Nonalcoholic steatohepatitis
NHANES	National Health and Nutrition Examination Survey
PUFA	Polyunsaturated fatty acid
RYGB	Roux-en-y gastric bypass
SFAs	Saturated fatty acids
TBILI	Total bilirubin
TGs	Triglycerides
TNF-α	Tumor necrosis factor alpha
VAT	Visceral adipose tissue
VLDL	Very low-density lipoprotein
VSG	Vertical sleeve gastrectomy
WHO	World Health Organization

M. E. Rinella (✉)
Department of Gastroenterology and Hepatology, Northwestern University Feinberg School of Medicine, 676 N. St. Clair, Arkes 14-005, Chicago, IL 60611, USA
e-mail: m-rinella@northwestern.edu

E. M. McCarthy
Center for Lifestyle Medicine, Northwestern Medicine, Chicago, IL, USA

Nonalcoholic Fatty Liver Disease (NAFLD): Impact on Public Health

NAFLD is the most common chronic liver disease in developed countries, affecting up to 30% of the adult population. Individuals with metabolic risk factors, particularly, the presence of obesity, insulin resistance, and diabetes, have a high prevalence of NAFLD estimated up to 80% and greater than 90% in patients with class III (body mass index, BMI ≥ 40 kg/m^2) obesity. NAFLD is characterized by the accumulation of lipids within hepatocytes that occurs in patients who do not abuse alcohol. It encompasses a spectrum that includes isolated hepatic steatosis (IHS), and when accompanied by inflammation and liver injury, it is referred to as nonalcoholic steatohepatitis (NASH). This distinction is important because NASH is much more likely than IHS to develop into cirrhosis (up to 30 vs. 3%, respectively), and its complications include liver failure and hepatocellular carcinoma (HCC). In contrast to the earlier held belief that NAFLD was a fairly benign condition, individuals with NAFLD and particularly NASH are actually at a higher risk for all-cause mortality. Death from cardiovascular disease (CVD) is the most common followed by malignancy and liver disease [1].

The apparent increase in cardiovascular risk in patients with NAFLD is in part mediated by common risk factors

© Springer International Publishing Switzerland 2016
J. I. Mechanick, R. F. Kushner (eds.), *Lifestyle Medicine*, DOI 10.1007/978-3-319-24687-1_29

Table 29.1 Risk factors associated with nonalcoholic fatty liver disease (NAFLD)

Major risk factors	Conditions with emerging association	Lifestyle risk factors
Abdominal obesity	Hypothyroidism	Physical inactivity
Insulin resistance[a]	Obstructive sleep apnea	Caloric excess
Type-2 diabetes	Hypopituitarism	Weight gain
Hypertriglyceridemia[a]	Hypogonadism	Carbohydrate-rich, high-sugar, high-fat diets
Older age	Polycystic ovary syndrome[b]	
Hypertension	Family history of diabetes	
	High-risk ethnic groups	
	Sex and menopausal status	

[a] Metabolic syndrome components include insulin resistance, obesity, hypertension, hypertriglyceridemia, and depressed high-density lipoprotein (HDL)-cholesterol
[b] It is unclear if this association extends beyond the common risk factor of insulin resistance

such as diabetes, insulin resistance, hypertension, dyslipidemia, obstructive sleep apnea, and others (Table 29.1). An in-depth discussion of this association is beyond the scope of this chapter and has been recently reviewed [2].

Visceral adipose tissue (VAT) is prominent, dysfunctional, and active in NASH. Increases in VAT contribute to a pro-inflammatory milieu through increased secretion of adipocytokines such as tumor necrosis factor alpha (TNF-α) and interleukin-6 (IL-6) and reduced secretion of adiponectin, which worsens insulin resistance and systemic inflammation. The pro-inflammatory signals, which stem from VAT lead to liver injury and the accumulation of fat within the liver. Because obesity is such an important factor in NAFLD and its associated comorbidities, weight loss is the cornerstone of any treatment approach.

Risk Factors and Disease Associations

How Does Obesity Promote Liver Injury in NAFLD and NASH?

Obesity, combined with host factors such as diet, sedentary lifestyle, and genetic predisposition, has been directly associated with increases in the prevalence of insulin resistance, type-2 diabetes, metabolic syndrome, and NAFLD. Obesity itself represents a chronic, inflammatory condition resulting from an imbalance of the normal homeostatic regulation of energy intake, storage, and utilization. In the setting of obesity, particularly central obesity, there is an expansion of the VAT compartment, which has profound effects on insulin resistance and systemic inflammation. The liver plays an important role in glucose and lipid metabolism as well as in the control of energy balance and body weight.

Energy balance is a major factor in liver fat accumulation. Although the liver is not meant to store fat, caloric excess and unmatched caloric expenditure can result in fat accumulation in the liver. While data are limited, some studies suggest that patients with NASH have increased caloric intake than healthy controls. Furthermore, overfeeding studies have shown that an increased intake of fat, glucose, or fructose can increase liver fat in young, healthy individuals [3].

Weight gain of more than 2 kg can result in elevated liver enzymes and the development of NAFLD after adjustment for age, gender, and baseline BMI [4]. The degree of weight gain also appears to be important with more significant weight gain associated with increased likelihood of developing NAFLD (Fig. 29.1).

Lean NAFLD

While most patients with NAFLD are obese, there is a subset of patients who are not. Lean patients with NASH can have the full spectrum of disease, including cirrhosis. The extent of excess abdominal fat required to produce a pro-inflammatory milieu is not known, though there are established differences in susceptibility to lesser degrees of obesity across ethnic groups. Adipose tissue insulin resistance is associated with increased liver fat content independent of obesity in humans. Weight gain even in nonobese subjects and the development of metabolic risk factors in lean individuals promotes the development of NAFLD [5]. Regardless of BMI, weight gain is a significant predictor of incident NAFLD.

Thresholds of lean individuals with "metabolic obesity" vary with different ethnic groups, and genetic background is associated with the development of NAFLD in nonobese (but often overweight) subjects. In the Dallas Heart Study, the prevalence of hepatic steatosis was 45% in Hispanics, 33% in non-Hispanic Caucasians, and 24% in African-Americans [6]. In US populations with a BMI below 25 kg/m², Hispanic origin correlates with the presence of NAFLD. In Asian populations (WHO-defined BMI categories for public health action in Asians: normal weight (18.5 to <23.0), moderate risk or overweight (23.0 to <27.5), and high risk or obese (≥27.5)) [7], despite a historically lower prevalence of metabolic risk factors and NAFLD, the incidence of NASH has increased dramatically and the prevalence of the disease is growing rapidly in this population [8]. Despite not having obesity as classified by BMI cutoffs for Caucasians (≥30 kg/m²), Asian individuals (≥27.5 kg/m²) often have central (visceral) adiposity, predisposing them to metabolic syndrome and insulin resistance [9]. Studies from Hong Kong Chinese

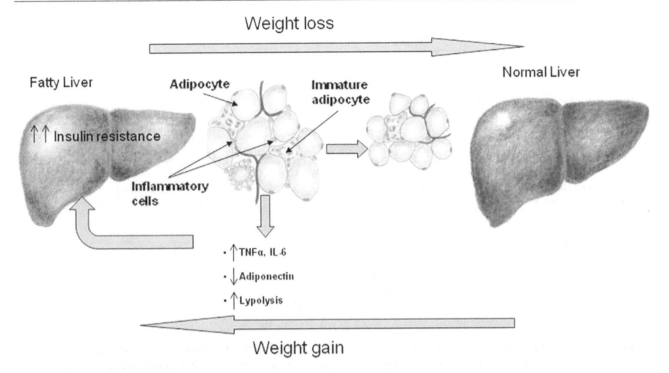

Fig. 29.1 Alterations in adipose and hepatic tissue related to weight change. Adipose tissue undergoes significant transformation during weight gain that is characterized by adipocyte hypertrophy and infiltration by macrophages. These changes lead to adipocyte apoptosis and secretion of proinflammatory cytokines. This chronic inflammatory state then promotes insulin resistance. Alternately, weight loss produces decreased fatty acid delivery and uptake in the liver and reduces intrahepatic triglyceride stores. In addition, weight loss reduces visceral adipose tissue (VAT) mass and thus reduces peripheral and hepatic insulin resistance via improved suppression of lipolysis and a reduction in the pro-inflammatory adipocytokine signal. *TNF-α* tumor necrosis factor alpha, *IL-6* interleukin-6, *MCP-1* monocyte chemoattractant protein-1. (Reprinted from Journal of the Academy of Nutrition and Dietetics, 112(3), McCarthy, E, The Role of Diet and Nutrient Composition in Nonalcoholic Fatty Liver Disease, 401-9, Copyright (2012), with permission from Elsevier)

and Asian Indians show that the odds ratio of clustering metabolic risk factors starts to increase at a BMI of about 23 kg/m^2 [9, 10]. Hence, there are different definition criteria for the diagnosis of metabolic syndrome among different ethnicities.

Sedentary Time/Inactivity

Patients with NAFLD generally engage in less than one half the amount of exercise performed by age- and sex-matched controls, with less than 80% not meeting current recommendations for physical activity (150 min or more of moderate-intensity physical activity per week) [11]. Globally in 2008, 31% of adults were insufficiently active (men 28% and women 34%). Decreased physical activity correlates with increased amounts of intrahepatic fat, decreased insulin sensitivity, and increased abdominal fat [12]. Furthermore, the amount of time patients are sedentary predicts higher levels of fasting insulin, independent of moderate- or vigorous-intensity activity. Low aerobic capacity is a stronger predictor of CVD and mortality compared with other risk factors. Individuals with biopsy-proven NAFLD who did not meet vigorous activity exercise guidelines of

≥75 min/week had greater odds of having NASH. Those who did not meet the guideline of moderate-intensity exercise of ≥150 min/week had an increased odds of having fibrosis, which suggests an increased risk of future cirrhosis [13].

Impact of Lifestyle Intervention

Promoting weight loss through lifestyle intervention is the cornerstone of treatment of NAFLD/NASH. The benefits of weight loss are clear; however, there are insufficient data to recommend a particular dietary approach or exercise prescription that would offer the optimal benefit to patients with NAFLD.

Energy expenditure exceeding intake promotes the use of energy stores. This can result in decreased fatty acid delivery and uptake in addition to increased beta-oxidation in the liver, hence reducing intrahepatic triglycerides (TGs). Moreover, weight loss reduces VAT mass and thus reduces peripheral and hepatic insulin resistance via the suppression of lipolysis and a reduction in pro-inflammatory adipocytokine signals. The extent of weight loss directly correlates with the degree of hepatic fat reduction, severity of NAFLD, and

Table 29.2 Recommended lifestyle intervention for patients with NAFLD and NASH

Dietary Recommendation	Include	Avoid
1. Weight loss ≥7–10% of initial body weight Maintain weight loss	Count calories daily 1200–1500 kcal/day <250 lb 1500–1800 kcal/day >250 lb	Weight gain High-calorie foods
2. Dietary restriction of calories (500–1000 kcal/day)		Empty calories
3. Low carbohydrate diet (<40–45%)	Vegetables (3–5 servings/day) Fruits (2–4 servings/day)	Simple carbohydrates, high-sugar foods
4. Replace calories with PUFA, MUFA	Nuts, avocado, olives Oily fish (salmon, tuna, mackerel, sardines)	Butter, margarine, cream sauces, and cream dressings
5. Avoid *trans* FA, limit saturated fats (7–10%)	Olive oil, olives	Fast food, fried foods
6. Consume zero-calorie beverages	Water is best	Sugar-sweetened beverages
	Wine (≤1 glass/day)	
	Coffee 1–2 cups/day	
7. Increase physical activity	Cardiovascular 5×/week Resistance training ≥2×/week 150–300 min/week at moderate or 75–150 min/week at vigorous intensity	Sedentary lifestyle

PUFA polyunsaturated fatty acid, *MUFA* monounsaturated fatty acid, *FA* fatty acid

need not be extreme (as little as 3–5%) to improve hepatic steatosis and liver enzymes [14]. However, more significant degrees of weight loss (7–10%) may be needed to improve necroinflammation, steatosis, lobular inflammation, and NAFLD activity scores [15, 16].

Bariatric surgery is the most effective therapy for obesity with significant weight loss and weight loss maintenance. The average weight loss is 40% for roux-en-y gastric bypass (RYGB), 35% for vertical sleeve gastrectomy (VSG), and 20% for adjustable gastric band (AGB). Bariatric surgery is an option in individuals with NAFLD and/or who have co-morbid conditions in addition to NASH. A comprehensive review discussing NAFLD/NASH and bariatric surgery is referenced here [17]. However, no randomized controlled trials have examined bariatric surgery as a treatment option for NAFLD or NASH. Results from several uncontrolled and small controlled studies indicate that weight loss (average 30% reduction in BMI and/or 60% excess weight loss) achieved through bariatric surgery reduces liver enzymes and improves NAFLD [18].

Weight loss is an effective treatment to improve the histology of NASH, provided sufficient weight reduction can be achieved and sustained. However, sufficient weight loss is difficult to achieve in most patients. In practical terms, patients should be assigned a calorie goal based on their starting weight: 1200–1500 calories per day (kcal/day) if the baseline weight is less than 250 pounds (lb) or 1500–1800 kcal/day if the baseline weight greater than 250 lb. These calorie goals have traditionally produced weight losses of 0.5–1.0 kg/week and 7–10% weight reduction from initial body weight [19].

Extreme and rapid weight loss should be avoided since it can result in hepatic decompensation, particularly if the patient has more advanced underlying liver disease, which is frequently under-recognized. Patients should be encouraged to make sustainable changes to their diets that will result in weight loss over the long term rather than embarking on a dramatically different diet they cannot maintain. Specific nutritional changes beyond weight loss are discussed below and reviewed in Table 29.2.

Metabolic Effects of Macronutrients with NAFLD

Carbohydrate Metabolism

Fatty acids accumulate in hepatocytes from multiple sources. In patients with NAFLD, the majority of hepatic TGs come from peripheral lipolysis; however, compared to control subjects, de novo lipogenesis (DNL) is also upregulated [20]. Carbohydrates are an important substrate for DNL, typically accounting for about 5% of the total fatty acid flux to the liver in healthy patients and approximately 10% in obese, hyperinsulinemic patients. However, in patients with NAFLD, the contribution of carbohydrates may contribute up to 25% of the substrate for DNL and therefore play a major role in hepatic lipid accumulation in NAFLD. Foods contain a variety of carbohydrates ranging from simple monosaccharides to disaccharides to large polymers of glucose that have differing rates of absorption and impact on hepatic lipid metabolism. Therefore, it is not just the quantity but also the type of carbohydrate ingested that may have differential effects on hepatic lipid accumulation in patients with NAFLD.

Fructose Metabolism in Fatty Liver

Distinctions between the metabolism of fructose and glucose may explain how excessive fructose consumption could

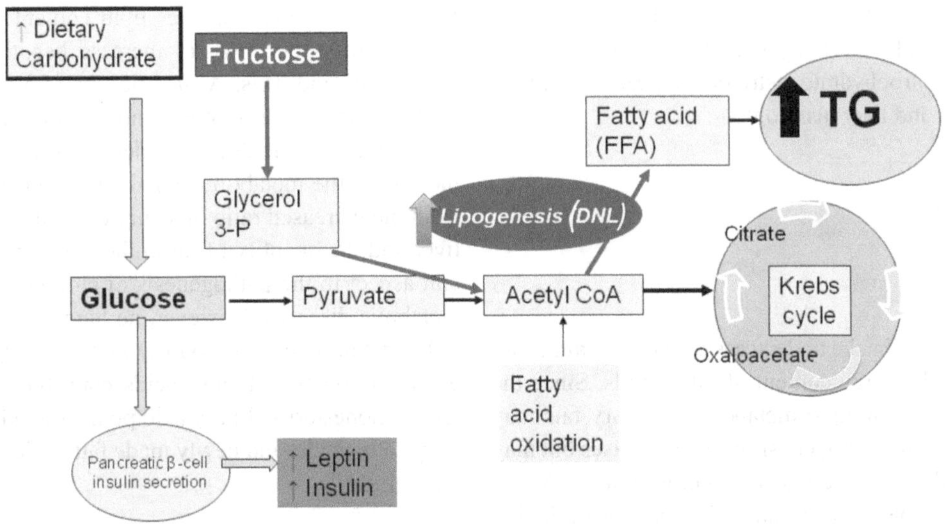

Fig. 29.2 Fates of glucose and fructose delivered to the liver and their introduction into the pathway of de novo lipogenesis (DNL). Of key importance is the ability of fructose to bypass the main regulatory step of glycolysis, the conversion of glucose-6-phosphate to fructose 1,6-bisphosphate, controlled by phosphofructokinase. While glucose metabolism is negatively regulated by phosphofructokinase, fructose can continuously enter the glycolytic pathway. Therefore, fructose can uncontrollably produce glucose, glycogen, lactate, and pyruvate. Unregulated fructose metabolism will promote the overproduction of triglycerides (TGs). The variations observed in gastrointestinal (GI) and appetite control of glucose and fructose can also be explained by differences in stimulation of insulin and leptin, important players in the long-term regulation of energy homeostasis. Fructose produces smaller insulin excursions upon consumption because it does not stimulate the secretion of insulin from pancreatic beta(β) cells, whereas glucose does. Insulin-regulated leptin will also have a reduced concentration and decreased effect on reducing appetite

have an adverse effect on the liver (Fig. 29.2). Energy appears to be central to any effect of fructose on body weight in controlled feeding trials. Sugar-sweetened beverage consumption correlates with the presence of metabolic syndrome. A high-fructose diet result in increase in intrahepatic fat [21, 22]. Daily fructose consumption ($\geq$7 servings/week), after adjustment for total caloric intake, was associated with a lower steatosis grade but a higher fibrosis stage as well as increased hepatic inflammation and injury in older subjects [23]. Fructose-sweetened beverages providing 25% of energy requirements (55% carbohydrate [CHO] total) produced dyslipidemia, insulin resistance, hepatic DNL, and an increase in postprandial TG when compared with glucose-sweetened beverages [24]. In hypercaloric trials, fructose-sweetened beverages have been associated with elevation in alanine aminotransferase (ALT) and intrahepatic lipids. However, data are inconsistent in hypercaloric trials. Isocaloric trials in which fructose are exchanged for glucose as beverages under energy-matched conditions have failed to show an effect [25–27]. In a systematic review, fructose intake and glucose intake had similar effects on liver fat and liver enzymes in healthy adults [28]. Comparing four equally hypocaloric diets containing different levels of sucrose or high-fructose corn syrup (HFCS) demonstrated reductions in all measures of adiposity and weight regardless of the type of sweetener [29]. In summary, the independent effects of fructose on the development and progression of NAFLD need to be further clarified.

Low-Carbohydrate Diets

Excess intake of refined carbohydrates (CHO) is associated with insulin resistance and obesity. Patients on low-carbohydrate diets produce more glucose from lactate or amino acids than those on low-calorie diets and derive less of their glucose from glycogen. Furthermore, a low-carbohydrate diet can favor the use of intrahepatic fat as substrate for energy rather than utilizing glycogen stores [30]. Therefore, low-CHO (40–45% CHO) hypocaloric diets in the short term reduce intrahepatic TG content, increase hepatic insulin sensitivity, improve liver histology, and decrease endogenous glucose production, in addition to promoting weight loss [31]. Compared to low-fat diets, low-CHO diets result in greater short-term (<6 months) weight loss, but both diets have similar long-term (>1 year) weight loss benefits [32]. While biochemically one could hypothesize that different types of carbohydrates would have differential effects on plasma lipids and NAFLD, longitudinal trials have failed to show differences in blood lipids or liver enzymes between a high-sugar diet and high-complex CHO diet [33]. However, given the observational nature of some of these studies, extrapolating the effects of differences in dietary macronutrient content is difficult as there could be many confounders—dietary and other. In an important proof of concept study by Browning et al. [34], patients were fed either a calorie-restricted (~1325 kcal/day, 50% CHO) or a carbohydrate-restricted diet (1550 kcal/day, ~20 g CHO/day or 8% CHO). Despite an intake of 200 cal more in the CHO-restricted group, both groups had a 4% weight loss, but the low carbohydrate group had a more significant reduction in hepatic fat [34]. Overall, carbohydrate restriction appears to improve intrahepatic TGs and liver histology.

Fat Metabolism

Low-Fat Diets

The link between fat intake and excessive weight gain is not limited to the high-energy content of fatty foods. Since the liver plays a key role in lipid metabolism, dietary fats may not only influence the pathogenesis of liver diseases but may also prevent and/or reverse disease manifestations. A few small human trials have noted that a high-fat isocaloric diet (60% of total calories) for at least 2 weeks increases liver fat by 35% [35]. However, well-controlled studies showed that when total fat intake ranges between 20–40% of the total energy intake, no major effect is observed on insulin sensitivity or body weight [36, 37]. A direct relationship between dietary fat and energy density has been questioned because many low-fat foods and diets displace fat with carbohydrates (often refined), leading to energy density values similar to those of their high-fat counterparts.

Monounsaturated Fatty Acids

Common MUFAs are palmitoleic acid (16:1 ω-7), cis-vaccenic acid (18:1 ω-7), and oleic acid (18:1 ω-9). The principal fatty acid esters present in a normal liver are palmitoleic acid (16:0, ω-7) and oleic acid (18:1, ω-9). Examples of foods high in MUFA include vegetable oils such as olive oil, canola oil, peanut oil, sunflower oil, and sesame oil. Other sources include avocados, peanut butter as well as many nuts and seeds.

An increase in MUFA intake, especially as a replacement for saturated fatty acids (SFAs), may offset the pro-inflammatory effects of SFA, decrease hepatic steatosis, and reduce insulin resistance. In individuals with diabetes, a high-fat diet (40% total fat, 40% CHO) with approximately 25% of the energy from MUFA, resulted in lower hepatic fat, plasma total cholesterol, very low-density lipoprotein (VLDL), and TG levels than did a low-fat, high-carbohydrate (~55% CHO, 30% fat) diet [38]. A meta-analysis suggests that a higher MUFA intake is associated with greater HDL and lower TGs as well as improved glycemic control in patients with diabetes [39]. Although data on MUFA are promising, no specific dietary recommendations have been determined for MUFA in patients with NAFLD.

Diets Low in SFAs

Greater than 10% of total energy from SFAs can contribute to insulin resistance, increase oxidative stress, decrease fatty acid oxidation, and potentially promote NASH [40].

Saturated fats increase liver lipid content as these dietary components are known to increase hepatic production of cholesterol and TGs. A diet rich in SFAs can cause liver dysfunction by promoting endoplasmic reticulum stress and apoptosis. The degree of desaturation of the fatty acids modulates the metabolic signaling and energy metabolism. Both the increased ratio of saturated to unsaturated fat in the liver and the quantity of fat in the liver represent an important aspect in the pathogenesis of chronic liver disease and metabolic diseases. However, no human studies have made a direct link between NAFLD and diets high in SFA. The potential sources of fatty acids contributing to fatty liver are the nonesterified fatty acid pool from adipose tissue, dietary fatty acids, and newly made fatty acids within the liver through DNL.

Polyunsaturated Fatty Acids

The two main families of polyunsaturated fatty acids (PUFAs) include omega (ω)-3 PUFA and omega (ω)-6 PUFA. ω-3 PUFA thought to promote increased fatty acid oxidation and reduced DNL includes the essential fatty acid, α-linolenic acid (ALA), which can be further metabolized to eicosapentaenoic acid (EPA) and docosahexaenoic acid (DHA). The ω-6 PUFA family comprises the essential fatty acid, linoleic acid (LA), and its primary metabolite, arachidonic acid (AA), which have more of a pro-inflammatory effect. Patients with NASH may have an imbalance in the increased ω-6:ω-3 ratio contributing to a pro-inflammatory state. PUFAs have positive effects on intrahepatic fat accumulation in patients with NAFLD [41]. Clinical trials have shown that the replacement of SFA and *trans* fatty acids with dietary PUFA reduces the incidence of coronary artery disease (CAD; [42]).

Omega-3 Fatty Acids

Low amounts of ω-3 PUFAs (eicosapentaenoic acid (C20:5ω3, EPA) and docosahexaenoic acid (C22:6ω3, DHA) are associated with an increase in oxidative stress, a decrease in fatty acid oxidation, and depletion of PUFA in the liver. ω-3 PUFAs are mostly produced in the liver under physiological conditions, therefore alterations in their metabolism during NAFLD could be both a consequence of reduced ω-3 intake and reduced ω-3 bioavailability.

Fish oil supplementation improves insulin sensitivity, decreases intrahepatic TGs, and increases adiponectin concentrations in the circulation and VAT in both animals and humans [43]. Consuming fatty fish rich in ω-3 PUFAs at least twice a week remains a key strategy for diabetes management and cardiovascular benefits. However, there is controversy over ω-3 supplementation because it has not been proven to induce any change in insulin sensitivity [44, 45].

In a systematic literature review of randomized control trials, six of the eight trials showed that PUFA supplementation significantly reduced hepatic fat but had no significant benefit on liver enzymes [46]. In NASH patients with diabetes who were fed an isocaloric diet, supplementation with PUFA's EPA (2.1 g) and DHA (1.4 g) did not improve liver enzymes or hepatic steatosis, while insulin resistance worsened [45]. Despite a strong theoretical rationale, a well-powered double-blind placebo-controlled trial of high- and low-dose EPA in patients with NASH failed to show benefit in liver enzymes, histology, or insulin resistance [47]. In summary, there is no evidence that ω-3 fatty acid supplements are beneficial in human NASH, therefore fish oil supplements are not specifically recommended as a therapy for NAFLD.

Omega-6 PUFAs

The ω-6 PUFAs include LA which can be found in vegetable oils such as soybean, safflower, maize, and rapeseed oils. Another ω-6 PUFA provided by the diet is AA, which can be found in meats, poultry, and eggs. Individuals with NASH have lower ω-6 ratios compared with healthy controls, a trend driven mainly by the change in AA levels [48]. The decrease in hepatic AA observed in NASH patients as well as a decreased EPA/AA ratio in NAFLD patients can be a possible link between NAFLD and CVD.

An ω-6 PUFA-rich diet (particularly linoleic) is associated with decreased risk of coronary heart disease (CHD; [49]). In one study, replacement of 10% of calories from SFA with ω-6 PUFA reduces the ratio of total cholesterol to high-density lipoprotein (HDL)-cholesterol to a greater extent than that observed with similar replacement with carbohydrate [49]. Based on lack of data, no conclusions can be made regarding whether increased ω-6 PUFA consumption, above the currently recommended levels (5–10% of energy), should be recommended in NAFLD patients [49, 50].

Protein Metabolism

While by a distinct mechanism than obesity, protein calorie malnutrition can result in hepatic steatosis. Available evidence suggests that whey protein and soy protein could prevent or ameliorate fatty liver, but these studies are exclusively limited to animals [51]. While there are theoretical benefits to a high-protein diets and limited animal data in fatty liver, recommendations regarding dietary protein as a disease modifier in NAFLD cannot be made at this time.

Other Dietary Factors Impacting NAFLD/NASH

Alcohol

CVD is the most common cause of death in patients with NAFLD. Landmark papers have shown that moderate wine consumption decreases metabolic risk factors as well as all-cause and cardiac mortality [52]. However, alcohol is a known hepatotoxin that is known to contribute to the burden of liver disease. A mounting body of evidence suggests that modest alcohol intake may not be harmful for patients with NAFLD or NASH and may even be protective. National Health and Nutrition Examination Survey (NHANES) indicated participants who consumed up to 10 g of wine (equivalent to one standard drink or about 100 ml) per day were half as likely to meet criteria for NAFLD. A meta-analysis of approximately 43,000 individuals determined that modest alcohol consumption is associated with a significant protective effect of 31% on the risk of having NAFLD and protection from NASH in patients with available histology [53]. Cross-sectional analyses have associated moderate alcohol consumption (≤20 g/d) with a reduction in liver steatosis (ultrasound) and NASH risk (biopsy). Despite these provocative results, it is too early to encourage moderate drinking in patients with NAFLD; however, a discussion of risks and potential benefits in selected patients is appropriate. In the setting of advanced NASH or NASH cirrhosis, complete abstinence should be stressed due to the risk of hepatic decompensation and risk of hepatocellular cancer potentiated by alcohol [54].

Coffee

Coffee consumption is associated with a reduction in NAFLD and liver fibrosis. Studies have linked coffee consumption with decreased hepatic fibrosis in patients with chronic liver disease, especially hepatitis C and HCC [55]. Coffee intake is inversely associated with advanced fibrosis among NAFLD patients with lower degrees of insulin resistance [56]. Aside from fibrosis, daily coffee consumption did not affect any of the other histologic features associated with NASH [57]. It is unclear which of the 1000+ substances in coffee could be beneficial; however, it does not appear to be correlated to the amount of caffeine. Moderate daily unsweetened coffee may be considered a reasonable adjunct to patients with NAFLD due to its low risk and potential benefit [58].

Vitamin E

An important study showed that therapy with vitamin E (rrr-alpha tocopherol) at 800 IU per day in patients with NASH resulted in histological improvement in a greater number of patients compared to placebo [59]. However, the study was limited to nondiabetic patients and therefore the conclusion cannot be extrapolated to patients with diabetes. In addition, there are concerns (albeit controversial) regarding the long-term safety of vitamin E given reports that it may increase all-cause mortality [60, 61]. Furthermore, treatment with vitamin E may be associated with an increased risk of developing prostate cancer as suggested by a recent trial of approximately 35,000 men [62]. There are insufficient data to recommend vitamin E for NASH patients with concomitant diabetes or cirrhosis. Importantly, there is no evidence that Vitamin E improves fibrosis, which may be the most relevant histological endpoint.

Physical Activity

General Statements

Exercise enhances insulin sensitivity, reduces the progression to type-2 diabetes, maintains weight loss, reduces visceral fat, improves measures of cardiac output and VO_{2max}, and favorably modifies the lipid profile independent of weight loss. Improvement in insulin sensitivity correlates with a reduction in total body fat, especially in visceral adiposity, which in turn reduces free fatty acid delivery to the liver. Regular physical activity may reduce hepatic fat content through several different mechanisms, including increased hepatic and muscle fatty acid oxidation, reduced postprandial hepatic lipogenesis, reduced fatty acid flux, and a reduction in pro-inflammatory signaling. Furthermore, increased lean mass (fat-free mass) increases glucose uptake, thus providing another mechanism by which exercise could protect against the development of fatty liver. However, to date only a few intervention studies have assessed the effect of exercise, either alone or in combination with diet, on hepatic fat content [16, 63]. Moreover, most of these studies included a combination of exercise and caloric restriction, making it difficult to independently assess the role of exercise.

Aerobic Versus Resistance Training

Regular increased aerobic exercise improves the metabolic parameters associated with NAFLD. Aerobic exercise reduces the relative risk of NAFLD and hepatic TG content by 21–35% [64]. Regular aerobic exercise >3 times/week for ≥30 min/session for 1–3 months reduced the risk of NAFLD, liver fat, and decreased liver enzymes in patients with NAFLD independent of obesity [65]. Endurance training (4×/week for 40 min) reduces waist circumference and blood pressure and increases HDL-cholesterol in patients with CVD which is relevant to NAFLD since CVD is the most common cause of morbidity and mortality in these patients [66].

Resistance exercise 2–3×/week for 8–12 weeks reduces liver fat independent of weight loss [67, 68]. Aerobic exercise is considered the treatment of choice, but resistance training can improve hepatic insulin resistance and decrease visceral fat regardless of weight loss.

Intensity and Duration of Exercise

Aerobic training for 30 min daily at 60–70% VO_{2max} improves insulin sensitivity, TGs, and liver enzymes. Moderate to vigorous activity of at least 150 min/week decreased the odds of developing fatty liver by 49% [69]. Vigorous activity and doubling the duration of vigorous exercise was associated with decreasing the odds of developing NASH. Patients who increased their physical activity by 60 min or more per week significantly reduced their weight and liver enzymes independent of body weight [70].

At this time, there is no consensus on the specific exercise prescriptions with regard to frequency, duration, intensity, or combination with resistance training in the NAFLD/NASH population. The World Health Organization (WHO) and American College of Sports Medicine (ACSM) recommend at least five sessions of physical activity for at least 150 min of moderate activity (but preferably 300 min) or 75 min of vigorous activity (but preferably 150 min) per week to achieve health benefits (see ACSM and WHO exercise guidelines; [71, 72]).

Behavior Therapy

Cognitive behavioral therapy (CBT) has been used in most of the interventions for weight loss. This therapy changes behaviors and cognitive processes, which underlie dietary habits in order to increase adherence to the intervention. The CBT approach produces an average weight loss of 0.5–1.0 kg/week, to a total weight loss of 8–10% with drop-out rates less than 20% [73]. Behavioral intervention in addition to weight loss and exercise results in improvement in liver enzymes [74]. The Diabetes Prevention Program [75] and the Look AHEAD study [76] compared CBT with standard nutritional treatment in NASH [15]. In a subgroup of the Look AHEAD cohort, participants in the lifestyle group lost more weight and had a larger decrease in percent liver fat [16]. At 12 months, 3% of subjects in the intensive lifestyle group developed fatty liver, compared with 26% in the controls [16]. Three areas of intervention (biological, cognitive, and environmental) have been proposed to improve the long-term maintenance of lifestyle modification [4]. A review using behavioral therapy for NAFLD recommends that unstructured exercise and self-monitoring programs be used to improve compliance.

Case Study

A 42-year-old Hispanic male was seen for evaluation of right upper quadrant pain of 6 months duration. He had obesity, class 1, with a BMI of 32 kg/m^2. Past medical history is no-

Table 29.3 Case study hepatic panel

Lab results

Component	Value	Reference range
ALB	4.7 g/dL	3.5–5.7 g/dL
ALT	62 unit/L	0–52 unit/L
AST	42 unit/L	0–39 unit/L
TBILI	0.6 mg/dL	0.3–1.9 mg/dL
ALKPHOS	49 units/L	30–115 units/L
Cholesterol	171 mg/dL	<200 mg/dL
LDL-cholesterol	107 mg/dL	<100 mg/dL
Glucose	96 mg/dL	<100 mg/dL

LDL-cholesterol low-density lipoprotein cholesterol, *ALB* albumin, *ALT* alanine aminotransferase, *AST* aspartate aminotransferase, *TBILI* total bilirubin, *ALKPHOS* alkaline phosphatase

Table 29.4 Case study risk factors for metabolic syndrome. (Weight: 230 lbs (104.5 kg), height: 5 ft 11 in. (71 in.))

Risk factor	Patient level	Defining level
Abdominal obesity	Waist circumference 41 in. (104 cm)	Men >102 cm[a] Women >88 cm
Triglycerides	171 mg/dL	<150 mg/dL
HDL-cholesterol	n/a	Men <40 mg/dl Women <50 mg/dl
Hemoglobin A1c	5.1%	5.7–6.4% pre-diabetes ≥6.5 diabetes

HDL-cholesterol high-density lipoprotein cholesterol

[a] 84 and 74 cm for males and females, respectively (Asian population)

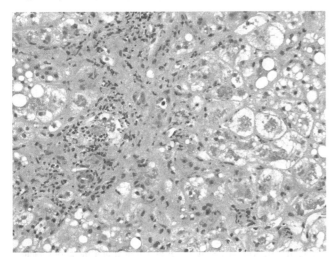

Fig. 29.3 A diagnosis of nonalcoholic steatohepatitis (NASH) was confirmed by liver biopsy which showed hepatic steatosis and liver injury (cellular ballooning and inflammation)

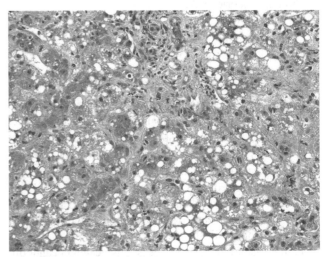

Fig. 29.4 A diagnosis of nonalcoholic steatohepatitis (NASH) was confirmed by liver biopsy and showed pericellular fibrosis

table for a mixed hyperlipidemia, but no evidence of diabetes or impaired fasting glucose.

Physical examination and laboratory analysis revealed hepatomegaly with an increased serum alanine aminotransferase concentration (55 U/L; Table 29.3). Obesity distribution (mid-circumference obesity), acanthosis nigricans, and adorso-cervical hump were noted on exam (Table 29.4). Serologic evaluation excluded the presence of other forms of liver disease, including viral and autoimmune etiologies, and the patient did not consume alcohol.

A diagnosis of NASH was confirmed by liver biopsy which showed hepatic steatosis and liver injury (cellular ballooning and inflammation; Fig. 29.3) in addition to pericellular fibrosis (Fig. 29.4).

Dietary Recall

Breakfast 6 a.m.: bagel, coffee with half/half and sugar, or cereal (granola), skim milk

Snack: Yoplait™ whip yogurt

Lunch 1:30 p.m.: sushi (vegetable roll) or grilled cheese panini on white, with potato chips and diet coke

Dinner: frozen pizza or frozen meal

Snack: Klondike bar×2 or popcorn (microwave) with butter

Drinks: water, seltzer, heifer, juice one cup per day

Biggest challenge with eating: overeating at night, eating out for lunch most days at work

Physical Activity Not Structured

Activities of preference: walking by the lake for 30 min 2×/week, yoga 1×/week.

He has a gym membership but does not use it.

Plan

Dietitian consultation.

Dietary therapy was initiated to promote weight loss with a goal of 10% weight reduction in 6 months.

RD visit: The diet chosen was the Mediterranean-style low-calorie diet for weight loss and healthy eating.

1. Decrease calorie intake:
   a. 2000 cal/day (based on Mifflin St. Jeor) [77]− 500 cal/day for weight loss = 1500 cal/day
   b. Track calories daily via online tracking program
   c. Weekly weights
2. Dietary macronutrient recommendations:
   a. Low simple sugar: Avoid high fructose and glucose in foods (in yogurt, cereal, bars, canned fruit, juice, syrups, agave, honey, sugar, high-fructose corn syrup, white sugar, and white breads)
   b. 40% carbohydrate intake = 150 g carbohydrate per day
   c. Low saturated fat: 12–16 g saturated fat (7–10%)
      i. Limit saturated fat = cheese, sour cream, mayo, high-fat meats (ribs, marbling), high-fat dairy, coconut milk, butter
   d. Increase MUFAs (nuts, seeds, olive/canola/peanut oil, and avocado) and PUFAs
      i. Plant sources of ω-3 PUFAs include flaxseed (ground), oils (canola, flaxseed, soybean), and nuts and other seeds (walnuts, butternuts, and sunflower)
3. General dietary recommendations:
   a. More fruits and vegetables (low calorie, high nutrient dense): 7–10 servings of fruits and vegetables each day
      i. Fresh or frozen fruits, vegetables. Any non-starchy vegetable including mushrooms, beets, cucumber, pepper, onion, celery, spinach, kale, broccoli, cauliflower, carrots
   b. Increase lean and vegetarian protein (low-saturated-fat protein sources)
   c. Two or more servings of seafood per week
      i. Fish high in ω-3 fatty acids include salmon, tuna, trout, mackerel, sardines, and herring
   d. Use 1–2 low-calorie meal replacements per day (frozen meals, shakes, and bars) for portion control
4. Activity recommendations:
   a. Increase activities of daily living
      i. Increase "less sedentary" time up to 2.5 h/day examples include walking, gardening, or dancing
      ii. Structured activity = 30–60 min of moderate intensity ≥5×/week or 20–60 min vigorous intensity ≥3×/week

Conclusion

In summary, weight loss, physical exercise, and dietary changes should be implemented on a long-term basis in all patients with NAFLD/NASH, regardless of the severity of their disease. Long-term lifestyle treatment of NAFLD optimally involves a multidisciplinary approach where physicians work together with trained lifestyle counselors (e.g., dietitians, psychologists, exercise physiologists, case managers, and nurse practitioners) to implement an effective and sustainable lifestyle modification program.

References

1. Adams LA, Sanderson S, Lindor KD, Angulo P. The histological course of nonalcoholic fatty liver disease: a longitudinal study of 103 patients with sequential liver biopsies. J Hepatol. 2005;42(1):132–8.
2. Trivedi IR. ME NAFLD and Cardiovascular Disease: Can the Real Association Be Determined? Curr Hepatol Rep 2014. 2014.
3. Capristo E, Miele L, Forgione A, et al. Nutritional aspects in patients with non-alcoholic steatohepatitis (NASH). Eur Rev Med Pharmacol Sci. 2005;9(5):265–8.
4. Centis E, Marzocchi R, Suppini A, et al. The role of lifestyle change in the prevention and treatment of NAFLD. Curr Pharm Des. 2013;19(29):5270–9.
5. Kim NH, Kim JH, Kim YJ, et al. Clinical and metabolic factors associated with development and regression of nonalcoholic fatty liver disease in nonobese subjects. Liver Int. 2014;34:604–11.
6. Browning JD, Szczepaniak LS, Dobbins R, et al. Prevalence of hepatic steatosis in an urban population in the United States: impact of ethnicity. Hepatology. 2004;40(6):1387–95.
7. Consultation WHOE. Appropriate body-mass index for Asian populations and its implications for policy and intervention strategies. Lancet. 2004;363(9403):157–63.
8. Chitturi S, Wong VW, Farrell G. Nonalcoholic fatty liver in Asia: firmly entrenched and rapidly gaining ground. J Gastroenterol Hepatol. 2011;26(Suppl 1):163–172.
9. Fan JG, Zhu J, Li XJ, et al. Fatty liver and the metabolic syndrome among Shanghai adults. J Gastroenterol Hepatol. 2005;20(12):1825–1832.
10. Park SH, Jeon WK, Kim SH, et al. Prevalence and risk factors of non-alcoholic fatty liver disease among Korean adults. J Gastroenterol Hepatol. 2006;21(1 Pt 1):138–143.

11. Zelber-Sagi S, Nitzan-Kaluski D, Goldsmith R, et al. Role of leisure-time physical activity in nonalcoholic fatty liver disease: a population-based study. Hepatology. 2008;48(6):1791–8.

12. Booth FW, Laye MJ, Lees SJ, Rector RS, Thyfault JP. Reduced physical activity and risk of chronic disease: the biology behind the consequences. Eur J Appl Physiol. 2008;102(4):381–390.

13. Kistler KD, Brunt EM, Clark JM, Diehl AM, Sallis JF, Schwimmer JB. Physical activity recommendations, exercise intensity, and histological severity of nonalcoholic fatty liver disease. Am J Gastroenterol. 2011;106(3):460–8. (quiz 469).

14. Harrison SA, Fecht W, Brunt EM, Neuschwander-Tetri BA. Orlistat for overweight subjects with nonalcoholic steatohepatitis: a randomized, prospective trial. Hepatology. 2009;49(1):80–6.

15. Promrat K, Kleiner DE, Niemeier HM, et al. Randomized controlled trial testing the effects of weight loss on nonalcoholic steatohepatitis. Hepatology. 2010;51(1):121–9.

16. Lazo M, Solga SF, Horska A, et al. Effect of a 12-month intensive lifestyle intervention on hepatic steatosis in adults with type 2 diabetes. Diabetes Care. 2010;33(10):2156–2163.

17. Mechanick JI, Youdim A, Jones DB, et al. Clinical practice guidelines for the perioperative nutritional, metabolic, and nonsurgical support of the bariatric surgery patient—2013 update: cosponsored by American Association of Clinical Endocrinologists, The Obesity Society, and American Society for Metabolic & Bariatric Surgery. Obesity (Silver Spring). 21(Suppl 1):S1–27.

18. Mechanick JI, Youdim A, Jones DB, et al. Clinical practice guidelines for the perioperative nutritional, metabolic, and nonsurgical support of the bariatric surgery patient—2013 update: cosponsored by American Association of Clinical Endocrinologists, the Obesity Society, and American Society for Metabolic & Bariatric Surgery. Endocr Pract. 2013;19(2):337–72.

19. Jeffery RW, Wing RR. Long-term effects of interventions for weight loss using food provision and monetary incentives. J Consult Clin Psychol. 1995;63(5):793–6.

20. Diraison F, Yankah V, Letexier D, Dusserre E, Jones P, Beylot M. Differences in the regulation of adipose tissue and liver lipogenesis by carbohydrates in humans. J Lipid Res. 2003;44(4):846–53.

21. Malik VS, Popkin BM, Bray GA, Despres JP, Hu FB. Sugar-sweetened beverages, obesity, type 2 diabetes mellitus, and cardiovascular disease risk. Circulation. 2010;121(11):1356–64.

22. Maersk M, Belza A, Stodkilde-Jorgensen H, et al. Sucrose-sweetened beverages increase fat storage in the liver, muscle, and visceral fat depot: a 6-mo randomized intervention study. Am J Clin Nutr. 2012;95(2):283–9.

23. Abdelmalek MF, Suzuki A, Guy C, et al. Increased fructose consumption is associated with fibrosis severity in patients with nonalcoholic fatty liver disease. Hepatology. 2010;51(6):1961–71.

24. Stanhope KL, Bremer AA, Medici V, et al. Consumption of fructose and high fructose corn syrup increase postprandial triglycerides, LDL-cholesterol, and apolipoprotein-B in young men and women. J Clin Endocrinol Metab. 2011;96(10):1596–1605.

25. Ha V, Jayalath VH, Cozma AI, Mirrahimi A, de Souza RJ, Sievenpiper JL. Fructose-containing sugars, blood pressure, and cardiometabolic risk: a critical review. Curr Hypertens Rep. 2013;15(4):281–97.

26. Silbernagel G, Machann J, Unmuth S, et al. Effects of 4-week very-high-fructose/glucose diets on insulin sensitivity, visceral fat and intrahepatic lipids: an exploratory trial. Br J Nutr. 2011;106(1):79–86.

27. Aeberli I, Gerber PA, Hochuli M, et al. Low to moderate sugar-sweetened beverage consumption impairs glucose and lipid metabolism and promotes inflammation in healthy young men: a randomized controlled trial. Am J Clin Nutr. 2011;94(2):479–85.

28. Chung M, Ma J, Patel K, Berger S, Lau J, Lichtenstein AH. Fructose, high-fructose corn syrup, sucrose, and nonalcoholic fatty liver disease or indexes of liver health: a systematic review and meta-analysis. Am J Clin Nutr. 2014;100(3):833–49.

29. Lowndes J, Kawiecki D, Pardo S, et al. The effects of four hypocaloric diets containing different levels of sucrose or high fructose corn syrup on weight loss and related parameters. Nutr J. 2012;11:55.

30. Volek J, Sharman M, Gomez A, et al. Comparison of energy-restricted very low-carbohydrate and low-fat diets on weight loss and body composition in overweight men and women. Nutr Metab. 2004;1(1):13.

31. York LW, Puthalapattu S, Wu GY. Nonalcoholic fatty liver disease and low-carbohydrate diets. Annu Rev Nutr. 2009;29:365–79.

32. Foster GD, Wyatt HR, Hill JO, et al. A randomized trial of a low-carbohydrate diet for obesity. N Engl J Med. 2003;348(21):2082–90.

33. Saris WH, Astrup A, Prentice AM, et al. Randomized controlled trial of changes in dietary carbohydrate/fat ratio and simple vs complex carbohydrates on body weight and blood lipids: the CARMEN study. The Carbohydrate Ratio Management in European National diets. Int J Obes Relat Metab Disord. 2000;24(10):1310–8.

34. Browning JD, Baker JA, Rogers T, Davis J, Satapati S, Burgess SC. Short-term weight loss and hepatic triglyceride reduction: evidence of a metabolic advantage with dietary carbohydrate restriction. Am J Clin Nutr. 2011;93(5):1048–52.

35. Westerbacka J, Lammi K, Hakkinen AM, et al. Dietary fat content modifies liver fat in overweight nondiabetic subjects. J Clin Endocrinol Metab. 2005;90(5):2804–2809.

36. Knopp RH, Walden CE, Retzlaff BM, et al. Long-term cholesterol-lowering effects of 4 fat-restricted diets in hypercholesterolemic and combined hyperlipidemic men. The dietary alternatives study. JAMA. 1997;278(18):1509–15.

37. Garg A, Grundy SM, Unger RH. Comparison of effects of high and low carbohydrate diets on plasma lipoproteins and insulin sensitivity in patients with mild NIDDM. Diabetes. 1992;41(10):1278–85.

38. Bozzetto L, Prinster A, Annuzzi G, et al. Liver fat is reduced by an isoenergetic MUFA diet in a controlled randomized study in type 2 diabetic patients. Diabetes Care. 2012;35(7):1429–1435.

39. Schwingshackl L, Hoffmann G. Monounsaturated fatty acids and risk of cardiovascular disease: synopsis of the evidence available from systematic reviews and meta-analyses. Nutrients. 2012;4(12):1989–2007.

40. Zivkovic AM, German JB, Sanyal AJ. Comparative review of diets for the metabolic syndrome: implications for nonalcoholic fatty liver disease. Am J Clin Nutr. 2007;86(2):285–300.

41. Masterton GS, Plevris JN, Hayes PC. Review article: omega-3 fatty acids—a promising novel therapy for non-alcoholic fatty liver disease. Aliment Pharmacol Ther. 2010;31(7):679–92.

42. Mensink RP, Zock PL, Kester AD, Katan MB. Effects of dietary fatty acids and carbohydrates on the ratio of serum total to HDL cholesterol and on serum lipids and apolipoproteins: a meta-analysis of 60 controlled trials. Am J Clin Nutr. 2003;77(5):1146–55.

43. Sofi F, Giangrandi I, Cesari F, et al. Effects of a 1-year dietary intervention with n-3 polyunsaturated fatty acid-enriched olive oil on non-alcoholic fatty liver disease patients: a preliminary study. Int J Food Sci Nutr. 2010;61(8):792–802.

44. Riccardi G, Giacco R, Rivellese AA. Dietary fat, insulin sensitivity and the metabolic syndrome. Clin Nutr. 2004;23(4):447–56.

45. Dasarathy S, Dasarathy J, Khiyami A, et al. Double-blind randomized placebo-controlled clinical trial of Omega 3 fatty acids for the treatment of diabetic patients with nonalcoholic steatohepatitis. J Clin Gastroenterol. 2014;49:137–44.

46. Parker HM, Johnson NA, Burdon CA, Cohn JS, O'Connor HT, George J. Omega-3 supplementation and non-alcoholic fatty liver disease: a systematic review and meta-analysis. J Hepatol. 2012;56(4):944–51.

47. Sanyal AJ, Abdelmalek MF, Suzuki A, Cummings OW, Chojkier M, Group E-AS. No significant effects of ethyl-eicosapentanoic acid on histologic features of nonalcoholic steatohepatitis in a phase 2 trial. Gastroenterology. 2014;147(2):377–84 e371.

48. Puri P, Baillie RA, Wiest MM, et al. A lipidomic analysis of nonalcoholic fatty liver disease. Hepatology. 2007;46(4):1081–90.
49. Harris WS, Mozaffarian D, Rimm E, et al. Omega-6 fatty acids and risk for cardiovascular disease: a science advisory from the American Heart Association Nutrition Subcommittee of the Council on Nutrition, Physical Activity, and Metabolism; Council on Cardiovascular Nursing; and Council on Epidemiology and Prevention. Circulation. 2009;119(6):902–7.
50. Czernichow S, Thomas D, Bruckert E. n-6 Fatty acids and cardiovascular health: a review of the evidence for dietary intake recommendations. Br J Nutr. 2010;104(6):788–96.
51. Yang HY, Tzeng YH, Chai CY, et al. Soy protein retards the progression of non-alcoholic steatohepatitis via improvement of insulin resistance and steatosis. Nutrition. 2011;27(9):943–8.
52. Alkerwi A, Boutsen M, Vaillant M, et al. Alcohol consumption and the prevalence of metabolic syndrome: a meta-analysis of observational studies. Atherosclerosis. 2009;204(2):624–35.
53. Sookoian S, Castano GO, Pirola CJ. Modest alcohol consumption decreases the risk of non-alcoholic fatty liver disease: a meta-analysis of 43 175 individuals. Gut. 2014;63(3):530–2.
54. Loomba R, Yang HI, Su J, et al. Synergism between obesity and alcohol in increasing the risk of hepatocellular carcinoma: a prospective cohort study. Am J Epidemiol. 2013;177(4):333–42.
55. Freedman ND, Everhart JE, Lindsay KL, et al. Coffee intake is associated with lower rates of liver disease progression in chronic hepatitis C. Hepatology. 2009;50(5):1360–9.
56. Gelatti U, Covolo L, Franceschini M, et al. Coffee consumption reduces the risk of hepatocellular carcinoma independently of its aetiology: a case-control study. J Hepatol. 2005;42(4):528–34.
57. Bambha K, Wilson LA, Unalp A, et al. Coffee consumption in NAFLD patients with lower insulin resistance is associated with lower risk of severe fibrosis. Liver Int. 2013;38:1250–8.
58. Corrado RL, Torres DM, Harrison SA. Review of treatment options for nonalcoholic fatty liver disease. Med Clin N Am. 2014;98(1):55–72.
59. Sanyal AJ, Chalasani N, Kowdley KV, et al. Pioglitazone, vitamin E, or placebo for nonalcoholic steatohepatitis. N Engl J Med. 2010;362(18):1675–85.
60. Miller ER 3rd, Pastor-Barriuso R, Dalal D, Riemersma RA, Appel LJ, Guallar E. Meta-analysis: high-dosage vitamin E supplementation may increase all-cause mortality. Ann Intern Med. 2005;142(1):37–46.
61. Bjelakovic G, Nikolova D, Gluud LL, Simonetti RG, Gluud C. Mortality in randomized trials of antioxidant supplements for primary and secondary prevention: systematic review and meta-analysis. JAMA. 2007;297(8):842–57.
62. Klein EA, Thompson IM Jr, Tangen CM, et al. Vitamin E and the risk of prostate cancer: the Selenium and Vitamin E Cancer Prevention Trial (SELECT). JAMA. 2011;306(14):1549–56.
63. Tamura Y, Tanaka Y, Sato F, et al. Effects of diet and exercise on muscle and liver intracellular lipid contents and insulin sensitivity in type 2 diabetic patients. J Clin Endocrinol Metab. 2005;90(6):3191–6.
64. Sullivan S, Kirk EP, Mittendorfer B, Patterson BW, Klein S. Randomized trial of exercise effect on intrahepatic triglyceride content and lipid kinetics in nonalcoholic fatty liver disease. Hepatology. 2012;55(6):1738–45.
65. Johnson NA, Sachinwalla T, Walton DW, et al. Aerobic exercise training reduces hepatic and visceral lipids in obese individuals without weight loss. Hepatology. 2009;50(4):1105–12.
66. Pattyn N, Cornelissen VA, Eshghi SR, Vanhees L. The effect of exercise on the cardiovascular risk factors constituting the metabolic syndrome: a meta-analysis of controlled trials. Sports Med. 2013;43(2):121–33.
67. Zelber-Sagi S, Buch A, Yeshua H, et al. Effect of resistance training on non-alcoholic fatty-liver disease a randomized-clinical trial. World J Gastroenterol. 2014;20(15):4382–92.
68. Cornelissen VA, Fagard RH, Coeckelberghs E, Vanhees L. Impact of resistance training on blood pressure and other cardiovascular risk factors: a meta-analysis of randomized, controlled trials. Hypertension. 2011;58(5):950–8.
69. Long M, Pedley A, Massaro JM. Non-alcoholic fatty liver disease is associated with lower levels of physical activity measured via Accelerometry: the Framingham Heart Study. Digestive Disease Week 2014. 2014; Chicago, Illinois.
70. George A St, Bauman A, Johnston A, Farrell G, Chey T, George J. Independent effects of physical activity in patients with nonalcoholic fatty liver disease. Hepatology. 2009;50(1):68–76.
71. Garber CE, Blissmer B, Deschenes MR, et al. American College of Sports Medicine position stand. Quantity and quality of exercise for developing and maintaining cardiorespiratory, musculoskeletal, and neuromotor fitness in apparently healthy adults: guidance for prescribing exercise. Med Sci Sports Exerc. 2011;43(7):1334–1359.
72. Organization WH. Global recommendations on physical activity for health 18–64 years old. 2014. Global recommendations on physical activity for health 2011. Accessed 8 July 2014.
73. Wing R. Behavioral weight control. In: Wadden TA, Stunkard AJ, editors. Handbook of obesity treatment. New York: Guilford; 2002. p. 301–316.
74. Shah K, Stufflebam A, Hilton TN, Sinacore DR, Klein S, Villareal DT. Diet and exercise interventions reduce intrahepatic fat content and improve insulin sensitivity in obese older adults. Obesity (Silver Spring). 2009;17(12):2162–8.
75. Diabetes Prevention Program Research G. The Diabetes Prevention Program (DPP): description of lifestyle intervention. Diabetes Care. 2002;25(12):2165–71.
76. Ryan DH, Espeland MA, Foster GD, et al. Look AHEAD (Action for Health in Diabetes): design and methods for a clinical trial of weight loss for the prevention of cardiovascular disease in type 2 diabetes. Control Clin Trials. 2003;24(5):610–28.
77. Frankenfield D, Roth-Yousey L, Compher C. Comparison of predictive equations for resting metabolic rate in healthy non-obese and obese adults: a systematic review. J Am Diet Assoc. 2005;105(5):775–89.

Gastroenterology Disease and Lifestyle Medicine

30

Gerald Friedman

Abbreviations

ADHD	Attention deficit hyperactivity disorder
BMI	Body Mass Index
CD	Crohn's disease
CMV	Cytomegalovirus
DNA	Deoxyribonucleic acid
EKG	Electrocardiogram
FISH	Fluorescence in situ hybridization
FODMAPs	Fermentable oligo-, di- and mono-saccharides and polyols
GERD	Gastroesophageal reflux disease
GI	Gastrointestinal
HIV	Human immunodeficiency virus
IBDs	Inflammatory bowel diseases
IBS	Irritable bowel syndrome
LES	Lower esophageal sphincter
NCGS	Non-celiac gluten sensitivity
NSAIDs	Nonsteroidal anti-inflammatory agents
n-3 FA	Omega-3 fatty acids
n-6 FA	Omega-6 fatty acids
PCR	Polymerase chain reaction
PUFA	Polyunsaturated fatty acids
RD	Registered dietitian
RNA	Ribonucleic acid
SCFA	Short-chain fatty acids
tTG	Tissue transglutaminase
tTG IgA	Tissue transglutaminase immunoglobulin A
tLESRs	Transient lower esophageal sphincter relaxations
T-RELP	Terminal restriction fragment length polymorphism
UC	Ulcerative colitis
UDCA	Ursodeoxycholic acid

G. Friedman (✉)
Division of Gastroenterology, Icahn School of Medicine at Mount Sinai, New York, NY, USA
e-mail: gfmd379@gmail.com

Introduction

Lifestyle medicine, emphasizing prevention as well as therapy, plays a fundamental role in the understanding and treatment of all gastroenterologic illnesses. This chapter will focus upon the central pathophysiologic features of specific gastrointestinal (GI) illnesses and identify lifestyle interventions, which can prevent or ameliorate the disease. A growing body of scientific evidence has demonstrated that lifestyle intervention in the treatment of chronic diseases can be as effective as medication without the risks and unwanted side effects.

Gastroesophageal Reflux Disease

The primary event in gastroesophageal reflux disease (GERD) is the movement of gastric juice from the stomach into the esophagus. The three dominant pathophysiologic mechanisms causing reflux include a hypotensive lower esophageal sphincter (LES), transient lower esophageal sphincter relaxations (tLESRs), and the presence of a hiatal hernia. Mucosal injury is related to the potency and frequency of refluxate and mucosal integrity. The frequency of tLESRs is increased by gastric distention or by assuming an upright position. Esophageal sphincter pressure can be reduced by a variety of factors including diet and drugs, such as smooth muscle relaxants. The diaphragm as well as the LES contributes to sphincter competence. The pinchcock effect of crural contraction is altered in the presence of a hiatus hernia. Obesity is a risk factor for GERD and erosive esophagitis. There is a significant correlation of body mass index (BMI) and waist circumference with intragastric pressure and the gastroesophgeal pressure gradient. Abdominal obesity has been associated with increased reflux symptoms [1]. Lifestyle changes recommended for reducing symptoms of GERD include weight reduction, reducing meal size, elimination or modification of selected dietary factors, and improved sleep hygiene (Table 30.1). Smoking should be

Table 30.1 Lifestyle changes for gastroesophageal reflux disease (GERD)[a]

Lifestyle change	Comment
Decrease alcohol, coffee, peppermint, chocolate	Improves LES pressure
Practice abdominal breathing exercises	
Decrease excessively hot liquids (such as tea), pepper and highly spiced foods, tomato paste, tomato juice	Improves esophageal mucosal health
Decrease soluble and insoluble fibers	Improves gastric emptying
Avoid large quantities of food at one sitting or within 3 h of bedtime	
Avoid tight-fitting garments	Decreases intragastric pressure
Use oral lozenges	Increases salivation, which neutralizes refluxed acid
Avoid smoking	
Elevate head of bed 6–8 in. such that the head and shoulders are higher than the stomach (can use blocks of wood under the legs of bed or a foam wedge under the mattress)	Reduces night-time reflux
Keep liquid antacid at bedside if needed	

[a] *LES* lower esophageal sphincter

avoided since smoking reduces the buffering effect of saliva, decreases LES pressure and reduces coughing episodes, which may increase reflux events.

Peptic Ulcer Disease and Gastritis

Three causal factors related to peptic ulcer disease include the presence of *Helicobacter pylori* infection, the use of nonsteroidal anti-inflammatory agents (NSAIDs), and psychological factors in selected subgroups of patients. *H. pylori* has been demonstrated to be the major cause of peptic ulcer and gastritis in humans and is present in over 90 % of duodenal ulcer patients [2]. Eradication of *H. pylori* significantly decreases the recurrence of duodenal ulcers. Epidemiologic studies reveal an increased incidence of *H. pylori* infection in the children of lower socioeconomic status in developing countries. The infection is usually acquired at an early age and last a lifetime. Risk factors relate to fecal-oral transmission, living conditions associated with overcrowding, number of siblings, bed sharing, and lack of running water. Lifestyle changes, emphasizing improvement in living conditions and hygiene facilities, have reduced the incidence of *H. pylori* infection in developing countries. Consumption of salted foods may increase the possibility of persistent infection and also increase the risk of gastric cancer [3]. NSAIDs act directly through inhibition of prostaglandin synthesis affecting the amount of gastric acid generated, the integrity of the mucosal barrier, the amount of bicarbonate and glutathione produced, and the rate of mucosal blood flow. NSAIDs are typically used for symptoms associated with musculoskeletal disease and headaches. In addition to analgesia, aspirin causes irreversible inhibition of normal platelet function. It is widely used for prophylaxis for thrombotic events such as myocardial infarction and stroke. The risks of gastrointestinal side effects from NSAIDs include caus-

ing peptic ulcers, which may lead to potential complications including bleeding or perforation [4]. Risks are greater with increased age, increased doses of NSAIDs, longer durations of therapy, and in those with a prior history of peptic ulcer disease. Lifestyle changes include avoiding the use of NSAIDs, using lower doses, or using alternative medications such as acetaminophen. Further preventive measures include behavior modification, joint protection, weight loss, and exercise. The pathogenesis of peptic ulcer is multifactorial, and psychodynamic factors are likely to play a role in a subset of patients. These factors need to be correlated with the pathophysiologic features noted above (*H. pylori*, NSAIDs, smoking, and alcohol). It has been noted that poorly tolerated stress or depressive symptoms at baseline increases the risk of ulcer development. Other psychosocial factors such as work-related stress and social problems are predictive of subsequent ulcer disease. Catastrophic societal conditions or natural disasters may play a role in the induction of peptic ulcer disease in certain subgroups of patients. Stress, anxiety, and depression have been known to impair ulcer healing. Lifestyle changes aided by psychiatrists, psychologists, or social workers may assist in appropriate integrative social adjustments.

Gallstone-Related Illnesses

Cholelithiasis is common among Western populations, occurring approximately 6 % in men and 9 % in women [5]. Prevalence rates among various ethnic populations reveal increased levels to be greater among Hispanic and Native American populations as opposed to Asian and African-American groups. Major risk factors include age, sex, pregnancy, oral contraceptives, estrogen replacement therapy, obesity, family history, hypertriglyceridemia, diabetes mellitus, rapid weight loss, post-bariatric surgery, prolonged total parenteral nutrition, certain drugs such as clofibrate and ceftriaxone, hemolysis, and Crohn's disease (CD). Conditions associated with gallbladder stasis promote stone formation by absorbing water causing enhanced bile acid concentration. Most patients with incidental gallstones will not develop symptoms and do not require therapy [6]. However, 15–25 % may develop biliary colic with right upper quadrant and right shoulder pain as well as the likeliness of recurrence predisposing patients to complications. Lifestyle changes may prevent the progression of biliary disease by noting the contributory causes and introducing prophylaxis. Prophylactic cholecystectomy is not indicated for most patients with silent gallstones [7]. Specific attention to individual risk factors may prevent further complications. In some instances the use of ursodeoxycholic acid (UDCA) may be effective in reducing the risk of further stone formation. This may be helpful as an adjunct to slow weight reduction in patients with obesity. In addition, increasing dietary consumption of coffee (2–4 cups/day), fiber, vegetable protein, nuts, calcium, vitamin C, and even alcohol, as well as increasing physical activity, reduces the risk for gallstones [8].

Pancreatitis

Acute pancreatitis is an inflammatory disease of the pancreas characterized by abdominal pain and elevated levels of pancreatic enzymes in the blood. Seventy-five percent of the cases of acute pancreatitis in the USA are due to gallstones and chronic alcoholism. Mechanical ampullary obstruction caused by small stones or transient reflux of bile into the pancreatic duct may occur during passage of gallstones. Small stones are associated with increased risk of pancreatitis. Other causes include hyperlipidemia, hypercalcemia, certain viral infections (e.g., cytomegalovirus, CMV; mumps; zoster; and human immunodeficiency virus, HIV), abdominal trauma, ischemia, and certain medications (e.g., metronidazole, tetracycline, furosemide, and thiazides). Prophylactic lifestyle modifications of etiologic factors are obviously related to antecedent triggering factors. Gallstone disease and its relationship to diabetes mellitus and obesity can be addressed as noted above. Chronic alcoholism noted by history requires appropriate attention and treatment. Metabolic evidence of hyperlipidemia should be treated by dietary control and statin medication. The etiology of hypercalcemia should be investigated to rule out hyperparathyroidism and other contributory factors. A medication history should be accurately obtained and suspicious medications known to induce pancreatitis eliminated. Drug-induced pancreatitis is classified based upon the number of cases reported, demonstration of a consistent latency period, and reaction with drug rechallenge [9]. The etiology of acute pancreatitis should focus

on prior symptoms of documentation of gallstones, alcohol use, history of hypertriglyceridemia, hypercalcemia, family history, and medication history [10]. In short, lifestyle components that are associated decreased risk for chronic pancreatitis, and by extension pancreatic cancer, include tobacco cessation, moderation to avoidance of alcohol consumption, and sufficient physical activity and healthy eating that reduces insulin resistance, dyslipidemia, and excessive body weight [11].

Celiac Disease and Non-celiac Gluten Sensitivity

Gluten is a complex of water-soluble proteins from wheat, rye, and barley [12]. Celiac disease is characterized by chronic inflammation of the proximal small bowel mucosa, which heals when gluten-containing foods are completely eliminated from the diet. The immunogenic peptides are resistant to digestion by proteases and are taken up by immune effector cells. Screening tests for celiac disease include antibodies against endomysium, tissue transglutaminase (tTG), and deaminated gliadin peptide. Overall, the tissue transglutaminase immunoglobulin A (tTG IgA) is the recommended test to screen with confirmation by small bowel biopsy. Non-celiac gluten sensitivity (NCGS) [13] comprises a variety of symptom complexes caused by gluten-containing foods. These patients have abdominal discomfort, bloating and flatulence as well as extra-intestinal symptoms such as headache, attention deficit hyperactivity disorder (ADHD), ataxia, or oral ulceration. In NCGS, screening tests and small bowel biopsies for gluten enteropathy are negative. Symptoms may improve or disappear with gluten withdrawal. Dietary lifestyle changes in both of these illnesses include strict adherence to a gluten-free diet monitored by a nutritionist or registered dietitian (RD) (Table 30.2).

Irritable Bowel Syndrome

Irritable bowel syndrome (IBS) is a GI disorder characterized by chronic, recurrent abdominal pain associated with altered stool frequency and consistency. The illness is not explained by structural or biochemical abnormalities. More than 20 % of the population report symptoms consistent with this disorder. IBS is the most common diagnosis noted among US GI practices [14]. The symptom onset and clinical relapses involve multifactorial triggers including genetic, environmental, and psychosocial components as well as a complex relationship with gut microbiota associated with a decrease in protective bacteria. Some cases trigger a subtle immune system activation, which compromises the critical epithelial barrier. Epidemiologically, there is a predominance of females affected, a family history of IBS,

Table 30.2 Gluten-containing and gluten-free grains, starches, and other carbohydrate sources

Gluten-containing foods	Gluten-free foods	
Barley	Amaranth	Sago
Bulgar	Arrowroot	Sorghum
Couscous	Buckwheat	Soy
Farina	Cassava	Tapioca
Graham flour	Corn	Yucca
Kamut	Flax	Wild rice
Rye	Legumes/dry bean/peas/lentils	
Semolina	Millet	
Spelt	Nuts	
Triticale	Potatoes	
Wheat	Quinoa	
Wheat germ	Rice	

and a history of functional abdominal pain in childhood. Multiple factors play a role in the pathophysiology of IBS. Gastrointestinal motor function, specifically increased frequency and irregularity of luminal contractions have been reported in diarrhea-prone IBS as well as prolonged transit time in constipation-prone IBS [15]. Visceral hypersensitivity is a frequent finding expressed as increased sensation in response to dietary and emotional stimuli. Selected hypersensitivity of visceral afferent nerves in the gut triggered by bloating or bowel distention engenders bowel symptoms. Intestinal inflammation, triggered by mucosal immune system activation, is characterized by alteration of specific immune cells and markers, particularly in patients with postinfectious IBS. Lymphocyte infiltration in the myenteric plexus and neuron degeneration have been reported. An increased number of mast cells have been demonstrated in the terminal ileum, jejunum, and colon in IBS patients. In addition, proinflammatory interleukins have been observed in IBS patients [16]. Postinfectious IBS has been reported based upon a history of acute diarrheal illness preceding the onset of IBS symptoms several months later. The diarrheal episodes have been reported in association with bacterial, viral, protozoan, and helminthes infections [17]. Alteration in fecal microflora reveal that fecal microflora of IBS patients differ from healthy controls. This dysbiosis has been confirmed by a detailed analysis of fecal microbiota in IBS and control patients and correlated the findings with key clinical and physiological parameters. An increased Firmicutes–Bacteroidetes ratio characterizes IBS patients [18]. Food sensitivity requires analysis, in large part due to the patient's observations that certain foods may trigger and perpetuate IBS symptoms. Some patients report worsening of symptoms after eating and perceive food intolerance to certain foods. There is evidence to support the role of impaired carbohydrate absorption. In particular, fermentable oligo-, di-, and mono-saccharides and polyols (FODMAPs) enter the small bowel and colon where they are fermented by colonic bacteria forming short-chain fatty acids (SCFA) and

gases (hydrogen, carbon dioxide, and oxygen) leading to abdominal bloating, cramps, and distention. Alternatively, diets low in FODMAP foods offer significant symptom relief to selected patients (Table 30.3; [19, 20]). Psychosocial factors may trigger abdominal pain and altered bowel function. Compared with controls, patients with IBS report more daily stressful events and exhibit increased anxiety, depression phobias, and somatization. Given the information noted above, IBS treatment provides a number of prescient areas whereby lifestyle interventions may be valuable. Since the two most significant features triggering IBS symptoms are food intake and psychosocial factors, lifestyle changes are directed to better nutrition, improved sleep hygeine, and stress reduction. Patients with IBS can initiate their evaluation by creating a 7-day written analysis of food intake and timing of symptoms. Two thirds of IBS patients complain of symptoms within 15 min of eating, and 90% are symptomatic within 3 h after a meal. Larger meals induce more symptoms than smaller meals. FODMAP foods should be reduced incrementally, the goal being gradual reduction in symptoms of bloating, distention, and pain. Consultation with an RD is recommended. Patients with IBS should have a minimum of 7–8 h of sleep nightly (adequate sleep will reduce the two major triggers of stress and food intake). Anxiety, depression, and stress can be reduced with an adequate exercise program as well as consultation with a psychiatrist, psychologist, or social worker when necessary.

Inflammatory Bowel Diseases

Ulcerative colitis (UC) and CD are chronic inflammatory disorders of the GI tract of unknown etiology and are collectively referred to as inflammatory bowel diseases (IBDs). These illnesses are thought to arise from dysregulation of both the innate and adaptive immune systems leading to an abnormal inflammatory response to commensal bacteria in a genetically susceptible individual. Etiologic hypotheses

Table 30.3 FODMAP (fermentable oligo-, di-, and mono-saccharides and polyols) food sources[a]

Free fructose	Lactose	Fructans	Polyols	Galacto-oligosaccharides
Apple	Milk	Peach	Apple	Legumes
Cherry	Ice cream	Persimmon	Apricot	Lentils
Mango	Custard	Watermelon	Pear	Chickpeas
Pear	Soft cheese	Artichokes	Cherry	
Watermelon		Beetroot	Avocado	
Asparagus		Brussels sprout	Plum/Prune	
Artichokes		Chicory	Nectarine	
Sugar snap peas		Fennel	Cauliflower	
Honey		Garlic	Mushroom	
		Leek	Snow peas	
		Onion		
		Peas		
		Wheat		
		Rye		
		Barley		
		Pistachios		
		Legumes		
		Lentils		
		Chickpeas		

[a] See [20]

include defective mucosal integrity associated with altered mucous, increased permeability, cellular starvation, and impaired restitution. Persistent infection is likely related to dysbiosis by aggressive commensals and a diminution of protective bacteria. UC involves an inflammatory process affecting separate segments of the colorectal area presenting as proctitis, proctosigmoiditis, left-sided colitis, or universal colitis. CD is a transmural disease, affecting any section of the GI tract, most commonly the small bowel and colon (small bowel alone—33%, Ileo-colic area—45%, colon only—20%). Epidemiologically, IBD may affect any age with peak incidence occurring at 15–30 years. The illnesses are essentially gender neutral, favoring Caucasians and Ashkenazi Jews. Environmental factors affecting IBD include cigarette smoking, urban living, diet, and oral contraceptives. A significant family history affects IBD as does the use of antibiotic therapy in early childhood. Clinical manifestations include persistent abdominal pain, nausea, emesis, fever, weight loss, and diarrhea (bloody diarrhea with UC; watery diarrhea with CD). Lifestyle risks for developing IBD include nutritional, environmental, and activity factors. The role of dietary was evaluated in Canadian children less than 20 years newly diagnosed with CD and compared with matched hospital controls [21]. The findings indicate that an imbalance in consumption of fatty acids, vegetables, and fruits is associated with CD risk. In addition, the ratio of long-chain omega-3 fatty acids (n-3 FA) to omega-6 fatty acids (n-6 FA) may also be related to the etiology of CD. A systematic review used guideline-recommended methodology to evaluate the association between pre-illness intake of nutrients and the risk of subsequent IBD diagnosis [22]. High intake of total fats, polyunsaturated fatty acids (PUFA),

n-6 FA, and meat are associated with an increased risk of CD and UC. In addition, high fiber and fruit intakes are associated with decreased CD risk, and high vegetable intake is associated with decreased UC risk.

In families where there is a history of IBD, the limited use of antibiotics and early introduction of dietary changes would be appropriate in asymptomatic children. The development and progression of IBD is multifactorial based upon host genotype, immune disequilibrium, and the composition of microbial communities resident in the GI tract. At birth the GI tract is essentially sterile and appropriate development of the immune system is dependent on GI colonization. Initial microbiome colonization occurs following vaginal delivery with transfer of maternal bacteria to the infant. Breast feeding also contributes bifidobacteria to the infant's developing commensal bacteria. Thus, a mature adult microbiome is established within 2–3 years. Specific bacteria activate host immune responses to facilitate their own survival and competitiveness by inducing host production of defensins to eliminate potential competing organisms. Furthermore, healthy GI microbiota enhance epithelial integrity, contribute protective mucous layers and immune system development, produce anti-inflammatory metabolites, and induce colonization resistance. Dysbiosis of GI bacteria in IBD has been reported in many studies and summarized by Nagalingam and Lynch [23]. Significant reductions in the abundance of members of the phylum *Firmicutes* have been noted in IBD patients. Their loss diminishes the production of SCFA reducing the nourishment of colonocytes and their anti-inflammatory activity. Lifestyle changes include reducing the use of antibiotics in infants and toddlers, except where medically indicated, as well as recommending dietary factors, which would enhance anti-inflammatory bacteria and prevent dysbiosis. The western diet is characterized by processed food and less vegetables, fruits, and fiber than in developing countries. Positive lifestyle dietary changes include the use of fiber and plant polysaccharides which are digested in the colon producing SCFA (acetate, propionate, and butyrate), which nourish colonocytes, providing energy, microbiome diversity, and less inflammation.

General Applications of the Microbiome Related to GI Illness and Immune Function

The role of the microbiome in human health and disease is important to the understanding of how bacteria contribute to health maintenance, how perturbations of the microbiome can engender disease, and how corrective action can ameliorate illness. The microbiome consists of groups of bacteria distributed throughout the body, including the oral cavity, nose, all skin surfaces, lungs, vagina, and all GI surfaces, particularly the colon [24]. Recent advances in the functional contributions of bacteria in humans have been accelerated by the discovery of new methods of analysis of bacterial communities, particularly the fecal microbiota. Molecular-based techniques use the bacterial 16rRNA gene as a marker of genetic diversity. Deoxyribonucleic acid (DNA) can be extracted, followed by polymerase chain amplification. Nucleic acid-based analytic methods useful in gut microbiota research include ribonucleic acid (RNA) dot blots for quantification of specific bacterial populations, fluorescence in situ hybridization (FISH) for detection and quantification of bacterial cells, terminal restriction fragment length polymorphism (T-RELP) for profiling and quantifying of the bacterial community, and polymerase chain reaction (PCR) combined with denaturing gradient gel electrophoresis (PCR/DGGE) for profiling the composition of bacterial communities for comparative analysis. Nucleic acid-based analysis of fecal samples enables descriptions to be made of the phylogenetic composition of the microbiome. It enables the genetic potential of the microbiota to be determined (metagenomics) as well as the expression of genes at a point of time to be revealed (transcriptomics) [25]. Using our current understanding of disease pathogenesis in IBD as a paradigm, functional genomics has revealed a complex interaction between host innate and adaptive immunity that provides protection against microbial invasion yet demonstrates tolerance to colonization with mucosal surfaces. The loss of mucosal tolerance in association with defective innate immunity leads to an unrestrained immune response characteristic of IBD. Societal changes in concert with environmental changes related to westernized diets, sedentary activity, smoking, alcohol, and drugs have contributed to dysbiosis and aberrant functional changes in the microbiome.

An expanding clinical trial evidence base has supported the use of probiotics in a variety of clinical scenarios. However, the answer is not simple with a variety of molecular targets, clinical endpoints, prebiotic (fiber and starch containing foods producing SCFA), probiotic, and symbiotic (pre- plus probiotic) formulations, and an underlying pathophysiology that is still elusive. Chatterjee et al. [26] found that *Lactobacillus acidophilus* LA-5 and *bifidobacterium* BB-12 did not decrease the incidence of antibiotic-associated diarrhea in children but did reduce the duration of diarrhea. These results are consistent with many other clinical investigations of antibiotic-associated and hospital-acquired diarrhea in adults and children. In a small randomized, controlled trial ($N=37$), Abbas et al. [27] found that *Saccharomyces boulardii* (750 mg/day × 6 weeks) and conventional ispaghula husk treatment improved inflammatory markers, histology, and quality of life in patient with IBS. Other clinical problems with evidence-based roles for probiotic intervention include cirrhosis [28], postgastrectomy [29], proton-pump inhibitor therapy [30], radiation enteritis [31], and travelers' diarrhea [32], and post-bariatric surgery [33] with research studies underway in obesity [34] and diabetes prevention and treatment [35]. In short, with a relatively low side-effect profile, the use of pre- and probiotic therapeutic strategies promises to be an important component of lifestyle medicine in the management of GI disease.

Case Report: Reflux esophagitis: A 62 y/o Caucasian male sanitation worker complains of chronic heartburn of increasing severity for the past 6 years, exacerbated by increased physical effort on the job. He has gained over 10 pounds over the past year and currently has a BMI of 38 kg/m^2. He has been a long-term one-pack-per-day cigarette smoker since age 20 and drinks 2–3 bottles of beer with lunch and evening meals. His past medical history is noncontributory except for an appendectomy at age 10. Family history: father, age 80, has hypertension and is on Dyazide once daily; mother, age 75, is in good health. Two siblings, brother, age 58, and sister, 56, are in good health. The patient has no allergies and is currently taking ibuprofen 400 mg twice daily for muscular discomfort. He states that his heartburn has increased after a heavy evening meal as well as at bedtime upon reclining; he is awakened frequently during the night with mid-chest burning, relieved, in part, by drinking milk or liquid antacid. Evaluation by his local internist reveals mild hypertension (BP = 145/85 mm Hg), elevated low-density lipoprotein(LDL)-cholesterol, and normal liver function tests; urinalysis is normal and stool guaiac is negative. Electrocardiogram (EKG) is unremarkable. Chest X-ray is negative. An upper GI series reveals a direct, sliding hiatus hernia; Upper GI endoscopy confirms evidence of the hiatus hernia and esophagitis. There is no biopsy evidence of Barrett's esophagus, and *H. pylori* is absent. He is placed on appropriate proton pump therapy as well as carefully explaining the following lifestyle changes:

1. Weight reduction and an exercise program are essential to reduce abdominal pressure causing reflux of acid into the lower esophagus.
2. Alcohol use is restricted to minimize the toxic impact of alcohol on the sensitive distal esophageal mucosa, and smoking must be discontinued since it lowers the LES pressure allowing acid to enter the esophagus.
3. Elevation of the head of the bed at night using 6–8 in. blocks or a foam wedge decreases acid reflux.
4. Eating several hours before bedtime is recommended to assure retained food and fluid from refluxing.
5. Reducing meal size is helpful as well as avoiding fats, peppermint, and chocolate aid in reducing reflux frequency.
6. Citrus drinks, spicy foods, tomato-based products, coffee, tea, and cola drinks should be moderated due to their direct impact upon the esophageal mucosa and the stimulation of acid secretory activity.
7. Excessively hot foods may further irritate the esophageal mucosa.
8. Medications, which decrease LES pressure including barbiturates, calcium channel blockers, diazepam, meperidine, morphine, prostaglandins E2, serotonin, and theophylline should be avoided when possible.

Follow-up appointment is scheduled for 1 month to test efficacy of symptom reduction and then perform repeat upper gastrointestinal (UGI) endoscopy in 6 months to evaluate reduced esophagitis and absence of Barrett's esophagus.

References

1. El-Serag HB, Ergun GA, Pandolfino J, et al. Obesity increases oesophageal acid exposure. Gut. 2007;56:749–55.
2. Marshall BJ, Warren JR. Unidentified curved bacilli in the stomach of patients with gastritis and peptic ulceration. Lancet. 1984;2:1311–5.
3. Lee SA, Kang D, Shim KN, et al. Effect of diet and Helicobacter pylori infection to the risk of early gastric cancer. J Epidemiol. 2003;13:162–8.
4. Allison MC, Howaston AG, Torrance CJ, et al., Gastrointestinal damage associated with the use of non-steroidal anti-inflammatory drugs. N Engl J Med. 1992;327:749–54.
5. Everhart JE, Khare M, Hill M, Maurer KR. Prevalence and ethnic differences in gall bladder disease in the United States. Gastroenterology. 1999;117:632–9.
6. Heaton KW, Braddon FE, Mountford RA, et al. Symptomatic and silent gallstones in the community. Gut. 1991;32:316–20.
7. Ransohoff DF, Gracie WA, Wolfenson LB, Neuhauser D. Prophylactic cholecystectomy or expectant management for silent gallstones. A decision analysis to assess survival. Ann Int Med. 1983;99:199–204.
8. Shaffer EA. Gallstone disease: epidemiology of gallbladder stone disease. Best Pract Res Clin Gastroenterol. 2006;20:981–96.
9. Badalov N, Baradarian R, Iswara K, et al. Drug-induced pancreatitis: an evidence-based review. Clin Gastroenterol Hepatol. 2007;5:648–61.
10. Forsmark CE, Baillie J. AGA Institute Councl Practice and Economics Committee, AGA Institute Governing Board. AGA Institute technical review on acute pancreatitis. Gastroenterology. 2007;132:2022.
11. Otsuki M, Tashiro M. Chronic pancreatitis and pancreatic cancer, lifestyle-related diseases. Intern Med. 2007;46:109–13.
12. Rostom A, Murray JA, Kagnoff ME. American Gastroenterological Association (AGA) Institute technical review on the diagnosis and management of celiac disease. Gastroenterology. 2006;131:1981–2002.
13. Mansueto P, Seidita A, D'Alcamo A, Carroccio A. Non-celiac gluten sensitivity: literature review. J Am Coll Nutr. 2014;33(1):39–54.
14. Brandt LJ, Chey WD, et al. American College of Gastroenterology Task Force on Irritable Bowel Syndrome, An evidence-based position statement on the management of irritable bowel syndrome. Am J Gastroenterol. 2009;104 Suppl 1:S1.
15. Chey WY, Jin HO, Lee MH, et al. Colonic motility abnormality in patients with irritable bowel syndrome. Am J Gastroenterol. 2001;96:1499–506.
16. Liebregts T, Adam B, Bredack C, et al. Immune activation in patients with irritable bowel syndrome. Gastroenterology. 2007;132:913–20.
17. Wang LH, Fang XC, Pan GZ. Bacillary dysentery as a causative factor of irritable bowel syndrome and its pathogenesis. Gut. 2004;53:1096–101.
18. Jeffery IB, O'Toole PW, Ohman L, et al. An irritable bowel subtype defined by species specific alterations in faecal microbiota. Gut. 2012;61:997–1006.
19. Chey WD. The role of food in the functional gastrointestinal disorders: introduction to a manuscript series. Am J Gastroenterol. 2013;108:694–7.
20. Gibson PR, Shepherd SJ. Food choice as a key management strategy for functional gastrointestinal symptoms. Am J Gastroenterol. 2012;107:657–66.
21. Amre AK, D'Souza S, Morgan K, Seidman G, et al. Imbalances in dietary consumption of fatty acids, vegetables, and fruits are associated with risk for Crohn's disease in children. Am J Gastroenterol. 2007;102:2016–25.
22. Hou JK, Abraham B, El-Serag H. Dietary intake and risk of developing inflammatory bowel disease: a systematic review of the literature. Am J Gastroenterol. 2011;106:563–73.
23. Nagalingam NA, Lynch SV. Role of microbiota in inflammatory bowel diseases. Inflamm Bowel Dis. 2012;18:968–80.
24. Sekirov I, Russell SL, Atunes CM, Finlay BB. Gut microbiota in health and disease. Physiol Rev. 2010;90:859–904.
25. Tannock GW. New Perceptions of the gut microbiota: implications for future research. Gastroenterol Clin N Am. 2005;41:361–82.
26. Chatterjess S, Kar P, Das T, et al. Randomised placebo-controlled double blind multicentric trial on efficacy and safety of Lactobacillus acidophilus LA-5 and bifidobacterium BB-12 for prevention of antibiotic-associated diarrhea. J Assoc Physicians India. 2013;61:708–12.
27. Abbas Z, Yakoob J, Jafri W, et al. Cytokine and clinical response to Saccharomyces boulardii therapy in diarrhea-dominant irritable bowel syndrome: a randomized trial. Eur J Gastroenterol Hepatol. 2014;26:630–9.
28. Bajaj JS, Heuman DM, Hylemon PB, et al. Randomised clinical trial: lactobacillus GG modulates gut microbiome, metabolome and endotoxemia in patients with cirrhosis. Ailment Pharmacol Ther. 2014;39:1113–25.

29. Aoki T, Asahara T, Matsumoto K, et al. Effects of the continuous intake of a milk drink containing Lactobacillus casei strain Shirota on abdominal symptoms, fecal microbiota, and metabolites in gastrectomized subjects. Scand J Gastroenterol. 2014;49:552–63.

30. Hegar B, Hutapea EI, Advani N, et al. A double-blind placebo-controlled randomized trial on probiotics in small bowel bacterial overgrowth in children treated with omeprazole. J Pediatr. 2013;89:381–7.

31. Shao F, Xin FZ, Yang CG, et al. The impact of microbial immune enteral nutrition on the patients with acute radiation enteritis in bowel function and immune status. Cell Biochem Biophys. 2014;69:357–61.

32. Virk A, Mandrekar J, Berbari EF, et al. A randomized, double blind, placebo-controlled trial of an oral symbiotic (AKSB) for prevention of travelers' diarrhea. J Travel Med. 2013;20:88–94.

33. Woodward GA, Encarnacion B, Downey JR, et al. Probiotics improve outcomes after Roux-en-Y gastric bypass surgery: a prospective randomized trial. J Gastrointest Surg. 2009;13:1198–204.

34. Mekkes MC, Weenen TC, Brummer RJ, et al. The development of probiotic treatment in obesity: a review. Benef Microbes. 2014;5:19–28.

35. Gomes AC, Bueno AA, de Souza RG, et al. Gut microbiota, probiotics and diabetes. Nutr J. 2014;13:60. doi:10.1186/1475-2891-13-60.

Glen B. Chun and Charles A. Powell

ADL	Activities of daily living
BMD	Bone mineral density
BMI	Body mass index
CF	Cystic fibrosis
CFA	Coefficient of fat absorption
CFTR	Cystic fibrosis transmembrane conductance regulator
COPD	Chronic obstructive pulmonary disease
DASH	Dietary approaches to stop hypertension
DIOS	Distal intestinal obstruction syndrome
DIP	Desquamative interstitial pneumonia
EELV	End-expiratory lung volume
EPI	Exocrine pancreatic insufficiency
ERV	Expiratory reserve volume
FE1	Fecal pancreatic elastase-1
FEV1	Forced expiratory volume at 1 s
FFM	Fat-free mass
FVC	Forced vital capacity
GI	Gastrointestinal
ILD	Interstitial lung disease
IM	Intramuscular
IPF	Idiopathic pulmonary fibrosis
MMA	Methylmalonic acid
NAC	N-acetyl cysteine
NREM	Non-rapid eye movement
OSA	Obstructive sleep apnea
PERT	Pancreatic enzyme replacement therapy
PLCH	Pulmonary Langerhans' cell histiocytosis
PMN	Polymorphonuclear leukocytes
PN	Parenteral nutrition
ppd	Pack per day
RBILD	Respiratory bronchiolitis-associated interstitial lung disease
REE	Resting energy expenditure
ROS	Reactive oxygen species
TST	Total sleep time

Introduction

Lifestyle medicine is an integral but often overlooked component in the management of chronic pulmonary disease. Contributing to this deficiency is the general lack of substantiating literature and specific evidence to guide pulmonologists on how to best address these crucial lifestyle issues. Typically, pulmonary disease lifestyle modifications predominantly and appropriately focus on smoking cessation given that:

- Smoking is the leading preventable cause of death and premature disease worldwide.
- Smoking is accountable for 20 % of deaths in men > 30 years of age and 5 % in women worldwide and in the USA.
- Smoking is responsible for more than 435,000 smoking-related deaths annually.
- For every death caused by smoking, approximately 20 % of smokers are afflicted with a smoking-related illness [1].

Pulmonary diseases tend to be systemic processes that affect multiple organ systems. For instance, pulmonary hypertension can cause right ventricular dysfunction and cor pulmonale; obstructive sleep apnea (OSA) can cause hypoxemia that worsens pulmonary hypertension, and OSA is associated with systemic hypertension and increased risk for ischemic strokes. Similarly, there are systemic effects of treatments for chronic pulmonary diseases. Steroids are an effective anti-inflammatory that are associated with glucose intolerance,

C. A. Powell (✉)
Division of Pulmonary, Critical Care and Sleep Medicine, Icahn School of Medicine at Mount Sinai, One Gustave L Levy Place, Box 1232, New York, NY 10029, USA
e-mail: Charles.Powell@mssm.edu

G. B. Chun
Division of Pulmonary, Critical Care and Sleep Medicine, Icahn School of Medicine at Mount Sinai, New York, NY, USA

© Springer International Publishing Switzerland 2016
J. I. Mechanick, R. F. Kushner (eds.), *Lifestyle Medicine*, DOI 10.1007/978-3-319-24687-1_31

hyperglycemia, body composition change, muscle loss, and bone loss; steroid-sparing agents are associated with immunosuppression, liver function abnormalities, and bone marrow suppression. Thus, an integrative approach to chronic pulmonary disease that accounts for these systemic effects can be highly effective and therapeutic. More specifically, a comprehensive lifestyle medicine approach for chronic pulmonary disease should focus on smoking cessation, nutrition, depression, physical activity, sexual dysfunction, behavior, and sleep hygiene.

Cystic Fibrosis

Cystic fibrosis (CF) is an autosomal recessive disease involving mutations in the cystic fibrosis transmembrane conductance regulator (CFTR) gene that affects multiple organ systems, such as the lungs, kidneys, and pancreas.[2] CF affects approximately 80,000 individuals worldwide [3]. According to the 2005 CF Foundation patient registry report, 23% of children with CF are below the 10th percentile weight-for-age and 22% of adults with CF have a body mass index (BMI) that is underweight. The malnutrition associated with CF is due to increased energy expenditure, increased micronutrient requirements, and nutrient malabsorption [4]. The energy expenditure of a patient with CF is determined by resting energy expenditure (REE; 60–70%), physical activity (10–25%), and diet-induced thermogenesis (10%) [5]. The majority of CF patients have a higher energy requirement—approximately 120–150% of normal requirements—due to increased resting energy expenditure and work of breathing resulting from obstructive and restrictive lung disease [6].

Approximately 80–90% of CF patients exhibit exocrine pancreatic insufficiency [3, 7, 8]. Decreased production and secretion of pancreatic enzymes lead to maldigestion and malabsorption of fat (and consequently fat-soluble vitamins [A, D, E, and K]) and protein. Approximately 20–30% of CF patients are predisposed to distal intestinal obstruction syndrome (DIOS), which is characterized by partial or complete fecal obstruction of the ileo-cecum. Impaired fat absorption in DIOS leads to significant malnutrition, failure to thrive, and steatorrhea [3]. Malnutrition in CF patients is also associated with worse overall general health, worse severity of pulmonary disease, and overall shorter life expectancy [4, 9].

CF patients have higher prevalence rates of osteoporosis and fractures. This is generally due to glucocorticoid therapy, malabsorption (leading to vitamin D undernutrition and secondary hyperparathyroidism), malnutrition, hypogonadism, decreased physical activity, and smaller skeletal frames [10]. Ferguson et al. [11] reported that a low bone mineral density (BMD) was associated with reduced vitamin D levels, despite oral supplementation of 400–800 IU vitamin D

daily. CF patients should have 25-hydroxyvitamin D levels measured routinely and then supplemented if low (< 30 ng/ml) [10], [12, 13]. The CF Foundation nutritional guidelines recommend the following: 400–500 IU vitamin D/day for children 12 months and younger, 800–1000 IU vitamin D/day for 1–10 years of age, and 800–1200 IU vitamin D/day for 11 years and older.

Patients with CF must be screened for exocrine pancreatic insufficiency (EPI) via fecal analysis either by calculation of the coefficient of fat absorption (CFA; the "gold standard") or by measurement of fecal pancreatic elastase-1 (FE1). EPI is treated with pancreatic enzyme replacement therapy (PERT) [14].

Vitamin B12 deficiency is seen in CF patients as another consequence of pancreatic insufficiency. The pathophysiology of B12 deficiency is due to a lack of cleavage of R proteins from the B12-intrinsic factor complex, leading to an inability of B12 to be absorbed in the terminal ileum. This deficiency is treated by initiation of PERT and vitamin B12 supplementation as guided by monitoring of vitamin B12 status [15, 16]. Vitamin B12 status is best assessed by measuring methylmalonic acid (MMA) [17]. When B12 levels are insufficient or deficient, MMA levels are abnormally elevated.

Mild vitamin deficiency states are usually not clinically evident. Hence, a prudent strategy to prevent subclinical abnormalities is to prevent these anticipated deficiencies. Consensus recommendations are to prophylactically provide supplemental vitamins based on the patient's risk status and clinical presentation. For patients at risk, we recommend biochemical testing (e.g., serum vitamin levels directly or with functional markers such as MMA) at baseline and follow-up after treatment (Table 31.1) [5].

Antioxidants may have a role in the treatment of CF. The production of reactive oxygen species (ROS) from persistent polymorphonuclear leukocytes (PMN)-dominated inflammation secondary to frequent recurrent pulmonary infections (specifically *Pseudomonas aeruginosa*) causes high levels of oxidative stress. The evidence to support the use of antioxidants in CF patients remains equivocal; however, some studies have shown improvements in pulmonary function (forced expiratory volume at 1 s (FEV_1) and forced vital capacity (FVC)) in CF patients treated with vitamin E, vitamin C, β-carotene, selenium, glutathione, and N-acetyl cysteine (NAC) [18].

Appetite stimulants, such as megestrol acetate (a progesterone steroid) and cyproheptadine hydrochloride (a serotonin and histamine antagonist), have been used to improve weight gain and appetite, without any proven significant benefit to pulmonary function [19–22]. Despite attempts to improve appetite and to control fat maldigestion and malnutrition with PERT, higher fat diets, and/or vitamin supple-

Table 31.1 Vitamin supplementation in cystic fibrosis[a]

Vitamins	Target population	Recommended dosages
A	Pancreatic insufficiency	4000–10,000 IU daily
D	Pancreatic insufficiency	400–800 IU daily
E	All CF patients	100–400 IU daily
K	Pancreatic insufficiency	1 mg daily to 10 mg per week
B12	Schilling Test <45 % after ileal resection pancreatic insufficiency	1000 µg intramuscular (IM) at least several times per week for 1–2 weeks, then weekly until clear improvement is shown, followed by monthly injections Alternative monitoring measurement: serum methylmalonic acid, homocysteine level, or both
Water soluble vitamins	Not indicated with normal diet	

[a] See reference [5, 17]

mentation, CF patients often require enteral tube feeding via a nasogastric or gastrostomy route in order to improve weight gain, nutritional status, lung function, and quality of life. More research is needed to compare tube feeding with oral supplementation and with normal diet [6]. Parenteral nutrition (PN) is recommended for infants and children after major gastrointestinal (GI) surgery or those who are severely ill and waiting for possible transplantation [5]. PN is also used for short-term support of adult patients with severe malnutrition who are unable to tolerate enteral nutrition support. PN is not generally considered a solution for long-term nutrition support in CF.

Physical activity is critical in the management of CF patients. Studies have shown that exercise therapy can lead to a slowed rate of decline in pulmonary function for CF patients [23].

Chronic Obstructive Pulmonary Disease

Chronic obstructive pulmonary disease (COPD) is a major global health issue. In 2020, COPD is projected to rank fifth in worldwide burden of disease and third in mortality. COPD is defined as a preventable and largely lifestyle-dependent disease [24]. COPD is characterized by persistent airflow obstruction (a mixture of small airways disease and parenchymal destruction) resulting from chronic inflammation and remodeling of the airways [25].

Among patients with COPD, low BMI has an independent adverse effect on all-cause mortality and COPD mortality [26]. Moreover, increasing BMI was found to have an association with decreased mortality in patients with severe COPD [26]. The prognostic advantage of mildly increased BMI in COPD, a phenomenon known as the "obesity paradox," is not fully understood [26, 27]. Conversely, obesity in COPD is associated with increased cardiovascular risk, related to a decrease in fat-free mass (FFM) and higher fat mass index, with redistribution of fat from subcutaneous to visceral areas [28]. Severe obesity presents the challenge of causing a restrictive physiology in pulmonary function in

these patients, along with a significant decrease in expiratory reserve volume (ERV) and end-expiratory lung volume (EELV) [29].

Malnutrition is prevalent in patients with COPD: 30–60 % in inpatients and 10–45 % in outpatients [30, 31]. Weight loss in patients with COPD has been found to be an independent negative determinant of survival, substantiating an imperative for achieving and maintaining a healthy weight in patient care [28]. Nutritional status is influenced by hormonal derangements in acute COPD exacerbations that cause elevated systemic levels of leptin and proinflammatory cytokines that reduce appetite and decrease dietary intake [31].

Patients with low body weights have significant physiological abnormalities compared to normal weight patients with COPD who have comparable respiratory mechanics and degree of airflow obstruction. Patients with lower body weights have a greater degree of gas trapping, lower diffusion capacity, and lower exercise capacity. These physiologic abnormalities are caused by the loss of body cell mass and the associated reduction in the mass of the diaphragm, and respiratory muscles, leading to decreased strength, and endurance [32].

Malnutrition also causes a decrease in immune status that further decreases airway defenses [32, 33]. To prevent hypercapnea, patients with COPD are often advised to limit carbohydrate consumption. This consequence of carbohydrate consumption can be overcome by consuming smaller meal portions throughout the day [31].

Patients with COPD should increase dietary intake of foods such as fruits and vegetables due to their rich antioxidant content (vitamin C, vitamin E, β-carotene, and carotenoids), which have been shown to be associated with improvement of pulmonary function [34–39]. Other studies have reported associations between antioxidants (specifically vitamin C and lycopene) and all-cause mortality in COPD individuals [37].

Vitamin D deficiency plays an important role in bone and calcium balance as well as having anti-inflammatory and anti-infectious properties. Oral supplementation of vitamin D (800–2000 IU/day) is recommended to achieve target serum levels >30 ng/dl along as is adequate elemental calcium from the diet and supplementation as needed [28]. There is also a role for adequate dietary fiber (>25 g/day, the highest quartile/quintile based on the European Food Safety Authority). Fiber has been reported to enhance lung function, lower the odds of developing COPD as well as to reduce the risk for respiratory symptoms in patients with COPD [24, 40, 41]. However, the evidence base for these studies is relatively small and more research is needed.

The most important lifestyle modification in COPD patients is smoking cessation. Cigarette smoking leads to increased ROS that may cause inflammatory stress-induced damage [42]. Smoking cessation in COPD patients remains the only treatment shown to be effective in slowing down the decline in FEV_1 [43] as well as decrease the frequency of early chronic respiratory symptoms in patients with COPD [44]. The Lung Health Study has shown that smoking cessation led to a small improvement in FEV_1 in the first year and a reduction in the rate of decline by approximately 50% in patients who sustained their abstinence from smoking. Significant smoking reduction (<5 cigarettes per day) is associated with a reduced FEV_1 decline [44, 45].

Physical activity is an important lifestyle modification for patients with COPD and is a strong predictor of all-cause mortality [46]. Exercise limitation in chronic pulmonary disease patients is the result of multiple factors including: ventilation constraints, gas exchange abnormalities, cardiac dysfunction, peripheral muscle dysfunction, mood disorders, and limited motivation. Exercise is strongly encouraged, though many patients are often too debilitated to maintain vigorous physical activity. Therefore, pulmonary rehabilitation has become an integral component in the management of COPD. Studies have proven the efficacy of a variety of outpatient pulmonary rehabilitation exercises such as interval training, strength training, upper limb training, and transcutaneous neuromuscular electrical stimulation [47]. One study has even shown that the use of progressive resistance training during hospitalization significantly improves lower-limb muscle strength, 6-min walk test distance, and health-care-related quality of life [48]. Pulmonary rehabilitation has been proven to be effective in improving symptoms, exercise tolerance, and quality of life. [47] Though the majority of studies have shown significant benefit of exercise training in moderate-to-severe COPD, there is recent evidence suggesting that early recognition and exercise training for mild-to-moderate COPD may improve exercise endurance, reduce hospitalizations, reduce symptoms, improve quality of life, and reduce health-care-related costs [49].

The prevalence of depression in COPD is 40% with 20% classified as moderate-to-severe [50]. Anxiety and depression correlate with health-related quality of life in COPD [51]. Depression can lead to further worsening of dyspnea due to hopelessness and decreased adherence with medical

and rehabilitation interventions [50, 52–54]. To date, there are no studies that convincingly demonstrate the efficacy of antidepressant medications on depression symptoms, dyspnea, or other physiological metrics specifically in COPD patients [50].

Sexual dysfunction is a major determinant of quality of life in patients with COPD that also needs to be addressed in routine lifestyle evaluations [55]. Male sexual dysfunction has been correlated with COPD disease activity in the absence of other known causes of sexual dysfunction [56]. Erectile dysfunction is the most common sexual dysfunction experienced in men with COPD older than the age of 55 years and leads to a significant negative impact on quality of life [57–59]. Sexual dysfunction is due to a combination of fear of dyspnea, reduced exercise tolerance, misconceptions, lack of understanding, and poor physical or mental health. Sexuality (including libido and performance) is negatively impacted by the use of noninvasive mechanical ventilation [60].

When evaluating patients with COPD, it is important to assess sleep quality and screen for sleep apnea and hypoxemia. The prevalence of sleep apnea in COPD patients is similar to the general population; however, hypoxemia during sleep is significantly more pronounced in the population with COPD [61]. Patient with COPD may develop hypoxemia when sleeping, which can be attributed to the chronic pulmonary disease rather than sleep apnea. Sleep hypoventilation is a common occurrence in patients with severe COPD and may contribute to chronic hypercapnic respiratory failure [62–64].

Asthma

Asthma is a chronic inflammatory disease, affecting the airways, and involving a complex imbalance of inflammatory cells and inflammatory mediators [65]. Over the past few decades, the prevalence of asthma has markedly increased. In the USA, the prevalence of asthma rose from 20.3 million in 2001 to 25.6 million in 2012 [66]. Globally, asthma affects 300 million people and is expected to affect 400 million by the year 2050 [66, 67].

Dietary change is one of the proposed environmental exposures that has led to a rising incidence of asthma over the past few decades. In particular, it is suspected that the westernization of the American diet has led to a chronic metabolic surplus and deficiency of micronutrients that are associated with increased inflammation. A western diet is more processed, "convenience oriented," and ultimately results in a state of chronic energy excess and decrease in fiber and micronutrients [65].

Recent studies have focused on asthma prevention by improving maternal nutrition during pregnancy. Despite a meta-analysis of clinical trials that did not demonstrate a strong association between eating patterns and asthma in adults or between maternal diet and childhood asthma or wheezing [66], current research continues to focus on the role of antioxidants, micronutrients, and fatty acid consumption by pregnant women in association with asthma outcomes in children [68–76]. A recent study has shown that reduced maternal iron status during pregnancy is adversely associated with childhood wheezing, lung function, and atopic sensitization [77]. Low antioxidant intake has been associated with higher asthma and allergy incidence; antioxidant supplementation may improve asthma control and lung function [78]. Currently, there is an ongoing clinical trial evaluating the implementation of the Dietary Approaches to Stop Hypertension (DASH) diet as adjunct therapy in uncontrolled asthma. This DASH diet study provides increased fruits and vegetables as a source for augmented antioxidant consumption while also monitoring symptoms, inflammatory markers, and pulmonary physiology [65]. In addition, the consumption of milk, wheat, and peanuts has been associated with reduced odds of childhood allergy and asthma [79].

Physical activity is important for the improvement of quality of life in patients with asthma. Exercise tolerance can be extremely limited due to dyspnea, which can lead to deconditioning and to a sedentary lifestyle [80]. In general, exercise should be recommended without concern for exacerbation [81]. Physical training protocols have been developed for patients with asthma with the overall goal of improving physical fitness. These programs include aerobic exercise, such as running, jogging, cycling, weight training, swimming, stretching, individually and in combination [80, 82]. Regular aerobic exercise has been found to improve asthma-related symptoms, lung function, and mental health [82, 83]. Water-based exercise has been proposed as a good exercise option for patients with asthma in order to improve muscle strength, cardiopulmonary fitness, flexibility, and body composition [80, 84]. Moreover, water-based exercise is beneficial to patients with asthma due to the temperature of the water and pollen-free air, which together facilitate air exchange. However, there are no conclusive studies to support the use of aquatic exercise in asthma for improvement of quality of life [80]. Central obesity has been associated with active asthma, possibly related to the effects of visceral adipose tissue deposition on pro-inflammatory mediators. These associations highlight the importance of diet and exercise in asthma [85].

Smoking is a preventable risk factor for patients with asthma. Namely, patients with asthma who smoke are at a higher risk of developing COPD than patients without asthma [86]. A review of data from Finland has found that exposure to smoking has been linked to higher incidence of several diseases, including asthma. The effects have been found to be greatest when smoking exposure occurs during pregnancy and in early childhood; however, larger and more comprehensive studies are needed to further corroborate this finding [87]. In a study by Gilliland et al. [88], regular smoking was associated with an increased relative risk (3.9) of new-onset asthma in children who reported smoking 300+ cigarettes per year compared to the nonsmokers.

Interstitial Lung Disease

Interstitial lung disease (ILD) includes a variety of disorders with a varying spectrum of underlying etiologies such as idiopathic, connective tissue disease related, and environmental exposure related. There is a subset of ILD that is directly associated with smoking exposure. These smoking-related ILDs include: desquamative interstitial pneumonia (DIP), respiratory bronchiolitis-associated interstitial lung disease (RBILD), and pulmonary Langerhans' cell histiocytosis (PLCH) [89–91]. Although DIP and RBILD are treated with steroids and PLCH is treated with corticosteroids or cytotoxic drugs, the mainstay initial therapeutic approach to smokers with these interstitial lung diseases is smoking cessation [90, 92, 93].

Progressive diminished exercise capacity is a hallmark of idiopathic pulmonary fibrosis (IPF). When evaluating IPF, there are several independent factors that can be used to predict mortality: age, hospitalizations, FVC, longitudinal change in FVC, 6-min walk distance as well as the longitudinal change in 6-min walk distance [94]. Recent studies show that pulmonary rehabilitation is beneficial to patients with ILD and that there is an improvement in quality of life and leg strength in patients with IPF who undergo an exercise-training program [95]. Patients who underwent pulmonary rehabilitation were found to have improved quality of life, less shortness of breath, and improved exercise tolerance (average improvement of 44 m in 6 min) [96–98]. The sustained benefit of pulmonary rehabilitation is unclear once the pulmonary rehab ceases.

OSA is a common comorbidity in patients with ILD. Therefore, it is recommended that patients with ILD should be screened for the presence of OSA [99]. Patients with ILD have been found to have persistently increased respiratory rates during sleep, disrupted sleep, and frequent arousals [100, 101]. Specifically, they often have an increase in arousals, an increase in N1 (non-rapid eye movement, NREM; light sleep stage) and N2 (NREM; less-activated brain waves stage) sleep, and a decrease in N3 (NREM; slow (delta) brain waves and deep sleep stage) and REM sleep [100, 102]. In a study by Perez-Padilla et al. [100], patients with ILD were found to be in N1 sleep 33.7% of their total sleep time (TST) compared to 13.5% of non-ILD controls and in REM 11.8% of their TST compared to 19.9% in non-ILD controls. The study also showed that the hypoxemia experienced during REM was more severe in those with more severe awake hypoxemia, which suggests the utility of nocturnal oximetry monitoring [100].

Clinical Case

A 65 y/o male with a history of COPD presents for progressively worsening dyspnea and reduced exercise tolerance. He has a history of COPD, diagnosed 5 years ago and an extensive smoking history, with multiple bouts of failed attempts at smoking cessation. His exercise tolerance is approximately 20 ft before having to stop due to significant dyspnea. He reports that his dyspnea has become so severe that he can no longer work and is having trouble with his activities of daily living (ADL). He smoked 1 pack per day (ppd) for 45 years and is currently down to 1/4 ppd. His most recent spirometry showed a severe obstructive ventilatory defect with a FEV_1 of 0.84 1 (25 % of his predicted value) and a 6-min walk test revealed a significant hypoxemia after his 3rd minute of ambulation that required 2 1 of supplemental oxygen to maintain an oxygen saturation (SaO_2) >90 % and a total distance of 125 m. Additional past medical history includes hypertension and hyperlipidemia. Family history was significant for lung cancer and COPD in his father. He denied any feelings of depression or anxiety. He reports that he has been steadily losing weight over the past few years despite having no significant change in diet or appetite. He has on average, 4–5 exacerbations that require either a course of steroids, antibiotics, or both. His current medications include: tiotropium (Spiriva), fluticasone propionate-salmeterol inhaled (Advair), and both an albuterol nebulizer and rescue inhaler.

Recommended lifestyle modifications included:

1. Pulmonary rehabilitation to increase exercise capacity and endurance.
2. Smoking cessation—counseling and consideration of nicotine replacement and pharmacologic agents (Bupropion or Varenicline).
3. Dietary evaluation and nutritional status monitoring. Suggest modifications to increase protein intake, decrease carbohydrates, and consume smaller, more frequent meals.
4. Medications—to help prevent recurrent exacerbations, suggest starting the patient on chronic macrolide therapy (Azithromycin 250 mg PO TIW) in addition to his maintenance inhaler regimen.
5. Supplemental oxygen therapy.
6. Screening for OSA and nocturnal hypoxemia.

A follow-up appointment was made for 6 weeks after the previous visit. He was sent to pulmonary rehabilitation

with some noted subjective and objective improvement in dyspnea. His exercise capacity improved from 20 ft to approximately 100 ft. Subjectively, he felt less dyspneic and stronger overall. His weight remained the same. However, he reported an increase in his appetite. The patient reported that he did not change his diet to a lower carbohydrate diet but was amenable to making the changes after this current visit. He was started on varenicline for smoking cessation and reported a decrease in smoking, cutting down to 1–2 cigarettes per day. Oxygen supplementation was started, specifically for use with exertion for which he feels better but reports not always using the oxygen. He was assessed for signs of OSA and was ordered for a polysomnography to diagnose OSA. Discussions were held regarding starting daliresp (a selective phosphodiesterase 4 (PDE4) inhibitor). Follow-up spirometry and 6-min walk test should be performed within 3–6 months.

References

1. Cahill K, et al. Pharmacological interventions for smoking cessation: an overview and network meta-analysis. Cochrane Database Syst Rev. 2013;5:Cd009329.
2. O'Sullivan BP, Freedman SD. Cystic fibrosis. Lancet. 2009;373(9678):1891–904.
3. Somaraju UR, Solis-Moya A. Pancreatic enzyme replacement therapy for people with cystic fibrosis. Cochrane Database Syst Rev. 2014;10:Cd008227.
4. Stallings VA, et al. Evidence-based practice recommendations for nutrition-related management of children and adults with cystic fibrosis and pancreatic insufficiency: results of a systematic review. J Am Diet Assoc. 2008;108(5):832–9.
5. Sinaasappel M, et al. Nutrition in patients with cystic fibrosis: a European Consensus. J Cyst Fibros. 2002;1(2):51–75.
6. Conway SP, Morton A, Wolfe S. Enteral tube feeding for cystic fibrosis. Cochrane Database Syst Rev, 2008;2:Cd001198.
7. Fieker A, Philpott J, Armand M. Enzyme replacement therapy for pancreatic insufficiency: present and future. Clin Exp Gastroenterol. 2011;4:55–73.
8. Bruno MJ, et al. Maldigestion associated with exocrine pancreatic insufficiency: implications of gastrointestinal physiology and properties of enzyme preparations for a cause-related and patient-tailored treatment. Am J Gastroenterol. 1995;90(9):1383–93.
9. Corey M, et al. A comparison of survival, growth, and pulmonary function in patients with cystic fibrosis in Boston and Toronto. J Clin Epidemiol. 1988;41(6):583–91.
10. Donovan DS Jr., et al. Bone mass and vitamin D deficiency in adults with advanced cystic fibrosis lung disease. Am J Respir Crit Care Med. 1998;157(6 Pt 1):1892–9.
11. Ferguson JH, Chang AB. Vitamin D supplementation for cystic fibrosis. Cochrane Database Syst Rev. 2012;4:Cd007298.
12. Stalvey MS, Clines GA. Cystic fibrosis-related bone disease: insights into a growing problem. Curr Opin Endocrinol Diabetes Obes. 2013;20(6):547–52.
13. Tangpricha V, et al. An update on the screening, diagnosis, management, and treatment of vitamin D deficiency in individuals with cystic fibrosis: evidence-based recommendations from the Cystic Fibrosis Foundation. J Clin Endocrinol Metab. 2012;97(4):1082–93.

14. Smyth AR, et al. European Cystic Fibrosis Society Standards of Care: best practice guidelines. J Cyst Fibros. 2014;13(Suppl 1):S23–42.

15. Gaskin KJ. Nutritional care in children with cystic fibrosis: are our patients becoming better? Eur J Clin Nutr. 2013;67(5):558–64.

16. Gueant JL, et al. Malabsorption of vitamin B12 in pancreatic insufficiency of the adult and of the child. Pancreas. 1990;5(5):559–67.

17. Stabler SP. Clinical practice. Vitamin B12 deficiency. N Engl J Med. 2013;368(2):149–60.

18. Ciofu O, Lykkesfeldt J. Antioxidant supplementation for lung disease in cystic fibrosis. Cochrane Database Syst Rev. 2014;8:Cd007020.

19. Chinuck R, et al. Appetite stimulants for people with cystic fibrosis. Cochrane Database Syst Rev. 2014;7:Cd008190.

20. Eubanks V, et al. Effects of megestrol acetate on weight gain, body composition, and pulmonary function in patients with cystic fibrosis. J Pediatr. 2002;140(4):439–44.

21. Homnick DN, Marks JH, Rubin BK. The effect of a first-generation antihistamine on sputum viscoelasticity in cystic fibrosis. J Aerosol Med. 2007;20(1):45–9.

22. Marchand V, et al. Randomized, double-blind, placebo-controlled pilot trial of megestrol acetate in malnourished children with cystic fibrosis. J Pediatr Gastroenterol Nutr. 2000;31(3):264–9.

23. Schneiderman-Walker J, et al. A randomized controlled trial of a 3-year home exercise program in cystic fibrosis. J Pediatr. 2000;136(3):304–10.

24. Fonseca Wald EL, et al. Dietary fibre and fatty acids in chronic obstructive pulmonary disease risk and progression: a systematic review. Respirology. 2014;19(2):176–84.

25. Vestbo J, et al. Global strategy for the diagnosis, management, and prevention of chronic obstructive pulmonary disease: GOLD executive summary. Am J Respir Crit Care Med. 2013;187(4):347–65.

26. Landbo C, et al. Prognostic value of nutritional status in chronic obstructive pulmonary disease. Am J Respir Crit Care Med. 1999;160(6):1856–61.

27. Ora J, et al. Effect of obesity on respiratory mechanics during rest and exercise in COPD. J Appl Physiol (1985). 2011;111(1):10–9.

28. Schols AM, et al. Nutritional assessment and therapy in COPD: a European Respiratory Society statement. Eur Respir J. 2014;44(6):1504–20.

29. O'Donnell DE, Ciavaglia CE, Neder JA. When obesity and chronic obstructive pulmonary disease collide. Physiological and clinical consequences. Ann Am Thorac Soc. 2014;11(4):635–44.

30. Collins PF, Stratton RJ, Elia M. Nutritional support in chronic obstructive pulmonary disease: a systematic review and meta-analysis. Am J Clin Nutr. 2012;95(6):1385–95.

31. Schols AM. Nutrition as a metabolic modulator in COPD. Chest. 2013;144(4):1340–5.

32. Ezzell L, Jensen GL. Malnutrition in chronic obstructive pulmonary disease. Am J Clin Nutr. 2000;72(6):1415–6.

33. Collins PF, Elia M, Stratton RJ. Nutritional support and functional capacity in chronic obstructive pulmonary disease: a systematic review and meta-analysis. Respirology. 2013;18(4):616–29.

34. Britton JR, et al. Dietary antioxidant vitamin intake and lung function in the general population. Am J Respir Crit Care Med. 1995;151(5):1383–7.

35. Chen R, et al. Association of dietary antioxidants and waist circumference with pulmonary function and airway obstruction. Am J Epidemiol. 2001;153(2):157–63.

36. Chuwers P, et al. The protective effect of beta-carotene and retinol on ventilatory function in an asbestos-exposed cohort. Am J Respir Crit Care Med. 1997;155(3):1066–71.

37. Ford ES, et al. Associations between antioxidants and all-cause mortality among US adults with obstructive lung function. Br J Nutr. 2014;112(10):1662–73.

38. Grievink L, et al. Dietary intake of antioxidant (pro)-vitamins, respiratory symptoms and pulmonary function: the MORGEN study. Thorax. 1998;53(3):166–71.

39. Schunemann HJ, et al. Lung function in relation to intake of carotenoids and other antioxidant vitamins in a population-based study. Am J Epidemiol. 2002;155(5):463–71.

40. Kan H, et al. Dietary fiber, lung function, and chronic obstructive pulmonary disease in the atherosclerosis risk in communities study. Am J Epidemiol. 2008;167(5):570–8.

41. Varraso R, Willett WC, Camargo CA Jr. Prospective study of dietary fiber and risk of chronic obstructive pulmonary disease among US women and men. Am J Epidemiol. 2010;171(7):776–84.

42. Zuo L, et al. Interrelated role of cigarette smoking, oxidative stress, and immune response in COPD and corresponding treatments. Am J Physiol Lung Cell Mol Physiol. 2014;307(3):L205–18.

43. Willemse BW, et al. Effect of 1-year smoking cessation on airway inflammation in COPD and asymptomatic smokers. Eur Respir J. 2005;26(5):835–45.

44. Simmons MS, et al. Smoking reduction and the rate of decline in FEV(1): results from the Lung Health Study. Eur Respir J. 2005;25(6):1011–7.

45. Ind PW. COPD disease progression and airway inflammation: uncoupled by smoking cessation. Eur Respir J. 2005;26(5):764–6.

46. Waschki B, et al. Physical activity is the strongest predictor of all-cause mortality in patients with COPD: a prospective cohort study. Chest. 2011;140(2):331–42.

47. Spruit MA, et al. An official American Thoracic Society/European Respiratory Society statement: key concepts and advances in pulmonary rehabilitation. Am J Respir Crit Care Med. 2013;188(8):e13–e64.

48. Borges RC, Carvalho CR. Impact of resistance training in chronic obstructive pulmonary disease patients during periods of acute exacerbation. Arch Phys Med Rehabil. 2014;95(9):1638–45.

49. O'Donnell DE, Gebke KB. Examining the role of activity, exercise, and pharmacology in mild COPD. Postgrad Med. 2014;126(5):135–45.

50. Yohannes AM, Alexopoulos GS. Pharmacological treatment of depression in older patients with chronic obstructive pulmonary disease: impact on the course of the disease and health outcomes. Drugs Aging. 2014;31(7):483–92.

51. Blakemore A, et al. Depression and anxiety predict health-related quality of life in chronic obstructive pulmonary disease: systematic review and meta-analysis. Int J Chron Obstruct Pulmon Dis. 2014;9:501–12.

52. Maurer J, et al. Anxiety and depression in COPD: current understanding, unanswered questions, and research needs. Chest. 2008;134(4 Suppl):43 s–56 s.

53. Whiteford HA, et al. Global burden of disease attributable to mental and substance use disorders: findings from the Global Burden of Disease Study 2010. Lancet. 2013;382(9904):1575–86.

54. Yohannes AM, Baldwin RC, Connolly MJ. Depression and anxiety in elderly outpatients with chronic obstructive pulmonary disease: prevalence, and validation of the BASDEC screening questionnaire. Int J Geriatr Psychiatry. 2000;15(12):1090–6.

55. Vincent EE, Singh SJ. Review article: addressing the sexual health of patients with COPD: the needs of the patient and implications for health care professionals. Chron Respir Dis. 2007;4(2):111–5.

56. Fletcher EC, Martin RJ. Sexual dysfunction and erectile impotence in chronic obstructive pulmonary disease. Chest. 1982;81(4):413–21.

57. Karadag F, et al. Correlates of erectile dysfunction in moderate-to-severe chronic obstructive pulmonary disease patients. Respirology. 2007;12(2):248–53.

58. Koseoglu N, et al. Erectile dysfunction prevalence and sexual function status in patients with chronic obstructive pulmonary disease. J Urol. 2005;174(1):249–52; discussion 252.

59. Collins EG, et al. Sexual dysfunction in men with COPD: impact on quality of life and survival. Lung. 2012;190(5):545–56.

60. Schonhofer B, et al. Sexuality in patients with noninvasive mechanical ventilation due to chronic respiratory failure. Am J Respir Crit Care Med. 2001;164(9):1612–7.

61. Sanders MH, et al. Sleep and sleep-disordered breathing in adults with predominantly mild obstructive airway disease. Am J Respir Crit Care Med. 2003;167(1):7–14.

62. Tarrega J, et al. Predicting nocturnal hypoventilation in hypercapnic chronic obstructive pulmonary disease patients undergoing long-term oxygen therapy. Respiration. 2011;82(1):4–9.

63. O'Donoghue FJ, et al. Sleep hypoventilation in hypercapnic chronic obstructive pulmonary disease: prevalence and associated factors. Eur Respir J. 2003;21(6):977–84.

64. Holmedahl NH, et al. Sleep hypoventilation and daytime hypercapnia in stable chronic obstructive pulmonary disease. Int J Chron Obstruct Pulmon Dis. 2014;9:265–75.

65. Ma J, et al. DASH for asthma: a pilot study of the DASH diet in not-well-controlled adult asthma. Contemp Clin Trials. 2013;35(2):55–67.

66. Lv N, Xiao L, Ma J. Dietary pattern and asthma: a systematic review and meta-analysis. J Asthma Allergy. 2014;7:105–21.

67. Masoli M, et al. The global burden of asthma: executive summary of the GINA Dissemination Committee report. Allergy. 2004;59(5):469–78.

68. Nurmatov U, Devereux G, Sheikh A. Nutrients and foods for the primary prevention of asthma and allergy: systematic review and meta-analysis. J Allergy Clin Immunol. 2011;127(3):724–33.e1–30.

69. Lange NE, et al. Maternal dietary pattern during pregnancy is not associated with recurrent wheeze in children. J Allergy Clin Immunol. 2010;126(2):250–5, 255.e1–4.

70. Martindale S, et al. Antioxidant intake in pregnancy in relation to wheeze and eczema in the first two years of life. Am J Respir Crit Care Med. 2005;171(2):121–8.

71. Litonjua AA, et al. Maternal antioxidant intake in pregnancy and wheezing illnesses in children at 2 y of age. Am J Clin Nutr. 2006;84(4):903–11.

72. Devereux G, et al. Low maternal vitamin E intake during pregnancy is associated with asthma in 5-year-old children. Am J Respir Crit Care Med. 2006;174(5):499–507.

73. Miyake Y, et al. Consumption of vegetables, fruit, and antioxidants during pregnancy and wheeze and eczema in infants. Allergy. 2010;65(6):758–65.

74. Miyake Y, et al. Maternal fat consumption during pregnancy and risk of wheeze and eczema in Japanese infants aged 16–24 months: the Osaka Maternal and Child Health Study. Thorax. 2009;64(9):815–21.

75. Camargo CA Jr, et al. Maternal intake of vitamin D during pregnancy and risk of recurrent wheeze in children at 3 y of age. Am J Clin Nutr. 2007;85(3):788–95.

76. Devereux G, et al. Maternal vitamin D intake during pregnancy and early childhood wheezing. Am J Clin Nutr. 2007;85(3):853–9.

77. Nwaru BI, et al. An exploratory study of the associations between maternal iron status in pregnancy and childhood wheeze and atopy. Br J Nutr. 2014;112(12):2018–27.

78. Moreno-Macias H, Romieu I. Effects of antioxidant supplements and nutrients on patients with asthma and allergies. J Allergy Clin Immunol. 2014;133(5):1237–44; quiz 1245.

79. Bunyavanich S, et al. Peanut, milk, and wheat intake during pregnancy is associated with reduced allergy and asthma in children. J Allergy Clin Immunol. 2014;133(5):1373–82.

80. Grande AJ, et al. Water-based exercise for adults with asthma. Cochrane Database Syst Rev. 2014;7:Cd010456.

81. Carson KV, et al. Physical training for asthma. Cochrane Database Syst Rev. 2013;9:Cd001116.

82. Avallone KM, McLeish AC. Asthma and aerobic exercise: a review of the empirical literature. J Asthma. 2013;50(2):109–16.

83. Pacheco DR, et al. Exercise-related quality of life in subjects with asthma: a systematic review. J Asthma. 2012;49(5):487–95.

84. Malkia E, Impivaara O. Intensity of physical activity and respiratory function in subjects with and without bronchial asthma. Scand J Med Sci Sports. 1998;8(1):27–32.

85. Sideleva O, et al. Obesity and asthma: an inflammatory disease of adipose tissue not the airway. Am J Respir Crit Care Med. 2012;186(7):598–605.

86. Lange P, et al. A 15-year follow-up study of ventilatory function in adults with asthma. N Engl J Med. 1998;339(17):1194–200.

87. Pietinalho A, Pelkonen A, Rytila P. Linkage between smoking and asthma. Allergy. 2009;64(12):1722–7.

88. Gilliland FD, et al. Regular smoking and asthma incidence in adolescents. Am J Respir Crit Care Med. 2006;174(10):1094–100.

89. Baumgartner KB, et al. Cigarette smoking: a risk factor for idiopathic pulmonary fibrosis. Am J Respir Crit Care Med. 1997;155(1):242–8.

90. Ryu JH, et al. Smoking-related interstitial lung diseases: a concise review. Eur Respir J. 2001;17(1):122–32.

91. Baumgartner KB, et al. Occupational and environmental risk factors for idiopathic pulmonary fibrosis: a multicenter case-control study. Collaborating Centers. Am J Epidemiol. 2000;152(4):307–15.

92. Vassallo R. Diffuse lung diseases in cigarette smokers. Semin Respir Crit Care Med. 2012;33(5):533–42.

93. Vassallo R, Ryu JH. Smoking-related interstitial lung diseases. Clin Chest Med. 2012;33(1):165–78.

94. du Bois RM, et al. 6-Minute walk distance is an independent predictor of mortality in patients with idiopathic pulmonary fibrosis. Eur Respir J. 2014;43(5):1421–9.

95. Vainshelboim B, et al. Long-term effects of a 12-week exercise training program on clinical outcomes in idiopathic pulmonary fibrosis. Lung. 2015;193(3):345–54. doi:10.1007/s00408-015-9703-0. Epub 2015 March 3.

96. Dowman L, et al. Pulmonary rehabilitation for interstitial lung disease. Cochrane Database Syst Rev. 2014;10:Cd006322.

97. Holland AE, et al. Short term improvement in exercise capacity and symptoms following exercise training in interstitial lung disease. Thorax. 2008;63(6):549–54.

98. Nishiyama O, et al. Effects of pulmonary rehabilitation in patients with idiopathic pulmonary fibrosis. Respirology. 2008;13(3):394–9.

99. Lancaster LH, et al. Obstructive sleep apnea is common in idiopathic pulmonary fibrosis. Chest. 2009;136(3):772–8.

100. Perez-Padilla R, et al. Breathing during sleep in patients with interstitial lung disease. Am Rev Respir Dis. 1985;132(2):224–9.

101. Bye PT, et al. Studies of oxygenation during sleep in patients with interstitial lung disease. Am Rev Respir Dis. 1984;129(1):27–32.

102. Won CH, Kryger M. Sleep in patients with restrictive lung disease. Clin Chest Med. 2014;35(3):505–12.

Lifestyle Medicine and HIV-Infected Patients

32

Vani Gandhi, Tiffany Jung and Jin S. Suh

J. S. Suh (✉)
Department of Medicine, Mount Sinai St. Luke's and Mount Sinai Roosevelt Hospitals, 1111 Amsterdam Avenue, New York, NY 10025, USA
e-mail: JSuh@chpnet.org

V. Gandhi · T. Jung
Spencer Cox Center for Health, Institute for Advanced Medicine, Mount Sinai St. Luke's and Mount Sinai Roosevelt Hospitals, Icahn School of Medicine at Mount Sinai, New York, NY, USA

Abbreviations

ART	Antiretroviral therapy
ACSM	The American College of Sports Medicine
BMI	Body Mass Index
CVD	Cardiovascular disease
FDA	Food and drug administration
HAART	Highly active antiretroviral therapy
HPA	Hypothalamic–pituitary–adrenal
MetS	Metabolic syndrome
NNRTIs	Non-nucleoside reverse transcriptase inhibitors
NRTIs	Nucleoside/nucleotide reverse transcriptase inhibitors
NFHL	Nutrition for healthy living
SAM	Sympathetic–adrenomedullary
SNAP EBT	Supplemental nutrition assistance program electronic benefits transfer
STDs	Sexually transmitted diseases
T2D	Type-2 diabetes

Introduction

HIV is a global public health problem affecting millions of individuals worldwide. By the end of 2013, this pandemic claimed over 39 million lives, and another 35 million people are now estimated to be living with HIV. The use of highly active antiretroviral therapy (HAART) has led to significant reduction in HIV-related morbidity and mortality [1]. Despite the effectiveness of ART, these medications have side effects that can affect quality of life and, in rare cases, lead to potentially life-threatening complications. HIV-infected patients are living longer and are now suffering from the same chronic diseases seen in the general population such as type-2 diabetes (T2D), hypertension, hyperlipidemia, and cardiovascular disease (CVD). It should be recognized that many of these conditions are exacerbated by HIV infection, as well as duration of ART use, underscoring the importance of lifestyle modifications to one's daily regimen. Clinicians should routinely inquire about their patients' diet, nutrition, and exercise habits; evaluate stressors and recommend practical strategies utilizing a multidisciplinary approach. Interventions should be individualized and referrals to appropriate specialists, such as nutritionists, exercise trainers, and counselors, should be considered when feasible.

Nutrition

Nutritional approaches to treating patients with HIV/AIDS have transitioned from clinicians managing malnutrition and wasting to managing obesity and metabolic syndrome (MetS). In the early days of HIV management, proper nutrition was often overlooked, as higher priority was placed on treatment of acute opportunistic infections and preventing progression of immune suppression [2]. In fact, it was common practice to encourage taking antiretroviral medications with unhealthy snacks, caloric drinks, and any other supplements to make it more palatable regardless of the nutritional pitfalls. Only recently has there been more focus on the benefits of proper nutrition in HIV care. Most patients are willing to change their lifestyle with appropriate counseling, education, and support. Currently, there are more than 25 Food and Drug Administration (FDA)-approved antiretroviral drugs in five different classes to treat HIV infection. Clinicians and patients should become familiar with drug-specific side effects, including lipid elevations, abnormalities in glucose metabolism, and increased CVD risks.

Several nutrition studies have been conducted in the general population, but few in HIV-infected patients. Most of the studies have focused on comorbid conditions common in HIV-infected patients, such as T2D, hypertension, and hyperlipidemia. HIV-infected patients often consume high levels of refined sugars, refined grains, processed meats, and other processed foods. Food is often an addiction that occurs after patients give up tobacco or other addictive substances. This is seen in the general population but often in HIV-infected patients due to increased prevalence of smoking and substance use [3]. Many patients with a previous history of tobacco or substance use make unhealthy choices, which may lead to adverse consequences.

MetS is also a complication associated with HIV disease and ART. It is a syndrome characterized by a cluster of components including insulin resistance, enlarged waist circumference, dyslipidemia, elevated blood pressure, impaired fasting glucose, and other risk features of CVD, including vascular inflammation and thrombosis. A high prevalence of MetS has been reported in various studies of HIV-infected patients. MetS increases the risk for development of CVD, T2D, cardiovascular mortality, and all-cause mortality. The Nutrition for Healthy Living (NFHL) study analyzed data from 567 subjects and found that MetS and high triglycerides were associated with an increased risk of death after 36 months of follow-up [4]. It is very important to screen HIV-infected patients for MetS and address all nutrition-related causes.

Although there is controversy regarding the definition as well as the pathogenesis of MetS in the HIV population, there is universal agreement regarding the benefit of nutritional intervention. A number of studies have shown that dietary factors play a major role in the development of MetS in HIV-infected patients [5, 6]. Mediterranean diets are considered as anti-inflammatory eating patterns and have traditionally been recommended to patients with MetS [7]. This eating pattern consists of the ample use of olive oil, along with plenty of fruits and vegetable, whole grains, legumes, nuts, fish, and moderate use of low-fat dairy products and mono- and omega-3 polyunsaturated fats. These diets are low in meat and other animal products. Patients with MetS should be referred to a registered dietitian and receive counseling about healthy nutrition and the benefits of increased physical activity [8]. A recent review by Botros et al. [9] showed that nutritional counseling and exercise interventions are effective for treating obesity and metabolic abnormalities in HIV patients.

Mediterranean diets are beneficial for most patients with MetS, though they do not differentiate between refined versus whole grains. The excess intake of refined grains in the form of bread and pasta may adversely affect the individual.

When grains are pulverized to flour, the effects on the metabolic profile are very different compared to consuming intact whole grains [10]. Thus, an example of a daily healthy eating pattern for HIV patients consists of 5–6 servings of vegetables, including leafy green vegetables, 2 servings of fruits (particularly berries), nuts (particularly almonds and walnuts), seeds (such as flax and pumpkin seeds), 2 servings of whole grains (such as brown rice), steel cut oatmeal, quinoa, and 1–2 servings of legumes. With this lifestyle intervention, patients progress extremely well and their metabolic parameters improve. Patients are also encouraged to try ginger, garlic, turmeric, pepper, cilantro, parsley, and other spices while cooking for overall anti-inflammatory effects and to improve flavor of food. Turmeric may have specific effects in HIV-infected patients [11]. Patients demonstrate overt improvements in glycemic and blood pressure control after implementing these dietary changes coupled with increased physical activity [12]. By following such a healthy diet, many HIV patients also have resolution or improvement of other conditions, such as irritable bowel syndrome, chronic diarrhea, other intestinal disorders, gastroesophageal reflux disease, asthma, chronic fatigue, and certain types of arthritis [13].

Numerous studies have also examined the benefits of fruits and vegetables in HIV-infected patients mainly for their fiber content and rich source of other phytonutrients [14]. Nuts are also extremely beneficial for patients as a preventive strategy for T2D, MetS, and even all-cause mortality [15]. A very large study in nurses and other health-care professionals showed that the frequency of nut consumption was inversely associated with total and cause-specific mortality [16]. There have been no studies on nut consumption in HIV-infected patients but there is expectation of significant, if not similar, benefits, considering the higher prevalence of vitamin and nutritional deficiencies seen in this cohort. Nuts are high in magnesium and fiber and can be part of healthy eating patterns in patients with HIV.

There is controversy regarding consumption of fat in patients with HIV. Presently, the evidence points to the benefit of a combination of good-quality fats. Nevertheless, a low-fat diet should not be recommended to HIV-infected patients, as many patients will merely increase refined carbohydrate intake. Fat is important for absorption of certain vitamins and production of certain hormones. Many low-fat products, including non-fat and low-fat yogurt are high in sugar content. Hence, it is important to counsel patients appropriately to choose olive oil, nuts, avocado, yogurt, and cold-water fish (e.g., salmon) to boost unsaturated fat intake.

Probiotics, probiotic yogurt, kefir, and other fermented foods are increasingly recognized as beneficial to health. Many patients report benefits due to addition of these foods in their diet [17]. Many HIV-infected patients consume prophylactic antibiotics for prevention of opportunistic infections. Patients with HIV are frequently treated with antibiotics for pneumonia, bronchitis, and other infections. Antibiotic use leads to proliferation of resistant bacteria and disruption of normal bacterial flora. Increased antibiotic exposure has been also associated with an increased risk of obesity, inflammatory bowel disease, and other conditions [18]. HIV infection causes damage and impairs the function of the gastrointestinal tract. HIV enteropathy is a condition characterized by pronounced CD4+ T cell loss, increased intestinal permeability, and microbial translocation, which lead to immune activation and disease progression. Probiotics may be beneficial in reducing diarrhea and other complications from prolonged antibiotic exposure on the gastrointestinal tract [19]. Probiotics may also improve immune function. González-Hernández et al. [20] have noted that the use of a symbiotic, which is a combination of probiotics and prebiotics, resulted in a decrease in harmful bacteria, interleukin-6, and an increase in CD4+ T cell counts.

Patients with chronic diarrhea or other gastrointestinal complaints may benefit from drinking 4 ounces of kefir daily, eating sauerkraut obtained from farmer's markets, or consuming a high-quality probiotic from a reputable company.

Patients without access to high-quality produce in their neighborhood stores due to limited choices or financial reasons should be referred to local farmer's markets, which accept Supplemental Nutrition Assistance Program Electronic Benefits Transfer (SNAP EBT) cards, and to pantries of various organizations serving patients with HIV. Such patients should be counseled to make better choices in choosing produce and educated about healthier ways to prepare food, such as steaming, to preserve nutrient content. Patients struggling to make changes should be supported during this process and advised to make incremental changes to their lifestyle.

Exercise

The health benefits of exercise and regular physical activity in T2D, dyslipidemia, and hypertension have been well documented in the literature. HIV disease is no exception. Patients with HIV may experience fatigue, body habitus changes, muscle wasting, and decreased quality of life. Exercise can help alleviate these symptoms. MacArthur et al. [21] showed that cardiopulmonary fitness in HIV-infected patients improved with aerobic exercise. Other physiological changes caused by exercise include improved body composition, such as decreased subcutaneous fat and abdominal girth, and increased strength. Additionally, conditions such as depression and anxiety seen in HIV-infected patients are also improved by exercise.

The American College of Sports Medicine (ACSM) issued physical activity guidelines in 2011 [22]. For cardiorespiratory exercise, adults should get at least 150 min of moderate intensity exercise per week. This can be done through 30–60 min of moderate intensity exercise 5 days a week or 20–60 min of high intensity exercise three times a week. For patients unable to do one continuous session, multiple shorter sessions (of at least 10 min) are acceptable to accumulate the desired amount of daily exercise. The ACSM guidelines also include guidance for resistance, flexibility, and neuromotor exercise.

In a 2009 review, Hand et al. [23] summarized the results of numerous studies of HIV-infected patients which examined both aerobic exercise and resistance training. In the studies employing aerobic exercise, the outcomes showed significant reductions in anxiety and depression as well as significant increases in maximal oxygen uptake (VO_{2max}) and decreases in body mass index (BMI), total cholesterol and triglycerides, body fat, and abdominal girth. In the same review, studies with resistance exercise also showed increases in VO_{2max} as well as in strength. The studies examining strength/resistance-only regimens were small and focused more on strength and did not examine overall fitness. As the HIV epidemic has shifted over the last several years towards a population with lower socioeconomic status, there are factors that predispose this group to higher rates of obesity. As guidelines have changed and treatment is now recommended for all, exercise becomes an effective non-pharmacologic way to help improve depression, dyslipidemias, and muscle weakness without the addition of yet another pill.

While HAART has improved the prognosis of HIV-infected persons, it has unfortunately been associated with body habitus changes, particularly for those individuals who were started on treatment early in the course of the epidemic. With older antiretroviral agents, patients reported increases in abdominal girth and thinning arms and legs. There have also been reports of dorsocervical fat pads. While the newer agents today are less likely to induce these changes, for those who received treatment earlier, the changes remained even after regimens were changed. Pharmacologic and non-pharmacologic interventions were explored. Segatto et al. [24] studied 42 HIV-infected persons on HAART. They found that more active subjects had a lower incidence of body habitus changes than more sedentary subjects. There are also case reports which document the beneficial effects of an aerobic and resistance exercise program on decreasing abdominal fat and increasing limb diameter via resistance training [25]. In the studies employing resistance training, strength training was performed 2–3 times a week, depending on the study protocol. The studies utilized weights, which exercised major muscle groups (i.e., chest press, leg press, lat pull downs, and knee extensions) in order to increase overall strength. The patients executed 2–3 sets with 8–10 repetitions. The weight of the repetition was determined to be 60–80% of one repetition max [23, 25].

Although exercise has been shown to improve quality of life and increase VO_{2max}, many clinicians may still hesitate to instruct their HIV-infected patients to exercise. Literature indicates that intense exercise (70–85% of maximal heart rate) or prolonged exercise (defined as 90 min or more by the ACSM) results in a decrease in CD4+ cells in a healthy person. In 1994, Ullum et al. [26] examined and reported the effects of acute exercise on immune response in a group of HIV-infected and seronegative individuals and concluded that although HIV can suppress features of the immune system, a patient can start an exercise program at high intensity, but not exhaustive exercise. In a more recent review of exercise and immune function, Walsh et al. [27] also concluded that acute intensive exercise can elicit a temporary decrease in CD4+ cells as well as a lymphocytosis. The decrease is proportional to intensity and duration; however, in a true resting state (i.e., greater than 24 h after last training session), circulating lymphocytes as well as T cell functions have returned to baseline. There are very few studies on exercise in HIV-infected patients on ART. Patients should consult with their medical provider before starting any formal exercise program.

As HIV treatments have become more potent and simpler to take, the population living with HIV has aged. As aging occurs, a small percentage of muscle mass is lost each decade along with a decrease in VO_{2max}. Both aerobic and resistance exercise can attenuate this response. Currently, there are limited data about the effects of exercise in an older population with HIV disease. Yahiaoui et al. [28] examined the research focused on older adults with frailty and their response to exercise to extrapolate findings to the older HIV-infected patients. Their study suggested that significant improvements could be gained in strength, balance, and range of motion exercises.

Engelson et al. [29] conducted a 12-week weight loss program with 18 HIV-infected obese (BMI 30) women. She reported moderate weight loss in the group with a short-term program of diet and exercise. No significant changes in CD4+ count or viral load were observed, and participants lost adiposity in both subcutaneous and visceral adipose tissue regions. Strength and fitness also improved in these women.

We have reported success engaging patients in an exercise and nutrition program [30]. For the past 3 years, we have been conducting a yearly 8–12-week program for HIV-infected patients who are overweight/obese. The goal is to help patients to lose weight and to counsel them about healthier nutrition and exercise habits. A secondary goal is to have them complete either a 5K or 4-mile race (either walking or running). Approximately 30% of our patients are able to accomplish this by the end of 12 weeks. Most have lost weight, but more importantly, they have learned about healthier eating choices and changed their lifestyle. Another important component of this program is that monthly meetings are made available to the participants who have completed the course. These meetings emphasize physical activity and reinforce the nutrition they have learned during the program in order to maintain weight loss and other benefits.

The exercise component of the program followed the ACSM guidelines for aerobic exercise—at least 150 min of moderate-intensity exercise per week. Each participant had this component tailored to their ability and need. Some were unable to initially meet the 150-min recommendation but each worked towards this goal. The participants were also instructed on resistance and flexibility exercises and advised to incorporate each of these into their routine two to three times a week. All participated in both the aerobic and resistance exercises.

Many HIV-infected patients have limited resources but would like to exercise for the health benefits. Some patients are involved in activities such as yoga and running. To help patients meet the ACSM goals for cardiorespiratory and resistance exercise, options that are relatively inexpensive can be recommended, such as using a pedometer to achieve 10,000 steps a day, joining a low-cost gym, searching YouTube for walking videos for the home, locating classes (yoga, aerobic, etc.) that are free or low-cost donation based, and using their own body weight (in place of more expensive equipment) for home-based resistance exercises.

More research is needed to determine if higher intensity exercise has a more deleterious effect on the immune system of an HIV-infected person compared with someone who is seronegative. Such studies should include women and standardize which immune markers are examined.

Multivitamins, Minerals, and Micronutrients

HIV-infected patients often have deficiencies of certain vitamins and minerals and need supplementation with a standard-dose multivitamin with minerals and micronutrients. Studies have shown that vitamin D insufficiency and accelerated bone loss is underestimated in this population [31]. Vitamin B12 deficiency due to poor absorption and decreased intrinsic factor secretion is also commonly encountered in patients with gastrointestinal disorders [32]. Certain patients may benefit from additional zinc, selenium, antioxidants, and other specific nutrients.

HAART and Food Interactions

There are specific interactions between antiretroviral medications and food. Clinicians should be aware of these possibilities and counsel patients appropriately. The most commonly known interaction is between grapefruit juice and protease inhibitors. Grapefruit juice can cause inhibi-

Table 32.1 HIV medications and food requirements

	Food requirements
Nucleoside/nucleotide reverse transcriptase inhibitors (NRTIs)	
3TC (lamivudine, *Epivir*)	May be taken with or without food
Abacavir (*Ziagen*)	May be taken with or without food
AZT (zidovudine, *Retrovir*)	May be taken with or without food, though taking with food may reduce nausea
Combivir (AZT+3TC)	May be taken with or without food, although taking with food may reduce nausea
d4T (stavudine, *Zerit*)	May be taken with or without food
Enteric-coated ddI (*Videx EC,* didanosine capsules)	Take on an empty stomach, at least 2 h before and 2 h after eating or drinking anything except water
Epzicom (3TC + abacavir)	May be taken with or without food
FTC (emtricitabine, *Emtriva*)	May be taken with or without food
Tenofovir (*Viread*)	Take with food
Trizivir (AZT + 3TC + abacavir)	May be taken with or without food
Truvada (tenofovir + FTC)	Take with food
Non-nucleoside reverse transcriptase inhibitors (NNRTIs)	
Efavirenz (*Sustiva*)	Take on an empty stomach
Etravirine (*Intelence*)	Take with or after food (within 2 h after a main meal or within half an hour after a snack)
Nevirapine (*Viramune*)	Take with or without food
Rilpivirine (*Edurant*)	Take with food
Protease inhibitors	
Atazanavir (*Reyataz*)	Take with or after food (within 2 h after a main meal or within half an hour after a snack)
Darunavir (*Prezista*)	Take with or after food (within 2 h after a main meal or within half an hour after a snack)
Fosamprenavir (*Lexiva*)	May be taken with or without food
Indinavir (*Crixivan*)	Take on an empty stomach, or with a light, low-fat snack, or at least 2 h after and 1 h before a meal
Lopinavir/ritonavir (*Kaletra*) tablets	May be taken with or without food
Lopinavir/ritonavir (*Kaletra*) liquid	Should be taken with food to increase its effectiveness
Ritonavir (*Norvir*)	May be taken with or without food
Saquinavir (*Invirase*) (must be taken with ritonavir)	Take within 2 h of food to increase its effectiveness
Tipranavir (*Aptivus*) (must be taken with ritonavir)	Take with or after food to reduce the incidence of side-effects
Fusion and entry inhibitors	
Maraviroc (*Selzentry*)	May be taken with or without food
T-20 (enfuvirtide, *Fuzeon*)	Administered by injection. No food restrictions
Integrase Inhibitors	
Raltegravir (*Isentress*)	May be taken with or without food
Elvitegravir (*Vitekta*)	May be taken with or without food
Dolutegravir (*Tivicay*)	Take with food
Single tablet regimens	
Atripla (efavirenz + FTC + tenofovir combined)	Take on an empty stomach (preferably at bedtime), to reduce the incidence of side-effects (particularly avoid taking it soon after a high-fat meal as this increases the risk of side-effects)
Complera (rilpivirine + tenofovir + emtricitabine)	Take with food
Stribild (elvitegravir + cobicistat + tenofovir + emtricitabine)	Take with food
Triumeq (dolutegravir + abacavir + lamivudine)	May be taken with or without food

tion of cytochrome P-450 3A4 in the small intestine and decrease drug metabolism. However, most patients currently do not consume enough grapefruit juice to cause sufficient interaction [33]. Most HIV medications do not have food requirements, but certain drugs do need to be taken on an empty stomach while others require food for proper absorption and attaining therapeutic serum concentrations (Table 32.1).

HAART and Herbal Therapies

HIV-infected patients often use dietary and herbal supplements without informing their primary care provider. While some dietary and herbal supplements may benefit specific patients, others, most notably garlic extract, milk thistle and St. John's wort, can interact with HAART and lead to adverse effects [34]. Patients should be routinely asked about the use of supplements and counseled appropriately.

Stress Management

HIV-infected patients are faced with an enormous amount of stress in their lives. For many, HIV-specific anxiety began while waiting for results of the HIV-confirmatory test and continued with daily reminders of taking antiretroviral medications to treat an incurable infection. To compound matters further, many newly diagnosed patients have existing psychiatric comorbidities, in particular, substance abuse and depression. The prevalence of depression is twice that of seronegative controls [35]. Other stressors may include a history of trauma, an inadequate food supply, and an unstable living situation. Stress can drive patients towards unhealthy behaviors such as tobacco, drug, and alcohol use, and consumption of unhealthy foods. Many HIV-infected patients are aware of stress in their lives and seek ways to manage it. Chronic stressors are known to be associated with suppression of cellular and humoral immunity [36]. Psychological stress affects immune function through central nervous system control of the hypothalamic–pituitary–adrenal (HPA) axis and sympathetic–adrenomedullary (SAM) axis. Hormones released from the HPA and SAM axes can then affect immune function [37]. Moreover, stress can lead to decreased adherence with medications leading to virologic rebound and progression of HIV/AIDS.

Clinicians and other health-care professionals should recognize that the stress of living with HIV can be alleviated by various lifestyle interventions. In severe cases, combination with both pharmacotherapy and psychotherapy may be required. Any intervention should be individualized on a case-by-case basis. Movement therapies, touch therapies, meditation, guided imagery, prayer, and expressive writing have demonstrated quality-of-life improvement through their ability to help patients manage stress, reduce pain, slow disease progression, and gain a sense of control over their lives [38, 39]. These therapies may differ in their mechanisms of action but may be effective and empowering for patients. Massage therapy may have a positive effect on immunological function and it improves quality of life for HIV-infected patients, especially if combined with other stress-management modalities, such as meditation and relaxation training [40]. Transcendental meditation and mindfulness meditation have been studied in HIV-infected patients, and benefits include decreased stress and improvement in health-related quality of life [41]. Acupuncture is widely used to reduce stress, decrease pain, and decrease side effects from HAART [42].

Clinicians should refer patients to therapists, psychologists, or other health-care professionals who are trained in stress-reduction techniques as described above. Patients may also be referred to in-person or online courses on mindfulness-based stress reduction. The Center for Mindfulness is an online resource and can assist clinicians in finding providers in their area (available at: http://www.umassmed.edu/cfm/). There may also be local yoga and meditation centers, which offer low-cost or donation-based classes. Clinicians should become familiar with these centers and refer patients as indicated. Utilizing a multidisciplinary approach to stress reduction can lead to an enhanced sense of well-being, boost immune function, and improve longevity in people living with HIV/AIDS.

Safe Sexual Practices for HIV-Infected Patients

Sexual contact remains the common route of HIV transmission worldwide. In HIV-infected patients, HAART can reduce but not eliminate the possibility of transmission. Sexual abstinence may be the choice for some, however not desirable or practical for most individuals. Patients should be counseled about safe sex practices and encouraged to use barrier protection, including male or female condoms and dental dams. Unfortunately, condoms can fail when used inconsistently, improperly, or due to breakage or slippage. Applying an oil-based lubricant can make condoms more susceptible to damage. Patients should be advised about correct use of latex or polyurethane condoms and to avoid use of lambskin condoms and nonoxynol-9. When used correctly and consistently, barrier protection is highly effective in preventing HIV infection, as well as other sexually transmitted diseases (STDs) including syphilis and hepatitis C. Risk assessment about sexual practices should be performed in a nonjudgmental manner and recommendations encouraging partner communication, prevention strategies, and healthy sexual habits should be provided [43–45].

Case Study

A 44-year-old male patient with HIV was referred because of difficulty losing weight and abnormal liver enzymes. He had tried several commercial diet plans without success. He also had significant abdominal lipodystrophy, which was attributed to HIV and antiretroviral therapy (ART). A plant-based diet was discussed and implemented, and he has lost more than 50 lbs in the past year. Currently, he eats oatmeal or

Table 32.2 Benefits of lifestyle medicine in HIV-infected patients

Resolution of diabetes, hypertension, hyperlipidemia
Weight loss in obesity
Illness prevention
Immunity booster
Increased energy
Improved mood
Pain management
Improvement in bowel disorders
Quality-of-life improvement

muesli for breakfast; brown rice, vegetables, and a smoothie with fruits, nuts, and flax seeds for lunch; and a large salad with fish with small portion of rice and a large serving of beans and vegetables for dinner. Ongoing discussions have resulted in participation with regular exercise programs, including walking stairs at work every day and now using weights for strength training. He has lost abdominal fat, as well as excessive fat around his face, chin, and neck. Overall, he reports increased energy and improved mood.

Conclusions

Lifestyle medicine is beneficial for patients with HIV and patients should receive counseling regarding healthy eating, exercise, stress management, and safe sexual practices to improve overall health. Lifestyle medicine can help HIV-infected patients with T2D, hypertension, hyperlipidemia, and obesity reverse or improve these conditions. Lifestyle medicine can also improve asthma, irritable bowel syndrome, and other conditions in HIV-infected patients. Health-care professionals taking care of HIV-infected patients should be aware of dietary approaches in the management of conditions and should refer patients to nutritionists, dieticians, and others trained in lifestyle medicine (Table 32.2).

References

1. Suh JS, Gandhi V. Management of HIV-infected patients. In: Rakel R, Bope E, editors. Conn's current therapy. 58th ed. Philadelphia: W.B. Saunders; 2006.
2. Suh JS, Sepkowitz KA. Treatment of HIV related opportunistic infections. In: Reese RE, Betts RF, editors. A practical approach to infectious diseases. 5th ed. Philadelphia: Lippincott Williams & Wilkins; 2003.
3. Hone-Blanchet A, Fecteau S. Overlap of food addiction and substance use disorders definitions: analysis of animal and human studies. Neuropharmacology. 2014;85:81–90.
4. Jarrett OD, Wanke CA, Ruthazer R, et al. Metabolic syndrome predicts all-cause mortality in persons with human immunodeficiency virus. AIDS Patient Care STDS. 2013;27(5):266–71.
5. Mondy K, Overton ET, Grubb J, et al. Metabolic syndrome in HIV-infected patients from an urban, Midwestern, US outpatient population. Clin Infect Dis. 2007;44:726–34.
6. Giugliano D, Esposito K. Mediterranean diet and metabolic diseases. Curr Opin Lipidol. 2008;19:63–8.
7. Knoops KT, de Groot LC, Kromhout D, et al. Mediterranean diet, lifestyle factors, and 10-year mortality in elderly European men and women: the HALE project. JAMA. 2004;292:1433–9.
8. Fitch KV, Anderson EJ, Hubbard JL, et al. Effects of a lifestyle modification program in HIV-infected patients with the metabolic syndrome. AIDS. 2006;20:1843–50.
9. Botros D, Somarriba G, Neri D, Miller TL. Interventions to address chronic disease and HIV: strategies to promote exercise and nutrition among HIV-infected individuals. Curr HIV/AIDS Rep. 2012;9(4):351–63.
10. Breen C, Ryan M, Gibney MJ, et al. Glycemic, insulinemic, and appetite responses of patients with type-2 diabetes to commonly consumed breads. Diabetes Educ. 2013;39(3):376–86.
11. Conteas CN, Panossian AM, Tran TT, Singh HM. Treatment of HIV-associated diarrhea with curcumin. Dig Dis Sci. 2009;54(10):2188–91.
12. Blanco F, San Román J, Vispo E, et al. Management of metabolic complications and cardiovascular risk in HIV-infected patients. AIDS Rev. 2010;12(4):231–41.
13. Catassi C, Bai JC, Bonaz B, et al. Non-Celiac Gluten sensitivity: the new frontier of gluten related disorders. Nutrients. 2013;5(10):3839–53.
14. Gil L, Lewis L, Martinez G, et al. Effect of increase of dietary micronutrient intake on oxidative stress indicators in HIV/AIDS patients. Int J Vitam Nutr Res. 2005;75(1):19–27.
15. Viguiliouk E, Kendall CW, Blanco Mejia S, et al. Effect of tree nuts on glycemic control in diabetes: a systematic review and meta-analysis of randomized controlled dietary trials. PLoS ONE. 2014;9(7):e103376.
16. Bao Y, Han J, Hu FB, et al. Association of nut consumption with total and cause-specific mortality. N Engl J Med. 2013;369:2001–11.
17. Floch MH, Walker WA, Madsen K, et al. Recommendations for probiotic use-2011 update. J Clin Gastroenterol. 2011;45(Suppl):S168–71.
18. Ungaro R, Bernstein CN, Gearry R, et al. Antibiotics associated with increased risk of new-onset Crohn's disease but not ulcerative colitis: a meta-analysis. Am J Gastroenterol. 2014;109(11)1728–38.
19. Hummelen R, Vos AP, van't Land B, et al. Altered host-microbe interaction in HIV: a target for intervention with pro- and prebiotics. Int Rev Immunol. 2010;29:485–513.
20. González-Hernández LA, Jave-Suarez LF, Fafutis-Morris M, et al. Synbiotic therapy decreases microbial translocation and inflammation and improves immunological status in HIV-infected patients: a double-blind randomized controlled pilot trial. Nutr J. 2012;11:90.
21. MacArthur RD, Levine SD, Birk TJ. Supervised exercise training improves cardiopulmonary fitness in HIV-infected persons. Med Sci Sports Exerc. 1993;25(6):684–8.

22. Garber CE, Blissmer B, Deschenes MR, Franklin BA, Lamonte MJ, Lee IM, Nieman DC, Swain DP. American College of Sports Medicine position stand. Quantity and quality of exercise for developing and maintaining cardiorespiratory, musculoskeletal, and neuromotor fitness in apparently healthy adults: guidance for prescribing exercise. Med Sci Sports Exerc. 2011;43(7):1334–59.

23. Hand GA, Lyerly GW, Jaggers JR, Dudgeon WD. Impact of aerobic and resistance exercise on the health of HIV-infected persons. Am J Lifestyle Med. 2009;3(6):489–99.

24. Segatto AF, Freitas IF Jr, Dos Santos, VR, Alves KC, Barbosa DA, Filho AM, Monteiro HL. Lipodystrophy in HIV/AIDS patients with different levels of physical activity while on antiretroviral therapy. Rev Soc Bras Med Trop. 2011;44(4):420–4.

25. Mendes EL, Andaki AC, Brito CJ, Cordova C, Natali AJ, Santos Amorim PR, de Oliveira LL, de Paula SO, Multimura E. Beneficial effects of physical activity in an HIV-infected woman with lipodystrophy: a case report. J Med Case Rep. 2011;5:430.

26. Ullum H, Palmo J, Halkjaer-Kristensen J. The effect of acute exercise on lymphocyte subsets, natural killer cells, proliferative responses, and cytokines in HIV-seropositive persons. J Acquir Immune Defic Syndr. 1994;7:1122–33.

27. Walsh NP, Gleeson M, Shephard RJ, et al. Position statement. Part one: immune function and exercise. Exerc Immunol Rev. 2011;17:6–63.

28. Yahiaoui A, McGough EL, Voss JG. Development of evidence-based exercise recommendations for older HIV-infected patients. J Assoc Nurses AIDS Care. 2012 23(3):204–19.

29. Engelson ES, Agin D, Sonjia K, et al. Body composition and metabolic effects of a diet and exercise weight loss regimen on obese HIV-infected women. Metabolism. 2006;55(10):1327–36.

30. Gandhi V, Lawrence N. It takes HEART: a multi-faceted weight loss program for people living with HIV. Global Adv Health Med. 2013;2(Suppl):1–3.

31. Kim JH, Gandhi V, Psevdos G Jr, Espinoza F, Park J, Sharp V. Evaluation of vitamin D levels among HIV-infected patients in New York City. AIDS Res Hum Retroviruses. 2012;28(3):235–41.

32. Herzlich BC, Schiano TD, Moussa Z, et al. Decreased intrinsic factor secretion in AIDS: relation to parietal cell acid secretory capacity and vitamin B12 malabsorption. Am J Gastroenterol. 1992;87(12):1781–8.

33. Dolton MJ, Roufogalis BD, McLachlan AJ. Fruit juices as perpetrators of drug interactions: the role of organic anion-transporting polypeptides. Clin Pharmacol Ther. 2012;92(5):622–30.

34. Henderson L, Yue QY, Bergquist C, Gerden B, Arlett P. St John's wort (Hypericum perforatum): drug interactions and clinical outcomes. Br J Clin Pharmacol. 2002;54(4):349–56.

35. Asch SM, Kilbourne AM, Gifford AL, et al. Underdiagnosis of depression in HIV: who are we missing? J Gen Intern Med. 2003;18:450.

36. Segerstrom SC, Miller GE. Psychological stress and the human immune system: a meta-analytic study of 30 years of inquiry. Psychol Bull. 2004:130:601–630.

37. Thornton LM, Andersen BL. Psychoneuroimmunology examined: the role of subjective stress. Cellscience. 2006:2:66–91.

38. Ironson G, Stuetzle R, Fletcher MA. An increase in religiousness/spirituality occurs after HIV diagnosis and predicts slower disease progression over 4 years in people with HIV. J Gen Intern Med. 2006;21:S62–8.

39. Rivkin ID, Gustafson J, Weingarten I, et al. The effects of expressive writing on adjustment to HIV. AIDS Behav. 2006;10:13–26.

40. Shor-Posner G, Miguez MJ, Hernandez-Reif M, et al. Massage treatment in HIV-1 infected Dominican children: A preliminary report on the massage therapy to preserve the immune system in children without antiretroviral medication. J Altern Complement Med. 2004;10:1093–5.

41. Chhatre S, Metzger DS, Frank I, et al. Effects of behavioral stress reduction Transcendental Meditation intervention in persons with HIV. AIDS Care. 2013;25(10):1291–7.

42. Phillips KD, Skelton WD, Hand GA. Effect of acupuncture administered in a group setting on pain and subjective peripheral neuropathy in persons with human immunodeficiency virus disease. J Altern Complement Med. 2004;10:449–55.

43. Koester KA, Maiorana A, Morin SF, et al. People living with HIV are receptive to HIV prevention interventions in clinical settings: a qualitative evaluation. AIDS Educ Prev. 2012;24(4):295–308.

44. Varghese B, Maher JE, Peterman TA, et al. Reducing the risk of sexual HIV transmission: quantifying the per-act risk for HIV on the basis of choice of partner, sex act, and condom use. Sex Transm Dis. 2002;29(1):38–43.

45. Conant M, Hardy D, Sernatinger J, et al. Condoms prevent transmission of AIDS-associated retrovirus. JAMA. 1986;255(13):1706.

Appendix: Lifestyle Medicine Checklist

	Item	Done/indicated (✓)	Not done/not indicated (×)	Action	Chapter
History	1			A focus on lifestyle	2, 3
	2			Assess eating patterns	11
	3			Assess physical activity patterns	8, 13
	4			Assess smoking and tobacco use	15
	5			Assess sleeping patterns	17
	6			Assess for alcohol misuse	16
	7			Utilize selected behavioral assessment instruments	6
Exam	8			Assess body composition (BMI, waist circumference)	7
Laboratory assessment	9			Cardiovascular and metabolic composite scores	5, 9
Management: preparation	10			Assess motivation and behavioral opportunities	14
	11			Assess community resources	18
	12			Assess transcultural considerations	19
	13			Assess attitude about using integrative medicine modalities	20
Management: specific recommendations	14			Cardiometabolic risk factors	21
	15			Obesity	12, 22
	16			Diabetes	23
	17			Depression	24
	18			Musculoskeletal disorder	25
	19			Fatty liver disease	26
	20			GI disease	27
	21			Chronic kidney disease	28
	22			Respiratory disease	29
	23			Neurodegenerative disease	30
	24			Cancer	31
	25			HIV	32
Adapt: office practice	26			Assess office system used to deliver lifestyle medicine	4, 10

BMI body mass index, *GI* gastrointestinal

J. I. Mechanick, R. F. Kushner (eds.), *Lifestyle Medicine,* DOI 10.1007/978-3-319-24687-1

Index

A

Accelerometer, 58
  ActiGraph, 80
  pedometer uses, 80
Acceptance and Commitment Therapy (ACT), 291
  goal of, 293
  treatment of choronic pain, 293
Acupuncture
  benefits of, 178
  manual, 178
  positive effect of, 178
  review of, 178
Adaptive stress responses, 305
Adipose
  tissues insulin, 322
AD *See* Alzheimer's disease (AD)
Aerobic vs. resistance training, 126
Alcohol, 146
  effect of, 275, 276, 284, 295, 296
  formal diagnosis of, 60
  harmful use of, 4, 9, 11, 12, 101, 135, 151, 156
  intake, 251, 252
  limited intake of, 270
  risk factors, 31
  safe and unsafe, 153
  unhealthy
    identify and treat, 152
  use and problems, 151
Alcohol use disorder (AUD), 153
Alzheimer's disease (AD), 300–304
  -diagnosis of, 306
  experimental model of
    degenration in, 303
  mouse model
    abnormailies in, 301
  mouse model of, 303
    study of, 304
  -patients cognitive abitlity, 306
  risk of, 301, 302, 304–306
  stages of, 300, 306
Assessment
  disordered eating, 57
  environmental factors and eating habits, 57
  general psychosocial functioning, 60
  of BED, 58
  of CVD, 45, 46, 51, 84, 85
  physical activity, 58
  psychiatric status and history, 59
  timing factors of, 62

Asthma, 2, 30, 90–93
Atherosclerotic cardiovascular disease (ASCVD), 83, 84
  models of, 85
  risk for, 87
Atherosclerotic cardiovascular risk, 45, 83, 86

B

Behavioral, 3, 4, 17–19, 21, 25, 35, 37, 55–57, 59, 61, 62
Behavior change, 17–20, 22, 24, 130, 131, 144, 177, 191, 193, 205, 228, 237
  stages of, 81
  theories of, 17
Behavior change counseling, 33, 34, 37
Behavior modification, 106, 129, 131, 133, 205, 228, 237
Behavior therapy, 26, 114, 129, 131
Binge eating disorder (BED), 58
Biomarkers, 13, 43, 44, 84, 103, 235, 258
Body composition, 186, 206, 207, 210, 211
  studies of, 199
Brief intervention, 142, 152–154, 156–158
Built environment, 25, 191, 192

C

CAM *See* Complementary and alternative medicine (CAM)
Cardiometabolic disease staging system, 42, 50, 261
Cardiometabolic risk, 4, 50, 245, 258
  assessment of, 48
  factors, 49, 210, 246
  lifestyle therapy
    benefits of, 248
    management of, 245, 248, 252, 255, 256
    mediterranean diet, 259
Cardiovascular disease (CVD), 11, 42, 58, 103
  risk of, 86, 122, 127, 163, 177, 184, 202, 224–228, 232, 235
CBT *See* Cognitive behavioral therapy (CBT), 26
CHD *See* Coronary heart disease (CHD), 42
Chronic care, 3, 5
  performance goals of, 93
Chronic care model, 89, 90, 92
  components of, 95, 191
Chronic kidney disease, 227, 250
Chronic obstructive pulmonary disease (COPD), 93
Chronic pain, 166
Clinical treatment, 136
CMC *See* Chronic care model (CMC), 89
Cognitive behavioral counseling, 132

© Springer International Publishing Switzerland 2016
J. I. Mechanick, R. F. Kushner (eds.), *Lifestyle Medicine*, DOI 10.1007/978-3-319-24687-1

Cognitive behavioral therapy (CBT), 152, 157, 165
Cognitive behavior therapy, 129, 130
    strategies of, 130
Cognitive therapy, 105, 129
Commercial programs, 106, 112, 116, 118
Communication, 3, 36
    methods of, 33, 37
    physician, study of, 33
    primer for lifestyle medicine counseling, 17
    quality of, 18
    risk, 41, 50, 51
    style of, 18, 19
Community engagement, 191
Community organization, 95, 191
Community partnership, 191, 193
Complementary and alternative medicine, 13, 35, 56, 171, 175, 193,
        194
    economics of, 179
    prevalence of, 172
Connected health, 36
Contextualization
    care of, 17, 18
    element of, 191
Counseling, 17
    aim of lifestyle, 18
    behavioral, 30
        evidence based, 141
        strategies, 22
    clinical, 19
    dietary, 56
    face to face, 112, 114
    higher doses of, 143
    lifestyle, 86, 105, 118
    Motivational Interviewing, process of, 22
    practical, 143
    strategies
        for obesity, 205
        smokeless tobacco, 147
        tobacco cessation benefits, 148
        waterpipe, 148
    supportive, 143, 145, 147
    telephone based, 106, 112, 114
    treatment for, 136
CVD See Cardiovascular disease (CVD), 41
Cystic fibrosis (CF), 223

D
Depression, 3, 4
Diabetes, 3, 10, 42, 93, 121, 163, 176–179, 194, 223, 224, 227–232
    American, 115
    and heart failure, 36
    duration of, 225
    management of, 95
    patients with, 20, 91, 93, 176, 193, 224, 232
    person with, 179, 225
    prevention, 87, 133, 195, 248, 249
    treatment of, 222
    types of, 223
Dialysis, 238
Diet, 10, 11, 13, 18, 25, 97, 105, 112, 114, 118, 129, 131, 206, 225,
        226, 249, 256, 259, 270, 273
    calorie-controlled, 103
    curriculum of, 133
    effect of, 2
    self-directed, 56
    self-reported, 103

    self-selected, 115
Diet and lifestyle, 222
Dietary energy intake, 204–207
    effect of, 114, 200, 211
    prevalence of, 98
    reduction of, 209, 256
Dietary patterns, 57, 100, 270
Dietary supplements, 172, 258, 274
Diet quality
    assessment of, 102, 103
Disease complexity, 2, 4
Dyslipidemia, 41, 46–48, 84, 123, 209, 225, 235, 237, 245–247,
        252–255, 257, 259
    treatment of, 42, 44, 252

E
Eating behavior, 55, 57, 62, 98, 119, 168, 228
E-cigarettes, 136, 147, 149, 277
Edmonton Obesity Staging System (EOSS), 42, 49, 202
Energy balance, 81, 203, 204, 206, 209, 233, 255, 259, 260, 269, 274
Energy density, 204, 206, 208
Energy medicine, 175
Exercise, 2, 13, 18

F
Fat, 101, 199, 202, 203, 210, 227, 233, 253, 256, 257
Fitness, 11, 32, 45, 85, 86, 122–125, 194, 195, 210, 212–214, 235,
        251, 259
Framingham Risk Score, 42, 43, 44, 51, 85, 177

G
Glycemic index (GI), 48, 188, 207, 225, 252, 256, 257, 258

H
Health promotion, 6, 29–31, 37, 83, 98, 99, 123, 174, 192
Healthy eating, 6, 24, 103, 187, 225, 273
    diet for, 330
    guidelines for, 97
    habits, 57, 113, 195
    pattern, 188, 195, 318
        HIV, 350
Healthy Eating Index (HEI), 315
Healthy meal plan, 225, 232, 235, 238, 239, 248, 252, 253, 254, 255,
        256, 257, 258, 259, 260, 261
Homeopathy, 178
Human, 3, 25, 98, 103, 121, 129, 132, 148, 184, 186, 194, 204, 206,
        211, 227, 254, 271, 274, 276, 277
Human immunodeficiency virus (HIV), 42, 74, 355, 349–355
Hypertension, 10
    benefits, 86
    causes of, 253
    chronic diseases, 157
    controlling on, 89
    dietary approaches for, 12, 48, 100–103, 185, 227, 232, 235, 239,
            250–253, 345
    dietary intervention for, 48
    impact of, 62, 258
    improvement in, 245, 260
    in diagnosis criteria, 47
    life therapy for, 248, 249
    management, 91, 249
    obesity, 93

primary strategies, 250
risk of, 164
treatment of, 251

I

Insomnia *See also* sleep disorders, 58, 161, 162, 164
    assessment of, 163
    causes of, 164
    chronic disorder, 164
    sleep pattern in, 163
    treatment, 165
Insulin resistance, 47, 50, 186, 223
    accurate measures of, 247
    assessment of, 48
    central role of, 238
    clinical manifestations of, 245, 248
    dyslipidemia of, 252, 261
    effect of intensity on, 126
    indicator of, 48
    prevailing degree of, 223
    risk for, 126, 187
    syndrome *See* metabolic syndrome (MetS), 46
    treatment of, 255
Integrative medicine, 13, 172
    affiliation of, 172
    aspect of, 172
    prevalence of use, 172
    role of, 180
    terminology in, 171
    therapies, 179
In vivo, 274

L

Lean, 101, 113, 115, 123, 124, 188, 199, 200, 203, 204, 208–211, 227, 246, 247, 249, 274, 275
    factor of, 203
Lifestyle, 1, 2, 4, 5, 6, 9–13, 19, 31, 33–36, 38, 44, 46, 48, 51, 55, 59, 60, 62, 78, 79
    application of, 37
    aspects of, 13
    behaviors, 9, 10, 13, 19, 20, 21, 187
    development of, 9
    medicine, 1, 5, 6, 9, 11, 13, 17, 23, 30, 31, 83, 87, 90, 95, 98
    modification, 46, 51, 60, 83, 125, 129, 131–133, 237, 249
    role of, 36
Lifestyle therapy, 202, 203, 211, 212, 221–224, 228, 231, 232, 235, 237–239, 245, 246, 249, 252, 255, 259, 262
    physical activity, 259
    treatment goals of, 248
Low calorie, 204, 209, 212, 227, 233, 238, 257, 260

M

Massage therapy, 175, 176, 178, 179
    prescription of, 176
    techniques, 176
Meal replacements (MR), 106, 112, 114–116, 118, 206, 208, 214, 233, 257
Measurement, 45, 57
Medical Nutrition Therapy (MNT), 224, 225, 228, 230, 237, 238, 314, 315
Metabolic syndrome, 2, 11, 42, 46, 48, 84, 177, 207, 222, 249
Method, 20, 21, 33, 37, 46

Mortality, 1–4, 9, 11–13, 32, 47, 48, 50, 77, 103, 122–125
Motivational interviewing, 20, 37, 145, 152

N

National dietary guidelines, 101
Naturopathic medicine, 176
Nonalcoholic fatty liver disease (NAFLD)
    diagnosis of, 329
    dietary factors impacting, 327
    impact on public health, 321
Non-communicable diseases, 3, 9
Nutrient density, 98, 103, 207, 208
Nutrition, 3–5, 12, 33, 57, 86, 97

O

Obesity, 2–4, 12, 22, 30, 33, 35, 47–51, 59–62
    degree of, 60
Overweight, 11, 33, 50, 56, 61, 83–85, 98, 105, 112, 118, 122, 123, 126

P

Pedometer, 78–81
    type of, 80
Physical activity, 5, 6, 11–13, 17, 23, 26, 34, 36
Positive airway pressure (PAP), 163, 167, 239
Prevention, 30, 47, 51, 85, 98, 103, 157, 222
    cancer, 36, 101, 270–275
        guidelines, 270
    challenges in, 5
    cardiovascular disease (CVD), 41, 44, 46, 101, 252, 259
    definition of, 30
    diabetes, 195
    disease, 29, 30, 37
        chronic, 3, 11, 103
        levels of, 30, 31
    illness, 13
    modification for, 144
    obesity of, 101
    physician, 34
    primary, 3, 30, 85, 87, 148
        risk of, 87
    relapse, 132, 144, 157
    role for, 2
    secondary, 30
    strategy for, 3, 9, 222, 238, 246, 260
    synergies in, 10
    T2D, 248, 257, 259, 260
    tertiary, 30
    weight regain of, 209, 235, 259
Preventive medicine, 4, 5, 11, 13, 29, 30, 33, 34, 37, 123, 172
Primary care, 18, 30, 35–37, 78, 79, 81, 89, 90–95
    model in, 92
    number of, 94
    pillars of, 92
    role of, 95
Primary care behavioral health, 35
Proteinuria, 236
Psychosocial status, 55

R

Referral to treatment, 157
Residual cardiovascular risk, 41, 46, 51
Residual risk
    factors, 6
    notion of, 4
Resistance training, 126
    benefits of, 210
    progressive, 188
Reynolds Risk Score, 42, 44, 45
Risk factor reduction, 247

S

Screening
    breast cancer, 34
    colorectal cancer, 152
    disease, 183
        coronary artery, 259
    hypertension, 152
    hypothyroidism, 57
    importance of, 151
    medical, 113, 118
    obesity, 275
    protocol, 154
    skin cancer, 34
Sedentary behaviors, 86, 211, 275
    detrimental effects of, 211
    reduction of, 211, 235, 239, 259, 260
Shared decision making, 18
Shift work
    definition of, 165
    disorder, 165
    treatment, 168
Sleep, 34, 36, 58
    basics of, 161
    diaries, 163
    disease risk, 163
    disorders, 161, 163
        classification of, 164
    disruption in, 59
    evaluation, 162
    habits, 163, 165
    hours of, 130
    hygiene, 165
    importance of, 161
    insufficient, 164, 168
    loss, 163, 166
        causes of, 161
    restriction, 166
    schedule, 162
    slow wave, 163, 165
    States
        non-rapid eye movement *see* slow wave sleep, 163
        rapid eye movement, 163
    study, 163
    time, 164
    treatment of, 168
Sleep apnea, 214
    improvements in, 231
    risk, 163
    severity, 168
Slow wave sleep, 165
Smoking, 11, 12
    cessation, 19, 33, 35, 41, 56, 78, 136
        pharmacotherapy, 143

cigarette, 12, 13
    effects of, 136
    rates of, 147
confer risk, 146
death, 276
health consequences of, 276
history, 261
patients, 143, 144
pregnancy risk, 145
prevalence of, 146
status, 45, 48, 123, 148
tobacco, 4
Smoking disparities, 135

T

Tobacco
    cessation, 6, 143
        benefits, 148
        PHS guidelines, 141
    control, strategies for, 276
    guidelines for, 136
    health consequences of, 33
    products, 83
        alternative, 136, 147
        smokeless, 276
    smoke effects, 136
    smokeless, 147
    treatment, 136, 148
        approaches, 136
        issues in, 147
        training programs, 34
    use
        causes, 144
        harmful consequences of, 276
        health risk of, 276
        rates of, 148
        societal and personal health burden of, 276
    users, 142
Transcultural
    effects, 186
    importance of, 184
    methodology for, 184
    principles of, 183
Treatment
    approaches, 171
    blood pressure, 42, 45
    disease, 10
    duration of, 136
    expectations for, 60
    goal, 156, 157, 224, 233
    intensity, 51
    patient course of, 19
    pharmacological, 136
    plans, 13
    strategies, 202, 205
    therapy, 50
Type-1 diabetes (T1D), 221
Type-2 diabetes (T2D), 238

U

Unhealthy alcohol use, 151–153, 156, 157
    pharmacologic treatment for, 157

V

Visceral adipose tissue (VAT), 202, 322, 323
Vital sign, 37, 78, 113

W

Weight loss, 11, 33, 48, 51, 60, 62, 105, 117, 205, 209, 228, 229, 232, 233, 237
    benefits of, 230

medicine-assisted, 231
Weight management, 6, 19, 41, 48, 49, 55, 116, 228
Wellness, 30, 31
    models of, 35
    of physicians, 34